Introduction to
# Chinese Internal Medicine

# World Century Compendium to TCM

Volume 1   Fundamentals of Traditional Chinese Medicine
*by Hong-zhou Wu, Zhao-qin Fang and Pan-ji Cheng*
*(translated by Ye-bo He)*
*(Shanghai University of Traditional Chinese Medicine, China)*
ISBN: 978-1-938134-28-9 (pbk)

Volume 2   Introduction to Diagnosis in Traditional Chinese Medicine
*by Hong-zhou Wu, Zhao-qin Fang and Pan-ji Cheng*
*(translated by Chou-ping Han)*
*(Shanghai University of Traditional Chinese Medicine, China)*
ISBN: 978-1938134-13-5 (pbk)

Volume 3   Introduction to Chinese Materia Medica
*by Jin Yang, Huang Huang and Li-jiang Zhu*
*(translated by Yunhui Chen)*
*(Nanjing University of Chinese Medicine, China)*
ISBN: 978-1-938134-16-6 (pbk)

Volume 4   Introduction to Chinese Internal Medicine
*by Xiang Xia, Xiao-heng Chen, Min Chen and Yan-qian Xiao*
*(translated by Ye-bo He)*
*(Shanghai Jiaotong University, China)*
ISBN: 978-1-938134-19-7 (pbk)

Volume 5   Introduction to Formulae of Traditional Chinese Medicine
*by Jin Yang, Huang Huang and Li-jiang Zhu*
*(translated by Xiao Ye and Hong Li)*
*(Nanjing University of Chinese Medicine, China)*
ISBN: 978-1-938134-10-4 (pbk)

Volume 6   Introduction to Acupuncture and Moxibustion
*by Ren Zhang (translated by Xue-min Wang)*
*(Shanghai Literature Institute of Traditional Chinese Medicine, China)*
ISBN: 978-1-938134-25-8 (pbk)

Volume 7   Introduction to Tui Na
*by Lan-qing Liu, Jiang Xiao and Gui-bao Ke (translated by Azure Duan)*
*(Yueyang Hospital of Integrated Traditional Chinese and Western Medicine, Shanghai University of Traditional Chinese Medicine, China)*
ISBN: 978-1-938134-22-7 (pbk)

World Century Compendium to TCM – Vol. 4

# Introduction to
# Chinese Internal
# Medicine

Xiang Xia
Xiao-heng Shen
Min Chen
Yan-qian Xiao
Shanghai Jiao Tong University , China

translated by

Ye-bo He

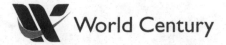
World Century

*Published by*

World Century Publishing Corporation
27 Warren Street
Suite 401-402
Hackensack, NJ 07601

*Distributed by*

World Scientific Publishing Co. Pte. Ltd.

5 Toh Tuck Link, Singapore 596224

*USA office:* 27 Warren Street, Suite 401-402, Hackensack, NJ 07601

*UK office:* 57 Shelton Street, Covent Garden, London WC2H 9HE

**Library of Congress Control Number:** 2013001662

**British Library Cataloguing-in-Publication Data**
A catalogue record for this book is available from the British Library.

**World Century Compendium to TCM**
**A 7-Volume Set**

**INTRODUCTION TO CHINESE INTERNAL MEDICINE**
**Volume 4**

ISBN 978-1-938134-34-0 (Set)
ISBN 978-1-938134-19-7 (pbk)


Typeset by Stallion Press
Email: enquiries@stallionpress.com


Printed in Singapore

# Contents

*Foreword to the English Edition*                                     ix
*Preface*                                                             xi

**Chapter 1    Common Ailments**                                      **1**
Week 1        Headache                                                1
              Vertigo                                                 11
              Insomnia                                                19
              Sweating Syndrome                                       26
              Aphtha                                                  33
              Diarrhea                                                40
Week 2        Constipation                                           49
              Bleeding                                                57

**Chapter 2    Diseases of the Respiratory System**                  **65**
              Cold                                                    65
              Bronchitis                                              72
              Bronchial Asthma                                        83
              Bronchiectasis                                          91
Week 3        Pneumonia                                              98
              Lung Abscess                                           105
              Pulmonary Tuberculosis                                 113
              Lung Cancer                                            122
              Chronic Cor Pulmonale                                  130

**Chapter 3    Cardiovascular Diseases**                             **139**
              Cardiac Arrhythmia                                     139
              Myocardial Disease                                     148

| | | |
|---|---|---|
| Week 4 | Viral Myocarditis | 155 |
| | Valvular Heart Disease | 163 |
| | Coronary Artery Disease | 170 |
| | Chronic Congestive Heart Failure | 179 |
| | Hypertension | 186 |
| | Cardioneurosis | 194 |
| **Chapter 4** | **Disorders of the Digestive System** | **201** |
| Week 5 | Reflux Esophagitis | 201 |
| | Esophageal Cancer | 207 |
| | Peptic Ulcer | 214 |
| | Chronic Gastritis | 221 |
| | Gastroptosis | 229 |
| | Irritable Bowel Syndrome | 234 |
| Week 6 | Intestinal Cancer | 240 |
| | Gastric Cancer | 248 |
| | Ulcerative Colitis | 254 |
| | Intestinal Tuberculosis | 264 |
| | Cirrhosis | 270 |
| | Primary Hepatic Carcinoma | 280 |
| Week 7 | Acute Pancreatitis | 289 |
| | Hepatic Encephalopathy | 296 |
| | Cholecystitis and Cholelithiasis | 303 |
| | Viral Hepatitis | 311 |
| | Bacillary Dysentery | 323 |
| **Chapter 5** | **Disorders of the Urinary System** | **333** |
| | Acute Glomerulonephritis | 333 |
| Week 8 | Chronic Glomerulonephritis | 341 |
| | Nephrotic Syndrome | 350 |
| | Pyelonephritis | 360 |
| | Renal Tuberculosis | 369 |
| | Urinary Calculosis | 377 |
| | Chronic Renal Failure | 385 |

**Chapter 6**    **Disorders of the Hematological System**                393
Week 9           Hypoferric Anaemia                                        393
                 Aplastic Anaemia                                          399
                 Leukemia (Chronic Granulocytic Leukemia)                  406
                 Leucopenia and Agranulemia                                413
                 Idiopathic Thrombocytopenic Purpura                       420
                 Anaphylactoid Purpura                                     426

**Chapter 7**    **Disorders of the Endocrine System**                     433
                 Hyperthyroidism                                           433
Week 10          Hypothyroidism                                            440
                 Benign Thyroid Tumor                                      446
                 Subacute Thyroiditis                                      451
                 Chronic Lymphocytic Thyroiditis                          456
                 Hypofunction of the Anterior Pituitary                   461
                 Chronic Adrenocortical Insufficiency                     467
                 Diabetes Insipidus                                       472
Week 11          Hypercortisolism                                         479
                 Idiopathic Edema                                         486
                 Female Climacteric Syndrome                              492

**Chapter 8**    **Neuropsychic Diseases**                                 501
                 Myasthenia Gravis                                         501
                 Progressive Muscular Dystrophy                            507
                 Trembling Palsy                                           514
Week 12          Bell's Paralysis                                          519
                 Ischemic Stroke                                           525
                 Hemorrhagic Stroke                                        533
                 Epilepsy                                                  542
                 Schizophrenia                                             550
                 Neurastheria                                              555
                 Senile Dementia                                           565

**Chapter 9**      **Connective Tissue Diseases**                           **573**
Week 13         Rheumatic Fever                                               573
                Rheumatoid Arthritis                                          581
                Systemic Lupus Erythematosus                                  587
                Dermatomyositis                                               596
                Scleroderma                                                   603
                Behcet Disease                                                610
Week 14         Sjogren's Syndrome                                            617

**Chapter 10**     **Metabolic Diseases**                                    **625**
                Diabetes                                                      625
                Osteoporosis                                                  633
                Simple Obesity                                                639
                Gout                                                          646
                Hyperlipemia                                                  653

*Index*                                                                       661

# Foreword to the English Edition

More than a decade has passed since the 1996 publication of the first book in the series *Learning Traditional Chinese Medicine in 100 Days*. The series contains 11 books, each of which discusses a different aspect of TCM. The contents of this series have been organized into bite-sized mini-chapters that aim to explain profound theories in simple language, thereby making it easy for readers to learn and consult in clinical practice. All of these books have been reprinted many times, with the highest print run reaching 100,000 copies.

From the end of the last century to the beginning of this century, the disease spectrum has undergone great changes. Accordingly, the application scope and methods of Chinese medicine have also changed. To ensure that readers can easily comprehend the content and be updated on the latest techniques in Chinese medicine, we invited many experts in this field to meticulously revise this series. The original format and style remain unchanged, but some obsolete techniques and contents have been deleted. In addition, new diseases and treatment methods have also been added. It is our sincere wish that the republication of this series will facilitate the spread and popularity of Chinese culture as well as Chinese medicine.

Shanghai Science & Technology Press

# Preface

Chinese internal medicine is a clinical subject which explains, using traditional Chinese theories, the etiology, pathology and therapeutic rules of the diseases or syndromes belonging to internal medicine. It is also the foundation for learning and research in other clinical branches of Chinese medicine, thus playing a vital role in traditional Chinese medicine (TCM).

Chinese internal medicine has had a long history. Its origin can be traced back several thousand years. As early as the Yin Dynasty, there were inscriptions on bones recording such internal diseases as heartache, headache and gastrointestinal diseases; in the Zhou Dynasty, Chinese medicine was divided into different branches and the "Ji Yi" is correspondent to the internist in modern times. Through long-term diagnostic and therapeutic practices, a rich collection of experience and theories in Chinese internal medicine has accumulated and this has gradually evolved into a complete, distinctive and effective clinical branch of TCM. In recent decades, Chinese internal medicine has also undergone significant developments, especially in the treatment of cardiac and cerebral vascular diseases, digestive tract diseases, renal diseases and autoimmune diseases.

In order to popularize Chinese internal medicine and enable readers to grasp its basic theories as well as diagnostic and therapeutic methods, we wrote this book in a language easily comprehensible by the layman. For ease of learning by modern doctors, we followed current clinical practice and outlined the contents with Western disease names. There are more than 80 diseases discussed in this book. For each disease, the Chinese syndrome differentiation and treatment as well as modern diagnostic key points are provided to make it more convenient for the readers to study and understand.

Readers are advised to work through the content in 100 days. Specifically, they should study 6~7 diseases in a week and complete the book in 14 weeks. A chronological reading of the book is recommended, in order that readers may proceed from preliminary understanding to relative familiarity and, in the end, to total mastery. We believe that Chinese internal medicine can only be practiced when diagnostic methods, syndrome differentiation and treatment rules are fully understood.

The study of each disease begins from its etiology, pathology and diagnostic key points, followed by the differentiated patterns and corresponding treatments. The respective points of caution at the end of each discussion provide crucial notes that readers should be familiar with for the particular disease covered. Finally, the questions forming the "Daily Exercises" are useful for readers to check their comprehension and recall of the material. Given the chance, readers should try to put the knowledge gleaned from this book into clinical practice, so that past knowledge can be tested and new clinical knowledge and skills can be learned.

This book is suitable for a general reader with interest in traditional Chinese medicine and with basic medical knowledge, as well as clinical TCM doctors, nursing personnel and TCM students.

Xia Xiang
Shen Xiao-heng
Chen Min
Xiao Yan-qian
May 2006

# CHAPTER 1

# Common Ailments

## Headache

## Week 1: Monday

Headache is a subjective symptom frequently encountered in the clinic. It may occur on its own or be experienced in a variety of acute or chronic diseases, such as hypertension, cerebrovascular accidents, brain tumor and angioneurotic headache. Headache discussed herein belongs to the category of miscellaneous internal diseases, marked by pain in the head.

### Etiology and Pathology

TCM holds that headache can be caused by either exogenous or endogenous factors. The former refers to pathogenic wind (the leading pathogen), cold, dampness and heat, while the latter refers to disorders of the liver, spleen and kidneys. In addition, traumatic injuries due to falls and knocks may affect the collaterals in the long run, bringing about obstruction of qi and blood in the vessels or collaterals, eventually leading to headache.

The pathological changes of headache are characterized by exogenous invasion of the six abnormal climatic factors into the vertex, obstructing the lucid yang and inducing headache. There are two factors attributed to the liver: The first is emotional depression resulting in transformation of stagnated liver qi into fire, which flames upward and disturbs the mind; the other is deficiency of liver yin resulting from either exuberance of fire or insufficiency of kidney water, both of which will lead to hyperactivity of liver yang, which harasses the clear orifices upwardly. There are similarly two factors attributed to the kidneys: The first is congenital deficiency or prolonged consumption of kidney essence, causing failed nourishment of the brain marrow and thereby triggering headache; the other is deficiency of yin involving yang, rendering the kidney yang debilitated and the lucid yang encumbered, finally bringing about headache. The remaining two factors attributed to the spleen are deficiency and excess. The former refers to malnutrition of the brain marrow and collaterals due to insufficient blood supply caused by irregular diet, overstrain, chronic diseases or childbirth (which makes the spleen and stomach become too weak to produce sufficient blood) and loss of blood; the latter refers to the clouding of the clear orifices and the encumbrance of lucid yang by phlegm and dampness, which ensue from malfunction of the spleen due to excessive intake of fatty and sweet food.

## Diagnostic Key Points

1. The patient has a history of hypertension or arteriosclerosis.
2. The pain may be in the temples or the vertex, or without a fixed location.
3. The onset is characterized by pricking, dull or distending pain.
4. Physical examination reveals no positive signs.

## Syndrome Differentiation

The following three types of headache described below are due to exogenous pathogenic factors:

## 1. Headache due to wind-cold

Symptoms: Headache by fits and starts, pain radiating to the nape and back, aggravation by wind, aversion to wind, intolerance of cold and absence of thirst; thin white coating on the tongue and floating pulse.

Analysis of symptoms: The head is the region where all yang meridians convene, so when pathogenic wind-cold attacks the body from the exterior, it will reach the vertex along the taiyang meridian, obstructing the lucid yang and triggering headache; the taiyang meridian dominates the superficies of the body, passes through the back and nape and arrives at the vertex, so the pain can radiate to the nape and neck; pathogenic wind-cold fetters the skin and muscles and stagnates the defensive yang, which explains the aversion to wind and intolerance of cold. Since there is no heat, thirst is absent; the thin white tongue coating and floating pulse are both manifestations of wind-cold in the exterior.

## 2. Headache due to wind-heat

Symptoms: Headache with distension or even a splitting sensation in the head, fever or aversion to wind, reddened eyes and flushed face, thirst with a desire to drink, constipation and yellowish urine, a reddened tongue with yellowish coating and floating, rapid pulse.

Analysis of symptoms: Heat is a yang pathogen marked by flaming up, so wind-heat attacks the yang collateral and disturbs the clear orifices upwardly, giving rise to distending headache or even a splitting sensation in the head; reddened eyes and a flushed face are attributable to a flaming up of pathogenic heat; wind-heat invades the defensive phase, bringing about fever and aversion to wind; abundant heat consumes body fluid, so there is thirst, constipation and yellowish urine; reddened tongue with yellowish coating and floating, rapid pulse are both manifestations of exuberant wind-heat.

## 3. Headache due to wind-dampness

Symptoms: Headache as if the head was being wrapped, heaviness in the limbs, a poor appetite, chest distress, difficulty in micturition and loose stools; white greasy tongue coating and soggy pulse.

Analysis of symptoms: Pathogenic wind-dampness invades the vertex and obstructs the clear orifices, so there is pressure around the head as if it is being wrapped by something; the spleen governs transformation and dominates the four limbs, so when turbid dampness is retained in the interior and encumbers the spleen yang, there will be heaviness in the limbs, poor appetite and chest distress. Since there is internal obstruction of pathogenic dampness, the small intestine may fail to separate the lucid from the turbid, with such symptoms as difficulty in micturition or loose stools; white greasy tongue coating and soggy pulse are both attributable to obstruction of turbid dampness in the interior.

The following four types of headache are due to endogenous pathogenic factors:

## 4. Headache due to hyperactivity of liver yang

Symptoms: Headache with dizziness, vexation, irascibility, insomnia at night which may be accompanied by hypochondriac pain, flushed face and a bitter taste in the mouth; thin and yellow tongue coating, as well as taut and forceful pulse.

Analysis of symptoms: All wind disorders, such as tremors and vertigo, are attributable to the liver, so when the liver qi is stagnated and the liver yang is hyperactive, the clear orifices will be affected, resulting in headache with dizziness; hyperactive liver fire can disturb the heart spirit, leading to vexation, irascibility and insomnia at night; stagnated liver qi and gallbladder qi produce fire and a predisposition to hyperactivity of the liver yang, marked by hypochondriac pain, a bitter taste in the mouth and a flushed face; thin and yellow tongue coating and taut and forceful pulse are both manifestations of hyperactive liver yang.

## 5. Headache due to deficiency of the kidneys

Symptoms: Headache with an empty sensation, often accompanied by dizziness or soreness and weakness of the waist, lassitude, nocturnal emissions, leukorrhea, tinnitus and poor sleep; reddish tongue with scanty coating and thin pulse.

Analysis of symptoms: The brain is known as the "sea of marrow" which is governed by the kidneys, so if the kidney essence is too deficient to nourish the brain marrow, there will be empty pain in the head, dizziness and tinnitus; the waist is the "house of the kidney", and if the kidneys are too weak, there will be nocturnal semen emission in males; the belt vessel becomes deficient, so it will fail to perform its function of controlling abnormal vaginal discharge in females; insomnia, reddish tongue with scanty coating and thin pulse are due to insufficiency of kidney yin.

## 6. Headache due to deficiency of blood

Symptoms: Headache with dizziness, palpitations and restlessness, lassitude, bright pale complexion and a pale tongue; thin white tongue coating, as well as thin and feeble pulse.

Analysis of symptoms: Deficient blood generates deficient fire, which attacks the head, leading to pain with dizziness; deficiency of blood brings about malnutrition of the heart spirit, so there are palpitations and feelings of uneasiness; deficiency of blood also involves qi, leading to symptoms of qi deficiency such as listlessness or lassitude; wan complexion, pale tongue with thin white coating, as well as thin and feeble pulse are all manifestations of blood deficiency.

## 7. Headache due to turbid phlegm

Symptoms: Headache with a befuddled mind, sensation of fullness and stuffiness in the chest, nausea with vomiting of sputum and saliva; white greasy tongue coating and slippery or taut, slippery pulse.

Analysis of symptoms: Dysfunction of the spleen in transportation and transformation may lead to internal obstruction of turbid phlegm which clouds the clear orifices and encumbers lucid yang, this is marked by headache with a befuddled mind; obstruction of turbid phlegm in the diaphragm can produce a sensation of fullness and stuffiness in the chest; adverse rising of turbid phlegm is characterized by nausea and vomiting of sputum and saliva; the white greasy tongue coating and slippery or taut, slippery pulse are caused by internal retention of phlegm and dampness.

## Differential Treatment

### 1. Headache due to wind-cold

Treatment principle: Dispersing wind and dispelling cold.

Prescription and herbs: Modified Chuanxiong Chatiao Powder.

Chuanxiong (Szechwan Lovage Rhizome) 9 g, Jingjie (Fineleaf Schizonepeta Herb) 9 g, Fangfeng (Divaricate Saposhnikovia Root) 9 g,

Qianghuo (Incised Notoptetygium Rhizome or Root) 12 g, Baizhi (Dahurian Angelica Root) 12 g, Xixin (Manchurian Wildginger) 6 g, Bohe (Peppermint) 6 g and Gancao (Liquorice Root) 6 g.

Modification: If pathogenic cold invades the jueyin channel, causing such manifestations as parietal headache and retching, Wuzhuyu (Medicinal Evodia Fruit) 9 g and Banxia (Pinellia Tuber) 9 g are added to warm the body, dissipate pathogens and reduce adverseness.

## 2. Headache due to wind-heat

Treatment principle: Dispersing wind and clearing heat.

Prescription and herbs: Modified Xiongzhi Shigao Decoction.

Chuanxiong (Szechwan Lovage Rhizome) 9 g, Baizhi (Dahurian Angelica Root) 12 g, Juhua (Chrysanthemum Flower) 9 g, Shengshigao (Unprepared Gypsum) 30 g, Huangqin (Baical Skullcap Root) 15 g, Bohe (Peppermint) 6 g and Zhizi (Cape Jasmine Fruit) 9 g.

Modification: If there is consumption of body fluid by intense heat, causing such manifestations as red and dry tongue and dry mouth with thirst, Zhimu (Common Anemarrhena Rhizome) 12 g, Shihu (Dendrobium) 15 g and Tianhuafen (Trichosanthin) 15 g are added to promote fluid production and quench thirst; for dry stools, oral and nasal sores and obstructed intestinal qi, Huanglian (Golden Thread) 3 g and Dahuang (Rhubarb) 9 g (decocted later) are added to bring down fire, cleanse the intestine and eliminate heat.

## 3. Headache due to wind-dampness

Treatment principle: Dispelling wind and eliminating dampness.

Prescription and herbs: Modified Qianghuo Shengshi Decoction.

Qianghuo (Incised Notoptetygium Rhizome or Root) 9 g, Duhuo (Doubleteeth Pubesscent Angelica Root) 9 g, Chuanxiong (Szechwan Lovage Rhizome) 9 g, Fangfeng (Divaricate Saposhnikovia Root) 9 g, Manjingzi (Shrub Chastetree Fruit) 12 g, Gaoben (Chinese Lovage) 12 g and Gancao (Liquorice Root) 6 g.

Modification: If there is internal obstruction by turbid dampness, causing such signs as chest distress, poor appetite and loose stools, Cangzhu (Atractylodes Rhizome) 12 g, Houpu (Magnolia Bark) 9 g, Chenpi (Dried Tangerine Peel) 9 g and Zhiqiao (Orange Fruit) 12 g are added to reduce dampness and relieve the middle energizer; for nausea and vomiting, Banxia (Pinellia Tuber) 9 g and Shengjiang (Fresh Ginger) 5 slices are used to bring down the adverse flow of qi and arrest vomiting.

## 4. Headache due to hyperactivity of liver yang

Treatment principle: Calming the liver and subduing yang.

Prescription and herbs: Modified Tianma Gouteng Decoction.

Tianma (Tall Gastrodis Tuber) 12 g, Gouteng (Gambir Plant) 15 g, Shijueming (Sea-ear Shell) 30 g, Huangqin (Baical Skullcap Root) 15 g, Zhizi (Cape Jasmine Fruit) 9 g, Niuxi (Two-toothed Achyranthes Root) 12 g, Duzhong (Eucommia Bark) 12 g, Sangjisheng (Chinese Taxillus Herb) 12 g, Yejiaoteng (Caulis Polygoni Multiflori) 30 g, Fushen (Indian Bread with Hostwood) 15 g, Muli (Oyster Shell) 30 g and Longgu (Os Draconis) 30 g.

Modification: If there is yin deficiency of the liver and kidneys, causing such manifestations as headache alleviated in the morning and aggravated in the evening or aggravated upon physical exertion, taut and thin pulse, as well as a red tongue, Shengdi (Dried Rehmannia Root) 12 g, Heshouwu (Fleeceflower Root) 15 g, Nuzhenzi (Glossy Privet Fruit) 12 g, Gouqizi (Barbary Wolfberry Fruit) 12 g and Huanliancao (Ecliptae Herba) 12 g are added to nourish the liver and kidneys; for relative hyperactivity of liver fire marked by severe headache, hypochondriac pain, a bitter taste in the mouth, flushed face, dry stools, reddish urine, yellowish tongue coating and rapid, taut pulse, it is advisable to add Longdancao (Radix Gentianae) 9 g, Xiakucao (Common Selfheal Fruit-Spike) 12 g and Yujin (Turmeric Root Tuber) 12 g so as to clear the liver and purge fire.

## 5. Headache due to deficiency of the kidneys

Treatment principle: Nourishing yin and supplementing the liver.

Prescription and herbs: Modified Dabuyuan Decoction.

Renshen (Ginseng) 9 g, Huaishanyao (Huaihe Common Yan Rhizome) 15 g, Shudi (Prepared Rhizome of Rehmannia) 12 g, Duzhong (Eucommia Bark) 12 g, Gouqizi (Barbary Wolfberry Fruit) 12 g, Danggui (Chinese Angelica) 12 g, Shanzhuyu (Asiatic Cornelian Cherry Fruit) 9 g and Zhigancao (Stir-baked Liquorice Root) 6 g.

Modification: If there is headache, intolerance of cold, pale complexion, lack of warmth in the limbs, pale tongue and thin, deep pulse, it is advisable to add decocted Fuzi (Prepared Common Monkshood Daughter) 9 g and Rougui (Cassia Bark) 6 g so as to warm and invigorate the kidney yang; if it is accompanied by exogenous invasion of pathogenic factors into the shaoyin channel, Mahuang (Ephedra) 6 g, Xixin (Manchurian Wildginger) 6 g and Fuzi (Prepared Common Monkshood Daughter) 9 g are used to warm the meridian and dissipate the cold.

## 6. Headache due to deficiency of blood

Treatment principle: Nourishing and regulating blood.

Prescription and herbs: Modified Supplementary Siwu Decoction.

Shengdi (Dried Rehmannia Root) 12 g, Baishao (White Peony Alba) 15 g, Danggui (Chinese Angelica) 12 g, Chuanxiong (Szechwan Lovage Rhizome) 10 g, Juhua (Chrysanthemum Flower) 9 g, Manjingzi (Shrub Chastetree Fruit) 12 g, Huangqin (Baical Skullcap Root) 12 g and Gancao (Liquorice Root) 6 g.

Modification: If deficiency of blood leads to insufficiency of qi, marked by lassitude aggravated upon physical exertion, sweating with shortness of breath, as well as intolerance of wind and cold, it is advisable to add Huangqi (Milkvetch Root) 15 g, Dangshen (Radix Codonopsis) 12 g and Xixin (Manchurian Wildginger) 6 g so as to invigorate qi and nourish blood, as well as to dissipate cold and stop pain; for insufficiency of liver blood with deficiency of liver yin, characterized by tinnitus, deficient restlessness, insomnia and dizziness, it is advisable to add Heshouwu (Fleeceflower Root) 15 g, Gouqizi (Barbary Wolfberry Fruit) 12 g, Huangjing (Solomonseal Rhizome) 12 g and Suanzaoren (Spine Date Seed) 12 g to supplement the liver and nourish the kidneys.

## 7. Headache due to turbid phlegm

Treatment principle: Dissolving phlegm and bringing down turbidity.

Prescription and herbs: Modified Banxia Baizhu Tianma Decoction.

Banxia (Pinellia Tuber) 9 g, Baizhu (Largehead Atractylodes Rhizome) 15 g, Tianma (Tall Gastrodis Tuber) 12 g, Chenpi (Dried Tangerine Peel) 9 g, Fuling (Indian Bread) 15 g, Houpu (Magnolia Bark) 6 g, Baijili (Tribulus Terrestris) 15 g, Manjingzi (Shrub Chastetree Fruit) 12 g, Gancao (Liquorice Root) 6 g, Dazao (Chinese Date) 7 dates and Shengjiang (Fresh Ginger) 3 slices.

Modification: If prolonged retention of turbid phlegm produces heat, marked by a bitter taste in the mouth, difficulty in defecation, yellow and greasy coating or slippery and rapid pulse, Baizhu (Largehead Atractylodes Rhizome) can be replaced with Huangqin (Baical Skullcap Root) 12 g, Zhuru (Bamboo Shavings) 9 g and Zhishi (Immature Orange Fruit) 9 g to promote flow of qi, dispel heat and dry dampness.

## Chinese Patent Medicine

1. Chuanxiong Chatiao Pill: 10 pills for each dose, 3 times a day (swallowed).
2. Quantianma Capsule: 2 pills for each dose, 3 times a day (swallowed).
3. Qiju Dihuang Pill: 4 pills for each dose, 3 times a day (swallowed).

## Simple and Handy Prescriptions

1. Shangyangjiao (Cornu Caprae Hircus Powder) 15~30 g (decocted first), Baijuhua (White Chrysanthemum Flower) 12 g and Chuanxiong (Szechwan Lovage Rhizome) 6 g are boiled in water. This decoction is used to treat headache due to upward disturbance of liver yang.
2. Zhichuanwu (Prepared Common Monkshood Mother Root) 6 g, Zhicaowu (Prepared Kusnezoff Monkshood Root) 6 g, Baizhi (Dahurian Angelica Root) 6 g, Jiangcan (Stiff Silkworm) 6 g and Shenggancao (Unprepared Liquorice Root) 9 g are ground up into fine powders,

packed into 6 bags and administered with green tea (1 bag a day at 3 different times). This therapy is used to treat obstinate headache due to wind-cold.

## Other Therapies

Dietary therapy: Juhuayu Decoction: 10 g of chrysanthemum flower from Hangzhou and a fresh river fish (250 g) are seasoned with cooking wine, ginger and onion and then boiled in water to make soup. The soup is used to treat headache due to hyperactivity of liver yang.

Hair-combing method: To comb the hair with a wooden comb 2~3 times a day, 10 minutes each time. The movements should be slow at first and then increased to a faster pace with use of stronger force. A course of treatment lasts 10 days.

## Cautions and Advice

1. Headache is a common ailment with multiple etiological factors that should be identified as early as possible, so that timely and appropriate treatment can be administered.
2. Patients should try to avoid emotional fluctuations, excessive excitation and overstrain.
3. They should also keep to a light diet and refrain from spicy, oily, fatty and sweet food.

## Daily Exercises

1. Concisely describe the different types of headache and compare their characteristics.
2. Explain how headache due to hyperactivity of liver yang can be diagnosed and treated.

# Vertigo

## Week 1: Tuesday

Vertigo refers to a condition of blurred vision and dizziness. In mild cases, the symptom will disappear when the patient closes his eyes; however, in severe cases, the patient may feel as if he were taking a vehicle or boat, incapable of standing still, along with nausea, vomiting, or even fainting. It can be a symptom in many internal diseases, such as hypertension, anaemia, cervical syndrome and Meniere's syndrome.

### Etiology and Pathology

Dizziness can be attributed to two aspects: Deficiency of the root (the primary aspect) or deficiency of the root (the primary aspect) complicated by excess of the branch (the secondary aspect). The former refers to the depletion of yin, deficiency of qi and blood, as well as insufficiency of marrow; the latter refers to consumption of liver yin complicated by hyperactivity of liver fire, or weakness of the spleen and stomach complicated by internal obstruction of turbid phlegm.

The pathological changes of vertigo are discussed as follows: Depletion of yin leads to hyperactivity of liver yang and internal stirring of liver wind, which disturb the clear orifices and make the patient feel dizzy. In addition, deficiency of qi can lead to stagnation of lucid yang while deficiency of blood may result in malnutrition of the brain, both of which will give rise to dizziness. Consumption of kidney essence (deficiency of the lower) predisposes the brain marrow to malnutrition (deficiency of the upper), eventually inducing dizziness. Finally, indulgence in fatty and sweet food, irregular diet or overstrain can also be detrimental to the spleen and stomach in terms of transformation and transportation, and consequently there will be transformation of water and food into damp-phlegm instead of essence or nutrients, with the former blocking the middle energizer and making the lucid yang unable to ascend and the turbid yin unable to descend, leading to dizziness.

## Diagnostic Key Points

1. The patient has a history of hypertension, anaemia, or cervical syndrome.
2. Symptoms of blurred vision and dizziness. In mild cases, vertigo will disappear when the patient closes his eyes; in severe cases, the patient may feel as if he was on a moving vehicle or boat and incapable of remaining stationary. There may also be nausea, vomiting, or even fainting.
3. Health examination shows occasional elevation of blood pressure or appearance of anaemia, or an absence of positive signs.
4. Blood test reveals a decrease in the number of hemoglobin molecules and red blood cells.

## Syndrome Differentiation

### 1. Hyperactivity of liver yang

Symptoms: Dizziness, tinnitus, headache with distension, aggravation by vexation, rage or physical strain, flushed face, irascibility, insomnia or dreaminess and a bitter taste in the mouth; red tongue with yellow coating and taut pulse.

Analysis of symptoms: Hyperactive liver yang attacks the upper orifices, leading to dizziness and headache; overstrain impairs the kidneys, while rage injures the liver, both of which will contribute to the hyperactivity of liver yang, marked by aggravation of dizziness and headache; ascent of yang reddens the face; hyperactivity of liver yang causes irascibility; flaming liver fire agitates the heart spirit, resulting in insomnia and dreaminess; bitter taste in the mouth, red tongue with yellow coating and taut pulse are all due to hyperactivity of liver yang.

### 2. Deficiency of qi and blood

Symptoms: Dizziness aggravated upon physical exertion and triggered by overstrain, pale complexion, lusterless lips and nails, withered hair, palpitations, insomnia, listlessness, reluctance to speak and reduced food intake; pale tongue and thin, feeble pulse.

Analysis of symptoms: Deficiency of qi can lead to stagnation of lucid yang while deficiency of blood may result in malnutrition of the brain, both of which will give rise to dizziness aggravated upon physical exertion; the heart controls blood and vessels and this is reflected by the complexion, so deficiency of qi and blood is manifested as pale face and lusterless lips and nails; the blood fails to nourish the heart, bringing about mental uneasiness, palpitations and insomnia; deficiency of qi is marked by listlessness, reluctance to speak and reduced food intake; the pale tongue and thin, feeble pulse are both manifestations of deficiency of qi and blood.

## 3. Insufficiency of kidney essence

Symptoms: Dizziness, listlessness, insomnia, dreaminess, forgetfulness, weakness and soreness of the waist and knees, nocturnal emissions and tinnitus. For relative deficiency of yin, there are manifestations of feverish sensation over the five centers (the palms, the soles, and the heart), red tongue and thin, rapid and taut pulse; for relative deficiency of yang, there is lack of warmth in the limbs, intolerance of cold, pale tongue and thin, weak and deep pulse.

Analysis of symptoms: Insufficiency of marrow and essence results in malnutrition of the brain, characterized by dizziness and listlessness; deficiency of the kidneys leads to failure of communication between the heart and kidneys, marked by insomnia, dreaminess, and forgetfulness; the waist is the "house of the kidneys", so if the kidneys are deficient, there will be weakness and soreness of the waist and knees; the kidneys open into the ear, so if the kidneys are deficient, frequent tinnitus will be felt; failure of the kidneys to control semen secretion results in nocturnal emission; relative deficiency of yin produces internal heat, with such signs as feverish sensation over the five centers (the palms, the soles, and the heart), red tongue and thin, rapid and taut pulse; relative deficiency of yang generates cold in the interior, with such manifestations as lack of warmth in the limbs, intolerance of cold, pale tongue and thin, weak and deep pulse.

## 4. Internal obstruction of turbid phlegm

Symptoms: Dizziness with a befuddled mind, chest distress, nausea, poor appetite and somnolence; white greasy tongue coating and soggy, slippery pulse.

Analysis of symptoms: Turbid phlegm encumbers lucid yang and makes it unable to ascend, with such signs as dizziness and heaviness of the head with a befuddled mind; internal obstruction of turbid phlegm leads to non-descent of turbid yin and impeded flow of qi, marked by chest distress and nausea; inactivation of spleen yang is responsible for inadequate eating and excessive sleeping; white greasy tongue coating and soggy, slippery pulse are both due to internal accumulation of turbid phlegm.

## Differential Treatment

### 1. Hyperactivity of liver yang

Treatment principle: Calming the liver and subduing yang, nourishing the liver and kidneys.

Prescription and herbs: Modified Tianma Gouteng Potion.

Tianma (Tall Gastrodis Tuber) 12 g, Gouteng (Gambir Plant) 15 g, Shengshijueming (Raw Sea-ear Shell) 30 g, Chuanniuxi (Szechwan Two-toothed Achyranthes Root) 12 g, Sangjisheng (Chinese Taxillus Herb) 12 g, Duzhong (Eucommia Bark) 12 g, Huangqin (Baical Skullcap Root) 12 g, Zhizi (Cape Jasmine Fruit) 9 g and Juhua (Chrysanthemum Flower) 9 g.

Modification: In cases of hyperactive liver fire, Longdancao (Radix Gentianae) 9 g and Mudanpi (Tree Peony Bark) 12 g are added to strengthen the action of removing liver heat; for constipation, Dahuang (Rhubarb) 9 g (decocted later) and Huanglian (Golden Thread) 3 g are added to dispel heat and dredge the intestines.

### 2. Deficiency of qi and blood

Treatment principle: Replenishing qi and blood, invigorating the spleen and the stomach.

Prescription and herbs: Modified Guipi Decoction.

Dangshen (Radix Codonopsis) 12 g, Huangqi (Milkvetch Root) 15 g, Baizhu (Largehead Atractylodes Rhizome) 12 g, Danggui (Chinese Angelica) 12 g, Fushen (Indian Bread with Hostwood) 10 g, Suanzaoren (Spine Date Seed) 12 g, Longyanrou (Longan Aril) 9 g, Yuanzhi (Thinleaf Milkwort Root) 6 g, Muxiang (Common Aucklandia Root) 9 g, Dazao (Chinese Date) 7 dates and Gancao (Liquorice Root) 6 g.

Modification: If the body and limbs feel cold and this is accompanied by vague abdominal pain, Guizhi (Cassia Twig) 9 g and Ganjiang (Dried Ginger) 6 g are added to warm the interior and reinforce yang; for severe deficiency of blood, Shudi (Prepared Rhizome of Rehmannia) 12 g, Ejiao (Donkey-hide Glue) 9 g (melted in decoction), Ziheche (Human Placenta Powder) 9 g (infused in water separately), as well as Renshen (Ginseng) and Huangqi (Milkvetch Root) in large quantities are added to produce qi and blood; if accompanied by pale complexion, listlessness, loose stools and tenesmus, Shengma (Rhizoma Cimicifugae) 9 g, Chaihu (Chinese Thorowax Root) 9 g and Chenpi (Dried Tangerine Peel) 9 g are added to move up the lucid and bring down the turbid.

## 3. Deficiency of kidney essence

Treatment principle: Tonifying the kidneys and nourishing yin for relative deficiency of yin, tonifying the kidneys and invigorating yang for relative deficiency of yang.

Prescription and herbs: Zuogui Pill for nourishing kidney yin, Yougui Pill for invigorating kidney yang.

Zuogui Pill: Shudi (Prepared Rhizome of Rehmannia) 12 g, Shanzhuyu (Asiatic Cornelian Cherry Fruit) 9 g, Huaishanyao (Huaihe Common Yan Rhizome) 12 g, Tusizi (Dodder Seed) 12 g, Chuanniuxi (Szechwan Two-toothed Achyranthes Root) 12 g, Guibanjiao (Tortoise Shell Gelatin) 9 g, Lujiaojiao (Deerhorn Glue) 9 g and Gouqizi (Barbary Wolfberry Fruit) 12 g.

Yougui Pill: Shudi (Prepared Rhizome of Rehmannia) 12 g, Shanzhuyu (Asiatic Cornelian Cherry Fruit) 9 g, Duzhong (Eucommia Bark) 12 g, Tusizi (Dodder Seed) 12 g, Rougui (Cassia Bark) 3 g, Fuzi (Prepared

Common Monkshood Daughter) 9 g (decocted first), Lujiaojiao (Deerhorn Glue) 9 g, Danggui (Chinese Angelica) 12 g, Huaishanyao (Huaihe Common Yan Rhizome) 12 g and Gouqizi (Barbary Wolfberry Fruit) 12 g.

Modification: In severe cases of internal heat due to deficiency of yin, marked by feverish sensation over the five centers (the palms, the soles, and the heart), red tongue and thin, rapid and taut pulse, Biejia (Stir-baked Turtle Shell) 9 g, Zhimu (Common Anemarrhena Rhizome) 12 g, Mudanpi (Tree Peony Bark) 9 g, Juhua (Chrysanthemum Flower) 9 g and Digupi (Chinese Wolfberry Root-Bark) 12 g are applied on the basis of the Zuogui Pill to nourish yin and dispel heat; for relatively severe dizziness due to deficiency of yin and floating of yang, Longgu (Os Draconis) 30 g and Muli (Oyster Shell) 30 g are used on the basis of the two prescriptions to nourish yin and subdue yang.

## 4. Internal obstruction of turbid phlegm

Treatment principle: Drying dampness and eliminating phlegm, subduing the liver to extinguish wind.

Prescription and herbs: Modified Banxia Baizhu Tianma Decoction.

Banxia (Pinellia Tuber) 9 g, Baizhu (Largehead Atractylodes Rhizome) 15 g, Chenpi (Dried Tangerine Peel) 6 g, Tianma (Tall Gastrodis Tuber) 12 g, Fuling (Indian Bread) 12 g and Gancao (Liquorice Root) 6 g.

Modification: In severe cases of dizziness and frequent vomiting, Daizheshi (Red Bole) 15 g, Zhuru (Bamboo Shavings) 9 g and Shengjiang (Fresh Ginger) 3 slices are added to check the adverse flow of qi and arrest vomiting; for gastric distension with a poor appetite, Sharen (Villous Amomum Fruit) 3 g and Kouren (Fructus Amomi Rotundus) 3 g are added to regulate the stomach with their aromatic flavors; for tinnitus and amblykusis, Congbai (Fistular Onion Stalk) 2 stalks, Yujin (Turmeric Root Tuber) 12 g and Shichangpu (Acorus Calamus) 12 g are added to activate yang for resuscitation; if accompanied by distending pain in the head and eyes, vexation and a bitter taste in the mouth, Huanglian (Golden Thread) 3 g and Huangqin (Baical Skullcap Root) 12 g are added to purge heat and dissolve phlegm.

## Chinese Patent Medicine

1. For dizziness due to hyperactivity of liver yang, infuse Tianma Gouteng Granule in warm boiled water and take 10 g for each dose.
2. Guipi Pill: 12 pills for each dose, 3 times a day orally. It is used to treat dizziness due to deficiency of qi and blood.

## Simple and Handy Prescriptions

1. Tianma (Tall Gastrodis Tuber) 10 g and Shijueming (Raw Sea-ear Shell) 30 g are boiled in water and taken twice a day to treat dizziness due to hyperactivity of liver yang.
2. Nuzhenzi (Glossy Privet Fruit) 12 g, Huanliancao (Ecliptae Herb) 15 g and Juhua (Chrysanthemum Flower) 9 g are boiled in water and taken twice a day to treat dizziness due to insufficiency of the liver and kidney.

## Other Therapies

Application method: Caojueming (Semen Cassia) 60 g and Shijueming (Sea-ear Shell) 10 g are ground up into powders, blended with strong tea and made into a paste, which is applied to the bilateral temples. It is used to calm the liver and subdue yang, as well as to treat dizziness due to hyperactivity of liver yang.

Dietary therapy: Roasted Chicken with Fleeceflower Root: First put 20 g of Shouwu (Fleeceflower Root) into the abdomen of a spring chicken, and then add the seasonings and roast the chicken with mild fire. This dish is used to nourish the liver and kidneys and supplement primordial qi, and effective in treating dizziness due to insufficiency of qi, blood, the liver and kidneys.

## Cautions and Advice

1. Patients should rest well, engage in moderate physical exercise and strike a balance between work and rest.

2. They should also maintain a peaceful mind and avoid emotional stimulation.
3. For those with upward disturbance of turbid phlegm, it is advisable to keep to a light diet.

## Daily Exercises

1. List the different types of vertigo.
2. Describe the clinical characteristics of vertigo due to hyperactivity of liver yang.

# Insomnia
## Week 1: Wednesday

Insomnia is a morbid condition marked by inability to have regular sleep. In mild cases, the patient often has difficulty falling asleep, and even if he manages to do so, tends to awaken and be unable to return to sleep, or only be able to sleep fitfully. In severe cases, the patient tosses and turns restlessly in bed and stays awake all night. Insomnia is nevertheless a symptom that seldom results in dire consequences. Also known as "sleeplessness" in TCM, it is often present in such disorders as depression, hypertension and climacteric syndrome, amongst others.

### Etiology and Pathology

Insomnia is a disorder featuring incoordination between yin and yang and the failure of yang to communicate yin, usually caused by emotional disturbance, imbalanced work and rest, physical weakness by chronic consumption, hyperactivity of the five emotions and improper diet.

The pathological changes of insomnia are discussed as follows: Mental or physical strain impairs the heart and spleen and consumes yin blood which fails to nourish the heart, bringing about a disquieted heart spirit. Prolonged weakness of the body or consumption of kidney yin due to chronic diseases may result in water (kidneys) failing to coordinate with fire (heart), hyperactivity of the heart yang or heart fire and five emotions and consequently, failure of the heart to communicate with the kidneys, marked by a restless spirit and uneasy mind. Furthermore, emotional disorder often stagnates qi and produces fire, disturbing the heart spirit and making it restless (the condition may also stem from hyperactivity of yang due to deficiency of yin). Finally, indigested food can cause disharmony of stomach qi and produce phlegm and heat which rise and disturb the mind, presenting as insomnia as a result.

### Diagnostic Key Points

1. In mild cases, the patient often has difficulty falling asleep, and even if he manages to do so, may suffer from excessive dreams, frequent awakenings and inability to return to sleep.

2. In severe cases, it is characterized by persistent sleeplessness at night and by weariness, listlessness and hypomnesis in the day.
3. Physical examination generally reveals no abnormalities.

## Syndrome Differentiation

### 1. Liver qi stagnation transforming into fire

Symptoms: Insomnia, irascibility, poor appetite, thirst, reddened eyes, a bitter taste in the mouth, yellowish or reddish urine and constipation; red tongue with yellow coating and rapid, taut pulse.

Analysis of symptoms: Worry and anger impair the liver and stagnate the liver qi which subsequently transforms into fire, disturbing the heart spirit and bringing about insomnia; the liver qi invades the stomach, resulting in poor appetite; stagnated liver qi transforms into fire, expressing in irascibility; the liver fire over-restricts the stomach, resulting in heat in the stomach and thirst; fire-heat attacks the upper body, presenting itself in reddened eyes and a bitter taste in the mouth; yellowish or reddish urine, constipation, reddened tongue with yellow coating and rapid, taut pulse are all attributable to heat.

### 2. Upward disturbance of phlegm and heat

Symptoms: Insomnia, vexation, chest distress with excessive phlegm, poor appetite with belching, nausea with acid regurgitation, a bitter taste in the mouth, heaviness of the head with dizziness, yellow greasy tongue coating and slippery rapid pulse.

Analysis of symptoms: Indigested food is retained in the stomach and produces dampness and phlegm, which further transforms into heat, disturbing the upper body and bringing about vexation and insomnia; phlegm and dampness obstruct the middle energizer and affect the functional activities of qi, leading to failure of the stomach qi to descend, with such signs as chest distress, poor appetite with belching, or nausea with acid regurgitation; lucid yang is blocked, so there is heaviness of the head with dizziness; the yellow and greasy tongue coating and slippery and rapid pulse are both due to internal retention of indigested food with phlegm and heat.

## 3. Hyperactivity of fire due to yin deficiency

Symptoms: Vexation, insomnia, palpitations, uneasiness, dizziness, tinnitus, forgetfulness, waist soreness, nocturnal emissions, feverish sensations over the five centers (the palms, the soles, and the heart), and dry mouth with scanty fluid; red tongue and thin, rapid pulse.

Analysis of symptoms: Insufficiency of kidney yin makes it unable to rise to communicate with the heart and consequently causes hyperactivity of heart fire and liver fire, which harass the spirit and lead to vexation, insomnia, palpitations, and uneasiness; consumption of kidney essence results in malnutrition of brain marrow, characterized by dizziness, tinnitus, and forgetfulness; since the kidneys are located in the waist, deficiency of the kidneys can cause soreness in the waist; the kidneys fail to control semen secretion, so there is nocturnal emissions; dry mouth, feverish sensation over the five centers, red tongue and thin, rapid pulse are all manifestations of fire exuberance due to deficiency of yin.

## 4. Deficiency of the spleen and stomach

Symptoms: Dreaminess, intermittent sleep, palpitations, forgetfulness, dizziness, lassitude, poor appetite, and lusterless complexion; pale tongue with thin coating and thin, feeble pulse.

Analysis of symptoms: The weak heart and spleen provide insufficient blood to nourish the heart, resulting in mental derangement, dreaminess, intermittent sleep, forgetfulness and palpitations; deficient qi and blood fail to nourish the brain, thus leading to failure of lucid yang to ascend, causing dizziness; the deficient blood is incapable of performing its nourishing function, so the complexion is lusterless and the tongue is pale; dysfunction of the spleen in transportation and transformation is responsible for poor appetite; lassitude and feeble pulse are attributable to insufficiency of qi and blood.

## 5. Qi deficiency of the heart and gallbladder

Symptoms: Insomnia, dreaminess, frequent waking, timidity, palpitations with susceptibility to fright, shortness of breath, lassitude, clear and profuse urine; pale tongue, and taut, thin pulse.

Analysis of symptoms: Deficiency of the heart leads to restlessness of the heart spirit, while deficiency of the gallbladder results in timorousness, so there is dreaminess with a tendency to wake up and palpitations with susceptibility to fright; shortness of breath, lassitude and clear, profuse urine stem from deficiency of qi; pale tongue and taut, thin pulse arise from insufficiency of qi and blood.

## Differential Treatment

### 1. Liver qi stagnation transforming into fire

Treatment principle: Dispersing the liver qi and purging heat, subduing the heart and tranquilizing the mind.

Prescription and herbs: Supplementary Longdan Xiegan Decoction.

Longdancao (Radix Gentianae) 9 g, Huangqin (Baical Skullcap Root) 12 g, Zhizi (Cape Jasmine Fruit) 9 g, Zexie (Oriental Waterplantain Rhizome) 12 g, Chuanmutong (Armand Clematis Stem) 5 g, Cheqianzi (Plantain Seed) 12 g (wrapped during decoction), Danggui (Chinese Angelica) 9 g, Shengdi (Dried Rehmannia Root) 12 g, Chaihu (Chinese Thorowax Root) 9 g, Fushen (Indian Bread with Hostwood) 9 g, Longgu (Os Draconis) 30 g, Muli (Oyster Shell) 30 g and Gancao (Liquorice Root) 6 g.

Modification: If there is chest distress, hypochondriac distension and frequent sighing, Yujin (Turmeric Root Tuber) 9 g, Qingpi (Green Tangerine Peel) 9 g and Foshou (Finger Citron) 6 g are added to disperse the liver qi and relieve depression.

### 2. Upward disturbance of phlegm and heat

Treatment principle: Dissolving phlegm and dispelling heat, harmonizing the middle energizer and tranquilizing the mind.

Prescription and herbs: Supplementary Huanglian Wendan Decoction.

Banxia (Pinellia Tuber) 9 g, Chenpi (Dried Tangerine Peel) 9 g, Fuling (Indian Bread) 12 g, Zhuru (Bamboo Shavings) 9 g, Zhishi (Immature Orange Fruit) 9 g, Beishumi (Northern Husked Sorghum) 12 g (wrapped during decoction), Huanglian (Golden Thread) 3 g, Shanzhi (Cape Jasmine Fruit) 9 g and Gancao ( Liquorice Root) 6 g.

Modification: For palpitations with fright, Zhenzhumu (Nacre) 30 g is added to relieve timorousness and calm the mind; if there is disorder of the stomach due to stagnation of phlegm and food, Shenqu (Massa Medicata Fermentata) 9 g, Shanzha (Hawthorn Fruit) 12 g and Laifuzi (Radish Seed) 12 g are added to remove stagnation and harmonize the stomach.

## 3. Hyperactivity of fire due to yin deficiency

Treatment principle: Replenishing yin to bring down fire, nourishing the heart to calm the mind.

Prescription and herbs: Modified Zhusha Anshen Pill.

Huanglian (Golden Thread) 3 g, Fushen (Indian Bread with Hostwood) 12 g, Shengdi (Dried Rehmannia Root) 15 g, Danggui (Chinese Angelica) 9 g, Maidong (Dwarf Lilyturf Tuber) 12 g, Gancao (Liquorice Root) 3 g, Suanzaoren (Spine Date Seed) 12 g and Baiziren (Chinese Arborvitae Kernel) 12 g.

Modification: For severe vexation, 9 g of Ejiao (Donkey-hide Glue, melted in decoction) and 2 yolks of Jizihuang (Hen Egg Yolk) are added to nourish yin and bring down fire; For deficiency of yin and floating of yang, marked by reddish and feverish complexion, dizziness, and tinnitus, Muli (Oyster Shell) 30 g, Guiban (Tortoise Shell) 9 g and Lingcishi (Magnetitum) 30 g are added to subdue yang with their heavy properties.

## 4. Deficiency of the spleen and stomach

Treatment principle: Invigorating the spleen and nourishing the heart, supplementing qi and replenishing blood.

Prescription and herbs: Modified Guipi Decoction.

Dangshen (Radix Codonopsis) 12 g, Baizhu (Largehead Atractylodes Rhizome) 15 g, Huangqi (Milkvetch Root) 15 g, Fushen (Indian Bread with Hostwood) 9 g, Longyanrou (Longan Aril) 9 g, Suanzaoren (Spine Date Seed) 12 g, Yuanzhi (Thinleaf Milkwort Root) 6 g, Muxiang (Common Aucklandia Root) 9 g and Gancao (Stir-baked Liquorice Root) 6 g.

Modification: For relatively severe insomnia, Wuweizi (Chinese Magnolivine Fruit) 9 g and Baiziren (Chinese Arborvitae Kernel) 12 g are added to nourish the heart and calm the spirit; Yejiaoteng (Caulis Polygoni Multiflori) 30 g, Hehuanpi (Silktree Albizia Bark) 12 g, Longgu (Os Draconis) 30 g and Muli (Oyster Shell) 30 g are added to tranquilize the mind.

## 5. Qi deficiency of the heart and gallbladder

Treatment principle: Supplementing qi and relieving timorousness, tranquilizing the spirit and calming the mind.

Prescription and herbs: Modified Anshen Dingzhi Pill.

Dangshen (Radix Codonopsis) 12 g, Fushen (Indian Bread with Hostwood) 15 g, Fuling (Indian Bread) 15 g, Yuanzhi (Thinleaf Milkwort Root) 3 g, Shichangpu (Acorus Calamus) 9 g, and Shenglongchi (Raw Fossilia Dentis Mastodi) 10 g.

Modification: For floating of yang due to deficiency of yin, marked by restlessness and insomnia, Zaoren (Semen Ziziphi Spinosae) 12 g, Chuanxiong (Szechwan Lovage Rhizome) 9 g, and Zhimu (Common Anemarrhena Rhizome) 12 g are added to nourish the blood and tranquilize the mind, as well as to dispel heat and relieve vexation; for those with severe fright, Lingcishi (Magnetitum) 30 g with its heavy properties is added to tranquilize the mind.

### Chinese Patent Medicine

1. Baizi Yangxin Pill: 12 pills for each dose, 3 times a day.
2. Fufang Zaoren Capsule: 2 capsules for each dose before sleep.
3. Zhenheling Tablet: 4 tablets for each dose, 3 times a day.

### Simple and Handy Prescriptions

1. Hehuanhua (Albizia Flower) 10 g, Zaoren (Semen Ziziphi Spinosae) 10 g, Yuanzhi (Thinleaf Milkwort Root) 3 g and Wuweizi (Chinese Magnolivine Fruit) 9 g are boiled in water and administered twice a day.

2. Huanglian (Golden Thread) 3 g, Zhizi (Cape Jasmine Fruit) 6 g, Lingcishi (Magnetitum) 30 g and Baihe (Lily Bulb) 12 g are boiled in water and taken twice a day to treat insomnia accompanied by irascibility.

## Other Therapies

Dietary therapy: Maidong Baihe Decoction: Maidong (Dwarf Lilyturf Tuber) 15 g, Baihe (Lily Bulb) 15 g, Lianzi (Lotus Seed) 15 g and Dazao (Chinese Date) 7 dates are used to calm the mind and relieve vexation after being boiled together in a proper amount of water.

Medicated pillow therapy: Put equal amounts of Heidou (Black Bean), Lingcishi (Magnetitum), Juemingzi (Cassia Seed) and Juhua (Chrysanthemum Flower) into a pillow to clear the heart and tranquilize the mind.

## Cautions and Advice

1. This disorder is closely related to emotions, so patients should disburden their minds of worries.
2. It is appropriate for patients to be quiet at night and to avoid immersion in a noisy or boisterous atmosphere, emotional fluctuation, as well as strenuous activities.
3. Patients should pay attention to their diet, refrain from strong tea or coffee and spicy or other food which may irritate their stomachs, as well as avoid smoking and alcohol consumption.
4. A healthy lifestyle and physical exercise will also help to strengthen the constitution.

## Daily Exercises

1. List the common causative factors of insomnia.
2. Explain how insomnia due to deficiency of the spleen and stomach can be diagnosed and treated.

# Sweating Syndrome

# Week 1: Thursday

Sweating syndrome is a disorder characterized by abnormal secretion of sweat. There are primarily five morbid conditions concerning perspiration. (1) Spontaneous sweating is the condition independent of external environmental factors, marked by frequent sweating in the daytime and aggravation upon physical exertion. (2) Night sweats is the condition marked by sweating during sleep and discontinuation of perspiration after waking up. (3) Collapse sweating is a critical condition, with presence of profuse perspiration or oily sweat accompanied by cold limbs and faint breath. (4) Yellowish sweating results in perspiration with yellowish sweat staining as named. (5) Shiver sweating occurs when the patient experiences chills and aversion to cold in acute febrile diseases. Clinically, the most common conditions are spontaneous sweating and night sweats. Abnormal perspiration can be experienced in many diseases, such as dysfunction of the autonomic nerve, hyperfunction of the thyroid, rheumatic fever, climacteric syndrome and tuberculosis.

## Etiology and Pathology

The causes of sweating syndrome are weakness of the body after diseases (which consume lung qi), invasion of pathogenic wind (which brings about disharmony between ying-nutrients and wei-defense), mental or physical overstrain and pathogenic heat (both of which deplete blood and exhaust yin), emotional disorders, hyperactivity of liver fire and internal damp-heat.

Its pathological changes are discussed as follows: Dysfunction of the defensive qi arises from insufficiency of lung qi with incompact skin and muscles, or from imbalance between ying-nutrients and wei-defense, marked by opening of the sweat pores and perspiration. Mental or physical overstrain depletes blood and consumes essence, or pathogenic heat exhausts yin, leading to internal production of deficient fire which drives the yin fluid out of the body via sweating. Emotional depression with stagnation of liver qi, indulgence in spicy and fatty food, or susceptibility to damp-heat can all contribute to the hyperactivity of liver fire and abundance of dampness and heat in the interior, which drive the yin fluid out of the body through perspiration.

## Diagnostic Key Points

1. With different clinical manifestations, the abnormal conditions of sweating are spontaneous sweating, night sweats, collapse sweating, yellowish sweating and shiver sweating.
2. Spontaneous sweating and night sweats may appear either alone or in combination with other symptoms in a certain disease.

## Syndrome Differentiation

### 1. Insecurity of lung-wei

Symptoms: Perspiration with aversion to wind, aggravation upon physical exertion, susceptibility to common cold, weariness and lusterless complexion; white and thin tongue coating and feeble, thin pulse.

Analysis of symptoms: Dysfunction of the defensive qi arises from insufficiency of lung qi with incompact skin and muscles, so there is perspiration with aversion to wind and susceptibility to common cold; physical exertion consumes qi and reduces the body's efficacy in controlling the secretion of sweat, leading to aggravated sweating; lusterless complexion, as well as thin and feeble pulse are manifestations of qi deficiency.

### 2. Disharmony between ying-nutrients and wei-defense

Symptoms: Local or general perspiration with aversion to wind, general soreness and alternated chills and fever; white, thin tongue coating and slow pulse.

Analysis of symptoms: Imbalance between ying and wei loosens the interstices of the skin, leading to perspiration with aversion to wind, general soreness, and alternated chills and fever; the white, thin tongue coating and slow pulse are manifestations of imbalance between ying and wei.

### 3. Hyperactivity of fire due to yin deficiency

Symptoms: Night sweats which may be accompanied by spontaneous sweating, feverish sensations over the five centers (the palms, the soles and the heart), or accompanied by hectic fever in the afternoon, flushed cheeks and thirst; reddish tongue with scanty coating and thin, rapid pulse.

Analysis of symptoms: Depletion of yin essence generates deficient fire in the interior, which drives the yin fluid out of the body, marked by sweating at night; deficient heat inside the body is responsible for feverish sensation over the five centers, hectic fever, and flushed cheeks; deficiency of yin gives rise to heat, which consumes body fluid and causes thirst; reddish tongue with scanty coating and thin, rapid pulse are manifestations of exuberant fire due to yin deficiency.

### 4. Stagnation and steaming of pathogenic heat

Symptoms: Profuse perspiration with sticky or yellowish sweat which may stain the clothes, reddish complexion with baking heat, restlessness, a bitter taste in the mouth and yellowish urine; thin and yellowish coating and rapid, taut pulse.

Analysis of symptoms: Hyperactivity of liver fire and exuberance of damp-heat in the interior lead to facial fever, restlessness, a bitter taste in the mouth and yellowish urine; heat drives the yin fluid out, leading to sweating; damp-heat steams inside, bringing about sticky or yellowish sweat (for stickiness and greasiness is characteristic of pathogenic dampness); thin and yellowish tongue coating and rapid, taut pulse are both due to accumulation of heat in the interior.

## Differential Treatment

### 1. Insecurity of lung-wei

Treatment principle: Replenishing qi to consolidate the superficies.

Prescription and herbs: Supplementary Yupingfen Powder.

Huangqi (Milkvetch Root) 15 g, Fangfeng (Divaricate Saposhnikovia Root) 9 g, Baizhu (Largehead Atractylodes Rhizome) 12 g, Fuxiaomai

(Blighted Wheat) 30 g, Nuodaogen (Glutinous Rice Root) 30 g, Dazao (Chinese Date) 5 dates and Gancao (Liquorice Root) 6 g.

Modification: For deficiency of qi, Dangshen (Radix Codonopsis) 12 g and Huangjing (Solomonseal Rhizome) 12 g are added to replenish qi and consolidate the superficies; if accompanied by deficiency of yin, with such signs of red tongue and thin, rapid pulse, Maidong (Dwarf Lilyturf Tuber) 12 g and Wuweizi (Chinese Magnolivine Fruit) 9 g are added to nourish yin and reduce sweat; for severe sweating, Longgu (Os Draconis) 30 g and Muli (Oyster Shell) 30 g are used to reduce sweat.

## 2. Disharmony between ying-nutrients and wei-defense

Treatment principle: Regulating ying and wei.

Prescription and herbs: Supplementary Guizhi Decoction.

Guizhi (Cassia Twig) 6 g, Baishao (White Peony Alba) 12 g, Dazao (Chinese Date) 5 dates, Shengjiang (Fresh Ginger) 3 slices and Gancao (Liquorice Root) 3 g.

Modification: For profuse sweating, Longgu (Os Draconis) 30 g and Muli (Oyster Shell) 30 g are added to reduce sweat; if accompanied by deficiency of qi, Huangqi (Milkvetch Root) 15 g is added to replenish qi and consolidate the superficies; if accompanied by deficiency of yang, Fuzi (Prepared Common Monkshood Daughter) 9 g (decocted first) is used to warm yang and reduce sweat.

## 3. Hyperactivity of fire due to yin deficiency

Treatment principle: Nourishing yin to bring down fire.

Prescription and herbs: Modified Danggui Liuhuang Decoction.

Shengdi (Dried Rehmannia Root) 15 g, Shudi (Prepared Rhizome of Rehmannia) 15 g, Danggui (Chinese Angelica) 9 g, Huanglian (Golden Thread) 3 g, Huangqin (Baical Skullcap Root) 9 g, Huangbai (Amur Cork-tree) 9 g and Huangqi (Milkvetch Root) 12 g.

Modification: For profuse sweating, Muli (Oyster Shell) 30 g, Fuxiaomai (Blighted Wheat) 30 g, and Nuodaogen (Glutinous Rice Root) 30 g are added to reduce sweat; for severe hectic fever, Qinjiao (Largeleaf Gentian

Root) 9 g, Yinchaihu (Stellaria Root) 9 g and Baiwei (Blackened Swallowwort Root) 12 g are added to subdue the deficient fever.

## 4. Stagnation and steaming of pathogenic heat

Treatment principle: Clearing the liver and purging heat, resolving dampness and harmonizing the ying phase.

Prescription and herbs: Modified Longdan Xiegan Decoction.

Longdancao (Radix Gentianae) 9 g, Huangqin (Baical Skullcap Root) 9 g, Zhizi (Cape Jasmine Fruit) 9 g, Chaihu (Chinese Thorowax Root) 9 g, Zexie (Oriental Waterplantain Rhizome) 12 g, Chuanmutong (Armand Clematis Stem) 6 g, Cheqianzi (Plantain Seed) 15 g (wrapped during decoction), Danggui (Chinese Angelica) 12 g, Shengdi (Dried Rehmannia Root) 12 g and Gancao (Liquorice Root) 6 g.

Modification: For relatively abundant damp-heat, Yinchen (Virgate Wormwood Herb) 30 g and Chifuling (Indian Bread Pink Epidermis) 12 g are added to dispel heat and eliminate dampness; for internal accumulation of damp-heat with mild fever, Huangqin (Baical Skullcap Root), Zhizi (Cape Jasmine Fruit) and Chuanmutong (Armand Clematis Stem), bitter in taste and cold in property, are used, while Cangzhu (Atractylodes Rhizome) 9 g and Shengyiyiren (Unprepared Coix Seed) 15 g are added to dispel heat and eliminate dampness.

## Chinese Patent Medicine

1. Yuping Feng Granule: 15 g for each dose, 3 times a day, for sweating due to deficiency of qi.
2. Ganlu Xiaodu Dan: 12 g for each dose, 3 times a day, for sweating due to stagnation and steaming of pathogenic heat.

## Simple and Handy Prescriptions

1. Huangqi (Milkvetch Root) 15 g, Dazao (Chinese Date) 5 dates and Fuxiaomai (Blighted Wheat) 15 g are boiled in water and administered twice a day for the treatment of spontaneous perspiration due to deficiency of qi.

2. Wumei (Smoked Plum) 10 plums, Fuxiaomai (Blighted Wheat) 15 g and Dazao (Chinese Date) 5 dates are boiled in water and taken twice a day for the treatment of night sweats due to deficiency of yin.
3. Wuweizi (Chinese Magnolivine Fruit) 10 g and Sangshenzi (Mulberry) 10 g are boiled in water and taken twice a day for the treatment of spontaneous perspiration and night sweats.

## Other Therapies

Application method: Yuliren (Chinese Dwarf Cherry Seed) 6 g and Wubeizi (Chinese Gall) 6 g are ground up into powders, blended into a paste with fresh pear juice and applied to the bilateral Neiguan (PC 6) acupoint. This is used to treat spontaneous perspiration. Wubeizi (Chinese Gall) and Wuweizi (Chinese Magnolivine Fruit) are ground up in equal quantities into fine powders, blended into a paste with a proper amount of 70% alcohol and applied to the center of the navel before a plastic film is placed over it. The paste should be changed once every 24 hours. Generally this therapy can take effect in 7~8 days. With the function of reducing sweat, it is effective for treating spontaneous perspiration and night sweats.

Dietary therapy: Qizao Porridge. Huangqi (Milkvetch Root) 30 g, Dazao (Chinese Date) 10 dates and Jiangmi (Rice Fruit) 100 g. First the milkvetch roots are immersed in water and simmered for a relatively long period, and then the condensed decoction is used to cook the rice fruit and red dates. The porridge can be taken twice a day for spontaneous perspiration with susceptibility to common cold.

## Cautions and Advice

1. For sweating due to other chronic diseases, the root cause(s) should be addressed in addition to stopping perspiration.
2. Patients with abnormal sweating are advised to keep a healthy diet, develop a healthy lifestyle, ward off wind and cold, to avoid catching flu or the common cold.
3. Patients with profuse sweating should change their undergarments regularly and keep themselves dry and clean.

## Daily Exercises

1. Describe the differences between spontaneous perspiration and night sweats in terms of their clinical characteristics.
2. Explain how spontaneous perspiration can be treated based on syndrome differentiation.

# Aphtha

## Week 1: Friday

Aphtha refers to an occurrence of ulcers or sores in the oral cavity (especially on the lingual surface and bucca cavioris), and it is characterized by intense spontaneous scorching pain. It can occur regardless of the seasons and usually afflicts young people and females. Under normal conditions, the ulcers or sores can be healed spontaneously, but in some cases, patients may experience frequent relapses and be afflicted over long durations — months, or even years. The occurrence of aphtha is closely related to viral infection, allergic response, gastrointestinal dysfunction, emotional factors, endocrine disturbance, microcirculation disturbance and immunological function. In TCM, it is also known as "mouth sores" and "mouth ulcers".

### Etiology and Pathology

The etiological factors of aphtha are mainly exogenous invasion of pathogenic toxins (which damage the viscera, turn into fire and attack the upper body), functional disorders of the viscera, as well as imbalance of yin, yang, qi and blood.

The pathological changes of aphtha are discussed as follows: Impairment of the stomach and intestine due to improper diet leads to stagnation of heat in the interior, which then moves upward and scorches the mouth and tongue, leading to sores or ulcers in the mouth. Both exogenous invasion of wind-heat into the body and invasion of pathogenic heat into the lung-wei can cause accumulation of pathogenic heat in the upper energizer, which scorches the mouth and tongue, presenting as aphtha; chronic disease consumes yin (or impairs yang), which brings about production of internal heat or even upward flaming of deficient fire (deficient yang also rejects yin and breaks the balance between yin and yang), consequently resulting in aphtha.

### Diagnostic Key Points

1. May afflict people of any age or gender, but females and young people are more susceptible.

2. With gray false membranes, the ulcers are deeply rooted and manifest themselves commonly on the lips, buccal cavioris, tongue margin and gums.
3. May occur repeatedly and persistently, usually re-triggered by emotional stress and overstrain.

## Syndrome Differentiation

### 1. Aphtha due to wind-heat

Symptoms: Canker sore(s), fever, aversion to wind, headache, sore throat, dry mouth, thirst, general pain and weariness, reddish urine, constipation, insomnia, vexation or irascibility, occasional cough with signs of heat and yellowish sputum; red tongue with yellow coating, rapid and floating pulse or tense and floating pulse.

Analysis of symptoms: These symptoms are caused by exogenous invasion of wind-heat, which damages the lung-wei and impairs the oral cavity. Pathogenic wind-heat invades the superficies, so there is syndrome of the exterior; pathogenic heat attacks the mouth, pharynx, and head, bringing about headache and sore throat; pathogenic heat consumes body fluid, leading to dry mouth, thirst, red urine and constipation; wind-heat invades the lungs, marked by occasional cough with signs of heat such as yellow sputum; red tongue with yellow coating and floating pulse are manifestations of external invasion of wind-heat.

### 2. Aphtha due to fire-heat

Symptoms: Canker sore(s) with scorching sensation, thirst, foul breath, vexation, insomnia, constipation, reddish urine, sore or dry throat; red tongue with yellow and greasy coating or yellow and dry coating, rapid and slippery pulse or rapid and taut pulse.

Analysis of symptoms: The symptoms are caused by internal abundance of fire and heat. Fire and heat scorch the upper energizer and burn the oral cavity, causing canker sore(s); pathogenic heat accumulates in the interior, bringing about general fever; pathogenic heat attacks the head and disturbs the mind, leading to vexation and insomnia; heat impairs body fluid, resulting in reddish urine, constipation, thirst and foul breath; red tongue with yellow coating, rapid and slippery pulse or rapid and taut pulse are due to internal abundance of fire and heat.

## 3. Aphtha due to yin deficiency

Symptoms: Canker sore(s), dry mouth, thirst with no desire for drinking, fatigue, feverish sensations in the palms and soles, difficulty in urination and defecation, vexation, palpitations, susceptibility to cold, red tongue with scanty coating and thin, rapid pulse.

Analysis of symptoms: Deficiency of yin produces internal heat and deficient fire, which attack the upper energizer and scorch the fine collaterals of the mouth and pharynx, resulting in canker sore(s), dry mouth and thirst with no desire for drinking; deficient fire flames up and troubles the mind, giving rise to vexation and palpitations; internal heat consumes body fluid, bringing about difficulty in urination and defecation; internal heat and deficient fire attracts external heat, causing susceptibility to common cold; the red tongue with scanty coating and thin, rapid pulse are manifestations of internal heat due to deficiency of yin.

## 4. Aphtha due to qi deficiency

Symptoms: Canker sore(s), pale complexion or facial edema, spontaneous perspiration, lassitude, intolerance of cold, cold limbs, poor appetite, loose stools, clear and profuse urine, susceptibility to common cold, pale tongue with white coating and thin and weak pulse.

Analysis of symptoms: Deficient qi fails to anchor yang and this leads to floating of the deficient yang, which is incapable of warming and activating the oral meridians or vessels, bringing about canker sore(s) and pale complexion; deficiency of inner qi results in lassitude; deficient qi fails to protect and consolidate the exterior, resulting in spontaneous perspiration, fatigue and susceptibility to cold; deficiency of qi leads to dysfunction of the spleen in transportation and transformation, with such signs as inadequate food intake and loose stools; pale tongue with white coating and thin, weak pulse are attributable to deficiency of qi.

## Differential Treatment

### 1. Aphtha due to wind-heat

Treatment principle: Dispersing wind and dispelling heat, purging fire and removing toxins.

Prescription and herbs: Modified Sangju Potion.

Sangye (Mulberry Leaf) 9 g, Juhua (Chrysanthemum Flower) 9 g, Bohe (Peppermint) 5 g, Lianqiao (Weeping Forsythia Capsule) 9 g, Xingren (Almond) 9 g, Jiegeng (Platycodon Root) 5 g, Banlange (Isatis Root) 30 g, Shandouge (Vietnamese Sophora Root) 15 g and Gancao ( Liquorice Root) 5 g.

Modification: For dry mouth with thirst, Tianhuafen (Trichosanthin) 15 g and Chuanshihu (Szechwan Dendrobium) 15 g are added to nourish yin, produce body fluid and quench thirst; in cases of restlessness and insomnia, Zhizi (Cape Jasmine Fruit) 9 g and Zhimu (Common Anemarrhena Rhizome) 9 g are added to clear the heart and relieve vexation.


### 2. Aphtha due to fire-heat

Treatment principle: Dispelling heat and purging fire.

Prescription and herbs: Modified Yunu Decoction and Daochi Powder.

Zhuye (Henon Bamboo Leaf) 9 g, Mutong (Caulis Hocquartiae) 5 g, Shengdi (Dried Rehmannia Root) 12 g, Maidong (Dwarf Lilyturf Tuber) 12 g, Zhimu (Common Anemarrhena Rhizome) 9 g, Shengshigao (Unprepared Gypsum) 30 g (decocted first), Lugen (Reed Rhizome) 30 g, Niuxi (Two-toothed Achyranthes Root) 12 g, and Gancao (Liquorice Root) 3 g.

Modification: For constipation, Dahuang (Rhubarb) 6 g is added to purge fire and promote defecation; in cases of insomnia and vexation, Huanglian (Golden Thread) 3 g, Dandouchi (Fermented Soybean) 15 g and Yejiaoteng (Caulis Polygoni Multiflori) 30 g are added to clear the heart, relieve vexation and improve sleep.

## 3. Aphtha due to yin deficiency

Treatment principle: Nourishing yin and dispelling heat, purging fire and relieving vexation.

Prescription and herbs: Modified Zhibai Dihuang Pill.

Zhimu (Common Anemarrhena Rhizome) 9 g, Huangbai (Amur Corktree) 9 g, Shengdi (Dried Rehmannia Root) 15 g, Shanzhuyu (Asiatic Cornelian Cherry Fruit) 9 g, Huaishanyao (Huaihe Common Yan Rhizome) 12 g, Fuling (Indian Bread) 15 g, Danpi (Cortex Moutan) 9 g, Zexie (Oriental Waterplantain Rhizome) 12 g, Zhihouwu (Prepared Fleeceflower Root) 15 g, Nuzhenzi (Glossy Privet Fruit) 12 g, Baihe (Lily Bulb) 15 g, Maidong (Dwarf Lilyturf Tuber) 12 g and Yuzhu (Fragrant Solomonseal Rhizome) 12 g.

Modification: For insomnia, Hehuanpi (Silktree Albizia Bark) 12 g and Yejiaoteng (Caulis Polygoni Multiflori) 30 g are added to calm the heart and tranquilize the mind; if it is accompanied by deficiency of qi and manifested as weariness, Huangqi (Milkvetch Root) 15 g and Taizishen (Heterophylly Falsesatarwort Root) 15 g are used to supplement qi and nourish deficiency.

## 4. Aphtha due to qi deficiency

Treatment principle: Supplementing qi, moving up yang and reinforcing healthy qi.

Prescription and herbs: Modified Buzhong Yiqi Decoction.

Dangshen (Radix Codonopsis) 12 g, Huangqi (Milkvetch Root) 15 g, Baizhu (Largehead Atractylodes Rhizome) 12 g, Danggui (Chinese Angelica) 9 g, Shengdi (Dried Rehmannia Root) 15 g, Chuanxiong (Szechwan Lovage Rhizome) 9 g, Baishao (White Peony Alba) 12 g, Shengma (Rhizoma Cimicifugae) 9 g, Chaihu (Chinese Thorowax Root) 9 g and Gancao (Liquorice Root) 5 g.

Modification: If accompanied by deficiency of yin and manifested as feverish sensation in the palms and soles and vexation, Maidong (Dwarf Lilyturf Tuber) 12 g, Zhimu (Common Anemarrhena Rhizome) 9 g, and

Danpi (Cortex Moutan) 9 g are added to nourish yin and dispel heat; for susceptibility to cold, Fangfeng (Divaricate Saposhnikovia Root) 9 g is used to dispel pathogenic wind in the exterior and, meanwhile, prevent wind from invading the interior.

## Chinese Patent Medicine

1. Tianwang Buxin Dan: 5 g for each dose, 3 times a day, used to treat aphtha due to deficient fire.
2. Huanglian Shangqi Tablet: 4~5 tablets for each dose, 3 times a day, used to treat aphtha due to excess fire.

## Simple and Handy Prescriptions

1. Zhuye (Henon Bamboo Leaf) 9 g and Shengshigao (Unprepared Gypsum) 30 g are boiled in water and used to treat aphtha due to exuberance of heart fire.
2. Maidong (Dwarf Lilyturf Tuber) 9 g, Tiandong (Cochinchinese Asparagus Root) 9 g, and Xuanshen (Figwort Root) 12 g are boiled in water and used to treat aphtha due to deficiency of yin.

## Other Therapies

Application method: Xixin (Manchurian Wildginger), ground up into powder and blended with vinegar, is applied to the umbilicus once a day for 4~5 consecutive days and discontinued when there is prurigo eruption; Wuzhuyu (Medicinal Evodia Fruit) is also ground up into powder, blended with vinegar and applied to the center of each sole once a day for 4~5 consecutive days.

Dietary therapy: Er Dong Porridge: Tiandong (Cochinchinese Asparagus Root) 9 g, Maidong (Dwarf Lilyturf Tuber) 9 g, Jiangmi (Rice Fruit) 100 g and sugar to taste are simmered into porridge and used to nourish yin, this porridge is best for aphtha due to deficiency of yin. Bamboo Leaf Porridge: Zhuye (Fresh Henon Bamboo Leaf) 20 g, Shengshigao (Unprepared Gypsum) 30 g, Jiangmi (Rice Fruit) 100 g and brown sugar to taste are made into porridge for dispelling heat and purging fire.

Topical therapy: Rinse the mouth with warm salt water before applying any of the following prescriptions such as Xilei Powder, Zhuhuang Powder, Xiguashuang Powder and Qingdai Powder onto the ulcer surface once every 1~2 hours.

## Cautions and Advice

1. Patients are advised to develop a healthy lifestyle and refrain from spicy and fried food and roasted meat.
2. They should drink plenty of water and eat more vegetables and fruits to promote bowel movements and prevent constipation.
3. They should also regulate their lifestyles, relieve stress and anxiety and avoid overstrain.

## Daily Exercises

1. Recall the different types of aphtha and their representative prescriptions.
2. Describe the pathogenetic characteristics of aphtha due to deficiency of yin.

# Diarrhea

# Week 1: Saturday

Diarrhea is a morbid condition marked by increased frequency of bowel movements, loose stools, or even watery fecal discharge. It can occur regardless of the seasons, but is more likely in summer and autumn. In addition, diarrhea is a common symptom of acute or chronic enteritis, functional disorder of the intestines, irritability of the colon and functional laxness. Clinically, this disease is divided into two types: acute diarrhea and chronic diarrhea.

### Etiology and Pathology

TCM holds that diarrhea can be caused by either exogenous or endogenous pathogenic factors. The former refers to the six abnormal climatic factors, particularly the pathogenic cold-dampness and summer-heat (with dampness playing a dominant role). The latter refers to deficiency of the spleen, or disorders of the liver and kidneys (most of which develop from spleen deficiency).

The pathological changes are discussed as follows: Invasion of exogenous pathogenic factors into the spleen and stomach leads to malfunction of the spleen in its ascending function and the stomach in its descending function, as well as dysfunction in transportation and transformation, with the mixing of lucid substances with turbid ones giving rise to diarrhea. Intake of fatty and sweet or raw and cold food, accidental intake of unsanitary food, or excessive intake of water and food may lead to internal retention of indigested food and malfunction of the spleen and stomach in transportation and transformation, as well as their ascending/descending functions, leading to diarrhea. Existing weakness of the spleen and stomach when coupled with emotional disorder, may lead to stagnation of the liver qi which restricts the spleen excessively, making it unable to transport and transform water and food, leading to diarrhea. Overstrain, internal damage and chronic diseases can weaken the spleen and stomach, leading to dysfunction in transportation and transformation, with the mixing of lucid substances and turbid ones giving rise to diarrhea. Decline of fire in mingmen (the life gate) due to senility results in failure of the spleen-earth to be warmed and disorder in transportation and transformation, causing diarrhea.

## Diagnostic Key Points

1. Increased frequency of bowel movements with loose stools.
2. Accompanying symptoms such as abdominal pain, rugitus, belching, poor appetite and fever in acute cases.
3. Routine stool test is normal or yields a small quantity of red blood cells and white blood cells.

## Syndrome Differentiation

### 1. Invasion of cold-dampness

Symptoms: Diarrhea with loose or even watery feces, abdominal pain with rugitus, gastric stuffiness and poor appetite; aversion to cold with fever, nasal obstruction, headache, and soreness of the limbs may also be present; white and thin or greasy tongue coating and slow and soggy pulse.

Analysis of symptoms: Invasion of exogenous pathogenic cold-dampness or wind-cold into the stomach and intestine, or excessive intake of raw and cold food, can lead to malfunction of the spleen in its ascending function and the stomach in its descending function, as well as dysfunction in transportation and transformation, with the mixing of lucid substances with turbid ones giving rise to loose stools; abundant cold-dampness in the interior obstructs the qi activities of the stomach and intestine, causing abdominal pain with rugitus; damp-cold encumbers the spleen, bringing about gastric stuffiness and poor appetite; aversion to cold, fever, nasal obstruction, headache and soreness of the limbs are due to wind-cold fettering the exterior; white greasy tongue coating and slippery, soggy pulse are manifestations of abundant cold-dampness in the interior.

## 2. Contraction of damp-heat (summer-heat)

Symptoms: Diarrhea with abdominal pain, urgent and unpleasant discharge of yellow-brown and fetid stools, burning pain in the anus, feverish dysphoria with thirst, scanty and yellowish urine; yellow and greasy tongue coating, rapid and soggy pulse or rapid and slippery pulse.

Analysis of symptoms: Pathogenic damp-heat or summer-heat affects the transporting and transforming functions of the spleen and stomach, giving rise to diarrhea with abdominal pain; heat exists in the intestine, causing urgent diarrhea; dampness and heat together result in unpleasant discharge of feces; damp-heat descends, bringing about burning pain in the anus, yellow-brown and fetid stools, as well as scanty and yellowish urine; feverish dysphoria with thirst, yellow and greasy tongue coating, rapid and soggy pulse or rapid and slippery pulse are all due to internal abundance of dampness and heat.

## 3. Retention of food in the stomach and intestine

Symptoms: Abdominal pain, rugitus, loose stools with the odor of rotten eggs, alleviation after fecal discharge, retention of indigested food, gastric and abdominal stuffiness and fullness, fetid and acidic regurgitation and poor appetite; turbid or thick greasy tongue coating and slippery pulse.

Analysis of symptoms: Improper diet leads to internal retention of indigested food in the stomach and intestine which fail to transport and transform normally, bringing about abdominal pain, rugitus, as well as gastric and abdominal stuffiness and fullness; retention of food causes adverse rising of turbid qi, so there is fetid and acidic regurgitation; indigested food descends, leading to loose stools with the odor of rotten eggs; the rotten and turbid substances are discharged with diarrhea, hence there is alleviation after defecation; thick and greasy tongue coating and slippery pulse are manifestations of internal retention of indigested food.

## 4. Liver qi affecting the spleen

Symptoms: Diarrhea with abdominal pain occurring together with depression, anger or emotional stress; frequent distending pain over the chest and hypochondria region, belching and poor appetite; pink tongue and taut pulse.

Analysis of symptoms: Emotional disorder or stress impedes the function of the liver in governing the free flow of liver qi which invades the spleen and causes dysfunction of this organ in transportation and transformation, hence there is diarrhea with abdominal pain; failure of the liver to promote the free flow of qi disrupts the functional activity of qi, giving rise to distension and fullness in the chest and hypochondria, belching and poor appetite; pink tongue and taut pulse are manifestations of liver hyperactivity and spleen deficiency.

## 5. Weakness of the spleen and stomach

Symptoms: Loose or watery stools, indigestion of water and food, increased frequency of bowel movements triggered by intake of oily food, reduced food intake, gastric and abdominal distension and discomfort, sallow complexion and weariness; pale tongue with white coating, thin and feeble pulse.

Analysis of symptoms: Weakness of the spleen and stomach leads to indigested water and food being mixed with turbid and lucid substances, giving rise to loose or watery stools; inactivation of spleen yang brings about dysfunction of the spleen in transportation and transformation, leading to reduced food intake, gastric and abdominal distension and discomfort, as well as increased frequency and duration of defecation triggered by intake of oily food; weakness of the spleen and stomach impairs their ability to produce sufficient qi and blood, causing sallow complexion and weariness; pale tongue with white coating and thin and feeble pulse are manifestations of a weak spleen and stomach.

## 6. Deficiency of kidney yang

Symptoms: Diarrhea before dawn with abdominal pain, fecal discharge following borborygmus with alleviation after defecation, cold body and limbs, weakness and soreness of the waist and knees; pale tongue with white coating and thin and deep pulse.

Analysis of symptoms: Because chronic diarrhea debilitates the kidney yang and makes it unable to warm the spleen and stomach (which leads to dysfunction in transportation and transformation) and since yang qi is inactivated and yin qi is still predominant before dawn, the result is abdominal pain and fecal discharge following borborygmus (also called "diarrhea before dawn"); after fecal discharge, the obstruction in the intestines is removed, hence the alleviation after defecation; cold body and limbs, weakness and soreness of the waist and knees, pale tongue with white coating and thin and deep pulse are attributable to insufficiency of spleen yang and kidney yang.

## Differential Treatment

### 1. Invasion of cold-dampness

Treatment principle: Relieving the exterior and dissipating cold, resolving dampness with aromatic flavor.

Prescription and herbs: Huoxiang Zhengqi San (Agastache Rugosa Healthy Qi-Invigorating Powder).

Huoxiang (Agastache Rugosa) 9 g, Zisu (Purple Common Perilla) 9 g, Baizhi (Dahurian Angelica Root) 6 g, Baizhu (Largehead Atractylodes Rhizome) 12 g, Fuling (Indian Bread) 15 g, Chenpi (Dried Tangerine Peel) 9 g, Banxia (Pinellia Tuber) 9 g, Houpu (Magnolia Bark) 6 g, Dafupi (Areca Peel) 6 g, Gancao ( Liquorice Root) 3 g and Dazao (Chinese Date) 5 dates.

Modification: If there are relatively severe exterior syndromes with fever and aversion to cold, Jingjie (Fineleaf Schizonepeta Herb) 9 g and Fangfeng (Divaricate Saposhnikovia Root) 9 g are added to strengthen the action of dispersing wind and dissipating cold; for relatively abundant dampness with chest distress, abdominal distension, scanty urine and weary limbs, Cangzhu (Atractylodes Rhizome) 6 g, Zhuling (Polyporus) 12 g and Zexie (Oriental Waterplantain Rhizome) 12 g are used to invigorate the spleen and eliminate dampness.

### 2. Contraction of damp-heat (summer-heat)

Treatment principle: Dispelling heat and eliminating dampness.

Prescription and herbs: Supplementary Gegen Qinlian Tang.

Huangqin (Baical Skullcap Root) 12 g, Huanglian (Golden Thread) 3 g, Gegen (Kudzuvine Root) 15 g, Fuling (Indian Bread) 15 g, Cheqianzi (Plantain Seed) 15 g (wrapped during decoction) and Jinyinhua (Honeysuckle Flower) 12 g.

Modification: For relative abundance of pathogenic dampness with manifestations of fullness and distension in the chest and abdomen as well as yellow and greasy tongue coating, Cangzhu (Atractylodes Rhizome) 9 g, Houpu (Magnolia Bark) 6 g and Chenpi (Dried Tangerine Peel) 9 g are added to dry dampness and relieve the middle energizer; for invasion of summer-heat and dampness, Huoxiang (Agastache Rugosa) 9 g, Heye (Lotus Leaf) 9 g, Xiangru (Haichow Elsholtzia Herb) 12 g and Biandouyi (Testa Dolichoris) 9 g are added to dispel summer-heat and resolve dampness.

### 3. Retention of food in the stomach and intestine

Treatment principle: Promoting digestion and removing stagnation.

Prescription and herbs: (Mainly) Baohe Pill.

Shanzha (Hawthorn Fruit) 9 g, Shenqu (Massa Medicata Fermentata) 9 g, Laifuzi (Radish Seed) 12 g, Fuling (Indian Bread) 15 g, Chenpi (Dried Tangerine Peel) 9 g, Banxia (Pinellia Tuber) 9 g and Lianqiao (Weeping Forsythia Capsule) 12 g.

Modification: For transformation of retained food into heat, Dahuang (Rhubarb) 9 g decocted later and Zhishi (Immature Orange Fruit) 9 g are used to treat diarrhea so as to resolve the stagnation, dispel heat and eliminate dampness; for impairment due to intake of raw or cold food, Ganjiang (Dried Ginger) 6 g and Roudoukou (Nutmeg) 9 g are added to warm the middle energizer and dissipate cold.

### 4. Liver qi affecting the spleen

Treatment principle: Suppressing the liver and reinforcing the spleen, regulating qi and checking diarrhea.

Prescription and herbs: (Mainly) Tongxie Yaofang Decoction.

Baizhu (Largehead Atractylodes Rhizome) 12 g, Baishao (White Peony Alba) 12 g, Fangfeng (Divaricate Saposhnikovia Root) 9 g, Chenpi (Dried

Tangerine Peel) 9 g, Chaihu (Chinese Thorowax Root) 9 g, Fuling (Indian Bread) 12 g, Zhixiangfu (Prepared Nutgrass Galingale Rhizome) 9 g and Gancao (Liquorice Root) 3 g.

Modification: For severe deficiency of the spleen with lassitude, gastric, and abdominal discomfort, Dangshen (Radix Codonopsis) 12 g, Huaishanyao (Huaihe Common Yan Rhizome) 15 g and Biandou (Hyacinth Bean) 12 g are added to replenish qi and invigorate the spleen; for poor appetite, Muxiang (Common Aucklandia Root) 9 g and Sharen (Villous Amomum Fruit) 3 g with their aromatic flavors are used to activate the spleen.

## 5. Weakness of the spleen and stomach

Treatment principle: Invigorating the spleen and nourishing the stomach, facilitating digestion and checking diarrhea.

Prescription and herbs: Modified Shenling Baizhu Powder.

Dangshen (Radix Codonopsis) 12 g, Fuling (Indian Bread) 15 g, Baizhu (Largehead Atractylodes Rhizome) 12 g, Huaishanyao (Huaihe Common Yan Rhizome) 15 g, Biandou (Hyacinth Bean) 12 g, Lianzi (Lotus Seed) 12 g, Shengyiyiren (Unprepared Coix Seed) 15 g, Sharen (Villous Amomum Fruit) 3 g, Jiegeng (Platycodon Root) 3 g and Gancao (Liquorice Root) 6 g.

Modification: For pain from abdominal cold and lack of warmth in the feet and hands, Fuzi (Prepared Common Monkshood Daughter) 9 g (decocted first), Ganjiang (Dried Ginger) 6 g and Rougui (Cassia Bark) 3 g are added to warm the middle energizer and dissipate cold; for chronic diarrhea with qi sinking of the middle energizer and anal prolapse, Huangqi (Milkvetch Root) 15 g, Shengma (Rhizoma Cimicifugae) 9 g and Chaihu (Chinese Thorowax Root) 9 g are used to replenish qi and move up yang.

## 6. Deficiency of kidney yang

Treatment principle: Warming the kidneys and invigorating the spleen, constricting the intestine and checking diarrhea.

Prescription and herbs: Supplementary Sishen Pill.

Buguzhi (Malaytea Scurfpea Fruit) 12 g, Roudoukou (Nutmeg) 12 g, Wuzhuyu (Medicinal Evodia Fruit) 3 g, Wuweizi (Chinese Magnolivine Fruit) 6 g, Paojiang (Prepared Dried Ginger) 6 g, Fuling (Indian Bread) 15 g and Baizhu (Largehead Atractylodes Rhizome) 12 g.

Modification: For intolerance of cold with cold limbs, Fuzi (Prepared Common Monkshood Daughter) 9 g (decocted first) and Ganjiang (Dried Ginger) 6 g are added to warm yang and dissipate cold; for chronic diarrhea with qi sinking of the middle energizer, Huangqi (Milkvetch Root) 15 g, Dangshen (Radix Codonopsis) 12 g, Hezirou (Medicine Terminalia Fruit) 9 g and Chishizhi (Red Halloysite) 9 g are added to replenish qi and invigorate the spleen, as well as astringe the intestine and check diarrhea.

## Chinese Patent Medicine

1. Xianglian Pill: 3 g for each dose, 3 times a day. It is used to dispel heat and eliminate dampness, applicable for diarrhea due to damp-heat.
2. Huoxiang Zhengqi Soft Capsule: 4 capsules for each dose, 3 times a day. It is used to resolve dampness with aromatic herbs, applicable for diarrhea due to exogenous pathogenic factors.
3. Jianpi Pill: 12 pills for each dose, 3 times a day. It is used to replenish qi and invigorate the spleen, applicable for diarrhea due to spleen deficiency.

## Simple and Handy Prescriptions

1. Shengjiang (Fresh Ginger) 9 g and Chenchaye (Old Tea Leaves) 9 g are boiled in water and taken several times in succession to treat watery diarrhea.
2. Huoxiangye (Fresh Agastache Rugosa Leaf) 10 g, Heye (Fresh Lotus Leaf) 10 g and Biandouye (Fresh Hyacinth Bean Leaf) 10 g are ground up into juice and infused in warm boiled water to treat sudden diarrhea due to summer-dampness.

## Other Therapies

Hot compress therapy: Crude salt 500 g is fried and dried in an iron pot over a strong fire and then wrapped and applied to the umbilicus, waist or back while it is still hot. This is used to warm the middle energizer and check diarrhea.

Dietary therapy: Shanyaoyu Soup. Huaishanyao (Huaihe Common Yan Rhizome) 300 g and river fish 250 g are decocted with sauces to taste and used to invigorate the spleen, reinforce the middle energizer and supplement qi so as to check diarrhea.

Skin scraping therapy: Scrape the bilateral sides of the spine and if there is chest distress and abdominal distension or agony, scrape the chest and abdomen so as to promote digestion, remove stagnation and check diarrhea due to food retention.

Vinegar-prepared egg therapy: Pound Shengjiang (Fresh Ginger) 50 g into juice and blend evenly with an egg and 15 ml of vinegar before ingesting. This therapy is used to promote digestion and resolve stagnation.

## Cautions and Advice

1. Diarrhea should be promptly addressed lest it develops into a chronic condition and results in problems of malnutrition and anaemia.
2. Patients should maintain a healthy diet, avoid indulgence in oily, fatty and sweet food and refrain from raw, cold and unsanitary food.
3. They are also advised to engage in physical exercise to strengthen their constitutions.

## Daily Exercises

1. Name the exogenous pathogenic factor most closely associated with diarrhea.
2. Describe the characteristics of diarrhea due to deficiency of kidney yang.
3. Explain how diarrhea due to weakness of the spleen and stomach can be diagnosed and treated.

# Constipation

## Week 2: Monday

Constipation is a morbid condition marked by retention of stools and difficult passage of stools. It may be caused by genetic disorders of the intestinal tract, but in most cases it is due to more straightforward factors:
Retention of food residues, reduced stress response of the intestinal tract,
lack of motive power for defecation, obstruction of the enteric cavity and
neuropsychosis can all lead to constipation.

### Etiology and Pathology

The etiological factors of constipation are external invasion of wind-heat,
insufficiency of body fluid, disorder of emotions, stagnation of qi movements, internal injury due to overstrain, weakness of the body and deficiency of qi and blood. All of these can result in malfunction of the large
intestine in transportation and, eventually, constipation.

The pathological changes of constipation are discussed as follows:
People with predominant yang in their constitution tend to accumulate
heat in the stomach and intestine, which consumes body fluid and reduces
moisture in the intestines, resulting in dry stools. Excessive worry and
contemplation, emotional depression, or a sedentary lifestyle can all lead
to stagnation of qi and dysfunction in the descending function and transportation, leading to internal retention of residues. Overstrain, internal
damage, chronic diseases, childbirth, senility, or physical deficiency can
all consume qi and blood, or even impair kidney essence and genuine yin
in the lower energizer, reducing body fluid and making stools drier.
Depletion of genuine yang leads to deficiency of body fluid which reduces
moisture in the intestine, resulting in constipation. A constitution deficient
in yang tends toward endogenous production of yin cold which stays
inside the stomach and intestine and blocks the movements of yang qi and
body fluid, affecting the smooth transportation of stools in the intestine
and resulting in constipation.

## Diagnostic Key Points

1. Difficult passage of dry and hard stools.
2. Decreased frequency of bowel movements, once in 2~3 days or more, with no regular patterns.
3. Possible presence of abdominal distension and pain.
4. Physical examination generally reveals no apparent abnormalities.

## Syndrome Differentiation

The following two types of constipation are due to excess:

## 1. Constipation due to accumulation of heat

Symptoms: Dry stools, scanty and reddish urine, flushed face, general fever which may be accompanied by abdominal distension and pain and dry mouth with foul breath; red tongue with yellow coating or yellow and dry coating, as well as slippery and rapid pulse.

Analysis of symptoms: The stomach is the "sea of water and food" and the intestine is the organ responsible for transportation, so if heat is accumulated in the intestine and consumes body fluid, the result will be dry stools; heat hidden in the spleen and stomach fumigates the upper part of the body, resulting in dry mouth with foul breath, flushed face and general fever; heat accumulates in the stomach and intestine and blocks the abdominal qi, with such symptoms as abdominal distension and pain; heat moves into the bladder, bringing about scanty and reddish urine; yellow and dry tongue coating is an indication of heat impairing yin and producing dryness; slippery and rapid pulse is a manifestation of excess in the body.

## 2. Constipation due to stagnation of qi

Symptoms: Frequent urges to have bowel movements foiled by difficult passage of stools, incessant belching, thoracic and hypochondriac stuffiness and fullness, or even abdominal distension and pain, as well as poor appetite; thin and greasy tongue coating and taut pulse.

Analysis of symptoms: Disorder of emotions leads to stagnation of liver qi and spleen qi, causing malfunction of the intestine in transportation and such manifestations as difficulty in defecation; obstruction of the intestine results in adverse rising of qi, leading to frequent belching with chest and hypochondriac stuffiness and fullness; internal retention of residues and stagnation of qi bring about gaseous distension in the abdomen; stagnation of qi in the stomach and intestine weakens the spleen in transportation, which is characterized by poor appetite; thin and greasy tongue coating and taut pulse are due to disharmony between the spleen and stomach with retention of dampness.

The following three types of constipation are due to deficiency:

## 3. Constipation due to deficiency of qi

Symptoms: Strong urges and excessive strain during bowel movements, sweating, shortness of breath, but inability to pass out even dry and hard stools, white complexion, weariness, or lassitude; pale and tender tongue with thin coating and weak pulse.

Analysis of symptoms: Deficiency of qi is due to impairment of the lungs and spleen, and the lungs are interiorly and exteriorly associated with the large intestine, so if the lung qi is deficient, the large intestine will exhibit disorder in transportation, resulting in unsuccessful discharge of fecal matter despite strong desire and great effort for defecation; insecurity of lung-wei leads to looseness of the skin and opening of the sweat pores, with such signs as sweating and shortness of breath during defecation; spleen deficiency is responsible for dysfunction in transportation and transformation, so there is insufficient qi and blood, giving rise to a white complexion and weariness; pale tongue with thin coating and weak pulse, as well as fatigue after defecation are manifestations of qi deficiency.

## 4. Constipation due to deficiency of blood

Symptoms: Dry and hard stools, dizziness, palpitations, lusterless complexion, colorless lips and nails; pale tongue and thin, unsmooth pulse.

Analysis of symptoms: Deficiency of blood leads to insufficiency of body fluid, which reduces moisture in the intestine and leads to dry stools; blood deficiency results in poor nourishment for the head, so the complexion is lusterless and the lips and nails lack color; the heart is also malnourished, as indicated by palpitations; similarly, deficient blood fails to nourish the brain, resulting in dizziness; pale tongue and thin, unsmooth pulse are manifestations of insufficient yin blood.

## 5. Constipation due to predominance of cold

Symptoms: Difficulty in defecation, clear and profuse urine, pale complexion, lack of warmth in the limbs, preference for heat and intolerance of cold, cold pain in the abdomen, or cold soreness in the waist and back; pale tongue with white coating, deep and slow pulse.

Analysis of symptoms: Deficiency of yang qi gives rise to production of cold from the interior which damages the intestine and causes difficulty in defecation; predominant yin cold in the interior blocks qi movements, causing preference for heat and intolerance of cold, with cold pain in the abdomen; the deficient yang is incapable of warming the body, giving rise to a lack of warmth in the limbs, cold soreness in the waist and back and clear and profuse urine; pale complexion and tongue, white coating, as well as deep, slow pulse, are all manifestations of internal cold due to deficiency of yang.

## Differential Treatment

### 1. Constipation due to accumulation of heat

Treatment principle: Dispelling heat and moistening the intestine.

Prescription and herbs: Modified Maziren Pill.

Shengdahuang (Unprepared Rhubarb) 9 g (decocted later), Zhishi (Immature Orange Fruit) 9 g, Houpu (Magnolia Bark) 6 g, Huomaren (Hemp Seed) 20 g (broken into pieces), Xingren (Almond) 12 g and Baishao (White Peony Alba) 10 g.

Modification: For massive accumulation of heat, Huanglian (Golden Thread) 3 g and Mangxiao (Sodium Sulfate) 9 g (infused into water) are added to dispel heat and dredge the intestine; if there is impairment of body fluid and dry mouth with thirst, Shengdi (Dried Rehmannia Root) 12 g, Xuanshen (Figwort Root) 15 g and Maidong (Dwarf Lilyturf Tuber) 12 g are added to nourish yin and produce fluid; for impairment of the liver by anger, coupled with irascibility and reddened eyes, Luhui (Herba Alose) 3 g and Zhizi (Cape Jasmine Fruit) 12 g are used to clear the liver and promote defecation.

## 2. Constipation due to stagnation of qi

Treatment principle: Smoothing qi and relieving stagnation, removing obstruction and promoting defecation.

Prescription and herbs: Modified Liumuo Decoction.

Muxiang (Common Aucklandia Root) 10 g, Wuyao (Combined Spicebush Root) 12 g, Chenxiang (Chinese Eaglewood) 3 g (swallowed), Shengdahuang (Unprepared Rhubarb) 9 g (decocted later), Binglang (Areca Seed) 12 g, Zhishi (Immature Orange Fruit) 12 g, Xiangfu (Nutgrass Galingale Rhizome) 12 g and Chaihu (Chinese Thorowax Root) 9 g.

Modification: For prolonged stagnation of qi transforming into fire, causing a bitter taste in the mouth, dry throat, yellow tongue coating and rapid, taut pulse, Huangqin (Baical Skullcap Root) 12 g and Zhizi (Cape Jasmine Fruit) 9 g are added to dispel heat and purge fire; if there is obstruction of the throat by phlegm and qi, Quangualou (Snakegourd Fruit) 12 g and Mangxiao (Sodium Sulfate) 9 g (infused into water) are added to dissolve phlegm and dredge the intestine.

## 3. Constipation due to deficiency of qi

Treatment principle: Supplementing qi and moistening the intestine.

Prescription and herbs: Modified Huangqi Decoction.

Huangqi (Milkvetch Root) 20 g, Dangshen (Radix Codonopsis) 12 g, Chenpi (Dried Tangerine Peel) 9 g, Huomaren (Hemp Seed) 20 g, Baimi (Whitish Honey) 12 g (infused into water) and Baizhu (Largehead Atractylodes Rhizome) 15 g.

Modification: For anal prolapse due to deficiency of qi, Shengma (Rhizoma Cimicifugae) 12 g, Chaihu (Chinese Thorowax Root) 9 g and Jiegeng (Platycodon Root) 6 g are added to supplement as well as move qi upward.

## 4. Constipation due to deficiency of blood

Treatment principle: Nourishing blood and replenishing yin, adding moisture and promoting defecation.

Prescription and herbs: Modified Runchang Pill.

Shengdi (Dried Rehmannia Root) 12 g, Danggui (Chinese Angelica) 12 g, Huomaren (Hemp Seed) 20 g, Taoren (Peach Seed) 10 g, Zhiqiao (Orange Fruit) 9 g, Shengshouwu (Fleeceflower Root) 15 g and Xuanshen (Figwort Root) 12 g.

Modification: For inadequacy of blood and internal heat due to deficiency of yin, resulting in feverish dysphoria, dry mouth, red tongue and scanty fluid, Zhimu (Common Anemarrhena Rhizome) 12 g and Dahuang (Rhubarb) 9 g are added to dispel heat; for severe depletion of yin, Maidong (Dwarf Lilyturf Tuber) 12 g and Yuzhu (Fragrant Solomonseal Rhizome) 12 g are added to nourish yin and add moisture; for deficiency of intestinal fluid, Baimi (Whitish Honey) 15 g infused into water and Yuliren (Chinese Dwarf Cherry Seed) 15 g are used to add moisture and promote defecation.

## 5. Constipation due to predominance of cold

Treatment principle: Warming yang to promote defecation.

Prescription and herbs: Jichuan Decoction plus Rougui (Cassia Bark).

Roucongrong (Desertliving Cistanche) 12 g, Niuxi (Two-toothed Achyranthes Root) 12 g, Danggui (Chinese Angelica) 12 g , Shengma (Rhizoma Cimicifugae) 3 g, Rougui (Cassia Bark) 3 g and Zhiqiao (Orange Fruit) 9 g.

Modification: For deficiency of qi with lassitude, Dangshen (Radix Codonopsis) 12 g and Baizhu (Largehead Atractylodes Rhizome) 15 g are added to replenish qi and invigorate the spleen; for apparent deficiency of kidney qi, Shudi (Prepared Rhizome of Rehmannia) 12 g, Shanzhuyu (Asiatic Cornelian Cherry Fruit) 9 g, Duzhong (Eucommia Bark) 12 g and Gouqizi (Barbary Wolfberry Fruit) 12 g are added to tonify the kidneys and supplement essence.

## Chinese Patent Medicine

1. Maren Soft Capsule: 2~3 capsules for each dose, twice a day. It is used to moisten the intestine and promote bowel movements.
2. Qing Ning Pill: 3 g for each dose, 3 times a day. It is used to dispel heat and promote bowel movements.

## Simple and Handy Prescriptions

1. Fanxieye (Senna Leaf) 6 g is added to boiled water and administered once a day for constipation due to dryness and heat.
2. Fried Laifuzi (Radish Seed) 6 g and Zaojia (Chinese Honeylocust Fruit) 1.5 g (ground up into powders) are added to boiled water and taken once a day for constipation due to stagnation of qi and phlegm.

## Other Therapies

Dietary therapy: Equal quantities of Heizhima (Black Sesame), Hutaorou (Walnut) and Guazhiren (Melon Seed) are ground up into fine powders, infused into water with a small amount of Baimi (Whitish Honey), and administered to nourish yin and supplement blood as well as moisten the intestine and promote bowel movements.

Exercise therapy: Strengthen the body with non-strenuous exercise in the morning, such as taijiquan (traditional Chinese shadow boxing) and jogging. This therapy can promote movement in the large intestine and improve symptoms.

Abdominal rubbing therapy: Rub the area around the umbilicus with both hands in a clockwise, circular fashion 36 times. It is effective for habitual constipation.

## Cautions and Advice

1. Patients should maintain regular bowel movements as this is closely involved in the treatment of many diseases. Regulating bowel movements plays an especially important role in the treatment of some diseases such as stroke, severe hypertension and myocardial infarction.
2. They should adopt a light diet and consume more vegetables or fruits.
3. Patients should also keep themselves in good spirits.

## Daily Exercises

1. List the etiological factors of constipation.
2. Describe the clinical characteristics of constipation due to qi stagnation.
3. Explain how constipation due to accumulation of heat can be diagnosed and treated.

# Bleeding
# Week 2: Tuesday

Bleeding refers to various forms of internal or external hemorrhage, peliosis and acute disseminated intravascular coagulation. All the morbid conditions due to extravasation of blood, marked by bleeding from the upper orifices such as the mouth and nose, from the lower orifices such as the urethral orifice and anus, and from the skin, may fall into this category. Bleeding discussed in this section refers to acute hemorrhages, a common internal disease, and include hematemesis, hemoptysis, hemafecia, hemuresis and hemorrhinia. In TCM, bleeding belongs to the category of "bleeding syndrome" which can be improved and halted if treated promptly and properly from both root and branch.

## Etiology and Pathology

There are a variety of causes for bleeding, such as invasion of pathogenic heat, impairment due to improper diet, disturbance by emotional disorder, or internal injury stemming from overstrain. Blood is governed by the heart, controlled by the spleen and stored by the liver, while qi is governed by the lungs. Hence bleeding disorders are mostly attributable to the heart, spleen, liver and lungs. Excess-type bleeding is primarily due to exuberance of fire, which drives the blood rampant while deficiency-type bleeding is mainly caused by deficiency of qi, which fails to control the blood.

The pathological changes are marked by damage of the vessels and the resultant bleeding is due to invasion of exogenous pathogenic factors, particularly pathogenic heat. Improper diet breeds damp-heat, which scorches the vessels and drives blood flow to be rampant, leading to hemorrhinia, hematemesis and hemafecia, amongst other conditions. Excessive intake of spicy or fatty food weakens the spleen and stomach, which fail to control the blood and consequently bring about extravasation. Hyperactivity of emotions gives rise to fire and generates wind, which force blood to deviate from the vessels. Furthermore, if overstrain debilitates qi, it will fail to control blood, with such manifestations as hemorrhinia, hematemesis, hemafecia and suggillation. If overstrain damages yin, there will be hyperactivity of fire and extravasation of blood resulting in hemorrhinia, hemuresis and suggillation.

## Diagnostic Key Points

1. An acute onset of profuse bleeding.
2. It is occasionally accompanied by hematemesis, hemoptysis, hemafecia, hemuresis, hemorrhinia, or subcutaneous bleeding.
3. Bleeding can be a symptom of many internal diseases, such as peptic ulcer, bronchiectasis and thrombopenia.

## Syndrome Differentiation

### 1. Upward attack of stomach fire

Symptoms: Hematemesis, hemoptysis and hemorrhinia with relatively large volumes of bright red blood, flushed face, thirst, constipation, red tongue with yellow coating and rapid, forceful pulse.

Analysis of symptoms: Abundant heat in the stomach gives rise to upward attack of stomach fire which drives blood to flow rampantly, marked by hematemesis, hemoptysis and hemorrhinia with bright red blood; the stomach fire consumes stomach fluid, with such signs as thirst and constipation; the stomach fire attacks the head, so the face is reddened; red tongue with yellow coating and rapid pulse are manifestations of abundant heat in the stomach.

### 2. Invasion of pathogenic heat

Symptoms: Hemoptysis, hemorrhinia, or hemafecia; dry mouth and throat, or general fever and cough with little sputum, or difficulty in defecation and abdominal pain; red tongue with scanty coating and rapid pulse.

Analysis of symptoms: Pathogenic wind, heat and dryness invade the body and damage the vessels, leading to hemoptysis, hemorrhinia, and hemafecia, amongst other conditions. If wind-heat attacks the upper energizer and stagnates the defensive qi in the exterior, there will be general fever and throat soreness; pathogenic heat invades the lungs and fetters the lung qi, leading to cough with little sputum; pathogenic heat damages body fluid, causing dryness in the mouth, nose and throat; if dampness and heat accumulate in the intestinal tract, there will be dysfunction in transportation and transformation, coupled with difficulty in defecation and abdominal pain due to stagnation of qi; the red tongue, scanty coating and rapid pulse are manifestations of pathogenic heat in the interior.

## 3. Exuberance of fire due to yin deficiency

Symptoms: (In most cases) repeated hemoptysis, hemorrhinia and hemuresis with small amounts of bright red blood, accompanied by dizziness, tinnitus, feverish sensations in the palms and soles, or hectic fever, night sweats, dry mouth and vexation; red tongue with scanty coating and thin, rapid pulse.

Analysis of symptoms: Deficiency of yin generates heat and fire in the interior, which scorch the vessels, leading to hemoptysis, hemorrhinia and hemuresis, amongst other conditions; deficiency of yin renders the body fluid too deficient to nourish the upper part, resulting in dry mouth and throat; deficiency of yin produces exuberant fire, coupled with feverish sensation in the palms and soles, or hectic fever and night sweats; deficiency of yin results in insufficient brain marrow, leading to dizziness and tinnitus; deficient fire disturbs the heart and triggers vexation; red tongue with scanty coating and thin, rapid pulse are manifestations of insufficiency of yin fluid due to exuberant fire.

## 4. Failure of qi to control blood

Symptoms: Chronic hemorrhinia, hematemesis, hemafecia and peliosis with large or small volumes of blood in dark red or light red color; pale complexion, weariness and dizziness; pale tongue and deficient, feeble pulse.

Analysis of symptoms: Deficient qi fails to control blood, leading to bleeding disorders such as hemorrhinia, hematemesis, hemafecia and peliosis; deficiency of qi also brings about insufficiency of blood, which fails to replenish the vessels, so the blood is dark red or light red in color; the vessels, tendons and bones are malnourished, with such signs as pale complexion, weariness and dizziness; the pale tongue and deficient, weak pulse are manifestations of insufficient qi and blood.

## Differential Treatment

### 1. Upward attack of stomach fire

Treatment principle: Clearing the stomach and purging fire, arresting bleeding.

Prescription and herbs: Modified Xiexin Decoction and Shihui Powder.

Shengdahuang (Unprepared Rhubarb) 6~9 g, Huanglian (Golden Thread) 3 g, Huangqin (Baical Skullcap Root) 9 g, Danpi (Cortex Moutan) 9 g, Daji (Japanese Thistle Herb) 15 g, Xiaoji (Field Thistle Herb) 15 g, Qiancao (Indian Madder Root) 12 g, Cebaiye (Chinese Arborvitae Twig and Leaf) 12 g, Zhimu (Common Anemarrhena Rhizome) 9 g, Niuxi (Two-toothed Achyranthes Root) 12 g and Baimaogen (Lalang Grass Rhizome) 15 g.

Modification: If there is relatively severe impairment of yin marked by thirst, Tianhuafen (Trichosanthin) 15 g, Shihu (Dendrobium) 15 g and Yuzhu (Fragrant Solomonseal Rhizome) 12 g are added to nourish the stomach and promote fluid production; for adverse rising of stomach qi with nausea and vomiting, Daizheshi (Red Bole) 15 g, Zhuru (Bamboo Shavings) 9 g and Xuanfuhua (Inula Flower) 9 g are added to harmonize the stomach and bring down qi.

### 2. Invasion of pathogenic heat

Treatment principle: Dispelling heat and removing toxins, cooling blood to arrest bleeding.

Prescription and herbs: Modified Xijiao Dihuang Decoction and Shihui Powder.

Xijiao (Rhinoceros Horn) 9 g (or Buffalo Horn 30 g), Shengdi (Dried Rehmannia Root) 15 g, Chishao (Red Peony Root) 12 g, Danpi (Cortex Moutan) 9 g, Zhizi (Cape Jasmine Fruit) 9 g, Shengdahuang (Unprepared Rhubarb) 9 g, Cebaiye (Chinese Arborvitae Twig and Leaf) 15 g, Zicao (Arnebia Root) 12 g, Lianqiao (Weeping Forsythia Capsule) 12 g, Daji (Japanese Thistle Herb) 15 g and Xiaoji (Field Thistle Herb) 15 g.

Modification: For relatively severe impairment of yin marked by apparent dryness in the mouth, nose and throat, Xuanshen (Figwort Root) 12 g and Maidong (Dwarf Lilyturf Tuber) 12 g are added to nourish yin and moisten the lungs; For relatively severe bleeding, Baimaogen (Lalang Grass Rhizome) 15 g, Oujie (Lotus Rhizome Node) 9 g and Qiancao (Indian Madder Root) 12 g are added to cool blood and stop bleeding; if accompanied by exterior syndrome of wind-heat, Jinyinhua (Honeysuckle Flower) 9 g and Niubangzi (Great Burdock Achene) 12 g are used to relieve the superficies with herbs pungent in flavor and cooling in property.

## 3. Exuberance of fire due to yin deficiency

Treatment principle: Nourishing yin and dispelling heat to arrest bleeding.

Prescription and herbs: Modified Qiangen Powder.

Shengdi (Dried Rehmannia Root) 12 g, Qiancao (Indian Madder Root) 12 g, Xuanshen (Figwort Root) 12 g, Ejiao (Donkey-hide Glue) 9 g (melted in decoction), Guiban (Tortoise Shell) 9 g, Nuzhenzi (Glossy Privet Fruit) 12 g, Huanliancao (Ecliptae Herba) 12 g, Danpi (Cortex Moutan) 9 g, Zhimu (Common Anemarrhena Rhizome) 9 g and Cebaiye (Chinese Arborvitae Twig and Leaf) 12 g.

Modification: For hectic fever with red cheeks, Qinghao (Sweet Wormwood Herb) 9 g, Biejia (Turtle Shell) 9 g and Digupi (Chinese Wolfberry Root-Bark) 15 g are added to dispel deficient heat; for night sweats, Nuodaogen (Glutinous Rice Root) 15 g, Fuxiaomai (Blighted Wheat) 30 g, Wuweizi (Chinese Magnolivine Fruit) 9 g and Muli (Oyster Shell) 30 g are added to astringe the skin and control perspiration.

## 4. Failure of qi to control blood

Treatment principle: Replenishing qi to invigorate the spleen, controlling blood circulation to arrest bleeding.

Prescription and herbs: Modified Guipi Decoction.

Dangshen (Radix Codonopsis) 12 g, Huangqi (Milkvetch Root) 15 g, Danggui (Chinese Angelica) 12 g, Baizhu (Largehead Atractylodes Rhizome) 12 g, Shudi (Prepared Rhizome of Rehmannia) 12 g, Longyanrou (Longan Aril) 9 g, Suanzaoren (Spine Date Seed) 12 g, Yuanzhi (Thinleaf Milkwort Root) 6 g, Zonglutan (Crinis Trachycarpi) 15 g, Dazao (Chinese Date) 9 g and Zhigancao (Stir-baked Liquorice Root) 6 g.

Modification: For more severe deficiency of yang characterized by intolerance of cold and cold limbs, Paojiang (Prepared Dried Ginger) 6 g, Aiye (Argy Wormwood Leaf) 9 g and Lujiaoshuang (Degelatined Deer-horn) 9 g are added to warm yang and stop bleeding; to reinforce the action of hemostasis, Xianhecao (Hairyvein Agrimonia Herb) 30 g, Qiancao (Indian Madder Root) 12 g and Ejiao (Donkey-hide Glue) 9 g are added.

## Chinese Patent Medicine

1. Guipi Pill: 8~10 pills for each dose, 3 times a day, used to stem bleeding due to failure of qi to control blood.
2. Zhibai Dihuang Pill: 8~10 pills for each dose, 3 times a day, used for bleeding due to deficient yin and exuberant fire.

## Simple and Handy Prescriptions

1. Dazao (Chinese Date) 4 dates and Oujie (Lotus Rhizome Node) 1 piece; at the beginning the Lotus Rhizome Node is boiled in water into a colloid substance, then the Chinese Dates are added for decoction. The Chinese dates can be eaten daily in moderation.
2. Lianqiao (Weeping Forsythia Capsule) 30 g is boiled in water and taken 3 times a day for bleeding due to pathogenic heat.
3. Sanqifen (Sanchi) 6 g, Xueyutan (Carbonized Hair) 6 g and Huaruishi (Ophicalcite) 20 g are ground up into fine powders, and taken 4 times a day for chronic hemoptysis with small volumes of blood.

4. Qingkailing Injection 30~40 ml is added to Glucose solution and administered intravenously for bleeding due to abundant heat.

## Other Therapies

Dietary therapy: Nuomi Ejiao Porridge: Ejiao (Donkey-hide Glue) 30 g, Nuomi (Glutinous Rice) 100 g and Hongtang (Brown Sugar) to taste. Glutinous Rice is decocted into a pot of porridge, and when it is ready, the pieces of Donkey-hide Glue are added and then the decoction is stirred while the glue pieces are decocted; after the water is boiled 2~3 times, add in the brown sugar. This porridge can nourish blood to stop bleeding as well as nourish yin and treat deficiency. Wuzhi Potion: Pear, Chinese Water Chestnut, Lotus Root, Dwarf Lilyturf Tuber and fresh Reed Rhizome are cleaned and ground up for extraction of juice, which is ingested in doses of 20~30 ml. This potion is effective in dispelling heat and producing fluid, quenching thirst and relieving vexation, as well as cooling blood to stop bleeding.

## Cautions and Advice

1. Profuse bleeding should be promptly addressed before the primary disorder is proactively diagnosed and treated.
2. Patients should pay attention to their diet: avoid spicy food, take plenty of food rich in vitamin C or K and avoid smoking and alcohol consumption.
3. Patients should also avoid overstrain and engage in moderate physical exercise so as to strengthen their constitution.

## Daily Exercises

1. List the common etiological factors of bleeding syndrome and explain their relationships with the viscera.
2. List the types of bleeding and describe their treatment principles and representative prescriptions.

# CHAPTER 2

# Diseases of the Respiratory System

## Cold
## Week 2: Wednesday

Cold is a catarrhal disorder of the upper respiratory tract stemming from invasion of viruses, clinically characterized by fever, nasal obstruction, runny nose, sneezing, cough, headache and general malaise. It can afflict people of any age, in any season, but outbreaks are more common in winter and spring. Cold is generally divided into two types: influenza and the common cold. The former is marked by sudden onset, strong infection and widespread outbreak; while the latter is characterized by a relatively slow onset, with no communicability and epidemicity. Common cold usually has a favorable prognosis, whereas influenza, if not promptly treated, can bring about other disorders, such as viral myocarditis. Influenza is regarded in TCM as a "seasonal epidemic disease", while common cold, a disorder due to "damage of wind" or "contraction of cold."

### Etiology and Pathology

The etiological factors of cold are the six abnormal climatic factors and seasonal epidemic viruses, particularly pathogenic wind. However, they often combine with other pathogens prevailing in different seasons to attack the human body. If the six climatic factors of the four seasons are in disorder, or the seasonal or non-seasonal pathogenic factors are in combination, the human body will become more susceptible to diseases. This is not confined to a particular season, and the disease that follows is often a severe and infectious one.

The pathological changes are explained as follows: Insufficiency of healthy qi and defensive qi fail to protect the exterior, and the six abnormal climatic factors take the chance to invade the body in combination with viruses through the mouth, nose, skin and hair, bringing about disharmony between the defensive qi and the exterior as well as failure of the lungs in performing their functions of dispersion and purification. In addition, lifestyle habits, exposure to excessively warm or cool environments and overstrain of the body can all loosen the skin and muscles, allowing exogenous pathogenic factors to enter the body and cause diseases. Furthermore, if the constitution is weak and the defensive qi is insufficient, the exterior will become vulnerable and more susceptible to pathogenic wind and cold. This disease can be divided into three patterns, based on body constitution and pathogenic factors: wind-cold, wind-heat and mixed summer-heat and dampness. For those with a body constitution of yang deficiency, they are susceptible to wind-cold; for those with yin deficiency, they are vulnerable to wind-heat and dry-heat; and for those with relative abundance of phlegm and dampness, they are liable to be invaded by external dampness.

## Diagnostic Key Points

1. Common cold is not associated with a history of epidemicity whereas influenza is.
2. Clinical manifestations are marked by nasal obstruction, runny nose, sneezing, cough, headache, aversion to cold, fever and general indisposition. Influenza with apparent toxic symptoms can be accompanied by high fever, vomiting and diarrhea.
3. Routine blood test is normal and may reveal decreased or increased (only on rare occasions) total number of white blood cells with normal or slight change in differential count.

## Syndrome Differentiation

### 1. Syndrome of wind-cold

Symptoms: Severe aversion to cold with mild fever, absence of sweat, headache, soreness in the limbs and joints, nasal obstruction with a low voice, frequent nasal discharging, scratchy throat, cough with thin and white phlegm, absence of thirst or presence of thirst with preference for hot drinks; white, thin and moist tongue coating and floating or tense pulse.

Analysis of symptoms: Pathogenic wind-cold fetters the skin and muscles and stagnates the defensive yang, so there is aversion to cold, fever and absence of sweat; lucid yang is encumbered, triggering headache and soreness in the limbs and joints; pathogenic wind-cold attacks the upper body and obstructs the lung qi, with nasal obstruction, nasal discharge, itchy throat and cough; pathogenic cold is a yin pathogen, explaining the absence of thirst or presence of thirst with preference for hot drinks; the white, thin and moist tongue coating, as well as tense and floating pulse are both manifestations of cold in the exterior.

## 2. Syndrome of wind-heat

Symptoms: Relatively severe fever with mild aversion to wind, inhibited sweating, distending pain in the head, cough, yellow or sticky sputum, dry throat, or red, swollen and painful tonsils, nasal obstruction with yellow and turbid discharge and thirst with preference for drinking; white, thin and slightly yellow tongue coating, red tongue tip and margin, as well as rapid and floating pulse.

Analysis of symptoms: Pathogenic wind-heat invades the exterior and stagnates in the muscular interstices, leading to disorder of the superficies, marked by fever with mild aversion to wind and unsmooth sweat excretion; pathogenic wind-heat disturbs the upper energizer, so there is distending pain in the head; pathogenic wind-heat fumigates the respiratory tract, resulting in dryness and swelling pain in the throat, thirst and turbid nasal discharge; pathogenic wind-heat also invades the lungs and inhibits their ability to purify, presenting as cough with yellow or sticky sputum; the white, thin and slightly yellow coating, red tongue tip and margin, as well as rapid and floating pulse are all due to invasion of wind-heat into the lung-wei.

## 3. Syndrome of summer-heat and dampness

Symptoms: Fever with slight aversion to wind, minimal sweating, soreness or heaviness of the limbs, dizziness and distending pain in the head, cough with sticky sputum, turbid nasal discharge, vexation with thirst, or sticky and greasy sensation in the mouth, mild thirst, chest distress, nausea and scanty reddish urine; yellow, thin and greasy tongue coating, as well as rapid and soggy pulse.

Analysis of symptoms: Catching of a cold in summer is due to invasion of pathogenic summer-heat which is mostly accompanied by dampness, and the combination of both may impair the exterior and the defensive qi, leading to such symptoms as aversion to wind, minimal sweating and soreness of the limbs; pathogenic summer-heat and wind often invade the upper orifices in combination with dampness, bringing about dizziness and distending pain in the head; pathogenic summer-heat scorches the lungs, resulting in cough with sticky sputum and turbid nasal discharge; summer-heat disturbs the interior and consumes body fluid causing vexation, thirst and scanty reddish urine; pathogenic damp-heat obstructs qi activity in the interior, presenting as chest distress, nausea, sticky and greasy sensation in the mouth, as well as mild thirst; the yellow, thin and greasy tongue coating, as well as rapid and soggy pulse are both manifestations of summer-heat accompanied by dampness.

## Differential Treatment

## 1. Syndrome of wind-cold

Treatment principle: Relieving the exterior with herbs pungent in flavor and warm in property.

Prescription and herbs: Modified Jingfang Baidu Powder.

Jingjie (Fineleaf Schizonepeta Herb) 9 g, Fangfeng (Divaricate Saposhnikovia Root) 9 g, Shengjiang (Fresh Ginger) 3 slices, Chaihu (Chinese Thorowax Root) 6 g, Bohe (Peppermint) 6 g, Qianhu (Hogfennel Root) 9 g, Chuanxiong (Szechwan Lovage Rhizome) 9 g, Zhiqiao (Orange

Fruit) 6 g, Qianghuo (Incised Notoptetygium Rhizome or Root) 9 g, Duhuo (Doubleteeth Pubesscent Angelica Root) 9 g, Fuling (Indian Bread) 12 g, Jiegeng (Platycodon Root) 6 g and Gancao ( Liquorice Root) 3 g.

Modification: For severe cold in the exterior, Mahuang (Ephedra) 6 g and Guizhi (Cassia Twig) 9 g are added to strengthen the cold-dissipating effect with their pungent and warm nature.

## 2. Syndrome of wind-heat

Treatment principle: Relieving the superficies with herbs pungent in flavor and cool in property.

Prescription and herbs: Modified Yinqiao Powder.

Jinyinhua (Honeysuckle Flower) 9 g, Lianqiao (Weeping Forsythia Capsule) 9 g, Jiegeng (Platycodon Root) 6 g, Bohe (Peppermint) 6 g, Zhuye (Henon Bamboo Leaf) 6 g, Jingjie (Fineleaf Schizonepeta Herb) 9 g, Niubangzi (Great Burdock Achene) 9 g, Dandouchi (Fermented Soybean) 9 g, Lugen (Reed Rhizome) 15 g and Gancao ( Liquorice Root) 6 g.

Modification: If there is relatively severe distending pain in the head, Sangye (Mulberry Leaf) 9 g and Juhua (Chrysanthemum Flower) 6 g are added to dispel heat and treat disorders of the head and eyes; for cough with excessive phlegm, Xiangbei (Bulbus Fritillariae Thunbergii) 9 g, Qianhu (Hogfennel Root) 9 g and Xingren (Almond) 12 g are added to dissolve phlegm and relieve cough.

## 3. Syndrome of summer-heat and dampness

Treatment principle: Relieving the exterior by dispelling summer-heat and eliminating dampness.

Prescription and herbs: Modified Jinjia Xiangru Potion.

Xiangru (Haichow Elsholtzia Herb) 6 g, Jinyinhua (Honeysuckle Flower) 9 g, Biandouhua (Fresh Flower of Hyacinth Bean) 9 g, Houpu (Magnolia Bark) 6 g and Lianqiao (Weeping Forsythia Capsule) 9 g.

Modification: If there is relative abundance of summer-heat, Huanglian (Golden Thread) 3 g, Qinghao (Sweet Wormwood Herb) 9 g, Heye (Fresh Lotus Leaf) 15 g and Lugen (Fresh Reed Rhizome) 30 g are added to dispel summer-heat and remove body heat; for dampness encumbering defense of the exterior, Doujuan (Semen Sojae Germinatum) 12 g, Huoxiang (Agastache Rugosa) 9 g and Peilan (Queen of the Meadow) 9 g are added to relieve the exterior and resolve dampness with their aromatic flavors; for relative abundance of dampness in the interior, Cangzhu (Atractylodes Rhizome) 9 g, Baikouren (Fructus Amomi Rotundus) 3 g, Banxia (Pinellia Tuber) 9 g and Chenpi (Dried Tangerine Peel) 6 g are added to harmonize the middle energizer and resolve dampness.

## Chinese Patent Medicine

1. Yinqiao Jiedu Tablet: 4 tablets for each dose, 3 times a day, to treat wind-heat cold.
2. Huoxiang Zhengqi Soft Capsule: 3 capsules for each dose, 3 times a day, to treat exogenous invasion of summer-heat and dampness.
3. Ganmao Tuire Chongji: 4.5~9 g for each dose, 3 times a day. It is applicable to treat all types of cold as well as influenza in the initial stage.

## Simple and Handy Prescriptions

1. Congbai (Fresh Fistular Onion Stalk) 5 sections and Shengjiang (Fresh Ginger) 5 slices are boiled in water and taken 3 times a day to relieve the exterior and dissipate cold. It is applicable to treat all types of cold.
2. Huangqin (Baical Skullcap Root) 9 g, Xuanshen (Figwort Root) 9 g and Lianqiao (Weeping Forsythia Capsule) 9 g are boiled in water and taken twice a day. It is used for high fever with a sore throat.

## Other Therapies

Dietary therapy: Huopei Donggua Decoction: Huoxiang (Unprepared Agastache Rugosa) 5 g, Peilan (Unprepared Queen of the Meadow) 5 g and Donggua (Chinese waxgourd) 500 g. First Huoxiang (Agastache Rugosa) and Peilan (Queen of the Meadow) are boiled in water, then 1 kg of the decoction is used to boil the Chinese waxgourd with salt to taste. It is used to treat cold in summer.

Hot application of medicine: Cangzhu (Atractylodes Rhizome) 30 g, Qianghuo (Incised Notoptetygium Rhizome or Root) 30 g, Kufan (Dried Alum) 10 g and Congbai (Fistular Onion Stalk) 3 pieces. The first three are ground up into crude powders and stir-fried, the powders are then mixed with the juice of Congbai (Fistular Onion Stalk). The mixture is applied to the umbilicus while it is still hot for dispersing wind and dissipating cold.

## Cautions and Advice

1. This disorder, if treated promptly and properly, can be quickly cured. However, for young children, elderly persons or those who have weakened immune systems, it is crucial to prevent the disease from transmission and complication.
2. The patients should keep warm and avoid wind exposure, so as to prevent relapses.
3. It is also advisable for the patients to drink plenty of boiled water and have proper rest.

## Daily Exercises

1. Briefly describe the clinical characteristics of cold.
2. Explain how cold due to wind-heat can be diagnosed and treated.

# Bronchitis

# Week 2: Thursday

Bronchitis is the inflammation of the mucous membranes of the trachea and bronchus due to bacterial/viral infection or physical/chemical factors, commonly marked by cough with sputum, discomfort or pain in the region behind the breast bone and panting or symptoms of common cold. It can be classified into two types, based on duration: acute bronchitis and chronic bronchitis. The former has a disease course of less than a month, with its pathological changes confined to the mucous membranes; while the latter has a disease course of two months or more, for at least two consecutive years, or of three successive months or more, for at least a year, with inflammation in the mucous membrane and its adjacent areas. Acute bronchitis can be found in any age group, whereas chronic bronchitis is mostly seen in adults. This disease is especially prevalent in winter and spring, but if treated promptly, can have a favorable prognosis. In TCM, this disease is closely associated with "cough", "phlegm and retained-fluid" and "panting syndrome".

## Etiology and Pathology

TCM holds that bronchitis is caused by either exogenous or endogenous pathogenic factors. The former refers to the six abnormal climatic factors which invade the pulmonary system; while the latter refers to the functional disorder of the viscera, disturbance of the internal pathogens and deficiency of the lungs.

The pathological changes of bronchitis are discussed as follows: Insufficiency of lung qi affects the ability of defensive qi to protect the exterior, allowing for invasion of the six abnormal climatic factors into the pulmonary system through the mouth, nose, skin and hair, leading to stagnation of lung qi and impairing the lung's functions of dispersion and descent; addiction to cigarettes and alcohol or indulgence in spicy and fire-provoking food will lead to consumption of body fluid and accumulation of phlegm in the airways, marked by adverse rising of lung qi such as cough with sputum and panting. Owing to the difference in exogenous pathogenic factors, there are several types of bronchitis resulting from wind-cold, wind-heat and wind-dryness. The functional disorders of the viscera may also involve the lungs. For instance, dysfunction of the spleen in transportation and transformation transforms the accumulated dampness into turbid phlegm which is detrimental to the lungs; insufficiency of kidney yang is responsible for failure of qi in reception; deficient mingmen fire fails to evaporate the water, which accumulates into phlegm or as retained fluid, obstructing the airways; depletion of kidney yin generates deficient fire which scorches the lung fluid and results in failure of the lungs to purify and disperse, as well as the adverse rising of lung qi, marked by panting and cough with production of sputum. In addition, the disorders of the lungs are also responsible for bronchitis. Chronic pulmonary diseases generally debilitate the lungs, exhaust qi and damage yin, resulting in failure of the lungs to govern qi and adverse rising of lung qi marked by cough with production of sputum.

## Diagnostic Key Points

1. Generally, there are symptoms of upper respiratory tract infection such as nasal obstruction, running nose, sore throat, headache, intolerance of cold and fever.
2. Cough is the main symptom. At the beginning there is dry cough, and 1~2 days later, production of sputum. Chronic bronchitis has a disease course of two months or more, for at least two consecutive years, or of three successive months or more, for at least a year.
3. Chest auscultation: Audible respiratory harshness, or even audible dry or moist rales. Chronic bronchitis patients may exhibit signs of emphysema.
4. X-ray test reveals no abnormalities or presence of thickening of pulmonary markings.

## Syndrome Differentiation

The following three patterns are generally seen in acute bronchitis.

## 1. Invasion of wind-cold into the lungs

Symptoms: Cough with white and thin sputum, itchy throat, which may be accompanied by nasal obstruction, runny nose, fever, headache, general malaise and intolerance of cold; white and thin tongue coating, floating pulse or tense and floating pulse.

Analysis of symptoms: Pathogenic wind-cold invades the lung and fetters the lung qi, leading to adverse rising of lung qi with cough; pathogenic wind-cold attacks the upper body and obstructs the lungs orifices, causing nasal obstruction, running nose and itchy throat; pathogenic cold stagnates the lung qi and impairs its function of dispersing the body fluid which accumulates into phlegm, marked by cough with white and thin sputum; pathogenic wind-cold encumbers the skin and muscles, with such signs as fever, headache, general indisposition and intolerance of cold; white thin tongue coating and floating pulse or tense and floating pulse are manifestations of wind-cold in the exterior.

## 2. Invasion of wind-heat into the lungs

Symptoms: Cough with rapid breathing, difficulty in expectoration of yellow and sticky sputum, often accompanied by yellowish nasal discharge, headache, soreness of the limbs, fever and mild aversion to wind; thin and yellow tongue coating, floating and rapid pulse or floating and slippery pulse.

Analysis of symptoms: Pathogenic wind-heat invades the lungs and impairs the lungs' ability in purification, resulting in cough with rough breathing; lung heat scorches the fluid, with such signs as dry mouth and sore throat; lung heat stagnates in the interior and transforms lung fluid into sputum, characterized by difficulty in expectoration of yellow and sticky sputum and yellow nasal discharge; pathogenic wind-heat invades the exterior and leads to disharmony between the defensive qi and the superficies, resulting in a syndrome of exterior-heat marked by fever and aversion to wind; yellow and thin tongue coating, as well as floating and rapid pulse are both manifestations of wind-heat in the exterior.

## 3. Impairment of the lungs by dry-heat

Symptoms: Dry or choking cough without sputum or with scanty sticky sputum, dry, itching or sore throat, dry nose, mouth and lips, (or accompanied by) nasal obstruction, headache, mild cold and fever; white and thin coating or yellow and thin coating, red and dry tongue, floating and rapid pulse or small and rapid pulse.

Analysis of symptoms: Pathogenic wind-dryness impairs the lungs and consumes lung fluid, so there is dry or choking cough; pathogenic dryness and heat scorches the lungs, marked by dryness in the throat, nose and mouth with sticky sputum hard to expectorate; external invasion of wind-dryness results in disorder of defensive qi, manifesting as nasal obstruction, headache, mild cold and fever; red and dry tongue as well as floating and rapid pulse are both due to invasion of dryness and heat.

The following four patterns are generally seen in chronic bronchitis.

## 4. Accumulation of phlegm and dampness in the lungs

Symptoms: Repeated cough with profuse white sputum, expectoration of sticky sputum, chest distress, gastric stuffiness, poor appetite and abdominal distension; white greasy tongue coating, taut and slippery pulse or soggy and slippery pulse.

Analysis of symptoms: Dampness in the spleen gives rise to phlegm which enters the lungs and stagnates the lung qi, resulting in cough with profuse sticky phlegm; impairment of the spleen in its function of transportation and transformation leads to internal obstruction of phlegm and dampness, characterized by chest distress and gastric stuffiness; deficiency of spleen qi results in digestive disorders, such as poor appetite and abdominal distension; white greasy tongue coating, as well as taut and slippery pulse or soggy and slippery pulse are attributable to internal accumulation of phlegm and dampness.

## 5. Stagnation of phlegm and heat in the lungs

Symptoms: Cough, rapid breathing, plenty of yellow and sticky phlegm, difficulty in expectoration, dry mouth and constipation; yellow or greasy tongue coating and slippery, rapid pulse.

Analysis of symptoms: Pathogenic heat accumulates in the lungs and scorches the body fluid into phlegm, leading to an adverse rising of lung qi marked by cough, shortness of breath, and yellow, sticky phlegm; phlegm and heat permeate in the interior, resulting in dry mouth or constipation; yellow or greasy tongue coating and slippery, rapid pulse are both attributable to internal accumulation of phlegm and heat.

## 6. Deficiency of qi and yin

Symptoms: Cough, shortness of breath, low or faint voice, feeble cough, expectoration of thin or scanty sputum, feverish dysphoria, dry mouth, discomfort in the throat and flushed complexion; pale tongue or red tongue with peeled coating and thin, rapid pulse.

Analysis of symptoms: Lung deficiency leads to insufficiency of lung qi, resulting in cough, shortness of breath and low or faint voice; qi fails to transform the fluid, leading to expectoration of thin sputum; insufficient lung yin generates deficient fire which flames up and results in cough with scanty sputum, feverish dysphoria, dry mouth, blocked throat and a flushed complexion; pale tongue or red tongue with peeled coating, as well as thin and rapid pulse are manifestations of deficiency of qi and yin.

## 7. Yang deficiency of the spleen and kidneys

Symptoms: Cough with panting, expectoration of thin sputum, chest distress, shortness of breath, or wheezy phlegm in the throat, palpitations upon physical exertion, intolerance of cold, cold limbs, swollen feet, poor appetite, weakness and soreness of the waist and knees; pale and enlarged tongue with white coating and thin, deep pulse.

Analysis of symptoms: Insufficiency of kidney yang or decline of fire from the life gate can lead to deficiency of spleen yang and impairment of the spleen and stomach in transportation and transformation, bringing about water and dampness which flow up to the lungs and obstruct the airways, resulting in dysfunction of the lungs in dispersion and descent and deficiency of kidney yang in receiving qi and leading to cough with panting and expectoration of thin sputum; deficiency of spleen yang and kidney yang fail to warm the body and promote digestion, presenting in intolerance of cold, cold limbs, swollen feet, poor appetite, or weakness and soreness of the waist and knees; pale and enlarged tongue with white coating and thin, deep pulse are manifestations of deficiency of spleen yang and kidney yang.

## Differential Treatment

### 1. Invasion of wind-cold into the lungs

Treatment principle: Dispersing wind and dissipating cold, diffusing the lung tissue and dissolving phlegm.

Prescription and herbs: Supplementary Sanao Decoction.

Mahuang (Ephedra) 6 g, Xingren (Almond) 10 g, Jingjie (Fineleaf Schizonepeta Herb) 10 g, Qianhu (Hogfennel Root) 10 g, Jiegeng (Platycodon Root) 6 g, Chenpi (Dried Tangerine Peel) 6 g and Gancao ( Liquorice Root) 6 g.

Modification: If accompanied by phlegm and dampness, cough with sticky sputum, chest distress and greasy tongue coating, Banxia (Pinellia Tuber) 9 g, Houpu (Magnolia Bark) 6 g and Fuling (Indian Bread) 12 g are added.

### 2. Invasion of wind-heat into the lungs

Treatment principle: Dispersing wind and dispelling heat, diffusing the lung tissue and dissolving phlegm.

Prescription and herbs: Modified Sangju Potion.

Sangye (Mulberry Leaf) 10 g, Juhua (Chrysanthemum Flower) 6 g, Xingren (Almond) 10 g, Bohe (Peppermint) 3 g, Lianqiao (Weeping Forsythia Capsule) 10 g, Jiegeng (Platycodon Root) 6 g, Lugen (Fresh Reed Rhizome) 30 g, Niubangzi (Great Burdock Achene) 10 g, Qianhu (Hogfennel Root) 10 g and Gancao ( Liquorice Root) 6 g.

Modification: For abundant heat in the lungs, Huangqin (Baical Skullcap Root) 12 g and Zhimu (Common Anemarrhena Rhizome) 9 g are added to clear and purge heat in the lungs; for soreness in the throat with hoarse voice, Shegan (Blackberrylily Rhizome) 9 g, Chishao (Red Peony Root) 10 g and Guajindeng (Franchet Groundcherry Persistent Calyx or Fruit) 12 g are added to dispel heat and alleviate discomfort in the throat.

### 3. Impairment of the lungs by dry-heat

Treatment principle: Dispersing wind and clearing the lungs, moistening and dissolving phlegm.

Prescription and herbs: Modified Sangxing Decoction.

Sangye (Mulberry Leaf) 10 g, Xingren (Almond) 10 g, Dandouchi (Fermented Soybean) 10 g, Nanshashen (Fourleaf Ladybell Root) 12 g, Xiangbei (Bulbus Fritillariae Thunbergii) 10 g, Xingren (Almond) 10 g, Gualoupi (Snakegourd Peel) 12 g, Zhizi (Cape Jasmine Fruit) 9 g, Huangqin (Baical Skullcap Root) 10 g and Lipi (Bretschneider Pear Pericarp) 10 g.

Modification: If there is abundant heat, Shigao (Gypsum) 30 g and Zhimu (Common Anemarrhena Rhizome) 12 g are added to clear and purge heat in the lungs; for relatively severe damage of fluid, Maidong (Dwarf Lilyturf Tuber) 12 g and Yuzhu (Fragrant Solomonseal Rhizome) 12 g are added to nourish the lung yin; for bloody sputum, Baimaogen (Lalang Grass Rhizome) 30 g are added to dispel heat and stop bleeding.

### 4. Accumulation of phlegm and dampness in the lungs

Treatment principle: Invigorating the spleen and drying dampness, dissolving phlegm to stop cough.

Prescription and herbs: Modified Erchen Decoction and Sanzi Yangqin Decoction.

Banxia (Pinellia Tuber) 9 g, Fuling (Indian Bread) 12 g, Chenpi (Dried Tangerine Peel) 6 g, Houpu (Magnolia Bark) 6 g, Gancao (Liquorice Root) 6 g, Cangzhu (Atractylodes Rhizome) 6 g, Suzi (Perillaseed) 9 g, Baijiezi (White Mustard Seed) 10 g and Laifuzi (Radish Seed) 12 g.

Modification: If there is abundant cold phlegm with white foam and intolerance of cold, Ganjiang (Dried Ginger) 6 g and Xixin (Manchurian Wildginger) 6 g are added to warm the spleen and dissolve phlegm; if chronic diseases debilitate the spleen and lead to listlessness, Dangshen (Radix Codonopsis) 12 g, Baizhu (Largehead Atractylodes Rhizome) 12 g and Zhigancao (Stir-baked Liquorice Root) 6 g are added to replenish qi and invigorate the spleen.

## 5. Stagnation of phlegm and heat in the lungs

Treatment principle: Dispelling heat, purifying the lungs, and dissolving phlegm to stop cough.

Prescription and herbs: Modified Sangbaipi Decoction.

Sangbaipi (White Mulberry Root-Bark) 10 g, Huangqin (Baical Skullcap Root) 12 g, Zhizi (Cape Jasmine Fruit) 10 g, Xiangbei (Bulbus Fritillariae Thunbergii) 9 g, Banxia (Pinellia Tuber) 9 g, Xingren (Almond) 12 g, Gualouren (Snakegourd Seed) 12 g and Suzi (Perillaseed) 9 g.

Modification: For severe general fever, Shigao (Gypsum) 30 g and Zhimu (Common Anemarrhena Rhizome) 12 g are added to dispel lung heat; for excessive sticky phlegm, Haihake (Clam Shell) 15 g is added to dissolve phlegm; for thirst with dry throat, Tianhuafen (Trichosanthin) 15 g is added to nourish yin and produce fluid; for inability to lie down due to dyspnea, vomiting of phlegm and constipation, Tinglizi (Herba Leonuri) 12 g, Dahuang (Rhubarb) 9 g (decocted later) and Mangxiao (Sodium Sulfate) 9 g (infused in water) are added to bring down qi and promote defecation.

## 6. Deficiency of qi and yin

Treatment principle: Nourishing the lungs to supplement qi, replenishing yin to produce fluid.

Prescription and herbs: Modified Shengmai Powder and Shashen Maidong Decoction.

Taizishen (Heterophylly Falsesatarwort Root) 15 g, Shashen (Root of Straight Ladybell) 12 g, Maidong (Dwarf Lilyturf Tuber) 12 g, Wuweizi (Chinese Magnolivine Fruit) 9 g, Baihe (Lily Bulb) 12 g, Ziwan (Tatarian Aster Root) 10 g, Kuandonghua (Common Coltsfoot Flower) 10 g and Sangbaipi (White Mulberry Root-Bark) 12 g.

Modification: For severe cough, Chuanbei (Tendrilleaf Fritillary Bulb) 9 g, Xingren (Almond) 10 g and Baibu (Stemona Root) 10 g are added to purify the lungs, dissolve the phlegm and stop cough; for hectic fever in the afternoon and feverish sensation in the palms and soles, Digupi (Chinese Wolfberry Root-Bark) 10 g and Yinchaihu (Starwort Root) 10 g are added to clear the lungs and bring down fire.

## 7. Yang deficiency of the spleen and kidneys

Treatment principle: Warming the kidneys and invigorating the spleen, receiving qi and alleviating panting.

Prescription and herbs: Modified Shenqi Pill and Liujunzi Pill.

Shufuzi (Prepared Common Monkshood Daughter) 9 g, Rougui (Cassia Bark) 5 g, Shudi (Prepared Rhizome of Rehmannia) 12 g, Shanzhuyu (Asiatic Cornelian Cherry Fruit) 6 g, Huaishanyao (Huaihe Common Yan Rhizome) 15 g, Fuling (Indian Bread) 12 g, Zexie (Oriental Waterplantain Rhizome) 10 g, Chenpi (Dried Tangerine Peel) 6 g, Banxia (Pinellia Tuber) 9 g, Dangshen (Radix Codonopsis) 15 g, Baizhu (Largehead Atractylodes Rhizome) 9 g and Gancao (Liquorice Root) 5 g.

Modification: For relative deficiency of kidney yin with dry mouth and throat, sore waist, and reddish urine, Fuzi (Prepared Common Monkshood Daughter) and Rougui (Cassia Bark) are replaced with Zhimu (Common Anemarrhena Rhizome) 9 g, Huangbai (Amur Cork-tree) 9 g and Maidong (Dwarf Lilyturf Tuber) 9 g to nourish yin and astringe the lungs; for failure of the kidneys to receive qi with panting aggravated upon exertion, sweating and cold limbs, Renshen (Ginseng) 9 g, Longgu (Os Draconis) 30 g, Muli (Oyster Shell) 30 g, Zishiying (Fluorite) 15 g, and Heixidan (Stannum Nigrum Pill) 6 g (wrapped during decoction) are added to receive qi and alleviate panting.

## Chinese Patent Medicine

1. Jizhi Syrup: 15 ml for each dose, 3 times a day, for acute bronchitis.
2. Qutanling: 30 ml for each dose, 3 times a day, for expelling phlegm.
3. Kuben Chuanke Tablet: 3 tablets for each dose, 3 times a day, for consolidating the kidneys and relieving panting.

## Simple and Handy Prescriptions

1. Chuanbeifen (Tendrilleaf Fritillary Bulb Powder) 3~6 g (per dose) is taken twice a day with warm boiled waterto treat cough with excessive phlegm.
2. Baoguoren (Ginkgo Seed) 3 g and Xingren (Almond) 3 g are boiled in water and taken once a day to treat body weakness due to chronic diseases.

## Other Therapies

Dietary therapy: Yiyiren (Coix Seed) 50 g and Xingren (Almond) 15 g, cleaned and pounded into pieces, are boiled in water into a pot of porridge. After a proper quantity of candy sugar is added, the porridge is taken in the morning and evening, respectively. It is used to treat chronic bronchitis marked by cough with profuse phlegm, poor appetite, and chest distress.

## Cautions and Advice

1. Bronchitis is a common and frequently encountered disease. It should be treated promptly to prevent development of persistent cough and chronic bronchitis.
2. Patients should keep warm, ensure the air they are exposed to is ventilated and fresh, and avoid exposure to hazardous toxic gases or substances.
3. It is also advisable for the patients to refrain from smoking.

## Daily Exercises

1. Describe the clinical characteristics of bronchitis.
2. Describe the pathological characteristics of bronchitis.
3. Explain how bronchitis due to accumulation of phlegm and dampness in the lungs can be diagnosed and treated.

# Bronchial Asthma

## Week 2: Friday

Bronchial asthma is a common hypersensitivity disease, clinically characterized by repeated expiratory dyspnea with wheezing rales. It can afflict people of any age, but is most common in children under the age of 12. It is prevalent in autumn and winter, less so in spring and rare in summer. Asthmatic attacks, if treated promptly, can generally have a favorable prognosis. It belongs to the category of "wheezing syndrome" in TCM.

## Etiology and Pathology

The root cause of bronchial asthma is phlegm lurking in the lungs. In addition, abrupt change of climate, improper diet, emotional disorder or overstrain can all trigger an asthmatic attack, bringing about obstruction of the airways by phlegm and adverse rising of lung qi.

The main pathological changes during the period of onset are caused by pathogenic factors triggering the "insidious" phlegm, which flows upward with the rising of qi and obstructs the airways, inhibiting respiration or the ascending and descending of qi, with manifestations of wheezing and panting.

## Diagnostic Key Points

1. There is generally an itchy sensation in the nose and throat, sneezing, cough and chest distress shortly before an asthmatic attack.
2. Asthmatic attacks commonly take place at night, marked by sudden chest distress, suffocation, instant dyspnea, expiratory flow retardation and such accompanying symptoms as wheezing with opened mouth and raised shoulders, wheezy phlegm in the throat and cough.
3. During the asthmatic attack, the chest is generally full and raised with hyper-resonant note during percussion and wheezing in the bilateral lungs during auscultation. For chronic asthma with prolonged bronchitis, dry or moist rales can be heard even during the remission period; if

there is complication of emphysema, the physical signs of emphysema can be observed.

4. X-ray test may indicate thickened bilateral pulmonary markings or increased brightness.

## Syndrome Differentiation

### 1. Asthma of cold (due to latent cold-phlegm in the lungs)

Symptoms: Shortness of breath, wheezy phlegm in the throat, fullness and tightness in the chest and diaphragm, mild cough, scanty sputum with difficulty in expectoration, bluish and lusterless complexion, absence of thirst, or presence of thirst with desire for hot drinks, susceptibility to cold and cold limbs with intolerance of cold; white and slippery tongue coating, taut and tense pulse or floating and tense pulse.

Analysis of symptoms: Cold phlegm hidden in the lungs, if triggered by inducing factors, can flow upward with the rising of qi, obstructing the throat with shortness of breath and wheezing; since the lung qi is stagnated, there is a feeling offullness and stuffiness in the chest and diaphragm, as well as mild cough with scanty sputum that is difficult cough out; predominant yin in the interior obstructs the flow of yang qi, so thecomplexion is bluish and lusterless and the body feels cold, particularly the; the etiological factor is cold instead of heat, this explains the absence of thirst and preference for hot drinks; invasion of exogenous factors often trigger the retained fluid in the interior, so it is susceptible to cold; white and slippery tongue coating, taut and tense pulse or floating and tense pulse are manifestations of predominant cold.

### 2. Asthma of heat (due to stagnated phlegm-heat in the lungs)

Symptoms: Fast and surging respiration, wheezy phlegm in the throat, thoracic and hypochondriac distension, paroxysmal chocking cough, difficulty in expectoration of turbid and sticky phlegm that is yellow or white in color, vexation, restlessness, sweating, red complexion, bitter taste in the mouth, thirst with desire for drinking and intolerance of cold; yellow and greasy tongue coating, red tongue, slippery and rapid pulse or slippery and taut pulse.

Analysis of symptoms: Stagnation of phlegm and heat in the lungs leads to failure of the lungs in their purifying function and adverse rising of lung qi, resulting in panting and rough breathing, wheezy phlegm in the throat, thoracic and hypochondriac distension and paroxysmal chocking cough; heat condenses the fluid into phlegm which is turbid, sticky and yellow or white and difficult to cough out; phlegmatic fire scorches the body, bringing about vexation, spontaneous perspiration, red complexion and a bitter taste in the mouth; the etiological factor is heat instead of cold, so there is thirst without intolerance of cold; red tongue with yellow and greasy coating, as well as slippery and rapid pulse are manifestations of abundant phlegm and heat in the interior.

The above-mentioned two types are observed during the period of asthmatic attack.

## 3. Asthma due to lung deficiency (deficiency of lung-wei)

Symptoms: Spontaneous perspiration, intolerance of wind, liability to catch a cold, susceptibility to climatic changes, sneezing before onset, nasal obstruction with a runny nose, shortness of breath with low voice, or slight wheezing in throat, expectoration of white and thin sputum and white complexion; white and thin coating on pale tongue, thin and feeble pulse or deficient and large pulse.

Analysis of symptoms: Weakness of defensive qi fails to protect the skin and muscles from the invasion of exogenous pathogenic factors, resulting in spontaneous perspiration, intolerance of wind, susceptibility to catch a cold and to climatic change; deficiency of the lungs prevents qi from transforming body fluid, bringing about phlegm and retained fluid in the lungs, marked by shortness of breath with low voice and expectoration of white and thin sputum; white complexion, pale tongue with white coating, as well as thin and deficient pulse are manifestations of deficiency of lung-wei.

## 4. Asthma due to spleen deficiency (deficiency of spleen qi)

Symptoms: persistently poor appetite, gastric stuffiness, loose stools, or diarrhea after eating fatty food; asthmatic attack often triggered by improper diet, accompanied by lassitude, shortness of breath and faint voice; thin and greasy or white and slippery coating on a pale tongue, as well as thin and soft pulse.

Analysis of symptoms: Deficiency of spleen leads to dysfunction in transformation, so there are poor appetite, gastric stuffiness, loose stool, or diarrhea due to intake of oily food, and asthmatic attack often triggered by improper diet; insufficiency of middle qi leads to lassitude, shortness of breath, and faint voice; pale tongue, thin and greasy coating or white and slippery coating, as well as thin and soft pulse, are all due to deficiency of spleen qi.

## 5. Asthma due to kidney deficiency (deficiency of primordial qi of the kidneys)

Symptoms: Usually shortness of qi aggravated by exertion, inhibited inhalation of qi, palpitations, tinnitus, soreness in the waist and legs, asthmatic attack follows overstrain; or intolerance of cold, cold limbs, spontaneous perspiration and pale complexion; tender and enlarged tongue with slightly white coating, thin and deep pulse; or red cheeks, feverish dysphoria, perspiration with sticky sweat, reddish tongue with scanty coating and thin or rapid pulse.

Analysis of symptoms: Chronic diseases debilitate the kidneys and impair them from receiving qi, leading to shortness of qi aggravated upon exertion and inhibited inhalation of qi; the essence is too deficient to nourish the brain, resulting in tinnitus, soreness in the waist and legs and asthmatic attack following overstrain; for deficiency of yang, cold manifestations can be seen, while for deficiency of yin, manifestations of internal heat can be observed.

The above-mentioned three types are seen in the remission period of asthma.

## Differential Treatment

### 1. Asthma of cold type

Treatment principle: Warming the lungs and dissipating cold, dissolving phlegm and relieving panting.

Prescription and herbs: Modified Shegan Mahuang Decoction.

Shegan (Blackberrylily Rhizome) 9 g, Mahuang (Ephedra) 9 g, Ganjiang (Dried Ginger) 6 g, Xixin (Manchurian Wildginger) 3 g, Banxia (Pinellia Tuber) 9 g, Ziwan (Tatarian Aster Root) 12 g, Kuandonghua (Common Coltsfoot Flower) 12 g, Wuweizi (Chinese Magnolivine Fruit) 9 g, Xingren (Almond) 12 g, Baiqian (Willowleaf Swallowwort Rhizome) 9 g, Jupi (Tangerine Pericarp) 9 g, Dazao (Chinese Date) 7 dates and Gancao (Liquorice Root) 6 g.

Modification: For difficulty in breathing when lying down accompanied by panting and abundant phlegm, Tinglizi (Herba Leonuri) 15 g is added to purge phlegm; for relatively severe cold in the exterior with fluid retention in the interior, Guizhi (Cassia Twig) 9 g and Ganjiang (Dried Ginger) 9 g are added to warm and ventilate yang qi; for severe deficiency of yang, Fuzi (Prepared Common Monkshood Daughter) 9 g and Buguzhi (Malaytea Scurfpea Fruit) 12 g are added to warm and invigorate the kidney yang.

## 2. Asthma of heat type

Treatment principle: Dispelling heat and dispersing lung qi, dissolving phlegm and relieving panting.

Prescription and herbs: Supplementary Dingchuan Decoction.

Mahuang (Ephedra) 9 g, Huangqin (Baical Skullcap Root) 15 g, Sangbaipi (White Mulberry Root-Bark) 15 g, Xingren (Almond) 12 g, Banxia (Pinellia Tuber) 9 g, Kuandonghua (Stir-baked Common Coltsfoot Flower) 12 g, Suzi (Stir-baked Perillaseed) 9 g (wrapped during decoction), Baoguo (Ginkgo Seed) 9 g (broken into pieces), Yuxingcao (Heartleaf Houttuynia Herb) 30 g, Dazao (Chinese Date) 7 dates and Gancao (Liquorice Root) 6 g.

Modification: For pathogenic cold in the exterior with abundant lung heat in the interior, Shigao (Raw Gypsum) 30 g is added to relive the muscles and dispel internal heat; for severe cold in the exterior, Guizhi (Cassia Twig) 9 g and Shengjiang (Fresh Ginger) 3 slices are added to relieve the exterior and dissipate cold.

## 3. Asthma due to lung deficiency

Treatment principle: Nourishing the lungs and consolidating the defensive phase.

Prescription and herbs: Supplementary Yupingfeng Powder.

Huangqi (Milkvetch Root) 15 g, Baizhu (Largehead Atractylodes Rhizome) 12 g, Fangfeng (Divaricate Saposhnikovia Root) 9 g, Guizhi (Cassia Twig) 9 g Baishao (White Peony Alba) 12 g Dazao (Chinese Date) 7 dates and Gancao (Liquorice Root) 6 g.

Modification: For deficiency of qi and yin marked by choking cough with scanty and sticky sputum, as well as red tongue, Beishashen (Coastal Glehnia Root) 12 g, Maidong (Dwarf Lilyturf Tuber) 12 g and (Fragrant Solomonseal Rhizome) 12 g are added to replenish qi and nourish yin.

## 4. Asthma due to spleen deficiency

Treatment principle: Invigorating the spleen and dissolving phlegm.

Prescription and herbs: Modified Liujunzi Decoction.

Dangshen (Radix Codonopsis) 12 g, Baizhu (Largehead Atractylodes Rhizome) 15 g, Fuling (Indian Bread) 12 g, Chenpi (Dried Tangerine Peel) 9 g, Banxia (Pinellia Tuber) 9 g, Gancao (Liquorice Root) 6 g and Dazao (Chinese Date) 7 dates.

Modification: For inactivation of spleen yang with cold body and limbs or loose stools, Guizhi (Cassia Twig) 9 g and Ganjiang (Dried Ginger) 6 g are added to warm the spleen and resolve fluid.

## 5. Asthma due to kidney deficiency

Treatment principle: Nourishing the kidneys and receiving qi.

Prescription and herbs: Modified Qiwei Duqi Pill.

Shudi (Prepared Rhizome of Rehmannia) 12 g, Shanzhuyu (Asiatic Cornelian Cherry Fruit) 9 g, Shanyao (Huaihe Plantain Herb) 15 g, Fuling (Indian Bread) 12 g, Danpi (Cortex Moutan) 9 g, Zexie (Oriental Water-plantain Rhizome) 12 g and Wuweizi (Chinese Magnolivine Fruit) 9 g.

Modification: For apparent deficiency of yang, Fuzi (Prepared Common Monkshood Daughter) 9 g, Guizhi (Cassia Twig) 9 g, Buguzhi (Malaytea Scurfpea Fruit) 12 g and Yinyanghuo (Epimedium Herb) 12 g are added to warm and invigorate the kidney yang; for deficiency of yin, Maidong (Dwarf Lilyturf Tuber) 12 g, Danggui (Chinese Angelica) 12 g and Guibanjiao (Tortoise Shell Gelatin) 9 g are used to nourish the kidneys and supplement essence; for inability of the deficient kidneys to receive qi, Hutaorou (Walnut) 12 g and Zishiying (Fluorite) 15 g are added to warm the kidneys and receive qi.

## Chinese Patent Medicine

1. Yupingfeng Granule: 1 small bag for each dose, 3 times a day.
2. Jingui Shenqi Pill: 10 pills for each dose, 3 times a day.
3. Guben Chuanke Tablet: 3 tablets for each dose, 3 times a day.

## Simple and Handy Prescriptions

1. Dilong (Angle Worm) Powder is capsulated and taken (3 g for each dose) twice a day to treat heat-type asthma.
2. Baiguo (Ginkgo Seed, broken into pieces with the shell) 7 seeds, Suzi (Perillaseed) 9 g and Xingren (Almond) 10 g are boiled in water and taken once a day for asthma with excessive phlegm and shortness of breath.

## Other Therapies

Dietary therapy: Sanren Porridge: Baoguo (Ginkgo Seed) 10 g, Yiyiren (Fresh Coix Seed) 30 g, Xingren (Almond) 10 g and Jiangmi (Rice Fruit) 50 g are boiled into porridge with candy sugar. The porridge is taken in the morning and evening to treat asthma with excessive phlegm and chest distress by dissolving phlegm and alleviating panting.

## Cautions and Advice

1. Bronchial asthma is a hypersensitivity disease commonly seen in the clinic. It should be promptly treated to prevent risk of suffocation.

2. Proper measures should be taken to prevent its occurrence, such as the methods for warding off cold and precautions for obviating exogenous pathogenic factors.
3. It is also advisable for patients to refrain from cigarettes and alcohol, avoid exposure to irritant gases or dust and pay attention to their diet.

## Daily Exercises

1. List the clinical characteristics of bronchial asthma.
2. Describe the basic pathological changes of bronchial asthmatic attack in the initial stage.
3. Explain how cold-type asthma and heat-type asthma can be differentiated.

# Bronchiectasis
# Week 2: Saturday

Bronchiectasis is a frequently encountered chronic purulent disease of the bronchus. It stems from chronic inflammation and suppuration of the bronchus and its adjacent tissues, presenting as cylindrical or cystic dilation of the lumens. Clinically it is marked by chronic cough with purulent sputum and repeated hemoptysis. About 80 % of patients with this disorder experience the initial onset before the age of 10 and in nearly 30 % of cases, there is a history of recurrent acute infection of the respiratory tract. If this disease can be promptly diagnosed and treated to bring the infection under control, a favorable prognosis is possible. In TCM, bronchiectasis is closely associated with "cough", "lung abscess" and "coughing up blood".

## Etiology and Pathology

TCM holds that bronchiectasis can be caused by either exogenous or endogenous pathogenic factors. The former refers to the six abnormal climatic factors which invade the pulmonary system and damage the lung collaterals; while the latter refers to the functional disorders of the viscera, which involve the lungs and damage the lung collaterals.

The pathological changes of bronchiectasis are discussed as follows: Insufficiency of healthy qi and insecurity of defensive qi allow for the six abnormal climatic factors to invade the pulmonary system, transform into heat and damage the lung collaterals, this is marked by cough with production of sputum and hemoptysis. Internal accumulation of phlegm and heat, if combined with exogenous pathogenic factors, may obstruct the lungs, impair their ability in purification and cause damage in the collaterals. Pathogenic heat scorches the fluid into phlegm which blocks the lung orifices and consequently disrupts the functional activities of qi and results in co-existence of phlegmatic heat and blood stasis, marked by foul and purulent sputum. Functional disorders of the viscera, such as hyperactivity of liver fire, may attack the lungs and impair their ability in purification, causing damage to the collaterals, marked by cough with blood. Furthermore, this disorder is apt to consume qi and exhaust yin because of its recurrent nature, bringing on deficiency of yin with heat in the lungs as well as deficiency of healthy qi with a lingering of pathogenic factors.

## Diagnostic Key Points

1. Prolonged cough and production of profuse purulent sputum, with the volume of sputum related to the body position. Static layering of the sputum indicates that there are three layers: foam, mucus and sediments of necrotic tissue.
2. Intermittent hemoptysis or absence of cough, with only repeated severe hemoptysis (also called dry bronchiectasis).
3. Recurrent lung infections, marked by repeated and protracted infestation in the same location.
4. Health examination reveals localized coarse and medium rales, or clubbed fingers or toes in some cases.
5. X-ray test reveals increased, thickened and disorganized lung markings in the lower field, or irregular lucent shadow and curly hair shadow.
6. Bronchography, pulmonary CT and fiber optic bronchoscopy reveal corresponding pathological changes in the lungs and bronchus.

## Syndrome Differentiation

## 1. Dryness and heat impairing the lungs

Symptoms: Cough with production of bloody sputum or hemoptysis, scratchy and sore throat, dry mouth and nose or general fever; red tongue with yellow and thin coating and floating and rapid pulse.

Analysis of symptoms: Pathogenic wind, heat and dryness impair the lungs and lead to failure of the lungs in purification and damage of lung collaterals, marked by cough with bloody sputum and itchy throat; pathogenic dryness and heat consume body fluid, drying the mouth and nose; red tongue with thin and yellow coating, as well as floating and rapid pulse are manifestations of fluid impairment due to pathogenic wind, heat and dryness.

## 2. Liver fire invading the lungs

Symptoms: Paroxysmal cough with blood-streaked sputum or pure blood in bright red color, chest and hypochondriac distending pain, restlessness, irascibility and a bitter taste in the mouth; red tongue with thin and yellow coating, as well as rapid and taut pulse.

Analysis of symptoms: Liver fire flames up and invades the lungs, leading to failure of the lungs in purification and damage to lung collaterals marked by cough and hemoptysis; the collaterals of the liver spread over the hypochondria, so if the liver fire is hyperactive and the collaterals are stagnated, there will be distending pain in the chest and hypochondria; the liver fire tends to flame up, causing a bitter taste in the mouth, restlessness and irascibility; the red tongue with thin and yellow coating, as well as rapid and taut pulse, is symptomatic of the predominant liver fire.

## 3. Phlegm and heat obstructing the lungs

Symptoms: Cough with yellow sticky sputum or blood-streaked phlegm, a bitter and dry sensation in the mouth, vague pain in the chest and hypo-chondria; red tongue with yellow and greasy coating, as well as slippery and rapid pulse.

Analysis of symptoms: Pathogenic heat stagnates in the lungs and pre-vents the lung qi from descending, resulting in cough with yellow sticky sputum; impairment of lung collaterals is manifested as blood-streaked sputum; phlegm and heat steams and stagnates inside the body, causing a bitter and dry sensation in the mouth; stagnation of phlegm and heat in the lungs results in disorder of the lung collaterals, with vague pain in the chest and hypochondria; red tongue with yellow and greasy coating, as well as slippery and rapid pulse are all due to stagnation of phlegm and heat in the lungs.

## 4. Deficiency of yin producing heat in the lungs

Symptoms: Cough with scanty sputum, blood-streaked sputum or repeated expectoration of bright-red blood, dry mouth and throat, red cheeks, feverish sensations over the five centers (the palms, the soles and the heart), hectic fever and night sweats; red tongue with scanty coating, as well as thin and rapid pulse.

Analysis of symptoms: Deficiency of yin leads to heat in the lungs and failure of the lungs in purification resulting in cough with scanty sputum; fire and heat scorch the lungs and damage the collaterals, causing the blood-streaked sputum or repeated expectoration of bright-red blood; deficient yin-fluid fails to moisten the upper energizer, characterized by dry mouth and throat; yin deficiency gives rise to abundant fire, with red cheeks, feverish sensation over the five centers (the palms, the soles and the heart), hectic fever and night sweats; the red tongue with scanty coating, as well as thin and rapid pulse are manifestations of yin deficiency with heat.

## Differential Treatment

### 1. Dryness and heat impairing the lungs

Treatment principle: Dispelling heat, moistening the lungs and soothing the collaterals to stop bleeding.

Prescription and herbs: Modified Sangxing Decoction.

Sangye (Mulberry Leaf) 9 g, Xingren (Almond) 12 g, Xiangbei (Bulbus Fritillariae Thunbergii) 12 g, Dandouchi (Fermented Soybean) 10 g, Zhizi (Cape Jasmine Fruit) 10 g, Nanshashen (Fourleaf Ladybell Root) 12 g, Baimaogen (Lalang Grass Rhizome) 30 g, Lugen (Reed Rhizome) 30 g, Lipi (Bretschneider Pear Pericarp) 12 g, Oujie (Lotus Rhizome Node) 12 g and Gancao (Liquorice Root) 6 g.

Modification: For more severe impairment of fluid, Maidong (Dwarf Lilyturf Tuber) 12 g, Xuanshen (Figwort Root) 12 g and Tianhuafen (Trichosanthin) 12 g are added to nourish yin and reduce dryness.

### 2. Liver fire invading the lungs

Treatment principle: Clearing the liver, purging the lungs and cooling blood to stop bleeding.

Prescription and herbs: Modified Xiebai Powder and Daiha Power.

Sangbaipi (White Mulberry Root-Bark) 10 g, Digupi (Chinese Wolfberry Root-Bark) 12 g, Huangqin (Baical Skullcap Root) 10 g, Longdancao (Radix Gentianae) 6 g, Haihake (Clam Shell) 15 g, Qingdai (Natural Indigo) 6 g, Huanliancao (Ecliptae Herba) 12 g, Shengdi (Dried Rehmannia Root) 12 g, Baimaogen (Lalang Grass Rhizome) 30 g, Xiaoji (Field Thistle Herb) 12 g and Gancao (Liquorice Root) 6 g.

Modification: For relative hyperactivity of liver fire with dizziness, reddened eyes, vexation and irascibility, Danpi (Cortex Moutan) 12 g and Zhizi (Cape Jasmine Fruit) 10 g are added to clear the liver and purge fire.

## 3. Phlegm and heat obstructing the lungs

Treatment principle: Dispelling heat, dissolving phlegm and cooling blood to stop bleeding.

Prescription and herbs: Modified Jingwei Decoction in *Qian Jin Yao Fang (Invaluable Prescriptions).*[1]

Lugen (Reed Rhizome) 30 g, Dongguaren (Chinese waxgourd seed) 15 g, Taoren (Peach Seed) 12 g, Yiyiren (Unprepared Coix Seed) 15 g, Jiegeng (Platycodon Root) 6 g, Huanglian (Golden Thread) 3 g, Xiangbei (Bulbus Fritillariae Thunbergii) 12 g, Banxia (Pinellia Tuber) 10 g and Gancao (Liquorice Root) 6 g.

Modification: For expectoration of yellow and sticky sputum, Sangbaipi (White Mulberry Root-Bark) 12 g and Gualouren (Snakegourd Seed) 12 g are added to dispel heat and dissolve phlegm; for obstruction of turbid phlegm in the lungs with cough, panting and chest fullness, Tinglizi (Herba Leonuri) 15 g is used to purge the phlegm in the lungs and dispel heat.

## 4. Deficiency of yin producing heat in the lungs

Treatment principle: Nourishing yin and moistening the lungs, soothing the collaterals to stop bleeding.

Prescription and herbs: Modified Baihe Guji Decoction.

---

[1]Written by Sun Simiao, Tang Dynasty Priest (581–682).

Shengdi (Dried Rehmannia Root) 12 g, Baihe (Lily Bulb) 12 g, Maidong (Dwarf Lilyturf Tuber) 12 g, Baishao (White Peony Alba) 15 g, Danggui (Chinese Angelica) 6 g, Xiangbei (Bulbus Fritillariae Thunbergii) 10 g, Xuanshen (Figwort Root) 12 g, Baimaogen (Lalang Grass Rhizome) 15 g, Huhuanglian (Figwort flower Picrorhiza Rhizome) 3 g, Qiancao (Indian Madder Root) 10 g and Gancao ( Liquorice Root) 6 g.

Modification: For repeated hemoptysis, Baiji (Common Bletilla Tuber) 12 g and Oujie (Lotus Rhizome Node) 10 g are added to cool blood and stop bleeding; for profuse bleeding, Ejiao (Donkey-hide Glue) 9 g and Sanqifen (Sanchi) 3 g (infused in water) are used to nourish the blood and stop bleeding.

## Chinese Patent Medicine

1. Yin Huang Tablet: 4 tablets for each dose, 3 times a day.
2. Compound Andrographolide Tablet: 4 tablets for each dose, 3 times a day.

## Simple and Handy Prescriptions

1. Baihe (Lily Bulb) 10 g, Baiji (Common Bletilla Tuber) 10 g, Nanshashen (Fourleaf Ladybell Root) 6 g, Baibu (Stemona Root) 6 g are boiled in water and separated into 2 portions to be taken at different times within a day . It can be administered over the long term.
2. Dahuang (Rhubarb) 10 g and Xiangbei (Bulbus Fritillariae Thunbergii) 10 g are boiled in water and separated into 2 portions to be taken at different times within a day. It is used for hemoptysis.
3. Baiji (Common Bletilla Tuber) 10 g, Ejiao (Donkey-hide Glue) 10 g, Sanqi (Radix Notoginseng) 3 g, Puhuang (Pollen Typhae) 6 g and Xiaoji (Field Thistle Herb) 30 g are boiled in water and separated into 2 portions to be taken a different times within a day. It is used for hemoptysis.

## Other Therapies

Dietary therapy: Baihe Yiyiren Decoction: Baihe (Lily Bulb) 100 g and Yiyiren (Coix Seed) 100 g are decocted together with crystal sugar to taste. It is used to moisten the lungs and dissolve phlegm.

Exercise therapy: Primarily taijiquan (traditional Chinese shadow boxing), combined with jogging and walking. This therapy is adopted to regulate yin and yang, as well as strengthen the constitution.

## Cautions and Advice

1. Prevent congestion of the airways by blood clots during severe hemoptysis; for those with expectoration of foul and thick sputum, postural drainage should be performed to discharge the sputum and saliva and ensure the respiratory tract is clear.
2. Patients below the age of 40 who have a healthy constitution can opt for excision of the pulmonary segment or lobes if treatment by drug administration is hard to control.
3. Patients should pay attention to nutrition, keep a balanced and healthy diet, refrain from spicy or other food which may irritate the stomach, as well as avoid cigarettes and alcohol.
4. Patients should also keep them selves in good spirits and avoid dramatic emotional fluctuations.

## Daily Exercises

1. List the clinical characteristics of bronchiectasis.
2. Explain how bronchiectasis due to invasion of liver fire into the lungs can be diagnosed and treated.

# Pneumonia

# Week 3: Monday

Pneumonia is an inflammatory disorder of the lung parenchyma due to a variety of pathogens (such as bacteria, viruses, fungi and parasites). Other factors, such as radioactive ray, chemical burn or supersensitivity, may also lead to pneumonia. Clinically, it is mainly characterized by chills, high fever, cough, expectoration of sputum and chest pain. Pneumonia can occur regardless of the four seasons, but is more prevalent in winter and spring. It is more common in young and middle-aged people, with males being more susceptible. If this disease is promptly diagnosed and treated, the prognosis is favorable. In TCM, pneumonia is in the category of, or closely linked to, "wind-warm disease", "cough" and "lung-heat disorder".

## Etiology and Pathology

TCM believes that pneumonia is often caused by overstrain or exposure to wind when one is drunk; under these circumstances, the body's healthy qi is insufficient and the defensive qi is weak, so pathogenic wind-heat or wind-cold will find their way to intrude, producing heat in the interior.

The pathological changes are explained as follows: The healthy qi and defensive qi are too weak to expel the exogenous pathogenic factors which damage the lungs and fetter the exterior, bringing about aversion to cold and fever. The lung qi is stagnated and fails to disperse, resulting in cough. The lungs fail to distribute body fluid, which accumulates into phlegm, marked by white and thin sputum if there is invasion of pathogenic cold, and white sticky sputum or yellow sputum if there is invasion of pathogenic heat or transformation of pathogenic cold into heat. Pathogenic factors obstruct the lung collaterals, giving rise to pain in the chest. Pathogenic heat scorches the lung collaterals, giving rise to hemoptysis. If pathogenic factors are predominant and the healthy qi fails to prevent them from developing into the ying (nutrient) phase and blood phase or even the pericardium, there can be exhaustion of genuine yin and depletion of yang qi.

## Diagnostic Key Points

1. Bacterial pneumonia is marked by sudden onset, chills, high fever, chest pain, cough and blood-streaked sputum; for widespread diffusion of the lesion, there might be shortness of breath and cyanosis. Other types of pneumonia have relatively mild symptoms.
2. The affected side demonstrates diminished breath sounds and moist rales, as well as dullness on percussion. Other areas may exhibit no physical signs.
3. Sputum examination or bacterial culture may help in differentiating between the different types of pneumonia.
4. Peripheral hemogram indicates an increase in the total number of white blood cells (WBC) and neutrophilic leukocytosis, with nuclear shift to the left or toxic granulations in the cytoplasm; normal or an increased number of WBC in mycoplasmal pneumonia; normal or a decreased number of WBC in viral pneumonia; an increased number of eosinophile granulocytes in fungal pneumonia; anaemia in friedlander pneumonia and fungal pneumonia.
5. X-ray test reveals large areas of dense shadow during the consolidation period of bacterial pneumonia; dotted, lamellar or evenly distributed shadows in viral or mycoplasmal pneumonia; scattered irregular shadows in the middle and lower part of the lungs in fungal pneumonia.

## Syndrome Differentiation

### 1. Invasion of wind-heat into the lungs

Symptoms: Fever, aversion to cold, headache, sore throat, cough with yellow and sticky sputum and chest pain; red tongue tip or margin with yellow coating and floating, rapid pulse; these symptoms are mostly observed during the early stage of bacterial pneumonia and in viral, mycoplasmal or fungal pneumonia.

Analysis of symptoms: Pathogenic wind-heat invades the exterior and stagnates in the muscular interstices, causing disorder of the superficies marked by fever and aversion to cold; pathogenic wind-heat disturbs the upper energizer, leading to headache; pathogenic wind-heat fumigates the respiratory tract, resulting in sore throat; pathogenic wind-heat invades the lungs and impairs their ability in purification, presenting as cough with yellow and sticky sputum; since the lung collaterals are damaged, there is pain in the chest; red tongue tip or margin with yellow coating, as well as floating and rapid pulse are manifestations of wind-heat attacking the lungs.

## 2. Accumulation of pathogenic heat in the lungs

Symptoms: Persistent fever unrelieved by sweating, cough, shortness of breath, flaring of nares, fast breathing, expectoration of yellow and sticky or rusty sputum, chest pain, thirst with restlessness, yellowish or reddish urine and dry stools; red tongue with yellow coating, as well as slippery and rapid pulse or surging and rapid pulse; these symptoms are mostly seen in bacterial pneumonia with large areas of consolidation.

Analysis of symptoms: Exterior pathogens invade the interior when they are not successfully expelled, causing heat in the lungs and stagnation of lung-wei, manifesting as persistent fever unrelieved by sweating; pathogenic heat stagnates the lung qi and gives rise to failure of the lungs in purification, resulting in cough, shortness of breath, nasal flaring, rough breathing and expectoration of yellow and sticky or rusty sputum; pathogenic heat damages the lung collaterals, causing pain in the chest; pathogenic heat consumes body fluid, marked by thirst, yellowish or reddish urine and dry stools; red tongue with yellow coating, slippery and rapid pulse or surging and rapid pulse are manifestations of accumulation of pathogenic heat in the lungs.

## 3. Invasion of heat-toxins into the interior

Symptoms: Persistent fever, cough, panting, blood-streaked sputum, restlessness, coma, delirium and thirst; deep red tongue with sallow and dry coating, thin and rapid pulse; these symptoms are mostly seen in severe pneumonia with complications.

Analysis of symptoms: Pathogenic heat invades the nutrient-blood and blocks the pericardium, causing persistent fever; toxic heat stagnates the lung qi and leads to failure of the lungs in purification, resulting in cough with panting; pathogenic heat damages the lung collaterals, marked by blood-streaked sputum; pathogenic heat disturbs the heart spirit, manifesting as restlessness or even coma and delirium; toxic heat scorches the fluid, bringing about thirst; dry and yellow coating on the deep red tongue, as well as thin and rapid pulse are manifestations of internal invasion of heat-toxins.

## 4. Extreme depletion of yang qi

Symptoms: Sudden fall in body temperature, oily cold sweat, pale complexion, cold limbs, bluish lips, shortness of breath, flaring of nares, dark tongue, as well as extremely thin and feeble pulse; these symptoms are mostly observed in pneumonia with shock or heart failure.

Analysis of symptoms: Internal invasion of heat-toxins results in depletion of healthy qi, consumption of yang qi and exhaustion of yin fluid, presenting as extremely unfavorable symptoms; since qi is poorly managed, there is shortness of breath and flaring of nares; because yin and yang are disassociated, there is a sudden dropping of body temperature with oily cold sweat; exhaustion of healthy qi affects smooth circulation of blood, marked by pale complexion and cyanosed lips; the dark tongue with extremely thin and feeble pulse is a sign of extreme depletion of yang qi.

## Differential Treatment

## 1. Invasion of wind-heat into the lungs

Treatment principle: Dispersing wind-heat, clearing the lungs and relieving the exterior.

Prescription and herbs: Modified Yinqiao Powder.

Jinyinhua (Honeysuckle Flower) 12 g, Lianqiao (Weeping Forsythia Capsule) 9 g, Zhuye (Henon Bamboo Leaf) 6 g, Jingjie (Fineleaf Schizonepeta Herb) 9 g, Bohe (Peppermint) 3 g, Dandouchi (Fermented Soybean) 12 g, Niubangzi (Great Burdock Achene) 9 g, Jiegeng (Platycodon Root) 3 g, Lugen (Reed Rhizome) 30 g and Gancao (Liquorice Root) 6 g.

Modification: If there is abundant heat in the interior and yellow sputum, Huangqin (Baical Skullcap Root) 12 g and Yuxingcao (Heartleaf Houttuynia Herb) 30 g are added to clear and purge heat in the lungs; for thirst with dry throat, Shashen (Root of Straight Ladybell) 12 g and Tianhuafen (Trichosanthin) 15 g are added to dispel heat and produce fluid.

## 2. Accumulation of pathogenic heat in the lungs

Treatment principle: Dispersing the lung tissue and dispelling heat, dissolving phlegm and bringing down adverseness.

Prescription and herbs: Modified Maxing Shigan Decoction and Jingwei Decoction.

Mahuang (Ephedra) 6 g, Xingren (Almond) 9 g, Shigao (Raw Gypsum) 30 g (decocted first), Gancao (Liquorice Root) 6 g, Lugen (Reed Rhizome) 30 g, Dongguaren (Chinese waxgourd Seed) 12 g, Taoren (Peach Seed) 9 g, Yiyiren (Unprepared Coix Seed) 15 g and Huangqin (Baical Skullcap Root) 12 g.

Modification: For abundance of phlegm and heat, Yuxingcao (Heartleaf Houttuynia Herb) 30 g and Quangualou (Snakegourd Fruit) 15 g are added to reinforce the effect of clearing the lungs and dissolving phlegm.

## 3. Invasion of heat-toxins into the interior

Treatment principle: Clearing the ying and opening orifices, eliminating toxins and dissolving phlegm.

Prescription and herbs: Modified Qingying Decoction.

Xijiao (Rhinoceros Horn) 3 g or Shuiniujiao (Buffalo Horn) 30 g, Shengdi (Dried Rehmannia Root) 20 g, Xuanshen (Figwort Root) 12 g, Maidong (Dwarf Lilyturf Tuber) 12 g, Danshen (Radix Salviae Miltiorrhiae) 12 g, Huanglian (Golden Thread) 6 g, Jinyinhua (Honeysuckle Flower) 12 g, Lianqiao (Weeping Forsythia Capsule) 12 g, Zhuye (Henon Bamboo Leaf) 9 g, Shichangpu (Acorus Calamus) 12 g and Tianzhuhuang (Tabasheer) 9 g.

Modification: For restlessness and delirium, Zixue Dan is added to dispel heat and extinguish wind; for appearance of coma, Angong Niuhuang Wan (Bezoar Uterus-Calming Pill) is administered nasally to dispel heat, open up the orifices and resuscitate the spirit.

## 4. Extreme depletion of yang qi

Treatment principle: Restoring yang and warming the extremities, nourishing qi and astringing yin.

Prescription and herbs: Shengfu Longmu Decoction and Shengmai Powder.

Renshen (Ginseng) 9 g, Fuzi (Prepared Common Monkshood Daughter) 9 g (decocted first), Maidong (Dwarf Lilyturf Tuber) 15 g, Wuweizi (Chinese Magnolivine Fruit) 9 g, Longgu (Os Draconis) 30 g (decocted first) and Muli (Oyster Shell) 30 g (decocted first).

Modification: For convulsions and spasms, Lingyangjiaofen (Antelope Horn Powder) 0.6 g (swallowed), Gouteng (Gambir Plant) 15 g is added to relieve convulsions and extinguish wind.

## Chinese Patent Medicine

1. Yinqiao Jiedu Tablet: 4 tablets for each dose, 3 times a day.
2. Baikejing Syrup: 10 ml for each dose, 3 times a day.

## Simple and Handy Prescriptions

1. Pugongying (Dandelion) 30 g, Baijiangcao (Dahurian Patrinia Herb) 45 g, Banzhilian (Barbated Skullcup Herb) 15 g and Huzhang (Giant Knotweed Rhizome) 30 g are boiled in water and separated into 2 portions to be taken at different times within a day. It is applicable to treat acute pneumonia.
2. Yu Xing Cao Decoction: Yuxingcao (Heartleaf Houttuynia Herb) 500 g is ground into 100 ml of solution and separated into 3 portions to be taken within a day. It is used for treating lobar pneumonia.

## Other Therapies

Aerosol inhalation: Yuxingcao Injection is administered to the respiratory tract through an ultrasonic nebulizer.

Scraping method: Scrape the chest, both sides of the spinal column and the scapular region with a coin dipped in vegetable oil or distillated spirits till the skin veins are congested. It is used to treat fever with coma.

Dietary therapy: Jinyinhua (Honeysuckle Flower) 9 g and Lugen (Fresh Reed Rhizome) 30 g are decocted with crystal sugar to taste and taken as tea. It is used to dispel heat and produce body fluid.

## Cautions and Advice

1. Patients who are old and weak or have immune system deficiency should take special care to prevent themselves from infection, transmission and complication of this disease.
2. Patients should keep out of the rain, avoid catching a cold and overstrain and refrain from alcohol and cigarettes.
3. They should also engage in regular physical exercise to improve their bodies' immunological functions.

## Daily Exercises

1. List the clinical characteristics of pneumonia.
2. Name the types of pneumonia and recall the treatment principles and representative prescriptions for each type.

# Lung Abscess
## Week 3: Tuesday

Lung abscess is a suppurative disorder of the pulmonary tissues due to multiple etiological factors. It is characterized by suppurative inflammation in the early stage and subsequently necrosis and abscess. Clinically, there are manifestations of high fever, cough and expectoration of profuse foul or purulent sputum. This disease is classified into two types: primary lung abscess and secondary lung abscess. The former, also called aspiration lung abscess, is concerned with aspiration and the abscesses are generally found in the posterior segments of the upper and lower lobes, with the right lung more frequently afflicted than the left. The latter is generally considered a hematogenous pulmonary abscess due to septicemia; secondary lung abscess may also stem from direct spread of infection in the adjacent organs or tissues, such as in the case of hepatic amoeba or subphrenic abscess. Chronic lung abscess, usually with a disease course of over 3 months, commonly afflicts middle-aged people, particularly the males. If it is promptly and thoroughly treated in the early stage, the prognosis is generally favorable. In TCM, lung abscess is closely associated with "Fei Yong" (lung carbuncle).

## Etiology and Pathology

The etiological factors of lung abscess are either exogenous or endogenous or a combination of both: Invasion of the exogenous pathogenic factors causes accumulation of heat in the lungs; improper diet produces damp-heat and phlegm in the interior; pre-existing phlegm-heat in the lungs, coupled with invasion of exogenous pathogenic factors into the body due to poor defensive function, can bring about co-existence of heat and stasis or heat and phlegm, and consequently, lung abscess.

The pathological changes of lung abscess are discussed as follows: Various pathogenic factors lead to the accumulation of heat in the lungs, which condenses fluid into phlegm, stagnating qi and blood in the lungs and rendering the lung collaterals obstructed and putrefied, marked by rupture of the abscess and discharge of pus. According to waxing and waning of healthy qi and pathogenic factors, the pathological process is divided into three stages: the initial stage, the abscess-forming stage, the pus-discharging stage and the recovery stage. The initial stage is marked by invasion of wind-heat or wind-cold into the lungs, which stagnates the lung qi and eventually gives rise to accumulation of heat in the lungs, putrefying the lung tissues and forming abscess in the long run. In the second stage, abundant toxic heat corrupts the lung tissues and blood, causing rupture of the abscess and expectoration of profuse foul and purulent sputum, or vomiting of pus and blood resulting from damage to the lung collaterals by toxic heat. The final stage is characterized by gradual ceasing of pus discharge and progressive disappearing of toxins, as well as the consumption of qi and yin, with simultaneous existence of excess and deficiency. After rupture, if the toxins are not completely eradicated, they will debilitate healthy qi and the disease may come and go, and last for a long time; in this case the manifestations of damaged qi and yin will become more conspicuous.

## Diagnostic Key Points

1. Abrupt high fever with intolerance of cold, cough and profuse foul, purulent sputum.
2. Increased number of white blood cells and neutrophilic granulocytes.
3. Thoracic X-ray examination reveals large areas of dense shadow, pus cavity and fluid level.

## Syndrome Differentiation

### 1. The initial stage

Symptoms: Aversion to cold, fever, cough with increased volume of white and foaming sputum, chest pain aggravated by cough, difficult breathing, dry mouth and nose; red tongue with thin and yellow coating and rapid, floating and slippery pulse.

Analysis of symptoms: Pathogenic wind-heat invades the interior and attacks the lungs, causing disharmony between the defensive qi and the superficies as well as a struggle between the healthy qi and pathogenic factors, manifesting as intolerance of cold and fever; pathogenic wind-heat invades the lungs and causes dysfunction of lung qi in dispersion and purification, bringing about cough with sputum and difficult breathing; pathogenic wind-heat invades the interior and attacks the lungs, rendering the lung qi unable to distribute fluid, resulting in an increased volume of white and sticky sputum; pathogenic wind-heat attacks the upper part of the body, characterized by dry mouth and nose; the stagnation of lung collaterals is responsible for chest pain aggravated by cough; red tongue with thin and yellow coating, as well as rapid, floating and slippery pulse are manifestations of external invasion of wind-heat.

## 2. The abscess-forming stage

Symptoms: Persistent ardent fever, frequent shivering, sweating, cough, shortness of breath, vomiting of yellow and thick sputum with pus and foul odor, pain in the chest and hypochondria, dry mouth, restlessness; red tongue with yellow and greasy coating, as well as slippery and rapid pulse.

Analysis of symptoms: Pathogenic heat invades the interior from the exterior and causes a struggle between healthy qi and pathogenic factors, resulting in ardent fever, shivering and sweating; accumulation of toxic heat in the lungs brings on adverse rising of lung qi and disorder of lung collaterals, causing cough, shortness of breath and chest pain; combat between turbid phlegm and stagnated heat leads to abscess, manifesting as vomiting of yellow and thick sputum with pus and foul odor; pathogenic heat disturbs the heart and consumes fluid, characterized by restlessness and dry mouth; red tongue with yellow and greasy coating, as well as slippery and rapid pulse are manifestations of exuberant heat.

## 3. The pus-discharging stage

Symptoms: Vomiting of profuse purulent sputum, sticky sputum or blood-streaked sputum with a foul odor, chest stuffiness and pain, or even panting with inability to lie flat, general fever and red complexion, thirst with desire for drinking; red tongue with yellow and greasy coating, as well as slippery and rapid pulse.

Analysis of symptoms: Internal ulceration of abscess and external discharge of pus is marked by putrefied blood and tissues, leading to the vomiting of large volumes of foul, purulent or even blood-streaked sputum; accumulation of pus and toxins in the lungs impede the flow of lung qi and obstruct lung vessels, characterized by thoracic stuffiness and pain; damage to the lung collaterals is responsible for blood-streaked blood; toxic heat scorches the interior and consumes body fluid, manifesting as general fever, red complexion and thirst; red tongue with yellow and greasy coating, as well as slippery and rapid pulse, are manifestations of internal accumulation of toxic heat.

## 4. The recovery stage

Symptoms: Fever that gradually subsides, alleviated cough, reduced volume of purulent blood, diminished foul odor, clear and thin sputum which may still be accompanied by vague pain in the chest and hypochondria, weariness, shortness of breath, spontaneous perspiration, night sweats, vexation and dry mouth; red tongue with thin and yellow coating, as well as thin, rapid and feeble pulse.

Analysis of symptoms: After rupture of the abscess, the toxins are eliminated, so the fever subsides, the cough is alleviated, there is less purulent blood and sputum turns thin and clear; prolonged accumulation of toxic heat in the lungs results in consumption of qi and yin, marked by shortness of breath, weariness, spontaneous perspiration, night sweats, dry mouth and vexation; impaired lung collaterals and unhealed ulcers are responsible for the vague pain in the chest and hypochondria; red tongue with thin and yellow coating, as well as thin, rapid and feeble pulse are manifestations of simultaneous impairment of qi and yin by lingering remnant pathogens.

## Differential Treatment

### 1. The initial stage

Treatment principle: Dispersing wind and diffusing the lung tissue, dispelling heat and removing toxins.

Prescription and herbs: Modified Yinqiao Powder.

Lianqiao (Weeping Forsythia Capsule) 20 g, Jinyinhua (Honeysuckle Flower) 12 g, Zhuye (Henon Bamboo Leaf) 6 g, Lugen (Reed Rhizome) 30 g, Jiegeng (Platycodon Root) 6 g, Xingren (Almond) 12 g, Niubangzi (Great Burdock Achene) 12 g, Baimaogen (Lalang Grass Rhizome) 30 g, Bohe (Peppermint) 9 g, Jingjie (Fineleaf Schizonepeta Herb) 9 g and Gancao (Liquorice Root) 6 g.

Modification: If there is severe fever, Huangqin (Baical Skullcap Root) 15 g and Yuxingcao (Heartleaf Houttuynia Herb) 30 g are added to strengthen the effect of dispelling heat and removing toxins; for expectoration of profuse sputum, Gualou (Snakegourd Fruit) 15 g and Xiangbei (Bulbus Fritillariae Thunbergii) 12 g are added to dissolve phlegm and relieve coughing.

## 2. The abscess-forming stage

Treatment principle: Resolving stasis and dissipating carbuncle, clearing the lungs and eliminating toxins.

Prescription and herbs: Supplementary Jingwei Decoction (recorded in *Invaluable Prescriptions*).

Lugen (Reed Rhizome) 30 g, Baimaogen (Lalang Grass Rhizome) 30 g, Yiyiren (Coix Seed) 30 g, Dongguaren (Chinese waxgourd Seed) 15 g, Taoren (Peach Seed) 12 g, Jiegeng (Platycodon Root) 6 g, Xingren (Almond) 10 g, Jinyinhua (Honeysuckle Flower) 15 g, Lianqiao (Weeping Forsythia Capsule) 20 g, Huangqin (Baical Skullcap Root) 12 g, Huanglian (Golden Thread) 6 g and Gancao (Liquorice Root) 6 g.

Modification: For cough with yellow, sticky phlegm, Sangbaipi (White Mulberry Root-Bark) 12 g, Gualou (Snakegourd Fruit) 12 g and Shegan (Blackberrylily Rhizome) 9 g are added to clear the lungs and dissolve phlegm; for stagnation of toxic heat with foul sputum, Xihuang Pill is used to dispel heat and dissolve phlegm, as well as cool blood and dissipate stasis.

## 3. The pus-discharging stage

Treatment principle: Dispelling heat and removing toxins, dissolving phlegm and discharging pus.

Prescription and herbs: Modified Supplementary Jiegeng Decoction.

Jiegeng (Platycodon Root) 15 g, Gancao (Liquorice Root) 9 g, Xiangbei (Bulbus Fritillariae Thunbergii) 12 g, Jinyinhua (Honeysuckle Flower) 15 g, Yiyiren (Coix Seed) 30 g, Tinglizi (Herba Leonuri) 15 g, Baiji (Common Bletilla Tuber) 15 g, Chenpi (Dried Tangerine Peel) 9 g, Taoren (Peach Seed) 10 g and Lugen (Reed Rhizome) 30 g.

Modification: For expectoration of sputum with difficult discharge of pus, Zaojiaoci (Gleditsiae Thorn) 12 g is used to dissolve phlegm and discharge pus; for inability to cough up sputum due to debilitation of the body, Huangqi (Milkvetch Root) 30 g is added to nourish qi and strengthen the healthy qi, as well as eliminate toxins and discharge pus; for cough with profuse blood, Oujie (Lotus Rhizome Node) 9 g, Danpi (Cortex Moutan) 12 g, Baimaogen (Lalang Grass Rhizome) 30 g and Sanqifen (Sanchi) 3 g (swallowed) are used to cool blood and stop bleeding.

## 4. The recovery stage

Treatment principle: Dispelling heat to nourish yin, replenishing qi to supplement the lungs.

Prescription and herbs: Modified Shashen Qingfei Decoction.

Beishashen (Coastal Glehnia Root) 15 g, Taizishen (Heterophylly Falsesatarwort Root) 15 g, Maidong (Dwarf Lilyturf Tuber) 12 g, Baihe (Lily Bulb)12 g, Xingren (Almond) 12 g, Xiangbei (Bulbus Fritillariae Thunbergii) 12 g, Huangqi (Unprepared Milkvetch Root) 30 g, Yiyiren (Coix Seed) 30 g, Dongguaren (Chinese waxgourd Seed) 20 g Jiegeng (Platycodon Root) 10 g, Baiji (Common Bletilla Tuber) 12 g and Gancao (Liquorice Root) 6 g.

Modification: For deficiency of blood, Danggui (Chinese Angelica) 9 g are added to nourish blood and activate collaterals; for severe deficiency of yin, Yuzhu (Fragrant Solomonseal Rhizome) 12 g are added to nourish yin and moisten the lungs; for remnant pus, toxins and purulent blood, Yuxingcao (Heartleaf Houttuynia Herb) 30 g, Baijiangcao (Dahurian Patrinia Herb) 15 g, Jinyinhua (Honeysuckle Flower) 15 g and Lianqiao (Weeping Forsythia Capsule) 15 g are added to eliminate toxins and discharge pus, as well as reinforce the healthy qi and expel pathogenic factors.

## Chinese Patent Medicine

1. Yinqiao Jiedu Tablet: 4 tablets for each dose, 3 times a day. It is used in the initial stage of lung abscess.
2. Qu Tan Ling Oral Solution: 30 ml for each dose, 3 times a day. It is used to clear the lungs and dissolve phlegm.

## Simple and Handy Prescriptions

1. Jinyinhua (Honeysuckle Flower) 15 g, Lianqiao (Weeping Forsythia Capsule) 15 g, Pugongying (Dandelion) 30 g, Yuxingcao (Heartleaf Houttuynia Herb) 30 g, Lugen (Reed Rhizome) 30 g and Baimaogen (Lalang Grass Rhizome) 30 g are boiled in water. A dose of the decoction is taken twice a day. It is used in the abscess-forming stage and pus-discharging stage of lung abscess to dispel heat and remove toxins, as well as dissolve phlegm and discharge pus.
2. Baiji (Common Bletilla Tuber) 200 g, Xiangbei (Bulbus Fritillariae Thunbergii) 50 g and Baihe (Lily Bulb) 50 g are ground up into fine powders and taken (6 g per dose) once in the morning and once in the evening. It is used in the recovery stage of lung abscess to astringe the lungs, nourish yin and dissolve phlegm.

## Other Therapies

Ultrasonic nebulization: Jiegeng (Platycodon Root), Chuanbei (Tendrilleaf Fritillary Bulb), Huangqin (Baical Skullcap Root), Gualoupi (Snakegourd Peel) and Gancao (Liquorice Root) (about 15~20 g of each) and Yuxingcao (Heartleaf Houttuynia Herb) 30~50 g are boiled in water (40 ml), which is condensed into 100 ml. Afterwards, 20 ml of the decoction is mixed with 20 ml of distilled water for ultrasonic atomizing inhalation (1~2 times a day). If it is combined with postural drainage, the effect for discharging pus and expelling phlegm is even better.

Dietary therapy: Baimuer Hongzao Porridge: Baimuer (Tremella) 50 g and Hongzao (Red Date) 15 dates are boiled in water till the Tremella becomes pasty. After adding crystal sugar to taste, the porridge can be taken to moisten the lungs and nourish deficiency. It is used in the recovery stage of lung abscess.

## Cautions and Advice

1. To completely cure upper respiratory infection, attention must be paid to oral infection, this is so that lung abscess will not be induced by aspiration of contaminated secretion into the lungs.
2. Dermal furuncles and carbuncles or extrapulmonary suppurative diseases should also be actively treated, so as to prevent hematogenous lung abscess.

## Daily Exercises

1. List the stages of lung abscess and describe their clinical characteristics.
2. Recall the treatment principle and prescription and herbs used to treat lung abscess in the pus-discharging stage.

# Pulmonary Tuberculosis

## Week 3: Wednesday

Pulmonary tuberculosis is an infectious disease of the lungs resulting from mycobacterium tuberculosis, clinically marked by cough, expectoration of sputum, hemoptysis, chest pain, hectic fever, night sweats and emaciation. It can occur regardless of the four seasons and afflict people of all ages, with the young and middle-aged being more susceptible. Pulmonary tuberculosis, if diagnosed and treated promptly, can be thoroughly cured. Not only can the TB bacilli be wiped out completely, the damaged tissues can also be repaired to an amazing extent. In TCM, pulmonary tuberculosis belongs to the category of "lung consumption".

## Etiology and Pathology

The etiological factors of pulmonary tuberculosis are either exogenous or endogenous: The former refers to the invasion of consumptive worms (tuberculomyces) into the lungs system; while the latter refers to the weakness of healthy qi, the insufficiency of qi and blood and the depletion of yin-fluid, all of which are favorable for the invasion of consumptive worms. The endogenous factors and exogenous factors are linked, i.e., consumptive worm invasion is the pathogenic factor, while deficiency of healthy qi is the foundation.

The pathological changes are discussed as follows: Invasion of consumptive worms into the lungs brings about damage to the lung tissue and consumption of lung yin, which eventually progress into a chronic condition marked by severe deficiency of yin and the ensuing exuberance of heat. Deficiency of yin may involve qi or even yang, leading to deficiency of yin and qi, or yin and yang. If the disease persists for a long time, the disorder of the lungs can spread to other organs, especially the kidneys and spleen and, in severe cases, there will be deficiency of the lungs, spleen and kidneys due to depletion of essence and blood. In this sense, it is evident that the core of this disease is deficiency of yin, which may also bring about exuberance of fire, deficiency of qi, or deficiency of yin and yang.

## Diagnostic Key Points

1. Long-term low-grade fever, night sweats, general indisposition, emaciation, cough, expectoration of sputum, hemoptysis and chest pain.
2. Slight dullness in the supraclavicular fossa, infraclavicular fossa and scapular region on percussion, as well as audible moist rales after coughing.
3. Tuberculin test and sputum bacillus tuberculosis test reveal positive results.
4. X-ray examination reveals fibrocalcific sclerosis, infiltrating foci, caseous necrosis and cavitary lesion.

## Syndrome Differentiation

### 1. Insufficiency of lung yin

Symptoms: Dry cough in short duration, blood streaked or dotted sputum in bright red color, hectic fever in the afternoon, vague pain in the chest, low fever, post meridiem feverish sensations in the palms and soles, dry skin with a burning sensation, dry mouth and throat, as well as mild night sweats; red tongue tip or margin with thin or scanty coating and thin and rapid pulse.

Analysis of symptoms: Invasion of consumptive worms into the lungs damages the lung body and causes consumption of lung yin, marked by dry cough and scanty sputum; since the lung collaterals are impaired, there is bloody sputum and a vague pain in the chest; deficiency of yin produces internal heat, leading to post meridiem low grade fever, feverish sensation in the palms and soles, as well as dry skin with a burning sensation; consumption of lung yin prevents body fluid from reaching the head, characterized by dry mouth and throat; deficiency of yin and excess of yang lead to excretion of fluid, presenting as mild night sweats; red tongue tip or margin with scanty coating, as well as thin and rapid pulse are all manifestations of yin deficiency.

### 2. Exuberance of fire due to yin deficiency

Symptoms: Choking cough, shortness of breath, scanty and sticky phlegm, frequent expectoration of bright red blood, hectic fever in the afternoon, bone-steaming sensation, red cheeks, feverish sensations over the five centers, profuse night sweats, vexation, insomnia, irascibility, dragging pain in the chest and hypochondria, nocturnal emission or consumption of essence in males, irregular menstruation in women, and gradual weight loss; purple-red and dry tongue with thin-yellow or peeled coating and thin-rapid pulse.

Analysis of symptoms: If the disease is prolonged, other organs will also be affected, leading to impairment of kidney yin and lung yin, as well as internal abundance of deficient fire which condenses body fluid into phlegm, marked by choking cough, shortness of breath and scanty sticky phlegm; deficient fire scorches the blood vessels, leading to the expectoration of bright red blood; deficiency of water leads to hyperactivity of fire, presenting as hectic fever in the afternoon, a feverish sensation over the five centers, a bone-steaming sensation and red cheeks; exuberant fire due to yin deficiency drives fluid out of the body and is marked by profuse night sweats; hyperactivity of fire in the heart and liver is responsible for vexation, insomnia and irascibility; obstruction of liver and lung collaterals causes dragging pain in the chest and hypochondria; relative exuberance of kidney fire ensuing from yin deficiency is characterized by nocturnal emission and seminal consumption in males; malnutrition of the thorough fare and conception vessels stemming from insufficiency of yin blood is marked by irregular menstruation in women; consumption of yin essence is manifested as emaciation; purple red tongue with thin and yellow or peeled coating, as well as thin and rapid pulse are manifestations of exuberant fire due to yin deficiency.

## 3. Consumption of qi and yin

Symptoms: Cough, lassitude, shortness of breath, low voice, occasional blood-streaked sputum in a slightly red color, low-grade fever, hectic fever in the afternoon, pale complexion, red cheeks, intolerance of wind and cold, co-existence of spontaneous perspiration and night sweats, inadequate food intake and loose stools; red and tender tongue with teeth marks on the margin, thin coating, and thin, rapid and feeble pulse.

Analysis of symptoms: Prolonged duration of this disease causes deficiency of the lungs and spleen, as well as qi and yin, marked by failure of the lungs in purification and governance of qi, with such signs as cough, low voice and shortness of breath; owing to the failure of qi to transform fluid, there is accumulation of phlegm; impairment of lung collaterals is manifested as sputum with light-red blood; deficient qi fails to defend the exterior and causes a sinking of yang into yin, presenting as fever, intolerance of wind and spontaneous perspiration; deficiency of yin produces internal heat, leading to night sweats and hectic fever; deficiency of the spleen leads to poor digestion, with inadequate food intake and loose stools; simultaneous impairment of qi and yin is characterized by pale complexion, red cheeks, red and tender tongue, as well as thin, rapid and feeble pulse.

## 4. Deficiency of yin and yang

Symptoms: Cough, gasping, shortness of breath, occasional presence of dark blood in the sputum, hectic fever, cold body, night sweats, spontaneous perspiration, hoarseness or loss of voice, facial edema and swollen limbs, palpitations, purple lips, cold limbs, diarrhea before dawn, erosion of the mucous membrane and tongue in the oral cavity, emaciation, involuntary emission and impotence in males and inadequacy or suppression of menses in females; red, dry and glossy tongue or pale tongue, weight gain, teeth marks on the margins, slightly thin and rapid pulse or deficient, large and feeble pulse.

Analysis of symptoms: Deficiency of yin involves yang and causes simultaneous impairment of the lungs, spleen and kidneys, marked by cough and gasping due to failure of the lungs to govern qi and the kidneys to receive qi; deficiency of yin results in dryness in the respiratorytract, causing hoarseness; damage to the lung collaterals is marked by bloody sputum; deficiency of the spleen and kidneys is responsible for facial edema, swollen limbs and diarrhea before dawn; since the heart is involved, palpitations and purple lips are also common; deficient fire flames upward, bringing about an erosion of the mucous membrane and tongue in the oral cavity; weakness of defensive qi is demonstrated in the cold body and spontaneous perspiration; deficiency of yin is characterized by hectic fever and night sweats; depletion of essence malnourishes the body, especially the thoroughfare vessel and the conception vessel, resulting in inadequacy or suppression of menses and emaciation in females; the fire from the life gate is subdued, leading to involuntary emission and impotence in males; the red, dry and glossy tongue or pale tongue, weight gain, teeth marks on the margins, slightly thin and rapid pulse or deficient, large and feeble pulse are all manifestations of deficiency of yin and yang.

## Differential Treatment

### 1. Insufficiency of lung yin

Treatment principle: Nourishing yin, moistening the lungs, and dissolving phlegm to stop cough.

Prescription and herbs: Modified Yuehua Pill.

Beishashen (Coastal Glehnia Root) 12 g, Tiandong (Cochinchinese Asparagus Root) 9 g, Maidong (Dwarf Lilyturf Tuber) 9 g, Shengdi (Dried Rehmannia Root) 12 g, Shudi (Prepared Rhizome of Rehmannia) 12 g, Baibu (Stemona Root) 9 g, Langan (Jecur Lutrae) 30 g, Chuanbei (Tendrilleaf Fritillary Bulb) 9 g, Ejiao (Donkey-hide Glue) 12 g (melted in decoction), Shensanqi (Panax pseudo-ginseng) 12 g, Fuling (Indian Bread) 12 g, Huaishanyao (Huaihe Common Yan Rhizome) 15 g and Baiji (Common Bletilla Tuber) 15 g.

Modification: For blood-streaked sputum, Xianhecao (Hairyvein Agrimonia Herb) 30 g, Oujie (Lotus Rhizome Node) 12 g and Baimaogen (Lalang Grass Rhizome) 30 g can be added to cool blood and stop bleeding; for low or hectic fever in the afternoon, Yinchaihu (Starwort Root) 9 g, Digupi (Chinese Wolfberry Root-Bark) 15 g and Gonglaoye (Ilecis) 30 g are added to dispel heat and relive hectic fever.

### 2. Exuberance of fire due to yin deficiency

Treatment principle: Nourishing yin to bring down fire, moistening the lungs to stop bleeding.

Prescription and herbs: Modified Baihe Guijin Decoction and Qinjiao Biejia Powder.

Baihe (Lily Bulb) 30 g, Maidong (Dwarf Lilyturf Tuber) 12 g, Xuanshen (Figwort Root) 9 g, Shengdi (Dried Rehmannia Root) 12 g, Shudi (Prepared Rhizome of Rehmannia) 12 g, Biejia (Turtle Shell) 20 g, Zhimu (Common Anemarrhena Rhizome) 12 g, Qinjiao (Largeleaf Gentian Root) 9 g, Yinchaihu (Starwort Root) 9 g, Digupi (Chinese Wolfberry Root-Bark) 15 g, Qinghao (Sweet Wormwood Herb) 15 g, Chuanbei (Tendrilleaf Fritillary Bulb) 9 g, Jiegeng (Platycodon Root) 9 g, Danggui (Chinese Angelica) 9 g, Baiji (Common Bletilla Tuber) 15 g and Gancao (Liquorice Root) 6 g.

Modification: For severe night sweats, Wumei (Smoked Plum) 9 g, Duanlonggu (Calcined Os Draconis) 30 g and Bietaogan (Persicae Immaturus) 12 g are added to astringe yin and alleviate perspiration; for expectoration of yellow and sticky sputum, Sangbaipi (White Mulberry Root-Bark) 12 g, Haihake (Clam Shell) 15 g and Yuxingcao (Heartleaf Houttuynia Herb) 30 g are added to clear the lungs and dissolve phlegm; for hemoptysis, Danpi (Cortex Moutan) 15 g, Zhizi (Cape Jasmine Fruit) 12 g and Zizhucao (Taiwan Beautyberry Leaf) 15 g are added to cool blood and stop bleeding.

### 3. Consumption of qi and yin

Treatment principle: Replenishing qi and nourishing yin, invigorating the spleen and supplementing the lungs.

Prescription and herbs: Modified Baozhen Decoction.

Dangshen (Radix Codonopsis) 9 g, Huangqi (Milkvetch Root) 15 g, Baizhu (Largehead Atractylodes Rhizome) 12 g, Fuling (Indian Bread) 12 g, Gancao (Stir-baked Liquorice Root) 6 g, Tiandong (Cochinchinese Asparagus Root) 9 g, Maidong (Dwarf Lilyturf Tuber) 9 g, Shengdi (Dried Rehmannia Root) 12 g, Shudi (Prepared Rhizome of Rehmannia) 12 g, Danggui (Chinese Angelica) 9 g, Baishao (White Peony Alba) 9 g, Digupi (Chinese Wolfberry Root-Bark) 12 g, Huangbai (Amur Cork-tree) 9 g, Zhimu (Common Anemarrhena Rhizome) 9 g, Yinchaihu (Starwort Root) 9 g, Chenpi (Dried Tangerine Peel) 9 g and Lianzixin (Lotus Plumule) 6 g.

Modification: For abdominal distension, loose stools and poor appetite, Dihuang (Rehmannia Root) and Maidong (Dwarf Lilyturf Tuber) are replaced with Chaobiandou (Fried Hyacinth Bean) 12 g, Yiyiren (Coix Seed) 15 g and Jianlianrou (Lotus Seed) 12 g so as to invigorate the spleen and supplement the lungs with their mild and sweet flavors; for expectoration of thin sputum, Ziwan (Tatarian Aster Root) 9 g, Kuandonghua (Common Coltsfoot Flower) 9 g and Suzi (Perillaseed) 9 g are added to warm and nourish the lungs and alleviate cough.

## 4. Deficiency of yin and yang

Treatment principle: Nourishing yin and invigorating yang, supplementing essence and replenishing blood.

Prescription and herbs: Modified Buqi Dazao Pill.

Renshen (Ginseng) 9 g, Huangqi (Milkvetch Root) 15 g, Huaishanyao (Huaihe Common Yan Rhizome) 15 g, Gouqizi (Barbary Wolfberry Fruit) 12 g, Guiban (Tortoise Shell) 30 g, Lujiaopian (Sliced Cornus Cervi) 6 g, Ziheche (Human Placenta Powder) 3 g (swallowed), Shudi (Prepared Rhizome of Rehmannia) 15 g, Danggui (Chinese Angelica) 9 g, Ejiao (Donkey-hide Glue) 12 g (melted in decoction) and Baishao (White Peony Alba) 12 g.

Modification: For relative deficiency of yin, Maidong (Dwarf Lilyturf Tuber) 12 g and Wuweizi (Chinese Magnolivine Fruit) 6 g can be added to nourish the lungs and tonify the kidneys; for diarrhea before dawn, Shudi (Prepared Rhizome of Rehmannia) and Ejiao (Donkey-hide Glue) are replaced with Weirouguo (Stir-baked Sarcocarp) 9 g and Buguzhi (Malaytea Scurfpea Fruit) 12 g to supplement kidney fire and warm spleen earth.

## Chinese Patent Medicine

1. Jade Screen Granule: 15 g for each dose, 3 times a day, to treat severe spontaneous perspiration.
2. Zhibai Dihuang Pill: 12 pills for each dose, 3 times a day, to treat night sweats due to deficiency of yin and exuberance of fire.

## Simple and Handy Prescriptions

1. Baiji (Common Bletilla Tuber) 15 g, Baibu (Stemona Root) 15 g, Muli (Oyster Shell) 15 g and Paoshanjia (Stir-baked Squama Manitis) 15 g are boiled in water, separated into 2 portions and taken at 2 different times within a day. It is used to moisten the lungs and alleviate cough as well as astringe yin and check bleeding.

2. Lucao (Cairo Morningglory Root or Leaf) 30 g, Baibu (Stemona Root) 15 g, Baiji (Common Bletilla Tuber) 15 g and Xiakucao (Common Selfheal Fruit-Spike) 15 g are boiled in water, separated into 2 portions and taken at 2 different times within a day. It is used to clear the lungs and stop bleeding.

## Other Therapies

Exercise therapy: Practice Taijiquan (traditional Chinese shadow boxing) or engage in other physical exercises to regulate qi, blood, yin and yang for rehabilitation.

Dietary therapy:

(1) Shuang Er Soup: Baimuer (Tremella) 50 g, Heimuer (Black Fungus) 30 g and Baihe (Lily Bulb) 30 g are boiled in water. Honey is added to the soup after it is ready. This therapy is used to nourish the lungs, reduce dryness and produce body fluid.

(2) Chongcai Laoya Soup: Dongchongxiacao (Chinese Caterpillar Fungus) 10 g, an aged duck and sauces to taste are made into soup. It is used to nourish the lungs and kidneys and supplement essence and blood.

## Cautions and Advice

1. This disease is a chronic one, so patients should not expect instant results but rather commit promptly to a treatment scheme that is holistic and chronological, with the proper amounts of drugs being administered throughout the whole period.

2. Patients should refrain from smoking; instead, they should keep indoor air ventilated or go outside to enjoy fresh air.
3. They should also maintain a nutritious and light diet and avoid too much spicy or other food that will irritate the stomach and produce fire or dryness.

## Daily Exercises

1. List the etiological factors of pulmonary tuberculosis.
2. Name the viscera that are most closely related to pulmonary tuberculosis.
3. Recall the types of pulmonary tuberculosis, their treatment principles and representative prescriptions.

# Lung Cancer
# Week 3: Thursday

Lung cancer, also called bronchiogenic cancer, arises from the bronchial mucous membrane. It is the most common type of primary malignant tumor in the lungs. Clinical manifestations depend on the sites of the tumor as well as the presence or absence of complications. In general, it is asymptomatic in the initial stage but presents with respiratory symptoms in the advance stage. Common complications are pulmonary atelectasis and pyogenic infection, as well as metastatic carcinomas from other organs. Lung cancer most frequently afflicts people above the age of 40, with the ratio of men to women being 5:1. This disease has a high death rate due to the unsatisfactory curative effect at the present time. Hence, early discovery, early diagnosis and early treatment are of utmost importance. In TCM, lung cancer is considered to be closely associated with "lung accumulation", "cough", "coughing up blood" and "chest pain".

## Etiology and Pathology

The etiological factors of lung cancer are pathogenic toxins, phlegm, dampness and toxic heat from the external environment which invade the lungs while the body is weak and subsequently accumulate into nodules in the chest.

The pathological changes of lung cancer are discussed as follows: Insufficiency of healthy qi incurs invasion of pathogenic factors into the lungs and these accumulate into nodules in the chest. Deficiency of the spleen produces phlegm and dampness, which glue to the invading exogenous pathogenic factors and eventually form nodules. Dysfunction of the kidneys, spleen and lungs (i.e., insufficiency of kidney qi, indigestion due to spleen deficiency, and lack of fluid in the lungs), if coupled with invasion of toxic heat, may bring about accumulation of body fluid into phlegm, which mixes with qi and blood and forms nodules. If the nodules form in the airway, there may be coughing (including the coughing up of sputum and sometimes blood) or even incessant hemoptysis due to damage of the lung collaterals. If the nodules are enlarged, they may obstruct the airway and impede the airflow, causing shortness of breath. If the disease is prolonged, marked by a sudden increase in accumulation of pathogens, obstruction of dampness and phlegm, and aggravation of toxins, there will be fever and subsequent deficiency of lung qi with aversion to cold and sweating. In conclusion, the root of this disease is deficiency from which excess stems; in other words, deficiency is the primary aspect, while excess is the secondary.

## Diagnostic Key Points

1. It generally afflicts males above 40 who have a long history of excessive tobacco smoking, a recent history of cough persistent for several weeks, repeated hemoptysis, recurrent obstructive pneumonia, or pulmonary atelectasis unaccountable for by other reasons.
2. Clinically, it is marked by cough (producing sputum and sometimes blood), chest pain and fever, or lung abscess and pleurisy, as well as supraclavicular lymphadenectasis or swelling of other superficial lymph nodes.
   (1) X-ray examination reveals unilateral enlargement of shadow in the hilum of the lung(s), or solitary round or nodular infiltrating focus in the lung(s); sometimes obstructive pneumonia, pulmonary atelectasis, widened hilum of the lung(s) and mediastinum, pleural or pericardial effusion and diaphragmatic paralysis.
   (2) CT scan reveals the overlapping anatomic sites on the chest radiograph, display more clearly the nodules indiscernible by X-ray chest examination and show the intruding scope of the tumors in the mediastinum, as well as the conditions of lymph node metastasis.
   (3) Sputum cytoscopy has a positive rate above 80% from 3~6 times of consecutive examinations.

## Syndrome Differentiation

### 1. Internal heat due to deficiency of yin

Symptoms: Unproductive cough, or expectoration of scanty and sticky sputum and sometimes bloody sputum, or dry mouth and throat, emaciation, hectic fever in the afternoon, feverish sensations over the five centers (the palms, the soles and the heart), night sweats, red cheeks, dry stools, yellow urine, and hoarse voice; red tongue with only a little fluid and little to no coating, as well as thin and rapid pulse.

Analysis of symptoms: Deficiency of lung yin produces blazing deficient fire and impairs the lung qi in descending and purifying, leading to unproductive cough or expectoration of scanty and sticky sputum; deficient fire scorches the lung collaterals, bringing about blood-stained sputum; deficient fire consumes body fluid, presenting as dry mouth and throat, as well as hoarse voice; depleted yin-fluid fails to moisten and nourish the five main internal organs and the skin and hair externally, which is marked by weight loss or even emaciation; hectic fever in the afternoon, feverish sensation over the five centers, red cheeks, night sweats, red tongue with only a little fluid and little to no coating, as well as thin and rapid pulse, are all manifestations of exuberant fire due to deficiency of yin.

### 2. Deficiency of qi and yin

Symptoms: Unproductive or productive cough, lassitude, sweating, shortness of breath, dry mouth, elevated body temperature, or hectic fever in the afternoon, feverish sensations in the palms and soles, occasional palpitations, poor appetite, gastric distension, dry or loose stools; red tongue with thin coating, or tender and enlarged tongue with teeth marks, as well as thin, rapid, and feeble pulse.

Analysis of symptoms: Insufficiency of lung qi impairs the functions of the lungs in dispersion and purification, and it is marked by unproductive or productive cough; insufficiency of lung qi also inhibits the lungs in governing qi, demonstrating as lassitude, shortness of breath, sweating and occasional palpitations; impairment of lung yin produces intense deficient heat, resulting in dry mouth, elevated body temperature, or hectic fever in the afternoon and feverish sensation in the palms and soles; weakness of the spleen leads to indigestion of food, with poor appetite, gastric distension, and dry or loose stools; the red tongue with thin coating, or tender and enlarged tongue with teeth marks, as well as thin, rapid and feeble pulse are all manifestations of deficiency of qi and yin.

### 3. Blood stasis due to stagnation of qi

Symptoms: Distending or pricking pain in the chest and hypochondria, cough, short and difficult breathing and sometimes dry stools; dark purple tongue with or without ecchymosis and taut or unsmooth pulse. Analysis of symptoms: Inhibited qi movements leads to obstruction of the collaterals, resulting in distending or pricking pain in the chest and hypochondria; qi stagnation and blood stasis result in failure of the lungs in purification, bringing about cough and shortness of breath; dark purple tongue with or without ecchymosis and taut or unsmooth pulse are manifestations of qi stagnation and blood stasis.

### 4. Stagnation of phlegm, dampness and blood

Symptoms: Cough with profuse sputum, shortness of breath, chest distress, or pain in the chest and hypochondria, or lobules below the costal region with unbearable pricking pain when pressure is applied, or fever with yellow, thick and sticky sputum; dark tongue with or without ecchymosis, or enlarged tongue, thick and greasy coating in white or yellow color, as well as taut, slippery and occasionally rapid pulse.

Analysis of symptoms: Accumulation of phlegm and dampness in the interior leads to stagnation of the lung qi, which fails to disperse body fluid and unblock the stasis, this is marked by cough with excessive sputum and pain in the chest and hypochondria; the ascending and descending of qi are impeded, so there is shortness of breath and chest distress; phlegm and stasis glue together, which bring about qi stagnation and blood stasis, with such signs as lobules below the costal region with unbearable pain when pressure is applied; stagnated phlegm and dampness produce heat, causing fever with yellow, thick and sticky sputum; the dark tongue with greasy coating as well as taut and slippery pulse are manifestations of stagnated phlegm, dampness and blood.

## Differential Treatment

### 1. Internal heat due to deficiency of yin

Treatment principle: Nourishing yin and moistening the lungs, dispelling heat and dissipating stagnation.

Prescription and herbs: Modified Yangyin Qingfei Decoction.

Nanshashen (Fourleaf Ladybell Root) 12 g, Shengdi (Dried Rehmannia Root) 12 g, Xuanshen (Figwort Root) 12 g, Maidong (Dwarf Lilyturf Tuber) 2 g, Baihe (Lily Bulb) 12 g, Zhimu (Common Anemarrhena Rhizome) 10 g, Danpi (Cortex Moutan) 12 g, Qinghao (Sweet Wormwood Herb) 12 g, Biejia (Turtle Shell) 12 g, Sangbaipi (White Mulberry Root-Bark) 12 g, Chuanbei (Tendrilleaf Fritillary Bulb) 10 g, Xingren (Almond) 10 g, Caoheche (Bistortae) 15 g, Banzhilian (Sun Plant) 15 g, Xianhecao (Hairyvein Agrimonia Herb) 15 g and Gancao (Freshe Liquorice Root) 6 g.

Modification: For severe and incessant expectoration of bloody sputum, Oujie (Lotus Rhizome Node) 12 g, Qiancaogen (Indian Madder Root) 15 g and Shensanqi (Panax pseudo-ginseng) 3 g are added to check bleeding; for severe night sweats, Nuodaogen (Glutinous Rice Root) 12 g and Bietaogan (Persicae Immaturus) 12 g are used to alleviate sweating.

### 2. Deficiency of qi and yin

Treatment principle: Replenishing qi and nourishing yin, dissolving phlegm and dissipating stagnation.

Prescription and herbs: Supplementary Shengmai Powder.

Huangqi (Milkvetch Root) 30 g, Taizishen (Heterophylly Falsesatarwort Root) 15 g, Maidong (Dwarf Lilyturf Tuber) 12 g, Shashen (Root of Straight Ladybell) 12 g, Wuweizi (Chinese Magnolivine Fruit) 6 g, Baihe (Lily Bulb) 12 g, Biejia (Turtle Shell) 15 g, Quangualou (Snakegourd

Fruit) 15g, Chuanbei (Tendrilleaf Fritillary Bulb) 10g, Baihuashecao (Hedyotic Diffusa) 15g, Shishangbai (Marchantia Polymorpha Lichen) 15g and Loufengfang (Honeycomb of Paper Wasps) 15g.

Modification: For dampness encumbering the spleen and stomach with gastric distension, nausea and vomiting, Cangzhu (Atractylodes Rhizome) 9g, Baizhu (Largehead Atractylodes Rhizome) 12g and Fangfeng (Divaricate Saposhnikovia Root) 9g are added to invigorate the spleen and resolve dampness; for dysfunction of the spleen qi and disharmony of stomach qi with poor appetite and nausea, Muxiang (Common Aucklandia Root) 6g, Sharen (Villous Amomum Fruit) 3g and Chenpi (Dried Tangerine Peel) 6g are used to invigorate the spleen, regulate qi and promote digestion.

### 3. Blood stasis due to stagnation of qi

Treatment principle: Promoting qi flow and activating blood, resolving stasis and softening hardness.

Prescription and herbs: Modified Xuefu Zhuyu Decoction.

Huangqi (Milkvetch Root) 30g, Danggui (Chinese Angelica) 10g, Shengdi (Dried Rehmannia Root) 15g, Taoren (Peach Seed) 10g, Honghua (Safflower) 9g, Chishao (Red Peony Root) 10g, Zhiqiao (Orange Fruit) 10g, Chaihu (Chinese Thorowax Root) 10g, Tianhuafen (Trichosanthin) 12g, Gualouren (Snakegourd Seed) 15g, Zhishanjia (Stir-baked Pangolin Scale) 12g, Ezhu (Zedoray Rhizome) 9g, Shijianchuan (Chinese Sage) 15g and Jiegeng (Platycodon Root) 6g.

Modification: For severe pricking pain in the chest and hypochondria, Xiangfu (Nutgrass Galingale Rhizome) 12g and Taoren (Peach Seed) 9g are added to regulate qi, activate blood and stop pain; for chest distress with greasy coating, Chenpi (Dried Tangerine Peel) 9g and Banxia (Pinellia Tuber) 9g are added to regulate qi and dissolve phlegm.

### 4. Stagnation of phlegm, dampness and blood

Treatment principle: Removing dampness and dissolving phlegm, dissolving stasis and dissipating stagnation.

Prescription and herbs: Modified Daotan Decoction.

Banxia (Pinellia Tuber) 10 g, Tiannanxing (Jackinthepulpit Tuber) 10 g, Fuling (Indian Bread) 12 g, Chenpi (Dried Tangerine Peel) 6 g, Zhishi (Immature Orange Fruit) 9 g, Taoren (Peach Seed) 12 g, Honghua (Safflower) 9 g, Shancigu (Edible Tulip) 15 g, Xingren (Almond) 12 g, Sangbaipi (White Mulberry Root-Bark) 15 g, Quangualou (Snakegourd Fruit) 15 g, Tieshuye (Fruticose Dracaena Leaf) 12 g, Banzhilian (Sun Plant) 15 g, Baihuashecao (Hedyotic Diffusa) 30 g, Quanxie (Scorpion) 3 g, Huangqi (Milkvetch Root) 30 g and Taizishen (Heterophylly Falsesatarwort Root) 15 g.

Modification: For pleural fluid with sensation of stuffiness, cough and wheezing, Tinglizi (Herba Leonuri) 15 g and Dazao (Chinese Date) 7 dates are added to purge the lungs and expel retained fluid; for pain in the chest and back, Weilingxian (Chinese Clematis Root) 12 g and Yanhusuo (Corydalis) 9 g are used to activate blood, regulate qi and stop pain.

## Chinese Patent Medicine

1. Pingxiao Capsule: 4~8 capsules for each dose, 3 times a day.
2. Kanglaite Injection: 100~200 ml for each dose, once a day through intravenous drip. A course of treatment generally spans 15~30 days.
3. Zhuling Duotang Injection (Polyporus Polysaccharide Injection): 4 ml for each dose, once a day or every other day for intramuscular injection. A course of treatment generally spans 15 days.

## Simple and Handy Prescriptions

1. Huangqi (Fresh Milkvetch Root) 15 g, Gouqizi (Barbary Wolfberry Fruit) 12 g, Nuzhenzi (Glossy Privet Fruit) 12 g, Taizishen (Heterophylly Falsesatarwort Root) 15 g, Tianmendong (Lucid Asparagus) 12 g and Honghua (Safflower) 6 g are boiled in water and separated into 2 portions to be taken at 2 different times within a day. It is used for lung cancer after radiotherapy.
2. Huangqi (Unprepared Milkvetch Root) 30 g, Baizhu (Largehead Atractylodes Rhizome) 15 g, Fangfeng (Divaricate Saposhnikovia

Root) 9 g, Longgu (Calcined Os Draconis) 30 g and Fuxiaomai (Blighted Wheat) 10 g are boiled in water and separated into 2 portions to be taken at 2 different times within a day. It is used for lung cancer after surgery with deficient sweating and weariness.

## Other Therapies

Dietary therapy:

(1) Asparagus Officinalis L. and Champignon: Asparagus Officinalis L. 200 g and Champignon 100 g, with gourmet power and salt added to taste, are stir-fried together and used for preventing cancer and eliminating the tumor.
(2) Lettuce and Champignon: Lettuce 400 g and Champignon 50 g, with sauces added to taste, are stir-fried together in an oil-pan and used for dispelling heat and dissolving phlegm, as well as preventing cancer and softening hardness.

## Cautions and Advice

1. Early diagnosis and timely treatment is crucial, if a surgery is appropriate, it should also be performed as soon as possible.
2. Patients should avoid cigarettes and alcohol, adopt a light diet and develop a regular and healthy lifestyle.
3. They should also engage in physical exercise so as to strengthen their constitution.

## Daily Exercises

1. Describe the pathological characteristics of lung cancer.
2. Explain how lung cancer due to internal heat from deficiency of yin can be diagnosed and treated.

# Chronic Cor Pulmonale
# Week 3: Friday

Chronic cor pulmonale (pulmonary heart disease) is an enlargement (hypertrophy or dilation) of the right ventricle of the heart as a response to increased pulmonary circulatory resistance or arterial hypertension resulting from chronic disorders of the lungs, thoracic cage or pulmonary arteries. Clinically, it is marked by repeated cough, wheezing, expectoration of sputum, edema and cyanosis. It can be divided into two types: compensation and decompensation. This disease mostly afflicts people who are above 40 years of age. It can occur regardless of the four seasons, but the acute onset usually takes place in winter and spring. Pulmonary heart disease is reversible at most stages of its pathological development; this means that the cardiac functions can be recovered to some extent through proper treatment. However, once it enters into the advanced phase, it may become life-threatening. In TCM, this disease is closely associated with "panting syndrome", "phlegm and retained-fluid", "lung distension" and "edema".

## Etiology and Pathology

The etiological factors of chronic pulmonary heart disease are insufficiency of healthy qi and repeated contraction of wind-cold, which damage the lungs and debilitate qi, causing retention of phlegm and fluid in the airway. Prolonged disorder of the lungs will inevitably involve the heart, leading to stagnation of blood in the lungs and impairment of heart qi.

The pathological changes are discussed as follows: Insufficiency of healthy qi and weakness of defensive qi allow invasion of pathogenic factors into the lungs, impairing its functions of dispersion and descent, leading to wheezing with cough. Repeated invasion of pathogenic factors damages the lung qi and causes retention of phlegm and fluid which, if left untreated, will inevitably debilitate the healthy qi and affect the heart, spleen and kidneys in the long run. Impairment of the heart is marked by deficiency of the heart qi and obstruction of the heart blood with such signs as palpitations, chest distress, dyspnea, cyanosis and dark tongue; impairment of the spleen leads to dysfunction of transportation and transformation, indigestion of water and food and production of phlegm and dampness in the interior which flow upward and attack the lungs, resulting in such symptoms as profuse expectoration of sputum; impairment of the kidneys is characterized by failure of the kidneys to control water, leading to adverse flow of water qi into the heart, with such symptoms as exacerbated palpitations and shortness of breath; if the kidneys are too deficient to receive the lung qi, there will be deficient panting. From the above analysis, it is evident that pulmonary heart disease is mainly attributed to the functional disorders of the lungs, heart, spleen and kidneys.

## Diagnostic Key Points

1. Patients have a history of chronic pulmonary diseases, functional compensation in the early stage and symptoms such as cough with sputum, debilitation and dyspnea; with the development of the disease, there may be right heart failure and respiratory failure marked by exacerbated palpitations, shortness of breath, cyanosis, headache, restlessness, delirium, spasms or even coma.
2. The early physical signs are emphysema, diminished breath sounds, audible dry or moist rales, unclear border of cardiac dullness, low and dull heart sounds, hyperactive pulmonary second heart sounds and, subsequently, distention of jugular veins, hepatomegalia, puffiness, ascites and accelerated heart rate.
3. Electrocardiogram reveals low voltage, clockwise rotation of the heart, pulmonary P wave, and right electrical axis deviation in the early stage; in the late stage, there is hypertrophy of the right atrium and right ventricle.
4. X-ray examination reveals a primary lesion in the lungs and enlarged right heart ventricle or even the entire heart.
5. Blood-gas analysis reveals hypoxemia and hypercapnia in different degrees during respiratory failure.

## Syndrome Differentiation

## 1. Accumulation of cold-phlegm in the lungs

Symptoms: Cough, panting and shortness of breath aggravated on exertion, chest distension, white and thin sputum, reduced food intake and lassitude; white, thin and greasy tongue coating, as well as taut and slippery pulse; these symptoms are mostly present in cases of pulmonary functional defect with respiratory tract infection.

Analysis of symptoms: Prolonged affliction debilitates the lungs and spleen, resulting in reduced food intake and lassitude; insufficiency of healthy qi, coupled with invasion of pathogenic cold, leads to stagnation of lung qi and upward flow of turbid phlegm, manifesting as cough, panting and excessive sputum; deficiency of the lungs is complicated by inhibition of qi movements due to phlegm, resulting in chest distension, cough and shortness of breath aggravated on exertion; the white, thin and greasy tongue coating, as well as taut and slippery pulse are manifestations of internal obstruction of cold phlegm.

## 2. Accumulation of heat-phlegm in the lungs

Symptoms: Cough with panting, yellow and thick sputum that is difficult to be expectorated, dry stools, yellowish or reddish urine and dry mouth; red tongue with yellow coating or yellow greasy coating, slippery and rapid pulse or rapid and taut pulse; these symptoms are commonly present in cases of pulmonary functional defect with respiratory tract infection.

Analysis of symptoms: Turbid phlegm accumulates in the lungs and transforms into heat, resulting in yellow and sticky sputum; the lung qi rises upward, presenting as accelerated breathing; heat consumes body fluid and the lungs fail to distribute this heat, with such signs as dry mouth and yellowish or reddish urine; the lungs are interiorly and exteriorly associated with the large intestine, so disorder of the lungs affects the large intestine, leading to dysfunction of the large intestine in transportation and transformation, this is marked by dry stools; red tongue with yellow or yellow-greasy coating and rapid-taut pulse or rapid-slippery pulse are manifestations of internal accumulation of phlegm and heat.

## 3. Clouding of the upper orifices by phlegm

Symptoms: Absent-mindedness, restlessness, apathy, lethargy and even coma, spasms of the limbs, cough, panting and expectoration of sputum; dark red or light purple tongue with white greasy or yellow greasy coating and thin, rapid and slippery pulse; these symptoms are mostly seen in pulmonary encephalopathy.

Analysis of symptoms: Phlegm obstructs the heart orifices as well as qi movements, resulting in symptoms such as absent-mindedness, restlessness, apathy, lethargy and even coma; turbid phlegm stirs the liver wind, manifesting as limb spasms; turbid phlegm obstructs the lungs and causes adverse rising of qi, with cough, panting and expectoration of sputum; dark red or light purple tongue is a sign of blood stasis in the heart, while white greasy or yellow greasy tongue coating, as well as thin, rapid and slippery pulse is suggestive of internal accumulation of turbid phlegm.

## 4. Qi deficiency of the lungs and kidneys

Symptoms: Cough with shortness of breath, aggravated upon physical exertion or even with opened mouth, raised shoulders and inability to lie flat, white and thin sputum with no strength to expectorate, chest distress, palpitations and sweating; pale or dark tongue and thin, rapid and deep pulse or knotted and intermittent pulse.

Analysis of symptoms: The deficient lungs fail to govern qi and deficient kidneys fail to receive qi, leading to shortness of breath, aggravated upon physical exertion or even with opened mouth, raised shoulders and inability to lie flat; insufficient lung qi fails to distribute body fluid, resulting in cough that is ineffective in removing sputum; the lung disease affects the heart and leads to deficiency of heart qi and inhibition of qi movements, with such signs as chest distress, palpitations and sweating; insufficient qi fails to promote the circulation of blood, bringing about pale or dark tongue; the thin, rapid and deep pulse or knotted and intermittent pulse is suggestive of deficient lung qi and kidney qi with blood stasis.

## 5. Yang deficiency of the spleen and kidneys

Symptoms: Facial edema and swollen limbs, palpitations, cough, panting, expectoration of clear and thin sputum, gastric stuffiness, poor appetite, cold body and limbs, weakness and soreness of the waist and knees, clear and profuse urine, loose stools; dark and enlarged tongue, white and slippery coating, as well as thin and deep pulse.

Analysis of symptoms: Weakness of yang qi brings about overflowing of water, marked by facial edema and swollen limbs; water and fluid attack the heart and lungs, leading to palpitations, cough, panting and expectoration of clear and thin sputum; deficiency of spleen yang gives rise to gastric stuffiness, poor appetite and loose stools; deficiency of kidney yang is responsible for the cold body and limbs, weakness and soreness of the waist and knees, as well as clear, profuse urine; dark and enlarged tongue with white and slippery coating, as well as thin and deep pulse are indicative of yang deficiency, water retention and blood stasis.

## Differential Treatment

## 1. Accumulation of cold-phlegm in the lungs

Treatment principle: Warming the lungs and dissolving phlegm.

Prescription and herbs: Modified Xiaoqinglong Decoction.

Mahuang (Ephedra) 9 g, Guizhi (Cassia Twig) 9 g, Xixin (Manchurian Wildginger) 6 g, Ganjiang (Dried Ginger) 6 g, Wuweizi (Chinese Magnolivine Fruit) 6 g, Banxia (Pinellia Tuber) 9 g, Chenpi (Dried Tangerine Peel) 6 g, Suzi (Perillaseed) 9 g and Gancao (Stir-baked Liquorice Root) 6 g.

Modification: If the patient presents with excessive phlegm, wheezing and fullness in the lungs, Baijiezi (White Mustard Seed) 15 g and Laifuzi (Radish Seed) 12 g are added to bring down qi and dissolve phlegm; for excessive sputum, reduced food intake and lassitude, Dangshen (Radix Codonopsis) 12 g, Baizhu (Largehead Atractylodes Rhizome) 15 g and Fuling (Indian Bread) 12 g are added to invigorate the spleen and nourish the lungs.

## 2. Accumulation of heat-phlegm in the lungs

Treatment principle: Clearing the lungs and dissolving phlegm, reducing adverseness and alleviating panting.

Prescription and herbs: Modified Sangbaipi Decoction.

Sangbaipi (White Mulberry Root-Bark) 12 g, Huangqin (Baical Skullcap Root) 15 g, Huanglian (Golden Thread) 3 g, Xiangbei (Bulbus Fritillariae Thunbergii) 9 g, Xingren (Almond) 9 g, Suzi (Perillaseed) 9 g, Zhuli (Succus Bambusae) 30 g (infused in water), Banxia (Pinellia Tuber) 9 g, Tianhuafen (Trichosanthin) 12 g and Dahuang (Rhubarb) 6 g (decocted later).

Modification: For excessive and sticky sputum, Haihake (Clam Shell) 15 g is added to clear the lungs and dissolve sputum.

## 3. Clouding of the upper orifices by phlegm

Treatment principle: Dissolving phlegm for resuscitation, extinguishing wind and activating blood.

Prescription and herbs: Modified Ditan Decoction combined with Zhibao Dan or Angong Niuhuang Pill (for oral or nasal administration).

Zhuli (Succus Bambusae) 30 g (infused in water), Banxia (Pinellia Tuber) 9 g, Dannanxing (Bile Arisaema) 9 g, Zhishi (Immature Orange Fruit) 9 g, Juhong (Red Tangerine Peel) 6 g, Changpu (Acorus Calamus) 9 g, Zhuru (Bamboo Shavings) 6 g, Fuling (Indian Bread) 12 g, Renshen (Ginseng) 9 g, Gancao (Liquorice Root) 3 g, Danshen (Radix Salviae Miltiorrhiae) 15 g, Taoren (Peach Seed) 9 g and Angong Niuhuang Wan (Bezoar Uterus-Calming Pill) 1 pill (dissolved in mouth).

Modification: For internal abundance of phlegm and heat, delirium, coma, red tongue with and yellow coating, Tinglizi (Herba Leonuri) 15 g and Tianzhuhuang (Tabasheer) 12 g are added to dissolve phlegm for resuscitation; for internal stirring of liver wind with spasms, Tianma (Tall Gastrodis Tuber) 12 g and Gouteng (Gambir Plant) 15 g are added to subdue the liver, extinguish wind and relieve spasms.

## 4. Qi deficiency of the lungs and kidneys

Treatment principle: Nourishing the lungs and tonifying the kidneys, eliminating dampness and dissolving sputum.

Prescription and herbs: Modified Bufei Decoction and Shenqi Pill.

Renshen (Ginseng) 9 g, Huangqi (Milkvetch Root) 15 g, Shudi (Prepared Rhizome of Rehmannia) 12 g, Wuweizi (Chinese Magnolivine Fruit) 9 g, Ziwan (Tatarian Aster Root) 12 g, Sangbaipi (White Mulberry Root-Bark) 9 g, Shanzhuyu (Asiatic Cornelian Cherry Fruit) 9 g, Fuling (Indian Bread) 12 g, Zexie (Oriental Waterplantain Rhizome) 9 g, Fuzi (Prepared Common Monkshood Daughter) 9 g, Guizhi (Cassia Twig) 6 g and Gancao (Stir-baked Liquorice Root) 6 g.

Modification: If there is deficiency of the spleen with accumulation of sputum and dampness, Chenpi (Dried Tangerine Peel) 9 g, Banxia (Pinellia Tuber) 9 g and Baizhu (Largehead Atractylodes Rhizome) 12 g are added to dry dampness and invigorate the spleen; for lung deficiency with cold, intolerance of cold and pale tongue, Ganjiang (Dried Ginger) 6 g is added to warm yang and resolve fluid; for severe manifestations of dyspnea and collapse, Shenfutang (Ginseng and Monkshood Decoction) and Gejiefen (Tokay Gecko Powder) 9 g, or Heixidan (Stannum Nigrum Pill) can be used to tonify the kidneys and receive qi, as well as revive yang and prevent collapse; if accompanied by damage of yin, low fever and reddish tongue with scanty coating, Maidong (Dwarf Lilyturf Tuber) 12 g and Yuzhu (Fragrant Solomonseal Rhizome) 12 g are added to nourish yin and moisten the lungs.

## 5. Yang deficiency of the spleen and kidneys

Treatment principle: Warming the kidneys and invigorating the spleen, resolving fluid and alleviating water retention.

Prescription and herbs: Modified Zhenwu Decoction.

Fuzi (Prepared Common Monkshood Daughter) 9 g, Guizhi (Cassia Twig) 12 g, Fuling (Indian Bread) 12 g, Baizhu (Largehead Atractylodes Rhizome) 12 g, Shengjiang (Fresh Ginger) 3 slices, Chishao (Red Peony Root) 12 g, Zexie (Oriental Waterplantain Rhizome) 15 g and Cheqianzi (Plantain Seed) 15 g (wrapped during decoction).

Modification: For severe blood stasis, Honghua (Safflower) 9 g and Zelan (Herba Lycopi) 12 g are added to resolve stasis and promote circulation of water; for severe swelling, Zhuling (Polyporus) 15 g, Heichou (Black Semen Pharbitidis) 9 g, Baichou (White Semen Pharbitidis) 9 g and Chenxiang (Chinese eaglewood Wood) 3 g are used to promote circulation of qi and expel water.

## Chinese Patent Medicine

1. Shuang Huang Lian Oral Liquid: 10 ml for each dose, 3 times a day. It can be used to dispel heat and remove toxins, applicable to pulmonary heart disease in the acute phase with lung infection.
2. Qu Tan Ling Oral Liquid: 30 ml for each dose, 3 times a day. It is applicable to pulmonary heart disease with excessive phlegm.

## Simple and Handy Prescriptions

Yuxingcao (Heartleaf Houttuynia Herb) 30 g, Jinyinhua (Honeysuckle Flower) 12 g, Qiancao (Indian Madder Root) 15 g and Danshen (Radix Salviae Miltiorrhiae) 12 g are boiled in water and separated into 2 portions to be taken at 2 different times within a day. It is used to clear the lungs, dissolve phlegm and activate blood.

## Other Therapies

Dietary therapy: Chongcao Laoya Soup: Chongcao (Cordyceps) 9 g, Huangqi (Milkvetch Root) 9 g and an aged duck are boiled together. This soup is effective for nourishing qi and blood and supplementing the lungs and kidneys.

## Cautions and Advice

1. Primary respiratory system diseases (such as chronic bronchitis and bronchial asthma) should be treated promptly as a fundamental measure for preventing pulmonary heart disease.

2. Patients should avoid exposure to pathogenic wind and cold, take initiative in preventing and treating common cold as well as other respiratory tract infections, and avoid various causative factors.

## Daily Exercises

1. Name the viscera which if malfunctioned, are most likely to be responsible for chronic pulmonary heart diseases. Briefly describe the etiological factors.
2. Describe the clinical characteristics, treatment principles and representative prescriptions of pulmonary heart disease due to qi deficiency of the lungs and kidneys.

# CHAPTER 3

# Cardiovascular Diseases

## Cardiac Arrhythmia
## Week 3: Friday

Cardiac arrhythmia refers to the impulse formation and/or abnormal conduction of the heart resulting from any cause, clinically characterized by palpitations, skipped heartbeat, chest distress, debilitation, dizziness, or even fainting. The simplest specific test for assessment of heart rhythm is the electrocardiogram, which can indicate various abnormal or irregular heartbeats. The most common clinical types of arrhythmia are premature beat, paroxysmal supraventricular or ventricular tachycardia, atrial fibrillation, atrioventricular block and sick sinus syndrome. Arrhythmia may sometimes afflict normal people with no history of heart diseases, but generally strikes those with organic heart diseases, such as coronary artery disease, myocarditis, cardiomyopathy, rheumatic heart disease, hypertensive cardiac damage, cardiac insufficiency, as well as drug intoxication due to throatwort. The factors triggering arrhythmia generally include organic disorders of the cardiac muscles, electrolyte disturbance, anoxia, agitation and addiction to tobacco, alcohol, or strong teas. Depending on the difference in etiological factors, arrhythmia varies considerably in prognosis. Functional arrhythmia usually has a favorable prognosis, whereas severe arrhythmia may pose a significant threat to life, with sudden death as the usual consequence. In TCM, arrhythmia is closely associated with "fright", "severe palpitations", "fainting" and "deficiency-consumption".

## Etiology and Pathology

The etiological factors of arrhythmia are sudden fright (which is usually observed in those who are timid), pre-existing phlegm and heat, coupled with depressed rage (which usually impairs the liver), severe or chronic diseases (which involve the heart, spleen and kidneys and impair qi, blood, yin and yang). All of these may disturb the heart spirit and malnourish or obstruct the heart, leading to palpitations.

The pathological changes are discussed as follows: People who are timid or deficient in heart spirit are susceptible to fright, which may impair the kidneys and deplete kidney essence; sudden rage impairs the liver and drives qi upward; deficiency of yin in the lower energizer and excess of fire in the upper energizer disturb the heart spirit, bringing on palpitations. Pre-existing phlegm and heat, coupled with such depressed rage, is responsible for failure of the stomach qi to descend and co-existence of phlegm and fire, which also disturb the heart spirit and bring on palpitations. People with chronic or severe diseases often present with impairment of the heart, spleen and kidneys, as well as disorders of qi, blood, yin and yang; deficiency of the spleen and stomach leads to inadequacy of both qi and blood, which fail to nourish and tranquilize the heart spirit; insufficiency of kidney yin is marked by water (kidneys) failing to coordinate fire (heart) which flames upward and disturbs the spirit; deficiency of heart yang and kidney yang causes internal retention of water and fluid, which flow upward and attack the heart, resulting in palpitations; stagnation or deficiency of qi often leads to obstruction of heart blood, which fails to nourish and tranquilize the heart spirit, predisposing the patient to palpitations.

## Diagnostic Key Points

1. Patients usually have a history of arrhythmia and/or heart diseases. Those experiencing the symptoms above for the first time should seek medical confirmation.
2. Chief clinical manifestations are palpitations, discomfort in the precordial region, skipped heartbeat, chest distress, debilitation, dizziness, or even fainting. Cardiac auscultation shows audible heart rate or abnormal

cardiac rhythm. The pulse is usually knotted, intermittent, abrupt, swift, soft, rapid, deep or unsmooth.

3. Laboratory examination: Both electrocardiogram and dynamic electrocardiogram demonstrate cardiac dysrhythmia.

## Syndrome Differentiation

### 1. Deficiency of the heart with timidity

Symptoms: Palpitations, susceptibility to fright or terror, restlessness, insomnia and dreaminess; white and thin tongue coating, rapid throbbing pulse, deficient taut pulse, or abrupt pulse.

Analysis of symptoms: Fright disturbs qi and the heart spirit, leading to palpitations; the heart fails to store the spirit, bringing about susceptibility to fright and terror, restlessness, insomnia and dreaminess; white and thin tongue coating, rapid throbbing pulse, deficient taut pulse, or abrupt pulse are all suggestive of deficiency of heart qi and gallbladder qi with disturbance of qi and blood.

### 2. Disturbance of the heart by phlegm-heat

Symptoms: Palpitations, vexation, profuse sputum, chest distress, poor appetite and nausea; yellow and greasy tongue coating, slippery and rapid pulse, or abrupt pulse.

Analysis of symptoms: Phlegm and heat disturb the heart and disquiet the heart spirit, leading to palpitations and vexation; phlegm and heat obstruct the stomach and block the downward flow of stomach qi, marked by excessive sputum, chest distress, poor appetite and nausea; yellow and greasy tongue coating, slippery and rapid pulse, as well as abrupt pulse are all manifestations of internal abundance of phlegm and heat.

### 3. Deficiency of the spleen and stomach

Symptoms: Palpitations, dizziness, lusterless complexion and lassitude; slightly red tongue, thin and feeble pulse, or thin and slow pulse, or knotted and intermittent pulse.

Analysis of symptoms: Deficiency of the spleen and stomach leads to insufficiency of qi and blood and malnutrition of the heart, leading to palpitations; qi fails to promote circulation of blood to the head, with such signs as dizziness and lusterless complexion; deficiency of qi and blood is responsible for lassitude; slightly red tongue, thin and feeble pulse, or thin and slow pulse, or knotted and intermittent pulse, are all indicative of deficiency of the spleen and stomach, as well as insufficiency of qi and blood.

## 4. Exuberance of fire due to yin deficiency

Symptoms: Palpitations and uneasiness, vexation, insomnia, dizziness, feverish sensations in the palms and soles, tinnitus and soreness in the waist; red tongue with little or no tongue coating, thin and rapid pulse or thin and abrupt pulse.

Analysis of symptoms: Insufficiency of kidney yin brings about water (kidneys) failing to coordinate fire (heart) and hyperactivity of heart fire which disturbs the heart spirit, marked by palpitations, vexation and insomnia; deficiency of yin in the lower energizer is manifested as waist soreness; disturbance of yang in the upper energizer is characterized by dizziness and tinnitus; feverish sensation in the palms and soles, red tongue with scanty or no tongue coating, thin and rapid pulse or thin and abrupt pulse are all attributable to exuberance of fire and deficiency of yin.

## 5. Yang deficiency of the heart and kidneys

Symptoms: Palpitations, uneasiness, chest distress, shortness of breath, pale complexion, cold body and limbs and sometimes nausea, poor appetite, stuffiness and fullness in the chest, oliguresis and dropsy of the lower limbs; white and slippery tongue coating, thin and deep pulse, or deep and slow pulse, or knotted and intermittent pulse.

Analysis of symptoms: Chronic diseases debilitate the body and lead to deficiency of heart yang and kidney yang, which fail to steam and transform the yin-water and result in retention of water and body fluid in the heart and lungs, leading to palpitations, chest distress and shortness of breath; the fluid is retained in the interior and obstructs the movements of qi, characterized by stuffiness and fullness in the chest, nausea and poor appetite; qi fails to promote the flow of water, with oliguresis and dropsy of the lower limbs; yang fails to warm the body, marked by pale complexion and cold body; white and slippery tongue coating, thin and deep pulse, or deep and slow pulse, or knotted and intermittent pulse, are all manifestations of deficiency of heart yang and kidney yang.

## 6. Obstruction of blood in the heart

Symptoms: Palpitations, chest distress and sometimes shortness of breath, weariness, heartache in fits and starts, or emotional depression, pricking pain in the chest, hypochondria and cyanosed lips and nails; dark purple tongue with ecchymosis on occasion, thin and unsmooth pulse, or knotted and intermittent pulse, or taut and knotted pulse.

Analysis of symptoms: Deficiency or stagnation of qi leads to obstruction of chest yang and heart vessels, inhibiting nourishment of the heart, coupled with palpitations and chest distress; deficiency of qi brings about blood stasis and contraction of heart collaterals, leading to shortness of breath, weariness and headache by fits and starts; qi stagnation and blood stasis in the liver meridian are marked by emotional depression and pricking pain in the chest and hypochondria; cyanosed lips and nails or dark purple tongue with ecchymosis on occasion are manifestations of blood stasis in the heart; thin and unsmooth pulse, knotted and intermittent pulse, or taut and knotted pulse is due to qi stagnation with blood stasis.

## Differential Treatment

## 1. Deficiency of the heart with timidity

Treatment principle: Relieving fright and calming the mind, nourishing the heart and tranquilizing the spirit.

Prescription and herbs: Anshen Dingzhi Pill and Ganmai Dazao Decoction.

Dangshen (Radix Codonopsis) 15 g, Fushen (Indian Bread with Hostwood) 15 g, Changpu (Acorus Calamus) 9 g, Yuanzhi (Thinleaf Milkwort Root)

6 g, Huangqi (Os Draconis) 30 g, Huaixiaomai (Huaihe Wheat) 30 g, Gancao (Stir-baked Liquorice Root) 9 g and Dazao (Chinese Date) 5 dates.

Modification: If there is insomnia and dreaminess, Suanzaoren (Spine Date Seed) 12 g and Baiziren (Chinese Arborvitae Kernel) 12 g are added to nourish the heart and tranquilize the spirit; for those susceptible to fright and terror, Cishi (Magnetite) 30 g (decocted first) and Hupofen (Amber Powder) 1.5 g (infused in water) are added to relieve fright and calm the mind.

## 2. Disturbance of the heart by phlegm-heat

Treatment principle: Dispelling heat and dissolving phlegm, tranquilizing the spirit and calming the mind.

Prescription and herbs: Supplementary Huanglian Wendan Decoction.

Huanglian (Golden Thread) 5 g, Zhiqiao (Orange Fruit) 12 g, Zhuru (Bamboo Shavings) 9 g, Chenpi (Dried Tangerine Peel) 9 g, Banxia (Pinellia Tuber) 9 g, Yuanzhi (Thinleaf Milkwort Root) 6 g, Suanzaoren (Spine Date Seed) 12 g and Gancao ( Liquorice Root) 5 g.

Modification: For excessive phlegm, constipation and restlessness, Qingmengshi (Chlorite Schist) 30 g is added to purge heat, dissolve phlegm and calm the mind.

## 3. Deficiency of the spleen and stomach

Treatment principle: Invigorating qi and nourishing blood, supplementing the heart and calming the spirit.

Prescription and herbs: Modified Guipi Pill.

Dangshen (Radix Codonopsis) 15 g, Huangqi (Milkvetch Root) 18 g, Baizhu (Largehead Atractylodes Rhizome) 12 g, Fushen (Indian Bread with Hostwood) 12 g, Danggui (Chinese Angelica) 9 g, Longyanrou (Longan Aril) 9 g, Suanzaoren (Spine Date Seed) 12 g, Yuanzhi (Thinleaf Milkwort Root) 6 g, Muxiang (Common Aucklandia Root) 6 g, Gancao (Stir-baked Liquorice Root) 6 g and Dazao (Chinese Date) 6 dates.

Modification: For palpitations with knotted or intermittent pulse, Zhigancao Decoction is taken for supplementing qi and nourishing blood so that the normal pulsation can be restored; in the late stage of febrile disease, the heart yin is consumed with the manifestation of palpitations and in this case Sheng Mai San (Pulsation-Restoring Powder) is used to replenish qi and nourish yin.

## 4. Exuberance of fire due to yin deficiency

Treatment principle: Nourishing yin and bringing down fire, supplementing the heart and calming the spirit.

Prescription and herbs: Modified Tianwang Buxin Pill.

Shengdi (Dried Rehmannia Root) 12 g, Xuanshen (Figwort Root) 9 g, Maidong (Dwarf Lilyturf Tuber) 12 g, Danggui (Chinese Angelica) 9 g, Danshen (Radix Salviae Miltiorrhiae) 12 g, Dangshen (Radix Codonopsis) 15 g, Fuling (Indian Bread) 15 g, Suanzaoren (Spine Date Seed) 12 g, Baiziren (Chinese Arborvitae Kernel) 12 g, Yuanzhi (Thinleaf Milkwort Root) 6 g, Wuweizi (Chinese Magnolivine Fruit) 6 g and Jiegeng (Platycodon Root) 3 g.

Modification: For the bitter taste in the mouth with vexation, Huanglian (Golden Thread) 5 g and Zhizi (Cape Jasmine Fruit) 9 g are added to clear the heart and purge fire; for feverish sensation in the palms and soles, nocturnal emission and waist soreness, Huangbai (Amur Cork-tree) 9 g and Zhimu (Common Anemarrhena Rhizome) 9 g are added to nourish the kidneys and purge fire.

## 5. Yang deficiency of the heart and kidneys

Treatment principle: Warming and invigorating heart yang, calming the mind and relieving fright.

Prescription and herbs: Supplementary Guizhi Gancao Huangqi Muli Decoction.

Guizhi (Cassia Twig) 9 g, Gancao (Stir-baked Liquorice Root) 9 g, Longgu (Os Draconis) 30 g (decocted first), Muli (Oyster Shell) 30 g (decocted first), Fupian (Radix Aconitilateralis Preparata) 9 g, Ganjiang (Dried Ginger) 3 g, Dangshen (Radix Codonopsis) 15 g and Maidong (Dwarf Lilyturf Tuber) 12 g.

Modification: If there is internal retention of water and fluid with palpitations, dizziness, gastric stuffiness, nausea, scanty urine, swollen limbs and dryness in the throat with no desire for drinking, Baizhu (Largehead Atractylodes Rhizome) 15 g, Fuling (Indian Bread) 15 g, Zexie (Oriental Waterplantain Rhizome) 15 g and Banxia (Pinellia Tuber) 10 g are added to warm yang, relieve edema and resolve retained fluid; for palpitations, chest distress with a sensation of suffocation, frequent fainting and slow pulse, Supplementary Mahuang Fuzi Xixin Decoction (Ephedra 9 g, Prepared Common Monkshood Daughter 12 g, Manchurian Wildginger 3 g, Ginseng 9 g and Chinese Angelica 9 g) are used to warm and activate heart yang, as well as nourish the heart qi.

## 6. Obstruction of blood in the heart

Treatment principle: Activating blood and resolving stasis, regulating qi and unblocking vessels.

Prescription and herbs: Taoren Honghua Decoction.

Taoren (Peach Seed) 9 g, Honghua (Safflower) 9 g, Danshen (Radix Salviae Miltiorrhiae) 15 g, Chuanxiong (Szechwan Lovage Rhizome) 9 g, Chishao (Red Peony Root) 12 g, Shengdi (Dried Rehmannia Root) 12 g, Danggui (Chinese Angelica) 9 g, Yanhusuo (Corydalis) 9 g, Xiangfu (Nutgrass Galingale Rhizome) 9 g and Qingpi (Green Tangerine Peel) 6 g.

Modification: If there is shortness of breath, weariness and palpitations, Huangqi (Milkvetch Root) 30 g, Dangshen (Radix Codonopsis) 15 g, Guizhi (Cassia Twig) 12 g and Gancao (Stir-baked Liquorice Root) 9 g are added to nourish the heart qi, warm the chest and dredge the vessels; for emotional depression with pricking pain in the chest and hypochondria, Chaihu (Chinese Thorowax Root) 9 g and Yujin (Turmeric Root Tuber) 9 g are added to soothe the liver and relieve depression.

## Chinese Patent Medicine

1. Zhen He Ling: 4 tablets for each dose, 3 times a day.
2. Tianwang Buxin Pill: 6 g for each dose, 3 times a day.

## Simple and Handy Prescriptions

Mahuang (Ephedra) 10 g, Fupian (Radix Aconitilateralis Preparata) 10 g and Xixin (Manchurian Wildginger) 3 g are boiled in water and taken once a day. It is applicable to treat sick sinus syndrome coupled with simple, slow heart rhythm.

## Other Therapies

Dietary therapy: A spring chicken and 10 longans are cooked in a steam boiler with salt, cooking wine and ginger. It is used to treat insufficiency of heart blood, with palpitations, shortness of breath, insomnia and dreaminess.

## Cautions and Advice

1. Arrhythmia is mostly present in organic heart diseases, so patients should focus their attention on treating the primary diseases and adopt an integrated treatment approach (featuring the combined use of traditional Chinese and Western medicine) to treat severe arrhythmia.
2. Patients should keep themselves in good spirits, avoid dramatic emotional fluctuations or tension and refrain from strong tea, coffee and alcohol.
3. It is also advisable for them to avoid overstrain and excessive food intake.

## Daily Exercises

1. List the pathological changes of arrhythmia.
2. Recall the common types and treatment principles of arrhythmia.
3. Describe how palpitations due to deficiency of the spleen and stomach and that due to yang deficiency of the heart and kidneys can be differentiated and treated. Explain how the prescriptions may be modified according to the specific changes.

# Myocardial Disease
# Week 3: Saturday

Myocardial disease refers to the dysfunction of the myocardium in contraction resulting from various complicated etiological factors, clinically marked by cardiac dilatation, shortness of breath on physical exertion, orthopnea, paroxysmal nocturnal dyspnea, edema of the lower limbs or palpitations, chest distress and angina pectoris. According to the difference in causative factors, this disease can be divided into two types: primary myocardial disease and secondary myocardial disease. In addition, depending on the pathology, it can also be classified into three types: dilated, hypertrophic and restrictive. Dilated myocardial disease is the most common one, while restrictive myocardial disease is seldom seen in China. Myocardial disease generally has a slow onset with varying durations. When it progresses into a state marked by pronounced dilation of the heart, severe heart failure or refractory arrhythmia, the prognosis can be extremely unfavorable. In TCM, this disease is closely associated with "palpitations", "chest bi-syndrome", "syndrome of panting" and "edema."

## Etiology and Pathology

The etiological factors of myocardial disease are either intrinsic or extrinsic: The former refers to the usual insufficiency of heart qi or deficiency of heart yang and kidney yang; while the latter refers to invasion of exogenous pathogenic factors, overstrain and improper treatment of chronic diseases. Generally speaking, this disease initially afflicts the heart and lungs and eventually involves the spleen and kidneys, causing obstruction of heart blood and overflowing of water and body fluid.

The pathological changes of myocardial disease are explained as follows: Deficiency of heart qi and lung qi predisposes a patient to blood stasis in the heart, marked by shortness of breath and chest distress and pain. Deficiency of qi with depletion of yin results in insufficient production of blood, which fails to nourish the heart and causes palpitations. Sluggish circulation of blood prevents it from nourishing the whole body, leading to lassitude. Prolonged affliction debilitates the healthy qi as well as the heart yang and kidney yang, bringing about obstruction of the heart vessels and exacerbation of chest distress and pain. Deficient yang fails to promote the flow of water and fluid, causing retention of these in the heart and lungs, with such signs as panting, shortness of breath aggravated at night, inability to lie flat and edema if the retained water and fluid reach the superficies.

## Diagnostic Key Points

1. Clinically the patients may present with progressive cardiac insufficiency, marked by symptoms of left heart failure such as shortness of breath on physical exertion, orthopnea and paroxysmal nocturnal dyspnea, or by symptoms of right heart failure such as decreased appetite, abdominal distension and edema. Angina pectoris does not respond to nitroglycerin. Health examination shows prominent enlargement of the heart even in a globular shape, palpable double apical impulses, audible cantering rhythm, ejection systolic murmur in the fifth intercostal space and the left sternal border, as well as holosystolic murmur in the mitral area and/or tricuspid area. In addition, there are various physical signs of heart failure, such as fine moist rales in the two lung bases, distention of the jugular vein, enlargement of the liver, dropsy in the abdomen and edema of the lower limbs.
2. Laboratory examination: Electrocardiogram shows hypertrophy and strain of the atriums and ventricles, myocardial damage, abnormal Q wave and various types of arrhythmia; X-ray examination indicates an enlarged heart and blood stasis in the lungs; ultrasonic cardiogram demonstrates an increase in the inner diameter of the heart chambers.
3. Myocardial disease should be differentiated from pericardial effusion, rheumatic heart disease, coronary artery disease, pulmonary heart disease and Keshan disease.

## Syndrome Differentiation

### 1. Deficiency of heart qi

Symptoms: Chest distress or pain, palpitations with shortness of breath aggravated upon physical exertion, pale complexion and lassitude; pale and enlarged or dark red tongue with white tongue coating and thin, knotted or intermittent pulse. This pattern is seen in the early stage of myocardial disease.

Analysis of symptoms: The heart controls blood and vessels, so if the heart qi is too deficient to promote the normal flow of blood, there will be obstruction of heart vessels marked by chest distress or pain; malnourishment of the heart brings about palpitations with shortness of breath aggravated upon physical exertion; prolonged deficiency of qi affects the heart yang, consumes the heart blood and slows down the blood flow, with the manifestations of pale complexion and lassitude; a pale and corpulent or dark red tongue with white tongue coating and thin, knotted or intermittent pulse are attributable to the insufficiency of heart qi with internal obstruction of blood stasis.

## 2. Deficiency of qi and yin

Symptoms: Chest distress, shortness of breath, lassitude, aggravation upon physical exertion, palpitations, poor sleep, dreaminess, dry mouth with less intake of water and sometimes dizziness and tinnitus; dark red tongue with thin or no tongue coating, as well as thin and unsmooth or thin and rapid pulse. This pattern is observed in the relatively stable period of myocardial disease.

Analysis of symptoms: Insufficiency of heart qi leads to inefficient pulsation and internal obstruction of heart blood, leading to chest distress, shortness of breath and lassitude; physical exertion consumes qi, triggering exacerbation of the symptoms; insufficiency of heart yin disturbs the spirit and is marked by palpitations; deficient fire disturbs the mind, giving rise to poor sleep and dreaminess; deficiency of yin with blood stasis is responsible for dry mouth without thirst; depletion of the liver and kidneys with malnutrition of the upper orifices is characterized by dizziness and tinnitus; a dark red tongue with thin or no tongue coating and a thin, unsmooth pulse are manifestations of deficiency of qi and yin with obstruction of the heart vessels; the thin and rapid pulse is a sign of internal heat due to deficiency of yin.

## 3. Deficiency of qi and yang

Symptoms: Chest distress, suffocative feeling and sometimes chest pain, palpitations with panting aggravated at night with inability to lie flat, chest and abdominal distension or fullness, poor appetite, scanty urine, dropsy in the legs and feet, intolerance of cold, lack of warmth in the limbs, dark and lusterless complexion and cyanosed lips; enlarged and pale or purple tongue with white and slippery tongue coating, as well as thin and deep or knotted and intermittent pulse. This pattern is observed in myocardial diseases with severe heart failure.

Analysis of symptoms: Deficiency of the heart qi and lung qi leads to inactivation of the chest yang and obstruction of the heart blood, leading to chest distress, suffocation, chest pain, dark and lusterless complexion and cyanosed lips; deficiency of heart yang and kidney yang leads to dysfunction of qi transformation and retention of water and fluid, which attack the heart and lungs and cause palpitations and panting, with inability to lie flat and aggravation at night because yang qi is diminished; obstruction of water and fluid in the middle energizer causes dysfunction of the spleen in transformation, characterized by thoracic and abdominal distension or fullness with poor food intake; water and fluid are retained in the lower energizer, manifesting as scanty urine and swelling of the legs and feet; declined yang qi fails to warm the body, leading to intolerance of cold and lack of warmth in the limbs; a corpulent, pale or purple tongue with white and slippery tongue coating and a thin and deep or knotted and intermittent pulse are manifestations of deficiency of qi and yang with blood stasis and fluid retention.

## Differential Treatment

### 1. Deficiency of heart qi

Treatment principle: Nourishing the heart qi, activating blood and unblocking vessels.

Prescription and herbs: Modified Shiquan Dabu Decoction.

Dangshen (Radix Codonopsis) 15 g, Baizhu (Largehead Atractylodes Rhizome) 12 g, Fuling (Indian Bread) 12 g, Shudi (Prepared Rhizome of Rehmannia) 9 g, Danggui (Chinese Angelica) 9 g, Baishao (White Peony Alba) 9 g, Chuanxiong (Szechwan Lovage Rhizome) 9 g, Guizhi (Cassia Twig) 9 g, Huangqi (Milkvetch Root) 15 g, Danshen (Radix Salviae Miltiorrhiae) 15 g, Yujin (Turmeric Root Tuber) 9 g and Gancao (Stir-baked Liquorice Root) 9 g.

Modification: If there are manifestations of distress and pain in the chest and white tongue coating, Gualoupi (Snakegourd Peel) 15 g and Xiebai (Longstamen Onion Bulb) 6 g are added to regulate qi, dissolve phlegm and relieve the chest; for ecchymosis on the tongue, Ruxiang (Prepared Boswellin) 6 g and Muoyao (Prepared Myrrh) 6 g are added to resolve stasis and stop pain.

## 2. Deficiency of qi and yin

Treatment principle: Supplementing qi and replenishing yin, activating blood and nourishing heart.

Prescription and herbs: Modified Shengmai Potion and Siwu Decoction.

Dangshen (Radix Codonopsis) 15 g, Maidong (Dwarf Lilyturf Tuber) 12 g, Wuweizi (Chinese Magnolivine Fruit) 6 g, Danggui (Chinese Angelica) 9 g, Chuanxiong (Szechwan Lovage Rhizome) 9 g, Shengdi (Dried Rehmannia Root) 12 g, Chishao (Red Peony Root) 12 g, Suanzaoren (Spine Date Seed) 12 g, Danshen (Radix Salviae Miltiorrhiae) 15 g, Huangqi (Milkvetch Root) 20 g and Gancao (Stir-baked Liquorice Root) 9 g.

Modification: If there is fright and profuse dreams, Longgu (Os Draconis) 30 g and Muli (Oyster Shell) 30 g are added to subdue the heart and calm the mind; for vexation with intolerance of heat, Huanglian (Golden Thread) 3 g and Zhimu (Common Anemarrhena Rhizome) 9 g are added to clear the heart and purge heat; for constipation, Huomaren (Hemp Seed) 9 g and Baiziren (Chinese Arborvitae Kernel) 9 g are added to nourish yin and promote defecation.

## 3. Deficiency of qi and yang

Treatment principle: Nourishing qi and warming yang, resolving stasis and draining water.

Prescription and herbs: Supplementary Zhenwu Decoction.

Renshen (Ginseng) 6 g, Huangqi (Milkvetch Root) 30 g, Fupian (Radix Aconitilateralis Preparata) 9 g, Baizhu (Largehead Atractylodes Rhizome) 15 g, Fuling (Indian Bread) 15 g, Zhuling (Polyporus) 15 g, Guizhi (Cassia Twig) 9 g, Danshen (Radix Salviae Miltiorrhiae) 15 g, Yimucao (Motherwort Herb) 30 g, Tinglizi (Herba Leonuri) 15 g (wrapped during decoction), Maidong (Dwarf Lilyturf Tuber) 12 g and Wuweizi (Chinese Magnolivine Fruit) 6 g.

Modification: If there is chest distress and pain as well as cyanosed lips, Danggui (Chinese Angelica) 9 g, Chuanxiong (Szechwan Lovage Rhizome) 9 g, Honghua (Safflower) 9 g and Yanhusuo (Corydalis) 12 g are added to activate blood and resolve stasis as well as regulate qi and stop pain; for severe edema with scanty urine, Zexie (Oriental Waterplantain Rhizome) 15 g and Dafupi (Areca Peel) 9 g are added to promote urination and relieve edema.

## Chinese Patent Medicine

1. Shengmaiyin Oral Liquid: 10 ml for each dose, 3 times a day.
2. Jingui Shenqi Pill: 6 g for each dose, 3 times a day.

## Simple and Handy Prescriptions

Shengshaishen (Dried Radix Ginseng) 6 g, Huangqi (Milkvetch Root) 15 g, Maidong (Dwarf Lilyturf Tuber) 12 g, Wuweizi (Chinese Magnolivine Fruit) 6 g, Danshen (Radix Salviae Miltiorrhiae) 15 g, Baizhu (Largehead Atractylodes Rhizome) 12 g and Fuling (Indian Bread) 12 g are boiled in water and taken once a day. This prescription is applicable for treating myocardial disease during the relatively stable period.

## Other Therapies

Dietary therapy:

(1) Xiyangshen (American Ginseng) 10 g, Baihe (Lily Bulb) 30 g, Yiner (White Fungus Gourd) 30 g and crystal sugar to taste are boiled in water and taken once a day for 5 consecutive days. It is used to treat myocardial disease marked by palpitations, vexation with feverish sensation and shortness of breath on exertion.

(2) Danggui (Chinese Angelica) 10 g, Fuling (Indian Bread) 15 g, Yangrou (Mutton) 250 g, Shengjiang (Fresh Ginger) 5 slices and Dazao (Chinese Date) 15 dates are used to make soup. It can be taken regularly for the treatment of myocardial disease with heart failure, edema and intolerance of cold.

## Cautions and Advice

1. Cardiomyopathy is a relatively refractory disease and patients may respond quickly to an integrated approach combining the use of traditional Chinese and Western medicine.
2. The chief etiological factors of myocardial disease such as viral infection should be prevented and treated. It is advisable for patients to engage in active physical exercises, ward off pathogenic factors and avoid long-term overstrain or adverse emotional stimulation. For pregnant women with hypertension, the high blood pressure should be addressed as early as possible.

## Daily Exercises

1. List the three types of myocardial disease.
2. Concisely describe the etiology and pathology of myocardial disease.
3. Explain how myocardial disease can be treated, based on syndrome differentiation.

# Viral Myocarditis
# Week 4: Monday

Viral myocarditis is an inflammatory disease of the heart caused by invasion of viruses. Its onset is triggered by acute viral infection, clinically marked by palpitations, chest distress and pain, shortness of breath, as well as abnormal changes on electrocardiogram. It can afflict people of any age or gender, but young people and males are particularly susceptible. It is prevalent in summer and autumn. The disease course is divided into three phases: acute phase (within 6 months), recovery phase (6 months ~1 year) and chronic phase (above 1 year). Most patients can recover from this disease, yet some may have signs of abnormal changes of the heart to varying extent, or electrocardiographic abnormalities. The state of the disease may be consistent throughout the entire course, marked by myocardial scar in most cases, resulting from an acute onset of myocarditis, called sequelae of myocarditis. Some cases of chronic myocarditis can evolve into myocardial diseases, but only a few patients may die in the acute phase from severe arrhythmia, acute heart failure or cardiac shock. In TCM, myocarditis is closely associated with "palpitations" or "severe palpitations", "chest bi-syndrome", "edema" and "deficiency-consumption".

## Etiology and Pathology

TCM holds that myocarditis is caused by invasion of exogenous pathogenic factors, unsanitary diet, overstrain, emotional disorders and, in particular, external contraction of pathogenic toxins, which damages the healthy qi and invade the pericardium.

The pathological changes are discussed as follows: Pathogenic toxins and heat invade the lung-wei, struggle with the healthy qi and finally seize the pericardium or heart vessels; furthermore, improper diet breeds phlegm and heat which obstruct the heart vessels and stagnate the heart blood; in either case, there is chest distress and pain, palpitations, shortness of breath and a knotted or intermittent pulse. Pathogenic toxins and cold congeal the heart vessels and obstruct the flow of blood, leading to chest distress and a slow pulse. Pathogenic factors damage the heart yang, resulting in retention of water which severely affects the heart, with such signs as palpitations, panting and swollen limbs. The pathogenic factors may diminish in strength with time, marked by deficiency of qi and yin or malnutrition of the heart spirit, with such signs as listlessness, palpitations, feverish sensation over the five centers (the palms, the soles and the heart) and a knotted or intermittent pulse.

## Diagnostic Key Points

1. Within 3 weeks after the occurrence of common cold or diarrhea (due to viral infection), the following manifestations may be present: chest distress, palpitations, shortness of breath and weariness. In severe cases, there is dyspnea, precordial pain, edema, fainting, or even death. Cardiac auscultation revealss low and dull cardiac sounds, anisorhythmia, tachycardia, or bradycardia.
2. Laboratory examination: Electrocardiogram reveals abnormal changes of the ST-T segment and various types of arrhythmia (including atrial, ventricular or junctional premature beat, as well as various conditions of conduction block); pronounced increase of serumal cardiac troponin I or troponin T, CK and Mb; Coxsackie virus antibody test is positive.

## Syndrome Differentiation

### 1. Invasion of pathogenic toxins into the heart

Symptoms: Fever with aversion to cold, headache, general malaise, nasal obstruction, sore throat and sometimes cough, palpitations, panting and chest distress and pain; red tongue with thin tongue coating and knotted, intermittent or abrupt pulse.

Analysis of symptoms: Pathogenic warm-heat invades the superficies and struggles with the healthy qi, bringing about fever with intolerance of cold; the defensive qi is stagnated, leading to headache, general indisposition, nasal obstruction, sore throat and sometimes cough; rampant pathogens debilitate the healthy qi, damage the heart vessels, and obstruct the circulation of qi and blood, marked by palpitations, panting, as well as chest distress and pain; a red tongue with thin coating and a knotted, intermittent or abrupt pulse are manifestations of pathogenic toxins invading the heart.

## 2. Retention of cold-toxins in the heart

Symptoms: Fever with intolerance of cold, absence of sweat, headache and general pain, soreness of bones and joints, chest distress or pain, palpitations and shortness of breath; a pale tongue with white and thin tongue coating and a slow pulse, or slow and tense pulse, or knotted and intermittent pulse.

Analysis of symptoms: Pathogenic wind-cold invades the body from the exterior and struggles with the healthy qi, marked by fever with intolerance of cold; pathogenic factors enfetter the muscles and skin and stagnate the meridian qi, leading to absence of sweat, headache, general pain and soreness in bones and joints; cold-toxins congeal the heart vessels and block the circulation of blood, with distress and pain in the chest, palpitations and shortness of breath; a pale tongue with white and thin tongue coating and a tardy, or tardy and tense, or knotted and intermittent pulse are manifestations of cold-toxins congealing the heart.

## 3. Co-existence of phlegm and stasis

Symptoms: Chest distress, palpitations, oppressed pain in the precordial region, a bitter and greasy taste in the mouth, or loose stools, red tongue with yellow and greasy or turbid and greasy coating and slippery or knotted-intermittent pulse.

Analysis of symptoms: Improper diet breeds abundant phlegm and heat which mix with blood stasis and obstruct the heart vessel, leading to chest distress, palpitations and oppressed pain in the precordial region. Obstruction of phlegm and heat in the middle energizer results in dysfunction of the spleen in transformation, marked by bitter and greasy taste in the mouth or loose stools; a red tongue with yellow and greasy or turbid and greasy coating, as well as a slippery or knotted-intermittent pulse are suggestive of abundant phlegm and heat obstructing the heart vessels.

## 4. Water retention affecting the heart

Symptoms: Chest distress, panting, inability to lie flat, lack of warmth in the limbs, cyanosed lips, abdominal distension and swollen limbs; a purple tongue with white greasy coating and a thin, deep pulse.

Analysis of symptoms: Pathogens debilitate the heart yang and give rise to edema which affects the heart, marked by chest distress, panting, inability to lie flat and cyanosed lips; internal retention of water qi is characterized by abdominal distension and swollen limbs; deficiency of yang qi is manifested as lack of warmth in the limbs; a purple tongue with white greasy coating and a thin, deep pulse are manifestations of blood stasis due to deficiency of yang.

## 5. Deficiency of qi and yin

Symptoms: Palpitations, chest distress, shortness of breath, weariness, or feverish sensations over the five centers (the palms, the soles and the heart), spontaneous perspiration and night sweats; red tongue with scanty fluid and thin tongue coating, as well as thin and feeble pulse or knotted and intermittent pulse.

Analysis of symptoms: Prolonged retention of pathogenic toxins in the heart damages the heart yin and heart qi, leading to malnutrition of the heart with the manifestation of palpitations; qi fails to promote circulation of blood, leading to sluggish flow of heart blood, marked by chest distress and shortness of breath; deficiency of qi and yin produces deficient heat, with such signs as weariness, feverish sensation over the five centers (the palms, the soles and the heart), spontaneous perspiration and night sweats; a red tongue with scanty fluid and thin coating, as well as a thin and feeble pulse or knotted and intermittent pulse are suggestive of deficiency of heart qi and heart yin.

## Differential Treatment

## 1. Invasion of pathogenic toxins into the heart

Treatment principle: Dispelling heat and removing toxins, dispersing and clearing the heart of pathogens.

Prescription and herbs: Modified Yinqiao Powder.

Jinyinhua (Honeysuckle Flower) 15 g, Lianqiao (Weeping Forsythia Capsule) 15 g, Maidong (Dwarf Lilyturf Tuber) 15 g, Banlange (Isatis Root) 15 g, Niubangzi (Great Burdock Achene) 12 g, Chishao (Red Peony Root) 15 g, Zhizi (Cape Jasmine Fruit) 9 g, Huanglian (Golden Thread) 3 g, Zhuye (Henon Bamboo Leaf) 9 g and Gancao ( Liquorice Root) 5 g.

Modification: If there is abundant heat, Shigao (Gypsum) 30 g (decocted first) is added to drastically dispel the interior heat; for feverish sensation and pain in the throat, Shengdi (Dried Rehmannia Root) 15 g, Xuanshen (Figwort Root) 15 g and Mabo (Puff-ball) 6 g are added to nourish yin, dispel heat and relieve pain in the throat; for diarrhea with abdominal pain, Baitouweng (Chinese Pulsatilla Root) 30 g and Qinpi (Ash Bark) 12 g are added to clear the intestine and eliminate toxins.

## 2. Retention of cold-toxins in the heart

Treatment principle: Expelling cold and pathogens, warming the heart vessels.

Prescription and herbs: Supplementary Mahuang Fuzi Xixin Decoction.

Mahuang (Ephedra) 9 g, Fupian (Radix Aconitilateralis Preparata) 9 g, Xixin (Manchurian Wildginger) 5 g, Guizhi (Cassia Twig) 9 g, Dangshen (Radix Codonopsis) 15 g, Danshen (Radix Salviae Miltiorrhiae) 15 g, Gancao (Stir-baked Liquorice Root) 9 g and Dazao (Chinese Date) 5 dates.

Modification: For cough with white sputum, Xingren (Almond) 9 g, Qianhu (Hogfennel Root) 9 g, Kuandonghua (Common Coltsfoot Flower) 9 g and Ziwan (Tatarian Aster Root) 9 g are added to disperse the lung tissue, dissolve phlegm and stop cough.

## 3. Co-existence of phlegm and stasis

Treatment principle: Dispelling heat and dissolving phlegm, activating blood and resolving stasis.

Prescription and herbs: Supplementary Xiaoxianxiong Decoction and Danshen Potion.

Huanglian (Golden Thread) 5 g, Banxia (Pinellia Tuber) 12 g, Gualou (Snakegourd Fruit) 20 g, Zhishi (Immature Orange Fruit) 10 g, Danshen (Radix Salviae Miltiorrhiae) 15 g, Chuanxiong (Szechwan Lovage Rhizome) 12 g, Taoren (Peach Seed) 9 g, Yujin (Turmeric Root Tuber) 15 g, Tanxiang (Sandalwood) 6 g (decocted later) and Sharen (Villous Amomum Fruit) 3 g (decocted later).

Modification: If there is poor appetite with greasy sensation in the mouth, Huoxiang (Agastache Rugosa) 9 g and Peilan (Queen of the Meadow) 9 g are added to dissolve the turbid substances and activate the spleen.

## 4. Water retention affecting the heart

Treatment principle: Warming yang and invigorating qi, reliving edema and activating blood.

Prescription and herbs: Shenfu Decoction and Linggui Zhugan Decoction.

Huangqi (Milkvetch Root) 30 g, Dangshen (Radix Codonopsis) 15 g, Fupian (Radix Aconitilateralis Preparata) 12 g, Guizhi (Cassia Twig) 10 g, Baizhu (Largehead Atractylodes Rhizome) 15 g, Fuling (Indian Bread) 15 g, Danshen (Radix Salviae Miltiorrhiae) 15 g and Maidong (Dwarf Lilyturf Tuber) 12 g.

Modification: For chest distress with excessive phlegm, Gualou (Snakegourd Fruit) 15 g, Xiebai (Longstamen Onion Bulb) 6 g and Banxia (Pinellia Tuber) 12 g can be added to dissolve phlegm and relieve the chest.

## 5. Deficiency of qi and yin

Treatment principle: Replenishing qi and nourishing yin, calming the heart and tranquilizing the mind.

Prescription and herbs: Modified Shengmai Potion and Guipi Decoction.

Huangqi (Milkvetch Root) 24 g, Taizishen (Heterophylly Falsesatarwort Root) 20 g, Maidong (Dwarf Lilyturf Tuber) 15 g, Wuweizi (Chinese Magnolivine Fruit) 6 g, Yuzhu (Fragrant Solomonseal Rhizome) 12 g,

Danggui (Chinese Angelica) 9 g, Fushen (Indian Bread with Hostwood) 15 g, Suanzaoren (Spine Date Seed) 12 g, Yuanzhi (Thinleaf Milkwort Root) 5 g and Gancao (Stir-baked Liquorice Root) 9 g.

Modification: For vague pain in the chest, Yujin (Turmeric Root Tuber) 10 g, Danshen (Radix Salviae Miltiorrhiae) 15 g and Jiangxiang (Rosewood) 5 g are added to regulate qi and activate blood; for spontaneous perspiration or night sweats, Longgu (Calcined Os Draconis) 30 g, Muli (Calcined Oyster Shell) 30 g (decocted first) and Fuxiaomai (Blighted Wheat) 15 g are added to subdue the heart and reduce sweating.

## Chinese Patent Medicine

1. Ningxinbao Jiaonang (Heart-Tranquilizing Capsule): 2 capsules for each dose, 3 times a day.
2. Shengmaiyin Koufuye (Pulse-Reviving Oral Liquid): 10 ml for each dose, 3 times a day.

## Simple and Handy Prescriptions

Xiyangshen (American Ginseng) 6 g, Maidong (Dwarf Lilyturf Tuber) 12 g and Wuweizi (Chinese Magnolivine Fruit) 5 g are boiled in water and taken as tea several times a day to treat chronic viral myocarditis.

## Other Therapies

Injection therapy: Huangqi (Milkvetch Root) Injection. 20 ml is added into 5 % Glucose (250 ml) for intravenous drip once a day. A course of treatment generally lasts 2~4 weeks. It is applicable to treat viral myocarditis in the acute or chronic phase.

Dietary therapy: A spring chicken, Longyanrou (Longan Aril) 10 g and Maidong (Dwarf Lilyturf Tuber) 15 g are boiled in a steam boiler with salt, cooking wine and ginger. This is appropriate for the treatment of viral myocarditis in the recovery or chronic phase.

## Cautions and Advice

1. Viral myocarditis should be promptly treated, ideally during the acute phase and patients must rest in bed and reduce the intensity of exercise for six months to facilitate recovery.
2. Common cold or diarrhea due to viral infection should be addressed early.
3. It is also advisable to avoid emotional stimulation.

## Daily Exercises

1. Concisely describe the pathological changes of viral myocarditis.
2. List the diagnostic key points of viral myocarditis.
3. Explain how viral myocarditis due to invasion of toxins into the heart and that due to deficiency of qi and yin can be differentiated and treated.

# Valvular Heart Disease
# Week 4: Tuesday

Valvular heart disease refers to the chronic valvular defects (stenosis and/ or insufficiency) due to a variety of factors, including inflammatory adhesion or fibrosis, ischemic necrosis, calcareous deposit and congenital development malformation. Hemodynamic changes may ensue subsequently and eventually lead to cardiac decompensation and congestive heart failure. Clinically, this disease is marked by palpitations, dyspnea, cough, hemoptysis and edema, in addition to some particular physical signs. It is divided into two major types: rheumatic valvular disease and non-rheumatic valvular disease. The former chiefly afflicts young and middle-aged people, with females being more susceptible than males, with a diminishing morbidity, while the latter mostly afflicts middle-aged and old people, with a rising morbidity. In TCM, valvular heart disease is closely associated with "heart bi-syndrome", "cough with blood", "panting syndrome", "palpitations" and "edema".

## Etiology and Pathology

The etiological factors of this disease are pathogenic wind-cold and damp-heat (which invade the viscera through the meridians and obstruct the heart vessels in combination) or weakness of the body due to senility coupled with improper life cultivation (which brings about obstruction of phlegm or blood in the heart vessels and damages the heart qi).

The pathological changes are discussed as follows: Pathogenic factors obstruct the heart vessels and stagnate the heart blood, leading to palpitations, chest distress and pain. The heart controls blood and has its luster reflected on the complexion, so obstructed heart vessels result in purple red cheeks and cyanosed lips. The heart and lungs are located in the upper energizer, if the heart blood is stagnated, the lung qi can also be inhibited, leading to retention of phlegm and blood or extravasation of blood marked by shortness of breath and cough with sputum or blood. The obstruction of heart blood, the debilitation of heart qi and the inactivation of heart yang affect the kidney yang and inhibit its transformation of cold water, which flows upward to attack the lungs and downward to impair the bladder, marked by palpitations, shortness of breath, gasping, peripheral coldness and difficulty in micturition. Decline of yang qi and exhaustion of yin fluid result in obstruction of the heart and lungs by blood stasis, with such critical signs as a depressive and stuffy sensation in the chest and heart, short or intermittent breath, coughing up bloody sputum, peripheral coldness and profuse perspiration.

## Diagnostic Key Points

1. Chief clinical manifestations are symptoms due to progressively aggravated left and right heart failure, such as palpitations on exertion, shortness of breath, nocturnal paroxysmal dyspnea, or even orthopnea, cough, hemoptysis and edema. Mitral stenosis is characterized by cyanosed cheeks and lips, the so-called "mitral facies". Cardiac auscultation shows special murmurs in the valves, such as diastolic blowing murmurs and systolic ejection murmurs in the mitral area.
2. Laboratory examinations: Chest X-ray, electrocardiogram, cardiac color ultrasonic wave and cardiac catheterization can all contribute to a definitive diagnosis.

## Syndrome Differentiation

### 1. Obstruction of heart blood

Symptoms: Purplish red cheeks, cyanosed lips and nails, palpitations, chest distress, or even chest pain, cough, expectoration, or perhaps hemoptysis, dizziness and weariness; a cyanosed tongue with or without ecchymosis and a thin, unsmooth pulse or knotted, intermittent pulse.

Analysis of symptoms: The heart controls blood and has its luster reflected on the complexion, so if the heart blood is stagnated, the result will be purplish red cheeks and cyanosed lips and nails; blood stasis in the heart weakens the heart yang and obstructs the heart vessels, resulting in palpitations, chest distress, or even chest pain; the heart and lungs are located in the upper energizer and so if the heart blood is obstructed, the lung qi will also be inhibited, leading to retention of phlegm and extravasation of blood, marked by cough with sputum or blood; unsmooth blood flow is responsible for the malnutrition of the body, with such signs as dizziness and weariness; the cyanosed tongue with or without ecchymosis and the thin, unsmooth pulse or knotted, intermittent pulse are manifestations of obstructed heart blood.

## 2. Exhaustion of qi and blood

Symptoms: Palpitations, chest distress, shortness of breath, profuse sweating, aggravation upon exertion and a pale complexion; a pale, enlarged tongue with teeth marks and a thin or soggy, feeble pulse.

Analysis of symptoms: Pathogenic factors impair the healthy qi, debilitate the heart qi and stagnate the heart blood, leading to palpitations, chest distress, shortness of breath and profuse perspiration aggravated on exertion; deficient blood fails to nourish the head, leading to pale complexion and dizziness; the pale, enlarged tongue with teeth marks and the thin or soggy, feeble pulse are manifestations of exhaustion of both qi and blood.

## 3. Yang deficiency of the heart and kidneys

Symptoms: A dark and lusterless complexion, palpitations, edema, cough, dyspnea with rapid respiration, or even inability to lie flat and lack of warmth in the feet and hands; a dark tongue with white, thin coating or white, slippery coating and a knotted, intermittent or thin, deep pulse.

Analysis of symptoms: Deficiency of heart yang and kidney yang results in cold water attacking the heart and lungs, leading to palpitations, cough, dyspnea with rapid respiration, or even inability to lie flat; dysfunction of qi transformation in the lower energizer gives rise to edema in the legs and feet; deficiency of yang fails to warm the body, leading to cold congealing the blood vessels, marked by a dark and lusterless complexion and lack of warmth in the feet and hands; the dark tongue with white, thin coating or white, slippery tongue coating and the knotted, intermittent pulse or thin, deep pulse are manifestations of deficiency of heart yang and kidney yang with cold congealing the blood vessels.

## Differential Treatment

### 1. Obstruction of heart blood

Treatment principle: Activating blood and resolving stasis.

Prescription and herbs: Modified Taohong Potion.

Guizhi (Cassia Twig) 12 g, Taoren (Peach Seed) 9 g, Honghua (Safflower) 6 g, Chuanxiong (Szechwan Lovage Rhizome) 9 g, Chishao (Red Peony Root) 12 g, Danggui (Chinese Angelica) 9 g, Danshen (Radix Salviae Miltiorrhiae) 15 g, Weilingxian (Chinese Clematis Root) 15 g, Yanhusuo (Corydalis) 12 g and Gancao (Stir-baked Liquorice Root) 9 g.

Modification: If there is cough and panting or even sticky sputum, Suzi (Perillaseed) 9 g, Xingren (Almond) 9 g and Banxia (Pinellia Tuber) 9 g are added to disperse the lung tissue, dissolve sputum and relieve panting; for hemoptysis, Cebaiye (Unprepared Chinese Arborvitae Twig and Leaf) 15 g and Shensanqi (Panax Pseudo-Ginseng Powder) 2 g (diffused in water) are added to clear the lungs, dissipate the stasis and stop bleeding.

### 2. Exhaustion of qi and blood

Treatment principle: Invigorating qi and nourishing blood.

Prescription and herbs: Modified Guipi Decoction.

Dangshen (Radix Codonopsis) 12 g, Huangqi (Milkvetch Root) 15 g, Danggui (Chinese Angelica) 9 g, Suanzaoren (Spine Date Seed) 12 g, Danshen (Radix Salviae Miltiorrhiae) 12 g, Guiyuanrou (Cassia Pulp) 9 g, Guizhi (Cassia Twig) 6 g, Maidong (Dwarf Lilyturf Tuber) 15 g, Gancao (Stir-baked Liquorice Root) 9 g and Dazao (Chinese Date) 5 dates.

Modification: If there are obvious manifestations of blood stasis, Taoren (Peach Seed) 9 g and Honghua (Safflower) 6 g are added to activate blood and resolve stasis; for severe palpitations, Longgu (Os Draconis) 30 g and Muli (Oyster Shell) 30 g (decocted first) are added to subdue the heart and tranquilize the spirit; if there is fever with a sore throat, Guiyuanrou (Cassia Pulp) and Guizhi (Cassia Twig) can be removed while Jinyinhua (Honeysuckle Flower) 12 g, Lianqiao (Weeping Forsythia Capsule) 12 g and Xuanshen (Figwort Root) 9 g are added to dispel heat and remove toxins, as well as nourish yin and relieve pain in the throat.

## 3. Yang deficiency of the heart and kidneys

Treatment principle: Warming yang to relieve edema.

Prescription and herbs: Modified Zhenwu Decotion.

Fupian (Radix Aconitilateralis Preparata) 15 g, Guizhi (Cassia Twig) 10 g, Huangqi (Milkvetch Root) 15 g, Baizhu (Largehead Atractylodes Rhizome) 12 g, Fuling (Indian Bread) 15 g, Tinglizi (Herba Leonuri) 15 g (wrapped during decoction), Fangji (Fourstamen Stephania Root) 12 g and Shengjiangpi (Fresh Ginger Peel) 5 g.

Modification: If there is chest distress with cyanosed lips, Danshen (Radix Salviae Miltiorrhiae) 15 g, Honghua (Safflower) 9 g and Tanxiang (Sandalwood) 6 g are added to activate blood and resolve stasis, as well as regulate qi and dredge the vessels; for gasping with inability to lie down and spontaneous perspiration, Shengshaishen (Dried Radix Ginseng) 6 g, Maidong (Dwarf Lilyturf Tuber) 12 g and Wuweizi (Chinese Magnolivine Fruit) 9 g are added to supplement the heart qi and astringe the heart yin; for panting, palpitations, extreme exhaustion, profuse sweat, cold limbs and an abrupt pulse due to decline of yang and depletion of yin, Hongshen (Red Ginseng) 9 g, coupled with certain western medicines, is decocted for prompt administration.

## Chinese Patent Medicine

1. Shexiang Baoxin Pill: 1 pill for each dose, 3 times a day.
2. Jingui Shenqi Pill: 6 g for each dose, 3 times a day.

## Simple and Handy Prescriptions

Shengshaishen (Dried Radix Ginseng) 6 g and Honghua (Safflower) 6 g are boiled in water and taken 3 times a day to treat valvular disease with palpitations, chest distress and fatigue.

## Other Therapies

Injection therapy: Shenmai Injection. 20 ml is added into 5% Glucose (250 ml) for intravenous drip. It is administered once a day, with two weeks making up a course of treatment. This is used to treat valvular disease due to exhaustion of both qi and blood, as well as deficiency of heart yang and kidney yang.

Dietary therapy: a. Ingredients: Duck meat 500 g, lean pork 250 g, edible mussels 25 g, Daylily 25 g and shelled shrimp 25 g. b. Method: Daylily, edible mussels and shelled shrimp are soaked in water till they are softened and the duck meat and pork are diced; afterwards they are boiled in a pressure cooker with condensed soup, ginger and cooking wine. The meat and the soup are consumed to treat rheumatic heart disease with severe heart failure.

## Cautions and Advice

1. Valvular heat disease is caused by various factors and eventually evolves into progressive heart failure with an unfavorable prognosis. For this reason, the etiological factors such as streptococcal infection should be promptly addressed to avoid acute rheumatic fever. Blood pressure, blood fat and blood sugar should be controlled and arteriosclerosis, valvular calcification and enlargement of the heart must be avoided. Syphilis must also be treated promptly, so that syphilitic heart disease can be prevented.
2. Patients should take warming measures to ward off cold, avoid living in damp places to prevent infection and refrain from unhealthy sexual activities.
3. Patients should keep themselves in good spiritspay attention to dietary nutrition and avoid a diet that is rich in oil, fat, sugar or salt. It is also advisable for them to avoid cigarettes and alcohol, balance work and rest and exercise regularly in order to strengthen their constitution.

## Daily Exercises

1. Briefly describe the pathological changes of valvular heart disease.
2. Explain how valvular heart disease due to obstruction of heart blood and that due to yang deficiency of the heart and kidneys can be differentiated and treated.

# Coronary Artery Disease
# Week 4: Wednesday

Coronary artery disease is a heart disease with restricted blood flow due to atherosclerosis occurring when the arteries become clogged and narrowed. Without adequate blood flow from the coronary arteries, the heart becomes starved of oxygen and the vital nutrients it needs to work properly. Clinically, the disease is marked by depression and pain in the precordial region which, in severe cases, may spread to the shoulders, back, throat and the medial side of the left upper arm. The pain may be paroxysmal or persistent. Severe, persistent pain is often accompanied by sweating, cold limbs, pale complexion, cyanosed lips and nails, or palpitations, shortness of breath, gasping, inability to lie down and even sudden death. Depending on the clinical characteristics, it can be classified into five types: latent or asymptomatic coronary artery disease, angina, myocardial infarction, ischemic myocardial disease and SD (sudden death). The middle-aged and the elderly are among the most susceptible to this disease. Cold, overeating, emotional disturbance or strenuous exercise may all create a predisposition to this disease. Coronary artery disease is among the most critical conditions of the heart and often poses a threat to life. Nevertheless, if it is diagnosed and treated in time, or addressed with effective preventive measures, the incidence rate can be reduced and the patient may have a relatively longer lifespan. In TCM, it is closely associated with "chest bi-syndrome", "chest pain", "genuine heart pain" and "heart pain with cold limbs".

## Etiology and Pathology

TCM believes that coronary artery disease is caused by either endogenous or exogenous pathogenic factors. The former refers to body weakness due to senility and insufficiency of qi, blood, yin and yang of the heart, spleen and kidneys; the latter refers to cold invasion, improper diet, emotional disorder and overstrain. In either case the blood flow in the heart will be impeded and the heart vessels may be congested, leading to the occurrence of this disease.

The pathological changes of coronary artery disease are discussed as follows: Old people usually have a weak body and their deficient kidney qi may fail to activate heart yang and nourish the heart vessels; overstrain and excessive contemplation consume qi and blood and damage the heart and spleen; in either case the heart qi will be weakened and the heart blood will be stagnated. Besides, yin cold can block the chest yang, inhibit qi movements and eventually obstruct the heart vessels. Moreover, emotional disorders often lead to failure of the liver to promote free flow of qi and result in qi stagnation, blood stasis and congested heart vessels. In conclusion, impairment of the heart, spleen and kidneys with insufficiency of qi, blood, yin and yang is the intrinsic cause of coronary artery disease, while obstruction of the heart vessels with pain and inactivation of chest yang by yin cold, turbid phlegm, or stagnated qi and blood are the extrinsic cause of coronary artery disease. In this sense, coronary artery disease is considered a disorder marked by deficiency of the root (the primary aspect) and excess of the branch (the secondary aspect).

## Diagnostic Key Points

1. The patients may present with typical angina attacks or myocardial infarction yet without evidence of severe lesion of the aortic valve, coronary artery embolization, or myocardial injury.
2. Electrocardiogram (ECG) in quiescent condition shows myocardial ischemia, or ECG exercise test demonstrates a positive result.
3. The patients above 40 might develop cardiac enlargement, heart failure, or arrhythmia, with apparent ischemic signs on resting electrocardiogram unaccountable by other reasons.
4. Most of the patients present with hypertension, hyperlipemia and diabetes.
5. Echocardiogram, myocardial zymogram determination, radioactive nuclide test and coronary arteriongraphy can be applied if necessary to make a definitive diagnosis.

## Syndrome Differentiation

### 1. Retention of cold in the heart vessels

Symptoms: Cold-induced heartache affecting the back, chest distress, palpitations, shortness of breath and body coldness; a dark tongue with white coating and a taut, tense pulse.

Analysis of symptoms: All sorts of yang receive qi in the chest and then move to the back, so if yin cold stagnates the chest yang and obstructs the heart vessels, there will be chest pain affecting the back; stagnation of chest yang and qi brings about chest distress, palpitations and shortness of breath; insufficiency of yang qi incurs cold which congeals the blood vessels, leading to physical coldness; a dark tongue with white coating and a taut, tense pulse are manifestations of insufficiency of yang qi with cold retention in the heart vessels.

## 2. Stagnation of qi and blood

Symptoms: Stuffy sensation and pain in the heart and chest, doleful expression or depressed rage, scurrying pain in the chest and hypochondria involving the shoulder and back (when stagnation of qi is the primary cause), pricking pain in the heart or chest aggravated at night, palpitations and disquietude (when stagnation of blood is the primary cause); a dark tongue with petechia or ecchymosis and a taut or unsmooth pulse.

Analysis of symptoms: Emotional disorder impairs the ability of the liver to promote free flow of qi, leading to stagnation of qi marked by a doleful expression or depressed rage and stuffy sensation in the heart and chest with pain; the liver qi is rampant, leading to scurrying pain in the chest and hypochondria involving the shoulder and back; stagnation of qi brings about blood stasis, leading to pricking pain in the heart or chest (since both blood and night pertain to yin, the pain is aggravated at night); obstruction of blood flow results in failure of the heart to be nourished, marked by palpitations and disquietude; the dark tongue with petechia or ecchymosis and taut or unsmooth pulse are manifestations of qi stagnation with blood stasis.

## 3. Obstruction of turbid phlegm

Symptoms: Chest distress and pain, shortness of breath, a fat and heavy body, weariness (especially the limbs) and sleepiness; turbid, greasy tongue coating and a slippery pulse.

Analysis of symptoms: The spleen governs transportation and transformation, so if the spleen is weak, there will be production of abundant phlegm which stagnates the chest yang and qi, leading to thoracic distress and pain, as well as shortness of breath; the spleen dominates the muscles and governs the ascent of lucid substances, when the spleen is encumbered by turbid phlegm and loses its ability to transform and ascend, the body becomes fat and heavy, accompanied by weariness (especially the limbs) and sleepiness; the turbid, greasy tongue coating and a slippery pulse are manifestations of internal abundance of turbid phlegm.

## 4. Deficiency of qi and yin

Symptoms: Stuffy sensation and vague pain in the chest, palpitations, shortness of breath, dizziness, weariness, night sweats or spontaneous perspiration, dry mouth and throat; a red tongue with thin or little tongue coating and teeth marks on the margins and a thin pulse or knotted, intermittent pulse.

Analysis of symptoms: Prolonged chest bi-syndrome brings about deficiency of qi and yin, malnutrition of the heart and obstruction of heart vessels, leading to a stuffy sensation and vague pain in the chest, palpitations and shortness of breath; deficient qi fails to promote blood, leading to dizziness and weariness; deficient qi fails to astringe the body fluid, leading to spontaneous perspiration; deficiency of yin produces internal heat, which gives rise to night sweats and dryness in the mouth and throat; a red tongue with teeth marks on the margins and a thin pulse or knotted, intermittent pulse are manifestations of deficiency of qi and yin.

## 5. Yang deficiency of the spleen and kidneys

Symptoms: Chest distress and pain, shortness of breath, physical coldness, listlessness, waist soreness, clear and profuse urine, or palpitations, swollen limbs and (in severe cases) chest pain affecting the back, coma, panting, cold limbs and sweating; a pale tongue with white tongue coating, a deep and feeble pulse or extremely feeble and faint pulse.

Analysis of symptoms: Yang deficiency of the spleen and kidneys leads to inactivation of chest yang and obstruction of heart blood, leading to chest distress and pain, shortness of breath, physical coldness, listlessness, waist soreness and clear, profuse urine; deficiency of yang results in adverse flow of water qi attacking the heart, leading to palpitations and swollen limbs; when the kidney yang is diminished, the yang qi is exhausted and the heart vessels are obstructed, leading to chest pain affecting the back, coma, panting, cold limbs and sweating; a pale tongue with white tongue coating, a deep and feeble pulse or extremely feeble and faint pulse are due to deficiency of spleen yang and kidney yang with extreme weakness of yang qi.

## Differential Treatment

### 1. Retention of cold in the heart vessels

Treatment principle: Dissipating cold and liberating yang, activating blood and unblocking obstruction.

Prescription and herbs: Modified Danggui Sini Decoction and Danshen Potion.

Danggui (Chinese Angelica) 9 g, Guizhi (Cassia Twig) 9 g, Chishao (Red Peony Root) 12 g, Gancao (Stir-baked Liquorice Root) 6 g, Danshen (Radix Salviae Miltiorrhiae) 15 g, Tanxiang (Sandalwood) 6 g, Honghua (Safflower) 6 g and Xixin (Manchurian Wildginger) 3 g.

Modification: If there is persistent chest pain and gasping with inability to lie flat, it is due to extreme yin-cold, so Wutou Chishizhi Pill (Sichuan Pepper, Monkshood, Prepared Common Monkshood Daughter and Dried Ginger.) and Shuhexiang Pill are added to warm the chest, dissipate cold, unlock obstruction and relieve pain.

### 2. Stagnation of qi and blood

Treatment principle: Regulating qi to relieve depression, activating blood to stop pain.

Prescription and herbs: Xuefu Zhuyu Decoction.

Chaihu (Chinese Thorowax Root) 9 g, Chishao (Red Peony Root) 12 g, Zhiqiao (Orange Fruit) 9 g, Danggui (Chinese Angelica) 9 g, Chuanxiong (Szechwan Lovage Rhizome) 9 g, Shengdi (Dried Rehmannia Root) 12 g,

Taoren (Peach Seed) 9 g, Honghua (Safflower) 6 g, Chuanniuxi (Shichuan Twotoothed Achyranthes Root) 9 g, Jiegeng (Platycodon Root) 3 g, Yanhusuo (Corydalis) 9 g and Gancao ( Liquorice Root) 3 g.

Modification: For scurrying pain in the chest and hypochondria, Xiangfu (Nutgrass Galingale Rhizome) 9 g and Yujin (Turmeric Root Tuber) 9 g are added to regulate qi and relieve depression; for pricking pain in the chest and heart, Sanqifen (Sanchi) 2~3 g, or Ruxiang (Boswellin) 6~9 g and Muoyao (Myrrh) 6~9 g are added to activate blood and relieve pain; for palpitations and disquietude with occasional premature beat, Danshen (Radix Salviae Miltiorrhiae) 15 g and Longchi (Fossilia Dentis Mastodi) 30 g are added to tranquilize the mind and calm disquietude.

## 3. Obstruction of turbid phlegm

Treatment principle: Dissolving phlegm and discharging turbidity, unblocking obstruction and freeing yang.

Prescription and herbs: Supplementary Gualou Xiebai Banxia Decoction.

Quangualou (Snakegourd Fruit) 15 g, Xiebai (Longstamen Onion Bulb) 6 g, Banxia (Pinellia Tuber) 9 g, Chenpi (Dried Tangerine Peel) 9 g, Fuling (Indian Bread) 15 g, Danshen (Radix Salviae Miltiorrhiae) 15 g and Sharen (Villous Amomum Fruit) 3 g.

Modification: If there is a greasy tongue coating and poor appetite, Cangzhu (Atractylodes Rhizome) 9 g is added to activate the spleen and resolve dampness; for heat resulting from prolonged stagnation of turbid phlegm with such signs as dry mouth and bitter taste, red tongue, yellow greasy tongue coating and rapid slippery pulse, Huanglian (Golden Thread) 3 g and Zhuru (Bamboo Shavings) 9 g are added to dispel heat and dissolve phlegm; for lassitude and sleepiness, Huangqi (Milkvetch Root) 15~30 g and Changpu (Acorus Calamus) 9 g are added to nourish qi, open the orifices and refresh the mind; for high blood-fat level, Puhuang (Pollen Typhae) 20 g (wrapped during decoction), Honghua (Safflower) 6~9 g and Shanzha (Hawthorn Fruit) 15~30 g are added to activate blood and reduce blood-fat.

## 4. Deficiency of qi and yin

Treatment principle: Replenishing qi and tonifying yin, nourishing blood and dredging vessels.

Prescription and herbs: Supplementary Shengmai Powder.

Huangqi (Milkvetch Root) 30 g, Dangshen (Radix Codonopsis) 15 g, Maidong (Dwarf Lilyturf Tuber) 15 g, Wuweizi (Chinese Magnolivine Fruit) 6 g, Yuzhu (Fragrant Solomonseal Rhizome) 9 g, Danggui (Chinese Angelica) 9 g, Chuanxiong (Szechwan Lovage Rhizome) 9 g, Danshen (Radix Salviae Miltiorrhiae) 15 g, Gancao (Stir-baked Liquorice Root) 9 g and Dazao (Chinese Date) 5 dates.

Modification: If there are palpitations and insomnia, Suanzaoren (Spine Date Seed) 12 g and Fushen (Indian Bread with Hostwood) 12 g are added to calm the heart and tranquilize the mind; for spontaneous perspiration, Nuodaogen (Glutinous Rice Root) 12 g and Fuxiaomai (Blighted Wheat) 15 g are added to nourish deficiency and reduce sweat; for night sweats, Zhimu (Common Anemarrhena Rhizome) 12 g is added to dispel heat and stop sweating; for progressively severe pain in the chest, Yanhusuo (Corydalis) 9 g and Wulingzhi (Faeces Trogopterorum) 9 g are added to regulate qi, activate blood and stop pain.

## 5. Yang deficiency of the spleen and kidneys

Treatment principle: Supplementing the spleen and kidneys with warmth, activating blood and unblocking vessels.

Prescription and herbs: Modified Jingui Shenqi Pill, Sijunzi Decoction and Danshen Potion.

Fupian (Radix Aconitilateralis Preparata) 9 g, Guizhi (Cassia Twig) 9 g, Shudi (Prepared Rhizome of Rehmannia) 9 g, Shanyao (Common Yan Rhizome) 12 g, Shanzhuyu (Asiatic Cornelian Cherry Fruit) 9 g, Fuling (Indian Bread) 15 g, Zexie (Oriental Waterplantain Rhizome) 15 g, Huangqi (Milkvetch Root) 30 g, Dangshen (Radix Codonopsis) 15 g, Baizhu (Largehead Atractylodes Rhizome) 15 g, Danshen (Radix Salviae Miltiorrhiae) 15 g and Tanxiang (Sandalwood) 6 g.

Modification: If there is coma, panting, or cold sweats and limbs, Shenfu Decoction (Ginseng 6~12 g and Radix Aconitilateralis Preparata 9~30 g) is used to resuscitate and warm the patient.

## Chinese Patent Medicine

1. Compound Danshen Dripping Pill: 10 pills for each dose, 3 times a day.
2. Shexiang Baoxin Pill: 1~2 pills for each dose, for sublingual administration during attacks.
3. Guanxin Suhexiang Pill: 1 pill for each dose, for sublingual administration when there is severe chest pain, sweating and cold limbs.

## Simple and Handy Prescriptions

Sanqifen (Sanchi Powder) is administered (2~4 pills for each dose) 3 times a day for repeated angina.

## Other Therapies

Acupoint Plaster-Application therapy: Warm-moxibustion plaster and Xianggui Huoxue Plaster are applied to the Xinshu (BL15), Jueyinshu (BL 14), or Danzhong (RN 17) acupoints.

Foot-bath therapy: Danggui (Chinese Angelica), Chuanxiong (Szechwan Lovage Rhizome), Chishao (Red Peony Root), Honghua (Safflower), Jixueteng (Henry Magnoliavine Stem or Root), Ruxiang (Boswellin), Muoyao (Myrrh), Sumu (Sappan Wood) and Guizhi (Cassia Twig) are boiled in water. The decoction is used for soaking the feet, for approximately 30 minutes each time.

Dietary therapy: Shanzha (Hawthorn Fruit) 30 g, Heye (Lotus Leaf) 30 g, Yiyiren (Coix Seed) 30 g and Jiangmi (Rice Fruit) 30 g are boiled to make porridge. This porridge can be taken regularly to reduce blood-fat and reduce body weight for patients with coronary artery disease.

## Cautions and Advice

1. Coronary artery disease, angina and myocardial infarction are mostly marked by sudden onset and severe consequences, particularly the latter, which is often life-threatening. So if there is an acute onset, patients should discontinue physical activities immediately, take first-aid medicines and seek medical attention without delay.
2. Patients should avoid the factors predisposing them to the acute onset of coronary artery disease, such as cold, overstrain, emotional hyperactivity and excessive eating and drinking.
3. Patients should also take initiative to treat hypertension, hyperlipemia and diabetes, engage in appropriate exercise and adopt a low-fat, low-salt and low-glucose diet, in addition to refraining from cigarettes and strong tea.

## Daily Exercises

1. List the five clinical types of coronary artery disease.
2. Explain why coronary artery disease is said to be marked by deficiency of the primary aspect and excess of the secondary aspect.
3. Explain how coronary artery disease due to qi stagnation with blood stasis and that due to obstruction of turbid phlegm can be differentiated and treated.

# Chronic Congestive Heart Failure
## Week 4: Thursday

Chronic congestive heart failure, or chronic cardiac insufficiency, abbreviated as heart failure, is an inevitable consequence in the late stage of almost every organic heart disease. It is clinically marked by symptoms or signs of left heart failure (due to pulmonary congestion) or right heart failure (due to venous congestion in systemic circulation). Cardiac insufficiency is divided into two phases: compensation phase and decompensation phase. Heart failure occurs in the decompensation phase and there are three degrees of severity (I~III). It is often triggered or aggravated by physical overstrain or emotional stimulation. This disease is generally poor in prognosis. In TCM, heart failure is closely associated with "fright with severe palpitations", "chest bi-syndrome", "dyspnea with cough", "edema" and "deficiency-consumption".

## Etiology and Pathology

Heart failure is often caused by chronic heart diseases or long-term debilitation of other organs involving the heart, with insufficiency of qi, blood, yin and yang of the viscera, as well as visceral dysfunction; if at this time the disease is coupled with invasion of exogenous pathogenic factors, overstrain, improper after-care, or emotional stimulation, the healthy qi may be further damaged and the heart can become more insufficient in capacity.

The pathological changes of heart failure are discussed as follows: Deficiency of heart qi and lung qi leads to stagnation of phlegm and blood, marked by chest distress, shortness of breath and cough with sputum or even blood. Deficiency of qi and yin results in obstruction of blood in the heart which drives out the heart spirit, causing palpitations aggravated upon physical exertion. Exuberance of deficient heat in the interior brings about night sweats, vexation, insomnia and flushed cheeks. Deficiency of heart yang and kidney yang causes an overflow of water and body fluid which attack the heart and lungs in the upper body (with such signs as palpitations and shortness of breath) and the bladder in the lower body (with such signs as scanty urine and edema). Prolonged affliction debilitates the healthy qi, as well as yin and yang, leading to extreme depletion of heart yang with a stuffy sensation in the heart or chest, sweating, cold limbs and an extremely feeble, faint pulse.

## Diagnostic Key Points

1. Chief clinical manifestations of left heart failure:
   (1) Symptoms (acute pulmonary edema): Exertional dyspnea, paroxysmal nocturnal dyspnea, orthopnea, weariness, or even cough, shortness of breath and expectoration of pink, frothy sputum.
   (2) Physical signs: Enlarged left ventricle, diastolic gallop in the apical region, fine rales in the two lung bases and retention of fluid in the chest.
   (3) X-ray examination: Enlarged heart and pulmonary congestion.
2. Chief clinical manifestations of right heart failure:
   (1) Symptoms: Abdominal distension, reduced appetite, scanty urine, profuse nocturnal urine and edema in the lower limbs.
   (2) Physical signs: Enlarged heart. If it involves primarily the right ventricle, there are accompanying symptoms such as heaving apex impulse, protodiastolic gallop near the left sternal border, fine rales in the two lung bases, hepatomegalia, engorgement of the jugular vein, positive hepatojugular reflux, edema in the lower limbs, retention of fluid in the chest and abdomen and cyanosis.
   (3) X-ray examination: Enlargement of heart shadow, superior vena cava and the right atrium and ventricle.
3. NYHA (New York Heart Association) cardiac functional grading.
Grade I: Unrestricted physical activities.
Grade II: Mild restriction of physical activities.
Grade III: Obvious restriction of physical activities, which is lower than the normal volume, with signs of weariness, panting, palpitations or angina.
Grade IV: Symptoms of restricted physical activities in any type or at any time, even when at rest.

## Syndrome Differentiation

### 1. Qi deficiency of the heart and lungs with blood stasis and phlegm

Symptoms: Palpitations, chest distress, shortness of breath aggravated upon physical exertion, cough, expectoration of white sputum or bloody sputum and lassitude; a dark red tongue with thin coating and a knotted, intermittent pulse.

Analysis of symptoms : The heart controls blood and the lungs govern qi, so if the heart and lungs are deficient, the qi fails to promote blood, leading to obstruction of heart vessels marked by palpitations, chest distress, shortness of breath and cyanosed lips and nails; physical exertion consumes qi, leading to exacerbation of symptoms upon exertion; the lungs fail in their dispersing and descending functions, leading to phlegm and retained fluid in the lungs, marked by cough with white sputum; blood stasis in the lung vessels is responsible for expectoration of bloody sputum; disorder of the child organ involves the mother organ, leading to deficiency of lung qi and spleen qi, marked by lassitude; the dark red tongue with thin coating and the knotted, intermittent pulse are both due to deficiency of heart qi and lung qi with retention of phlegm and blood.

### 2. Deficiency of qi and yin with internal obstruction of heart blood

Symptoms: Palpitations aggravated upon physical exertion, lassitude, dizziness, night sweats, red cheeks, vexation and insomnia; a slightly red tongue and a knotted, intermittent pulse or thin, rapid pulse.

Analysis of symptoms: Deficiency of qi and yin leads to obstruction of blood in the heart, as well as malnutrition of the heart, resulting in palpitations aggravated upon physical exertion and lassitude; malnutrition of the clear orifices brings about dizziness; deficiency of yin produces internal heat, leading to night sweats and red cheeks; heat disturbs the heart spirit, with such signs as vexation and insomnia.

### 3. Yang deficiency of the heart and kidneys with retention of blood stasis and fluid

Symptoms: Palpitations, chest distress, shortness of breath, cough with white frothy sputum, intolerance of cold, cold limbs, sore waist, scanty urine, pale or cyanosed complexion and general dropsy; a dark purple tongue with white coating and a thin, deep pulse or knotted, intermittent pulse.

Analysis of symptoms: Deficiency of heart yang brings about obstruction of heart vessels, marked by palpitations, chest distress and cyanosed complexion; deficiency of kidney yang leads to malnutrition of the kidneys, causing waist soreness; cold congeals the blood vessels, marked by intolerance of cold with cold limbs; internal accumulation of water and fluid affects the heart and lungs, resulting in shortness of breath and cough with white frothy sputum; retention of water and fluid in the bladder results in dysfunction of qi transformation, with scanty urine; retention of water and fluid in the skin and muscles is responsible for general dropsy; the dark purple tongue with white coating and a thin, deep pulse or knotted, intermittent pulse are attributable to deficiency of heart yang and kidney yang with blood stasis and edema.

## Differential Treatment

### 1. Qi deficiency of the heart and lungs with blood stasis and phlegm

Treatment principle: Nourishing the heart and supplementing the lungs, activating blood and dissolving phlegm.

Prescription and herbs: Modified Yangxin Decoction.

Dangshen (Radix Codonopsis) 15 g, Huangqi (Milkvetch Root) 20 g, Gancao (Stir-baked Liquorice Root) 9 g, Guizhi (Cassia Twig) 9 g, Danggui (Chinese Angelica) 9 g, Chuanxiong (Szechwan Lovage Rhizome) 9 g, Banxia (Pinellia Tuber) 9 g and Fuling (Indian Bread) 15 g.

Modification: If the patient presents with dark red cheeks and cyanosed lips and nails, Taoren (Peach Seed) 9 g, Honghua (Safflower) 9 g and

Yimucao (Motherwort Herb) 15 g are added to activate blood and resolve stasis; for expectoration of white sputum, panting with suffocating sensation and inability to lie down, Tinglizi (Herba Leonuri) 15 g (wrapped during decoction) and Sangbaipi (White Mulberry Root-Bark) 15 g are added to purge the lungs and drain the retained fluid.

## 2. Deficiency of qi and yin with internal obstruction of heart blood

Treatment principle: Supplementing qi and astringing yin, activating blood and nourishing the heart.

Prescription and herbs: Modified Shengmai Potion and Zhigancao Decoction.

Dangshen (Radix Codonopsis) 15 g, Maidong (Dwarf Lilyturf Tuber) 15 g, Wuweizi (Chinese Magnolivine Fruit) 5 g, Gancao (Stir-baked Liquorice Root) 9 g, Guizhi (Cassia Twig) 9 g, Shengdi (Dried Rehmannia Root) 12 g, Suanzaoren (Spine Date Seed) 15 g and Danshen (Radix Salviae Miltiorrhiae) 15 g.

Modification: If the patient presents with apparent internal heat, feverish dysphoria, night sweats and palpitations due to deficiency of yin, Huanglian (Golden Thread) 3 g and Zhimu (Common Anemarrhena Rhizome) 9 g are added to dispel deficient heat; for swollen feet, Huangqi (Milkvetch Root) 15 g, Baizhu (Largehead Atractylodes Rhizome) 12 g and Fangji (Fourstamen Stephania Root) 15 g are added to invigorate the spleen, supplement qi and remove water.

## 3. Yang deficiency of the heart and kidneys with retention of blood stasis and fluid

Treatment principle: Warming yang and invigorating qi, resolving blood stasis and expelling retained fluid.

Prescription and herbs: Modified Zhenwu Decoction and Tingli Dazao Xiefei Decoction.

Fupian (Radix Aconitilateralis Preparata) 15 g, Ganjiang (Dried Ginger) 5 g, Guizhi (Cassia Twig) 9 g, Baizhu (Largehead Atractylodes Rhizome)

15 g, Fuling (Indian Bread) 15 g, Zelan (Herba Lycopi) 15 g, Yimucao (Motherwort Herb) 30 g, Tinglizi (Herba Leonuri) 15 g (wrapped during decoction) and Dazao (Chinese Date) 3 dates.

Modification: If there is lassitude, Huangqi (Milkvetch Root) 30 g and Dangshen (Radix Codonopsis) 15 g are added to replenish qi; for abdominal distension, reduced food intake and nausea, Dafupi (Areca Peel) 9 g, Chenpi (Dried Tangerine Peel) 9 g and Banxia (Pinellia Tuber) 9 g are added to invigorate the spleen and promote flow of qi, as well as relieve distension and reinforce the stomach; for palpitations with a suffocating sensation, restlessness, profuse sweat and a thin, deep and feeble pulse due to deficiency of yin and yang with extreme depletion of heart yang, Shenfu Longmu Decoction, coupled with Western medicines, can be used to restore yang and nourish yin.

## Chinese Patent Medicine

1. Jisheng Shenqi Pill: 6 g for each dose, 3 times a day.
2. Compound Danshen Dripping Pill: 10 pills for each dose, 3 times a day.

## Simple and Handy Prescriptions

Shengshaishen (Dried Radix Ginseng) 6 g, Fupian (Radix Aconitilateralis Preparata) 9 g, Maidong (Dwarf Lilyturf Tuber) 15 g and Honghua (Safflower) 6 g are boiled in water and taken 3 times a day. It is used a long period of time for chronic heart failure.

## Other Therapies

Injection therapy: 20 ml of Shenmai Injection is added into 250 ml of 5% Glucose for intravenous drip. It is administered once a day with a proper dripping rate. This injection is used to treat various types of heart failure. For those with diabetes, insulin should be added.

Dietary therapy: Yangrou (Mutton) 250 g, Guipi (Cinnamon Bark) 3 g, Huangqi (Milkvetch Root) 50 g and Danggui (Chinese Angelica) 9 g. First the mutton is sliced and stir-fried and then the Guipi (Cinnamon Bark),

Huangqi (Milkvetch Root) and Danggui (Chinese Angelica) are boiled thoroughly in water. Before serving, ginger, cooking wine, salt and gourmet power are added. This dish can be consumed repeatedly and used to treat chronic heart failure with declined yang qi and adverse flow of water qi which attacks the heart.

## Cautions and Advice

1. Chronic congestive heart failure is attributed to the disorder of haemodynamics and the abnormal activation of nerrohumor factors resulting from progressive development of a variety of organic heart diseases. For this reason, the primary diseases should be proactively addressed and the Western medicines for heart failure are also indispensable.
2. When there is heart failure and infection, the latter should be promptly treated and arrhythmia, electrolyte disturbance or acid-base metabolism disorder must be dealt with, so as to prevent exacerbation of heart failure.
3. Patients should take a good rest, avoid overstrain and adopt a light, low-salt diet. They should also be aware of various pathogenic factors in their daily lives, such as pathogenic wind-cold, to prevent the occurrence of heart failure.

## Daily Exercises

1. List the etiological factors of heart failure.
2. Recall the diagnostic key points of left and right heart failures.
3. Explain how heart failure can be treated based on syndrome differentiation.

# Hypertension

# Week 4: Friday

Hypertension is a syndrome due to the elevation of systemic arterial blood pressure. Hypertension is classified as either primary hypertension or secondary hypertension. The former comprises most cases, while the latter is secondary to other diseases and is also called symptomatic hypertension. Hypertension is clinically marked by elevated levels of blood pressure, dizziness, headache, chest distress and weariness, in addition to the organic lesions of the heart, brain and kidneys. The occurrence of hypertension is closely related to heredity, age, occupation, environment and eating or living habits. Besides, emotional stress and strenuous activities may also create a predisposition to sudden elevation of blood pressure. The middle-aged or elderly are the most vulnerable to this disease. If the patients' conditions are complicated by damage to the heart, brain and kidneys, the prognosis can be unfavorable. In TCM, hypertension belongs to the category of "dizziness" or "headache".

## Etiology and Pathology

The etiological factors of hypertension are long-term emotional stress, anger, worry or excessive contemplation (which lead to stagnated liver qi transforming into fire), or unrestricted intake of alcohol and fatty or sweet food (which give rise to turbid phlegm in the interior), or overstrain, excessive sexual activity and senility (which debilitate the body and consume the essence of the liver and kidneys). In a word, the above-mentioned factors can all result in imbalance between yin and yang of the liver and kidneys, as well as disturbance of the upper orifices, thereby creating a predisposition to this disease.

The pathological changes are discussed as follows: Prolonged stagnation of liver qi makes it transform to fire, marked by hyperactivity of liver yang and internal stirring of wind which disturbs the clear orifices upwardly, with such signs as headache, dizziness, irascibility and a bitter taste in the mouth. Improper diet damages the spleen and stomach, leading to accumulation of dampness and phlegm in the interior which inhibits the lucid yang from ascending and the turbid yin from descending, with such signs as dizziness, heaviness of the head and chest distress. The kidneys can be impaired by overstrain and excessive sexual activity, or become debilitated with aging; when the kidney essence is depleted, there will be deficiency of liver yin and kidney yin and the ensuing hyperactivity of deficient yang, marked by a vague pain in the head, dizziness, tinnitus and soreness in the waist. If the disease persists, the collaterals will be affected, leading to obstruction of blood vessels by blood stasis, presenting as headache with pricking sensation, chest distress with stabbing pain, numbness in the hands and feet, cyanosed tongue and unsmooth pulse. If deficiency of yin involves yang, leading to deficiency of yin and yang of the liver and kidneys, with yin failing to nourish and yang failing to warm, there will be dizziness, emaciation, lassitude and profuse nocturnal urination. If the liver yang suddenly goes rampant, generating wind and stirring blood, the heart spirit will be disturbed and the upper orifices may be clouded, marked by stroke or coma.

## Diagnostic Key Points

According to the standards in China released in 2004 for prevention and treatment of hypertension, it can be classified as follows:

| Classification | Systolic pressure mmHg | Diastolic pressure mmHg |
|---|---|---|
| Normal | <120 | <80 |
| Prehypertension | 120~139 | 80~89 |
| Stage 1 (mild) | 140~159 | 90~99 |
| Stage 2 (moderate) | 160~179 | 100~109 |
| Stage 3 (severe) | ≥180 | ≥110 |
| Isolated systolic hypertension | ≥140 | <90 |

## Syndrome Differentiation

## 1. Hyperactivity of liver yang

Symptoms: Headache with a distending sensation, dizziness, restlessness, irascibility, sleeplessness at night, (or accompanied by) hypochondriac pain, facial redness and a bitter taste in the mouth; a red tongue with thin, yellow coating and a taut, forceful pulse.

Analysis of symptoms: All wind disorders and dizziness can be attributed to the liver, so if the liver fails to promote free flow of qi, there will be hyperactivity of liver yang and internal stirring of wind, which disturb the upper orifices upwardly, leading to headache with distending sensation and dizziness; exuberance of liver fire brings about a disquieted heart spirit, leading to restlessness, irascibility and sleeplessness at night; the liver qi and gallbladder qi are stagnated into fire, which flames upward and results in hypochondriac pain, facial redness and mouth bitterness; a red tongue with thin, yellow coating and a taut, forceful pulse are manifestations of hyperactivity of liver yang.

## 2. Internal obstruction of phlegm and dampness

Symptoms: Headache with a heavy sensation, dizziness, chest distress, nausea, poor appetite and sleepiness; a white greasy tongue coating and a soggy, slippery pulse.

Analysis of symptoms: Phlegm and dampness encumbers the lucid yang, leading to headache with heavy sensation, dizziness and sleepiness; Obstruction of qi activity manifests itself as chest distress; non-descending of turbid yin is marked by nausea; deficiency of spleen and stomach gives rise to poor appetite; a white greasy tongue coating and a soggy, slippery pulse are suggestive of dampness in the interior.

## 3. Internal retention of blood stasis

Symptoms: Dizziness, headache with pricking pain, or chest distress with stabbing pain; cyanosed lips and tongue with petechia and ecchymosis, as well as a thin or unsmooth pulse.

Analysis of symptoms: If the disease persists, the collaterals will be affected, leading to obstruction of blood stasis in the vessels, marked by dizziness, headache with pricking pain or chest distress with stabbing pain; cyanosed lips and tongue with petechia and ecchymosis and a thin or unsmooth pulse are indicative of blood stasis in the interior.

## 4. Yin deficiency of the liver and kidneys

Symptoms: Vague pain in the head, dizziness, tinnitus, feverish sensations over the five centers (the palms, the soles and the heart) and weakness and soreness of the waist and legs; a reddish tongue with scanty tongue coating and a thin pulse or thin, rapid pulse.

Analysis of symptoms: Deficiency of liver yin and kidney yin leads to floating of deficient yang to the head, leading to vague pain in the head, dizziness and tinnitus; deficiency of yin gives rise to internal heat, marked by feverish sensation over the five centers (the palms, the soles and the heart); the waist is the "house of the kidneys" and the kidneys control the bones, so if the kidneys are deficient, there will be weakness and soreness of the waist and legs; a reddish tongue with scanty tongue coating and a thin pulse are due to exhaustion of liver yin and kidney yin and a thin, rapid pulse is attributable to internal heat with deficiency of yin.

## 5. Deficiency of yin and yang

Symptoms: Dizziness, forgetfulness, emaciation, dry mouth, lassitude, or frequent nocturnal urination and weakness and soreness of the waist and legs; a reddish tongue with thin coating and a thin, weak pulse.

Analysis of symptoms: Insufficiency of kidney essence results in malnutrition of the brain and the upper orifices, leading to dizziness and forgetfulness; malnutrition of the body is responsible for emaciation; the body fluid is insufficiently produced, marked by dry mouth; deficiency of yin involves yang and debilitates it, presenting as lassitude; dysfunction of qi transformation is manifested as frequent nocturnal urination; the deficient kidneys are located in the lower energizer, leading to weakness and soreness of the waist and legs; a reddish tongue with thin coating and a thin, weak pulse are caused by deficiency of yin and yang.

## Differential Treatment

### 1. Hyperactivity of liver yang

Treatment principle: Calming the liver and subduing yang.

Prescription and herbs: Modified Tianma Gouteng Potion.

Tianma (Tall Gastrodis Tuber) 9 g, Gouteng (Gambir Plant) 15 g, (decocted later) Shijueming (Sea-ear Shell) 30 g (decocted first), Huangqin (Baical Skullcap Root) 9 g, Zhizi (Cape Jasmine Fruit) 9 g, Niuxi (Twotoothed Achyranthes Root) 9 g, Duzhong (Eucommia Bark) 9 g, Sangjisheng (Chinese Taxillus Herb) 12 g, Yejiaoteng (Caulis Polygoni Multiflori) 30 g, Fushen (Indian Bread with Hostwood) 12 g and Zhenzhumu (Nacre) 30 g (decocted first).

Modification: If the patient presents with severe headache, hypochondriac pain, a bitter taste in the mouth, flushed complexion, constipation and reddish urine due to relative exuberance of liver fire, Longdancao (Radix Gentianae) 6 g, Xiakucao (Common Selfheal Fruit-Spike) 12 g and Yujin (Turmeric Root Tuber) 9 g are added to clear the liver and purge fire.

### 2. Internal obstruction of phlegm and dampness

Treatment principle: Dissolving phlegm and expelling dampness.

Prescription and herbs: Modified Banxia Baizhu Tianma Decoction.

Tianma (Tall Gastrodis Tuber) 9 g, Baizhu (Largehead Atractylodes Rhizome) 12, Banxia (Pinellia Tuber) 9 g, Fuling (Indian Bread) 12 g, Chenpi (Dried Tangerine Peel) 6 g, Zexie (Oriental Waterplantain Rhizome) 15 g, Daizheshi (Red Bole) 30 g (decocted first) and Shengjiang (Fresh Ginger) 5 g.

Modification: If there is tinnitus and amblykusis, Yujin (Turmeric Root Tuber) 9 g and Changpu (Acorus Calamus) 9 g are added to free yang and open the orifices; for vexation with a bitter taste in the mouth, Huanglian (Golden Thread) 3 g and Zhuru (Bamboo Shavings) 9 g are used to dispel heat and dissolve phlegm.

## 3. Internal retention of blood stasis

Treatment principle: Activating blood and resolving stasis.

Prescription and herbs: Modified Tongqiao Huoxue Decoction.

Taoren (Peach Seed) 9 g, Honghua (Safflower) 6 g, Chuanxiong (Szechwan Lovage Rhizome) 9 g, Chishao (Red Peony Root) 15 g, Congbai (Fistular Onion Stalk) 5 g, Shengjiang (Fresh Ginger) 5 g, Shexiang (Musk) 0.3 g, Gancao ( Liquorice Root) 3 g, Yujin (Turmeric Root Tuber) 9 g, Changpu (Acorus Calamus) 9 g, Baizhi (Dahurian Angelica Root) 9 g and Xixin (Manchurian Wildginger) 3 g.

Modification: For headache with distending pain, Baijili (Tribulus Terrestris) 9 g and Lingyangjiaofen (Antelope Horn Powder) 0.6 g (swallowed) are added to subdue the liver and extinguish wind; if it is accompanied by stroke as a lingering effect, supplementary Buyang Huanwu Decoction (Milkvetch Root 30 g, Chinese Angelica 9 g, Szechwan Lovage Rhizome 9 g, Red Peony Root 15 g and Angle Worm 9 g) are used to activate blood, dredge collaterals and expel wind; for chest distress with pricking pain, Yanhusuo (Corydalis) 9 g and Wulingzhi (Faeces Trogopterorum) 9 g are added to regulate qi, activate blood and stop pain.

## 4. Yin deficiency of the liver and kidneys

Treatment principle: Nourishing the liver and kidneys.

Prescription and herbs: Modified Dabuyuan Decoction.

Shudi (Prepared Rhizome of Rehmannia) 12 g, Shanyao (Common Yan Rhizome) 12 g, Shanzhuyu (Asiatic Cornelian Cherry Fruit) 9 g, Gouqizi (Barbary Wolfberry Fruit) 12 g, Taizishen (Heterophylly Falsesatarwort Root) 15 g, Danggui (Chinese Angelica) 9 g, Duzhong (Eucommia Bark) 9 g, Niuxi (Twotoothed Achyranthes Root) 9 g, Baijili (Tribulus Terrestris) 9 g and Juhua (Chrysanthemum Flower) 9 g.

Modification: For feverish dysphoria and night sweats, Huangbai (Amur Cork-tree) 9 g and Zhimu (Common Anemarrhena Rhizome) 9 g are added to nourish yin and purge fire.

## 5. Deficiency of yin and yang

Treatment principle: Regulating and nourishing yin and yang.

Prescription and herbs: Supplementary Jingui Shenqi Pill.

Shudi (Prepared Rhizome of Rehmannia) 15 g, Shanyao (Common Yan Rhizome) 15 g, Shanzhuyu (Asiatic Cornelian Cherry Fruit) 10 g, Danpi (Cortex Moutan) 10 g, Zexie (Oriental Waterplantain Rhizome) 12 g, Fuling (Indian Bread) 12 g, Rougui (Cassia Bark) 3 g (decocted later), Fupian (Radix Aconitilateralis Preparata) 10 g, Gouqizi (Barbary Wolfberry Fruit) 12 g, Duzhong (Eucommia Bark) 12 g and Sangjisheng (Chinese Taxillus Herb) 12 g.

Modification: For tinnitus and deafness, Cishi (Magnetite) 30 g (decocted first) and Wuweizi (Chinese Magnolivine Fruit) 6 g are added to anchor the floating yang; for proteinuria, Huangqi (Milkvetch Root) 30 g, Buguzhi (Malaytea Scurfpea Fruit) 12 g and Luxiangcao (Pyrolae) 15 g are added to replenish qi and nourish the kidneys so as to reduce proteinuria.

## Chinese Patent Medicine

1. Longdan Xiegan Pill: 6 g for each dose, 3 times a day.
2. Qiju Dihuang Pill: 6 g for each dose, 3 times a day.

## Simple and Handy Prescriptions

Garden lettuce seeds 25 g are crushed into pieces, boiled in water and afterwards administered several times a day.

## Other Therapies

Medicated pillow therapy: Yejuhua (Wild Chrysanthemum Flower), Sangye (Mulberry Leaf), Shigao (Gypsum), Baishao (White Peony Alba), Chuanxiong (Szechwan Lovage Rhizome), Cishi (Magnetite), Manjingzi (Shrub Chastetree Fruit), Qingmuxiang (Common Aucklandia Root) and Chansha (Excrementum Bombycis) are combined in equal quantities to make a medicated pillow, which should be used for more than 6 hours every 24 hours.

Foot-bath therapy: Gouteng (Gambir Plant) 30 g is wrapped in a cloth and boiled in water, into which a little borneol is added. The decoction is put into a washbasin and mixed with warm water for foot bathing, 30 minutes at a time, with 10 days forming a course of treatment.

Dietary therapy: Wild celery 250 g is boiled in water for 2 minutes and then mixed with a small quantity of oil and salt to be taken for hypertension with obesity.

## Cautions and Advice

1. Hypertension is a common disease and if uncontrolled, will affect the heart, brain and kidneys, causing severe complications. Hence, this disease should be promptly diagnosed and treated with routine hypotensive drugs.
2. Blood pressure should be regularly tested and a diet that is low in salt, fat and sugar should be adopted. It is advisable for patients to engage more actively in physical exercises, keep themselves in good spirits and avoid becoming obese.

## Daily Exercises

1. Concisely describe the etiology and pathology of hypertension.
2. Recall the diagnostic criteria of hypertension.
3. Explain how hypertension due to hyperactivity of liver yang, deficiency of liver yin and kidney yin, and internal obstruction of turbid phlegm (3 patterns) can be differentiated and treated.

# Cardioneurosis

# Week 4: Saturday

Cardioneurosis is a syndrome marked by functional disorder of the cardiovascular system due to dysfunction of the nerves. It is an uncommon type of neurosis and clinically this disease manifests itself as symptoms of the cardiovascular system or concomitant symptoms of neurosis. Generally there is no evidence of organic heart lesions, but this disease can be simultaneously present with or ensue from organic heart diseases. Emotional factors play a significant role in the occurrence of this disease, such as anxiety, agitation and psychic trauma. In addition, physical overstrain is also an inducing factor. Cardioneurosis is commonly reported in young or middle-age people. Females, especially those experiencing menopause, are more vulnerable to this disease than males. The clinical manifestations are various and may be characterized by alternated aggravation and alleviation. In some cases, physical activities are severely impeded. It is believed in TCM that this disease has a close relation with "fright with severe palpitations", "chest bi-syndrome" and "syndrome of depression".

## Etiology and Pathology

Cardioneurosis is mostly caused by emotional factors, such as fright (as is usually seen in those with deficiency of heart qi and timorousness), anger (which impairs the liver qi and drives liver fire upward) and emotional depression (which leads to stagnation of liver qi and internal disturbance of phlegmatic fire). In addition, stagnation of qi and stasis of blood also impair the blood vessels and disquiet the heart spirit. Furthermore, chronic or severe disease, overstrain and an excessive sexual life may all damage the heart, spleen and kidneys and consume qi and blood (yin), leading to malnourishment of the heart and failure of the spirit to be stored.

The pathological changes are discussed as follows: Deficiency of heart qi and gallbladder qi makes the body vulnerable to panic attacks, marked by a disquieted spirit, fright or fluster. Intense anger predisposes the body to an upward flaming of liver fire or stagnation of liver qi which invades the spleen and causes phlegm; the phlegm, coupled with fire, disturbs the heart spirit and leads to fright, restlessness, chest distress and insomnia. Stagnation of qi with blood stasis results in obstruction of the chest collaterals or cardiac vessels, marked by chest distress and pain. Furthermore, simultaneous impairment of the heart and spleen, co-existence of deficient qi and blood, or concurrent deficiency of the heart yin and kidney yin (which brings about upward disturbance of deficient fire) can all lead to malnourishment of the heart to be nourished and failure of the spirit to be stored, marked by palpitations and insomnia.

## Diagnostic Key Points

1. Chief clinical manifestations: Functional disorder of the cardiovascular system, marked by palpitations, precordial pain, shortness of breath and excessive ventilation; neurotic symptoms, such as insomnia, anxiety, profuse sweating and dizziness.
2. Generally no evidence of organic heart diseases.

## Syndrome Differentiation

### 1. Stagnation of liver with deficiency of gallbladder

Symptoms: Emotional depression, timorousness, fright, frequent palpitations, poor and restless sleep, stuffiness and distension in the chest and hypochondria, or pain in the chest without a fixed location, the pain is often related to emotions; a red tongue with white, thin coating and a taut pulse.

Analysis of symptoms: Stagnation of liver qi leads to unsmooth functional activities of qi, characterized by emotional depression with stuffiness and distension in the chest and hypochondria; stagnation of qi results in blood stasis, while free flow of qi promotes blood circulation, leading to pain in the chest without fixed location which is often induced by emotional factors; deficiency of heart qi and gallbladder qi brings about a disquieted spirit, with timidity, fright, palpitations, or poor and restless sleep as the result; the red tongue with white, thin coating and taut pulse are due to stagnation of the liver with deficiency of gallbladder.

## 2. Internal disturbance of phlegm and fire

Symptoms: Palpitations with vexation, stuffy sensation in the thoracic or gastric region, or corpulence, excessive dreams during sleep, a bitter taste in the mouth, oral dryness with inadequate drinking and profuse sputum; red tongue with yellow, greasy coating or turbid, greasy tongue coating and rapid, slippery pulse.

Analysis of symptoms: Internal abundance of turbid phlegm is manifested as corpulence and excessive sputum; if the phlegm impedes qi activities, there will be a stuffy sensation in the thoracic or gastric region; internal disturbance of phlegm and fire gives rise to palpitations with vexation and profuse dreams during sleep; phlegm and fire damage yin, leading to bitter taste in the mouth and oral dryness with inadequate drinking; the red tongue with yellow, greasy coating or turbid, greasy tongue coating and rapid, slippery pulse are attributable to internal disturbance of phlegm and fire.

## 3. Deficiency of the spleen and stomach

Symptoms: Palpitations, dizziness, vague pain in the chest, a white complexion, listlessness, insomnia and forgetfulness; reddish tongue with thin coating and thin, feeble pulse.

Analysis of symptoms: Deficiency of the spleen and stomach leads to concurrent depletion of qi and blood, so the heart becomes malnourished, marked by palpitations and vague heartache; the spirit has no place to hide, leading to insomnia; the heart blood fails to nourish the brain, bringing about dizziness and forgetfulness; the blood fails to nourish the face, leading to a pale complexion; concurrent deficiency of qi and blood cannot invigorate the body, leading to listlessness; the reddish tongue with thin coating and thin, feeble pulse are manifestations of deficiency of the spleen and stomach with concurrent depletion of qi and blood.

## 4. Exuberance of fire due to deficiency of yin

Symptoms: Palpitations, uneasiness, vexation, insomnia, fright, irascibility, dizziness, tinnitus, feverish sensations in the palms and soles, soreness in the waist, nocturnal emissions, dry mouth with scanty fluid; red tongue with little or no coating and thin, rapid pulse.

Analysis of symptoms: Insufficiency of kidney yin leads to the condition in which water (kidneys) fails to coordinate fire (heart), resulting in internal disturbance of heart fire and disquietude of the heart spirit, marked by palpitations, uneasiness, vexation, insomnia, fright and irascibility; the lower energizer (the kidneys) is deficient in yin-fluid, leading to symptoms of waist soreness and nocturnal emissions; the upper energizer is disturbed by the deficient yang, leading to dizziness and tinnitus; the feverish sensation in the palms and soles, dry mouth with scanty fluid, red tongue with little or no coating and thin, rapid pulse are all manifestations of fire exuberance due to yin deficiency.

## Differential Treatment

### 1. Stagnation of liver with deficiency of gallbladder

Treatment principle: Relieving stagnation and tranquilizing the mind.

Prescription and herbs: Modified Chaihu Shugan Powder and Ganmai Dazao Decoction.

Chaihu (Chinese Thorowax Root) 9 g, Baishao (White Peony Alba) 12 g, Zhiqiao (Orange Fruit) 9 g, Chuanxiong (Szechwan Lovage Rhizome) 9 g, Xiangfu (Nutgrass Galingale Rhizome) 9 g, Huaixiaomai (Huaihe Wheat) 30 g, Gancao (Stir-baked Liquorice Root) 9 g and Dazao (Chinese Date) 5 dates.

Modification: For palpitations with poor sleep, Yejiaoteng (Caulis Polygoni Multiflori) 30 g, Hehuanhua (Albizia Flower) 15 g and Zaoren (Fried Semen Ziziphi Spinosae) 12 g are added to nourish the heart and calm the spirit; for restlessness, vexation and fright, Baihe (Lily Bulb)15 g, Zhimu (Common Anemarrhena Rhizome) 9 g and Cishi (Magnetite) 30 g (decocted first) are added to clear the liver and relieve convulsion.

### 2. Internal disturbance of phlegm and fire

Treatment principle: Dispelling fire and dissolving phlegm.

Prescription and herbs: Modified Huanglian Wendan Decoction.

Huanglian (Golden Thread) 3 g, Zhuru (Bamboo Shavings) 9 g, Huangqin (Baical Skullcap Root) 12 g, Banxia (Pinellia Tuber) 9 g, Chenpi (Dried

Tangerine Peel) 6 g, Fuling (Indian Bread) 12 g, Gancao ( Liquorice Root) 3 g and Zhishi (Immature Orange Fruit) 9 g.

Modification: If the patient presents with severe chest distress, Gualou (Snakegourd Fruit) 15 g, Xiebai (Long Stamen Onion Bulb) 6 g and Yujin (Turmeric Root Tuber) 9 g are added to dissolve phlegm and relieve chest discomfort; for palpitations and dreaminess, Mengshi (Phlopopitum) 30 g and Yuanzhi (Thinleaf Milkwort Root) 5 g are used to relieve fright, calm the mind and dissolve phlegm.

### 3. Deficiency of the spleen and stomach

Treatment principle: Nourishing the heart and invigorating the spleen.

Prescription and herbs: Modified Guipi Decoction.

Huangqi (Milkvetch Root) 20 g, Dangshen (Radix Codonopsis) 15 g, Baizhu (Largehead Atractylodes Rhizome) 12 g, Fushen (Indian Bread with Hostwood) 12 g, Yuanzhi (Thinleaf Milkwort Root) 6 g, Suanzaoren (Spine Date Seed) 9 g, Longyanrou (Longan Aril) 9 g, Danggui (Chinese Angelica) 9 g, Gancao (Stir-baked Liquorice Root) 6 g and Dazao (Chinese Date) 5 dates.

Modification: If the patient presents with relatively severe insomnia, Wuweizi (Chinese Magnolivine Fruit) 6 g and Baiziren (Chinese Arborvitae Kernel) 9 g are used to nourish the heart and calm the spirit; if the patient has a poor appetite, Shanzha (Hawthorn Fruit) 15 g and Chenpi (Dried Tangerine Peel) 6 g are added to invigorate the stomach and facilitate digestion.

### 4. Exuberance of fire due to deficiency of yin

Treatment principle: Nourishing yin and purging fire.

Prescription and herbs: Modified Tianwang Buxin Pill.

Shengdi (Dried Rehmannia Root) 9 g, Maidong (Dwarf Lilyturf Tuber) 9 g, Tiandong (Cochinchinese Asparagus Root) 9 g, Xuanshen (Figwort Root) 9 g, Danshen (Radix Salviae Miltiorrhiae) 15 g, Danggui (Chinese Angelica) 9 g, Huangbai (Amur Cork-tree) 9 g and Zhimu (Common Anemarrhena Rhizome) 9 g.

Modification: If there is relatively severe feverish dysphoria and insomnia, Huanglian (Golden Thread) 3 g, Zhizi (Burnt Cape Jasmine Fruit) 9 g, Longgu (Os Draconis) 30 g and Muli (Oyster Shell) 30 g are added to dispel heat and relieve vexation as well as tranquilize the mind and calm the spirit.

## Chinese Patent Medicine

1. Xiaoyao Pill: 6 g for each dose, 3 times a day.
2. Zheheling Tablet: 4 tablets for each dose, 3 times a day.
3. Zhusha Anshen Pill: 6 g for each dose, 3 times a day.
4. Tianwang Buxin Dan: 6 g for each dose, 3 times a day.

## Simple and Handy Prescriptions

1. Haixiaomai (Huaihe Wheat) 30 g, Baihe (Lily Bulb) 30 g, Gancao (Stir-baked Liquorice Root) 6 g and Dazao (Chinese Date) 10 g are boiled in water and taken twice a day. It is used to treat patients with cardioneurosis marked by palpitations and restlessness, especially women experiencing menopause.
2. Taizishen (Heterophylly Falsesatarwort Root) 15 g, Maidong (Dwarf Lilyturf Tuber) 15 g and Wuweizi (Chinese Magnolivine Fruit) 9 g are boiled in water and taken twice a day. It is used to treat cardioneurosis with symptoms such as listlessness, shortness of breath, palpitations and liability to sweat.

## Other Therapies

Immersion bath therapy: The patient lies on his back and immerses himself in a tub filled with water (36°~37° Celsius) till the region below the ensiform process of sternum is submerged. This should be done once a day, for 15~20 minutes.

Dietary therapy:

(1) Longyanrou (Longan Aril) 30 g, Danggui (Chinese Angelica) 10 g and lean pork 100 g are boiled in a casserole with a proper amount of

water. This is used to treat cardioneurosis with palpitations, chest distress, weariness and weakness of the body.

(2) Baihe (Lily Bulb) 30 g, Shengdi (Dried Rehmannia Root) 15 g and Jiangmi (Rice Fruit) 100 g are made into porridge and taken for the treatment of cardioneurosis marked by palpitations, insomnia and restlessness.

## Cautions and Advice

1. The key to preventing this disease is avoiding emotional stimulation and keeping a healthy and stable mental state.
2. Patients should avoid mental or physical overstrain and strike a balance between rest and sleep.

## Daily Exercises

1. List the etiological factors of cardioneurosis.
2. Explain how cardioneurosis can be treated based on syndrome differentiation.

# CHAPTER 4

# Disorders of the Digestive System

## Reflux Esophagitis
## Week 5: Monday

Reflux esophagitis refers to the inflammation, erosion, ulceration or fibrous degeneration of the esophageal mucosa induced by the reflux of contents from the stomach and duodenum. It is a gastroesophageal reflux disease, clinically marked by a burning sensation or pain behind the breast bone or below the xiphoid process, acid regurgitation, vomiting, dysphagia, or even haematemesis, hemafecia and anaemia. In TCM, reflux esophagitis is closely associated with "stomachache", "chest pain", "acid regurgitation", "stomach upset", "vomiting" and "difficult swallowing".

### Etiology and Pathology

The location of this disease is in the esophagus, but the cause of it is closely linked to the liver, gallbladder, spleen and stomach. In the initial stage, it may be caused by failure of the liver to maintain a normal flow of qi, which invades the stomach and drives the stomach qi upward. If the liver qi is persistently stagnated, it will transform into fire and damage yin; if the spleen qi is persistently debilitated, it will fail to control the blood, with various bleeding syndromes; furthermore, if the general qi is persistently stagnated, there will be accumulation of blood stasis inside the esophagus, thereby bringing about this disease.

## Diagnostic Key Points

1. Burning sensation or pain behind the breast bone or below the xiphoid process, acid regurgitation, vomiting, dysphagia, or even haematemesis, hemafecia and anaemia.
2. Esophageal acidimetry: Positive.
3. Intraesophageal pH < 4.
4. Intraesophageal manometry: Functional defects of the lower esophageal sphincter.
5. Endoscopy is of great diagnostic value to this disease.

## Syndrome Differentiation

### 1. Adverse qi flow of the liver and stomach

Symptoms: Frequent burning pain in the thoracic and gastric region that is aggravated when lying flat, distension and fullness in the chest and hypochondria, frequent belching, regurgitation of acid or bitter fluid; white and thin tongue coating and a taut pulse.

Analysis of symptoms: The liver fails to maintain the normal flow of qi, so the rebellious qi invades the stomach and causes pain; the qi disorder is marked by migration over the liver-dominated area, the hypochondria, causing distension and fullness in the chest and hypochondria; inhibited functional activity of qi prevents the stomach qi from descending normally, resulting in belching and acid regurgitation; the taut pulse is a sign of liver disease and stagnation of liver qi.

### 2. Stagnation of heat in the liver and stomach

Symptoms: Frequent burning pain in the thoracic and gastric region that is aggravated upon swallowing, dry mouth and throat, preference for cold drink, a bitter taste in the mouth, acid regurgitation, vomiting of bloody fluid, dry stools; red tongue with scanty fluid and rapid pulse.

Analysis of symptoms: Persistently stagnated liver qi transforms into fire which scorches the liver and invades the stomach, leading to the burning pain in the chest and hypochondria; the liver heat and gallbladder fire attack the upper energizer, causing the dry mouth and throat, the bitter taste in the mouth and acid regurgitation; heat scorches the stomach collaterals, bringing about the vomiting of bloody fluid; stagnated heat consumes fluid, inhibiting the moistening of the large intestine, with dry stools as the result; the red tongue is a sign of stagnated heat (which consumes fluid and makes it inadequate) and the rapid pulse is suggestive of heat.

## 3. Blood stasis due to deficiency of qi

Symptoms: Vague burning pain in the thoracic and gastric region, or pricking pain, a sense of obstruction when swallowing food and in severe cases, vomiting triggered by intake of water or soup even in small quantities, weariness, feeble limbs, poor appetite and loose stools; a dark tongue with possible ecchymosis and a deep, slow and unsmooth pulse.

Analysis of symptoms: Prolonged affliction debilitates the spleen qi, inhibiting its function to promote blood circulation, so there is retention of blood marked by burning pain in the thoracic and gastric region or pricking pain as an accompanying symptom; internal accumulation of blood stasis in the esophagus brings about a sense of obstruction when swallowing food and prompts vomiting after food intake; the spleen dominates the four limbs and muscles, so a weak spleen results in feeble limbs; deficiency of spleen qi is marked by poor appetite and loose stools; a dark tongue with possible ecchymosis and a deep, slow and unsmooth pulse are manifestations of blood stasis due to deficiency of qi.

## Differential Treatment

### 1. Adverse qi flow of the liver and stomach

Treatment principle: Soothing the liver and regulating qi, harmonizing the stomach and bringing down qi.

Prescription and herbs: Modified Chaihu Shugan Powder.

Chaihu (Chinese Thorowax Root) 6 g, Foshou (Finger Citron) 9 g, Zhiqiao (Orange Fruit) 15 g, Xiangfu (Nutgrass Galingale Rhizome) 12 g, Chenpi (Dried Tangerine Peel) 6 g, Gancao (Liquorice Root) 6 g, Baishao (White Peony Alba) 9 g, Chuanxiong (Szechwan Lovage Rhizome) 6 g and Xuanfuhua (Intussusceer) 12 g.

Modification: If the patient presents with severe pain, Chuanlianzi (Szechwan Chinaberry Fruit) 9 g and Yanhusuo (Corydalis) 9 g can be added to reinforce the pain-relieving effect.

## 2. Stagnation of heat in the liver and stomach

Treatment principle: Clearing the liver and purging fire, harmonizing the stomach and bringing down qi.

Prescription and herbs: Modified Huagan Decoction and Zuojin Pill.

Baishao (White Peony Alba) 9 g, Danpi (Cortex Moutan) 9 g, Zhizi (Cape Jasmine Fruit) 9 g, Chenpi (Dried Tangerine Peel) 6 g, Qingpi (Green Tangerine Peel) 6 g, Huanglian (Golden Thread) 3 g and Wuzhuyu (Medicinal Evodia Fruit) 2 g.

Modification: If the pain is alleviated, Chaihu (Chinese Thorowax Root) 6 g, Baishao (White Peony Alba) 12 g, Baizhu (Largehead Atractylodes Rhizome) 12 g and Fuling (Indian Bread) 12 g are added to relieve depression and invigorate the spleen.

## 3. Blood stasis due to deficiency of qi

Treatment principle: Supplementing qi and invigorating the spleen, resolving stasis and reversing the adverse rising of qi.

Prescription and herbs: Modified Buqi Yunpi Decoction and Tongyou Decoction.

Dangshen (Radix Codonopsis) 15 g, Huangqi (Milkvetch Root) 15 g, Baizhu (Largehead Atractylodes Rhizome) 12 g, Fuling (Indian Bread) 9 g, Banxia (Pinellia Tuber) 9 g, Chenpi (Dried Tangerine Peel) 6 g, Shengjiang (Fresh Ginger) 3 slices, Shengdi (Dried Rehmannia Root)

12 g, Shudi (Prepared Rhizome of Rehmannia) 12 g, Danggui (Chinese Angelica) 9 g, Taoren (Peach Seed) 9 g and Honghua (Safflower) 3 g.

Modification: If there is severe stasis, Danshen (Radix Salviae Miltiorrhiae) 9 g, Shensanqi (Radix Notoginseng) 9 g and Chishao (Red Peony Root) 9 g are added to activate blood and remove stasis.

## Chinese Patent Medicine

1. Zuojin Pill: 4.5 g for each dose, twice a day.
2. Yushu Pellet: 0.6 g for each dose, twice a day.

## Simple and Handy Prescriptions

1. Meiguihua (Rose Flower) 6 g is first immersed in water over a strong fire until it is boiled and then decocted over aslow fire for half an hour. Finally, crystal sugar is added. The decoction is used for esophagitis due to qi stagnation with phlegm.

## Other Therapies

Dietary therapy:

(1) A big fresh carp is stuffed with Chenpi (Dried Tangerine Peel) 9 g and Gongdingxiang (Flos Caryophylli) 3 g and boiled in clear water to make soup. The fish and soup are consumed at different times in a consecutive manner. It is used to treat esophagitis in early stage.
(2) 200 ml of warmed cow's milk or warmed soyabean milk is taken twice a day, in the morning and evening.

## Cautions and Advice

1. Patients should avoid lying flat after meals and should raise their heads and chests during sleep as well as loosen their belts so as to reduce abdominal pressure.

2. They should also adopt a light, low-fat diet and have more meals a day but less food for each meal; the drinks and food consumed should not be too hot, sour or sweet and consumption of cigarettes, alcohol or coffee is prohibited.

## Daily Exercises

1. Recall the diagnostic key points of reflux esophagitis.
2. Briefly describe the different patterns of reflux esophagitis.

# Esophageal Cancer
# Week 5: Tuesday

Esophageal cancer refers to the malignancy of the squamous cells lining the inside of the esophagus, clinically marked by progressive dysphagia and pain in the region posterior to the sternum. This disease frequently occurs in the three physiological narrows of the esophagus, with the middle segment being the most common, the lower part less common and the upper part the least common. In TCM, esophageal cancer corresponds to "obstructive ingestion".

## Etiology and Pathology

The location of this disease is the esophagus which is governed by the stomach qi. The main pathological changes are stenosis of the esophagus and the mechanism is closely associated with disorders of the stomach, spleen, liver and kidneys. The branches (secondary aspects) of this disease are qi stagnation, phlegm accumulation and blood coagulation, while the root (primary aspect) lies in deficiency of the healthy qi. In many cases, excessive worry and contemplation exhaust the spleen and stagnate the spleen qi, which then fails to distribute the body fluid, leading to the accumulation of phlegm and obstruction by phlegm and qi inside the esophagus. Outbursts of depressed rage damages the liver, causing depression of the liver, stagnation of qi and accumulation of blood, all of which may contribute to the obstruction of the esophagus. Alcohol abuse and excessive intake of fatty and sweet food causes a predisposition to esophageal stenosis by producing turbid phlegm. Indulgence in spicy or dry-natured food can lead to an inadequacy of body fluid and blood and the resultant pharyngeal dryness. Furthermore, chronic diseases often involve the kidneys in the end, bringing about deficiency of yin and yang and posing a serious threat to life.

## Diagnostic Key Points

1. In the early stage, there are such symptoms as obstructing sensation after ingestion of food, pain in the region posterior to the sternum or below the xiphoid process, sense of food retention or foreign body

obstruction, throat dryness or striction and the resultant reflux of food and progressive dysphagia; in the late stage there is a hoarse voice, esophageal bleeding and cachexia.

2. X-ray barium meal examination shows stiffened esophageal wall and a narrowed, irregular esophageal lumen; retention of barium at the point where the tumor arises from and thinned stream of barium throughout the narrowed segment.
3. Esophagofiberoscope makes it possible to examine the morphous of the tumors under direct observation and also make it available for biopsy.
4. The positive result of exfoliative cytological examination on the esophageal mucosa may serve as a definitive diagnosis.
5. CT scan on the esophagus reveals the size of esophageal tumors, the scope of invasion and the degree of infiltration.

## Syndrome Differentiation

### 1. Obstruction of mixed phlegm and qi

Symptoms: Obstructing sensation during ingestion of food, stuffiness and sensation of fullness in the chest which is aggravated by emotional stimulation, vomiting of sputum and saliva, dry mouth and throat, belching and hiccuping; a slightly red tongue with thin, greasy coating and a thin, taut and slippery pulse.

Analysis of symptoms: Simultaneous obstruction of phlegm and qi gives rise to an obstructing sensation while ingestion, stuffiness and fullness in the chest is aggravated by emotional stimulation and the vomiting of sputum and saliva; retained phlegm and qi block the upward flow of fluid, or stagnated heat consumes the fluid, bringing about dryness of the mouth and throat; belching and hiccuping are suggestive of the adverse rising of stomach qi; a slightly red tongue with thin, greasy coating and a thin, taut and slippery pulse are manifestations of stagnated qi, phlegm and heat.

### 2. Accumulation of heat with depletion of yin

Symptoms: Difficulty in swallowing, scorching pain in the chest and diaphragm, difficult ingestion of solid food (but not water and soup), progressive weight loss, thirst, dry stools, a feverish sensation over the five centers (the palms, the soles and the heart), hectic fever and night sweats; reddish or fissured tongue with scanty coating and thin, rapid and taut pulse.

Analysis of symptoms: The yin fluid of the stoma is too deficient to moisten the esophagus, leading to difficulty in swallowing that is accompanied by burning pain; thirst and dry stools are due to the depletion of fluid in the stomach and intestine as a result of an accumulation of heat; the feverish sensations over the five centers (the palms, the soles and the heart), hectic fever and night sweats are attributable to the deficiency of kidney yin ensurng from the insufficiency of stomach fluid; a reddish or fissured tongue with scanty coating and a thin, rapid and taut pulse are indicative of accumulated heat with depletion of yin.

## 3. Obstruction of the diaphragm by blood stasis

Symptoms: Pricking pain behind the sternum in a fixed location, difficulty in swallowing, or instant vomiting after ingestion (with the ejected contents resembling red soyabean milk), dry and stiff stools, severe emaciation, dry skin and muscles and a dark, lusterless complexion; cyanosed tongue with greasy coating and thin, unsmooth pulse.

Analysis of symptoms: Internal accumulation of blood stasis leads to esophageal obstruction, so there is a pricking pain behind the sternum, difficulty in swallowing, or instant vomiting after ingestion; the collaterals are damaged and the blood is oozing out, so the ejected contents resemble red soyabean milk; chronic disease consumes the yin blood and dries the intestinal tract, bringing about the dry and stiff; long-term poor food intake depletes the source of qi and blood, resulting in severe emaciation with dry skin and muscles; the dark, lusterless complexion, cyanosed tongue with greasy coating and thin, unsmooth pulse are all attributable to internal accumulation of blood stasis.

## 4. Decline of yang qi

Symptoms: Long-term poor intake of water and food, listlessness, physical coldness, shortness of breath, regurgitation of clear fluid, facial edema and swollen limbs, gastric and abdominal distension and a grayish-white complexion; pale tongue with white coating and thin and feeble pulse or thin and deep pulse.

Analysis of symptoms: Chronic disease consumes the yin fluid, which also affects the yang qi in the end, leading to weakness of the spleen yang and depletion of the source for production and transformation, giving rise to a long-term poor intake of water and food, listlessness and regurgitation of clear fluid; the kidney yang is declined, bringing about facial edema and swollen limbs, as well as gastric and abdominal distension; the primordial yang is debilitated, giving rise to a grayish-white complexion, coldness of the body, shortness of breath, pale tongue with white coating and thin and feeble pulse or thin and deep pulse.

## Differential Treatment

### 1. Obstruction of mixed phlegm and qi

Treatment principle: Regulating qi and relieving depression, moistening the mouth and throat and dissolving phlegm.

Prescription and herbs: Modified Qige Powder.

Danshen (Radix Salviae Miltiorrhiae) 9 g, Yujin (Turmeric Root Tuber) 9 g, Sharen (Villous Amomum Fruit) 3 g, Beishashen (Coastal Glehnia Root) 9 g, Chuanbei (Tendrilleaf Fritillary Bulb) 3 g, Fuling (Indian Bread) 12 g, Heyedi (Hindu Lotus Leaf-base) 5 leaf-bases, Gualou (Snakegourd Fruit) 12 g, Chenpi (Dried Tangerine Peel) 6 g and Xiakucao (Common Selfheal Fruit-Spike) 9 g.

Modification: For vomiting with sputum and saliva, belching, or severe hiccups, Xuanfuhua (Intussusceer) 12 g, Daizheshi (Red Bole) 30 g, Zhuru (Bamboo Shavings) 9 g and Jiangbanxia (Ginger-prepared Pinellia Tuber) 9 g are added to reinforce the action of dissolving phlegm and curbing vomiting.

### 2. Accumulation of heat with depletion of yin

Treatment principle: Nourishing yin to produce fluid.

Prescription and herbs: Wuzhi Anzhong Potion.

Lizhi (Pear Juice), Ouzhi (Lotus Root Juice) and Niuru (Cow's Milk) are added to a small amount of Shengjiangzhi (Fresh Ginger Juice) and Jiucaizhi (Chinese Chive Juice). The mixed juices are taken in a small quantity for each dose, but at many different times within a day.

Modification: If there is severe consumption of yin and fluid, equal quantities (9 g each) of Xuanshen (Figwort Root), Maidong (Dwarf Lilyturf Tuber), Beishashen (Coastal Glehnia Root), Shengdi (Dried Rehmannia Root), Shudi (Prepared Rhizome of Rehmannia) and Shihu (Dendrobium) are added to simultaneously nourish the stomach and kidneys.

## 3. Obstruction of the diaphragm by blood stasis

Treatment principle: Dissolving phlegm and breaking nodules, relieving stagnation and resolving stasis.

Prescription and herbs: Modified Banxia Houpu Decoction and Tongyou Decoction.

Banxia (Pinellia Tuber) 9 g, Houpu (Magnolia Bark) 9 g, Zisu (Purple Common Perilla) 9 g, Fuling (Indian Bread) 12 g, Shengdi (Dried Rehmannia Root) 12 g, Danggui (Chinese Angelica) 9 g, Taoren (Peach Seed) 9 g, Honghua (Safflower) 6 g and Gancao (Liquorice Root) 6 g.

Modification: If there is severe blood stasis, Shensanqi (Panax Pseudo-Ginseng) 9 g, Sanleng (Common Burreed Tuber) 9 g and Ezhu (Zedoray Rhizome) 9 g are added to resolve stasis and dissipate stagnation.

## 4. Decline of yang qi

Treatment principle: Replenishing qi to invigorate the spleen, warming yang to nourish the kidneys.

Prescription and herbs: Supplementary Buqi Yunpi Decoction and Yougui Pill.

Dangshen (Radix Codonopsis) 15 g, Huangqi (Milkvetch Root) 15 g, Baizhu (Largehead Atractylodes Rhizome) 9 g, Fuling (Indian Bread) 12 g, Banxia (Pinellia Tuber) 9 g, Chenpi (Dried Tangerine Peel) 6 g, Shudi (Prepared Rhizome of Rehmannia) 12 g, Shanzhuyu (Asiatic

Cornelian Cherry Fruit) 6 g, Danggui (Chinese Angelica) 9 g, Gouqizi (Barbary Wolfberry Fruit) 12 g, Lujiaojiao (Deerhorn Glue) 12 g, Rougui (Cassia Bark) 3 g, Fuzi (Prepared Common Monkshood Daughter) 9 g, Duzhong (Eucommia Bark) 9 g and Gancao (Liquorice Root) 6 g.

Modification: If there is severe vomiting, Xuanfuhua (Intussusceer) 12 g, Daizheshi (Red Bole) 30 g and Jiangzhuru (Ginger-prepared Bamboo Shavings) 9 g are added to curb vomiting.

## Chinese Patent Medicine

1. Chansu Pill: 5 pills for each dose, twice a day. It is administered with warm boiled water.
2. Pingxiao Capsule: 8 capsules for each dose, 3 times a day. It is administered (only the powders contained in the capsule are taken) with warm boiled water.

## Simple and Handy Prescriptions

1. Weilingxian (Chinese Clematis Root) 50 g, Banzhilian (Barbated Skullcup Herb) 50 g, Shijianchuan (Chinese Sage) 50 g and Jixingzi 50 g are decocted into medicated juice. The juice is made into porridge to be taken within a day at different times.
2. Liushen Pill (100 pills) and Yushu Pellet (30 g) are ground up into fine powders and then glutinous rice and honey are added so the mixture can be made into, pills. They are orally administered 4 times a day for 5 consecutive days.

## Other Therapies

Dietary therapy:

(1) Goose blood 100 ml is taken while it is hot. It is administered once a day for 10 consecutive days. The goose blood can also be made into soup with pepper added to taste. If goose blood is not available, chicken blood or duck blood is also applicable.

(2) Equal quantities of Nuomi powder (Glutinous Rice) and Shanyao powder (Common Yan Rhizome) are mixed evenly with white sugar and a little pepper. It can be consumed several times.

If the disease is discovered early, surgery should be performed as early as possible once it is considered appropriate after evaluating the patient's condition.

## Cautions and Advice

1. Patients should take more meals a day but eat smaller amounts at each meal. The food should be soft, semi-fluid, or totally fluid and at a moderate temperature and the same applies for the herbal decoction mentioned above.
2. Patients should also consume more fresh food that is rich in protein and vitamins.

## Daily Exercises

1. Concisely introduce the diagnostic key points of esophageal cancer.
2. Explain how esophageal cancer can be treated based on syndrome differentiation.

# Peptic Ulcer

# Week 5: Wednesday

Peptic ulcer refers primarily to the open sores that develop on the inside lining (the mucous membrane) of the esophagus, stomach and the upper portion of the small intestine (the duodenum) due to caustic action of the gastric digestive juice. Clinically it is characterized mainly by repeated, periodic and rhythmic pain in the middle and upper belly that is associated with food intake. It may also be accompanied by acid regurgitation, gastric upset, belching, nausea, vomiting and even hematemesis, hemafecia, perforation, pyloric obstruction and cancerization. This disease can afflict people of any age, especially young and middle-aged males. In TCM, it is closely related to "stomachache", "vomiting" and "acid regurgitation".

## Etiology and Pathology

This disease arises from the stomach and may also be indirectly attributed to the liver and spleen. Excessive worry, contemplation or anger may encumber the liver and stagnate qi and since the liver fails to maintain the normal flow of qi, the stomach will be affected by the outburst of depressed liver qi; the stomach fails in its descending function, and the result is stomach pain. If the liver qi is persistently stagnated, it can transform into fire which subsequently damages yin, thereby aggravating the stomach pain and prolonging the disease course. Besides, long-term stagnation of qi can also hamper the smooth circulation of blood or cause internal accumulation of blood stasis, bringing about persistent or lingering pain. Further more, stomach pain often stems from deficiency of the middle energizer which is due to innate weakness of the spleen and stomach, overstrain, or damage to the spleen and stomach by chronic diseases.

## Diagnostic Key Points

1. Repeated, periodic and rhythmic pain in the middle and upper belly. The ache due to gastric ulcer usually takes place within 1 hour after meals at the right side of the middle and upper belly, the left side of the

subxiphoid, or the region below the xiphoid process. The ache due to duodenal ulcer generally occurs between meals in the middle and upper belly, or the right side of the region above the umbilicus. The ache is marked by a dull, scorching pain when the stomach is empty.

2. Other symptoms or physical signs: Possible acid regurgitation, gastric upset, abdominal distension, belching, nausea and vomiting. During the onset, there may be localized pain in the middle and upper belly.
3. Endoscopy is a definitive diagnostic approach to peptic ulcer.
4. X-ray barium meal examination shows mainly crater or niche sign and occasionally deformity or irritation of the duodenum.
5. Gastric analysis may point to an increase of basal acid output (BAO) in patients with peptic ulcer.
6. A positive result may suggest helicobacter pylori infection.

## Syndrome Differentiation

### 1. Liver qi invading the stomach

Symptoms: Distension, fullness or pain in the gastric cavity which may involve the hypochondria, alleviation after belching, aggravation on emotional depression, acid regurgitation, chest distress, frequent sighing and poor appetite; a white tongue with thin coating and a taut pulse.

Analysis of symptoms: Emotional depression may encumber the liver and stagnate qi and since the liver fails to maintain the normal flow of qi, the stomach will be affected by the outburst of depressed liver qi; the stomach fails in its descending fuction and the result is stomach pain; the disorder of qi is characterized by migration, so there is pain involving the hypochondria and alleviation after belching; functional disorder of qi leads to failure of the stomach qi to descend normally manifested as chest distress, frequent sighing, acid regurgitation and poor appetite; the taut pulse points to disorder of the liver with pain.

### 2. Stagnation of heat in liver and stomach

Symptoms: Intense scorching pain in the gastric cavity triggered by intake of food, acid regurgitation, dry sensation or a bitter taste in the mouth, restlessness, irascibility and constipation; a red tongue with yellow coating and a rapid, taut pulse.

Analysis of symptoms: If the liver qi is persistently stagnated, it will transform into fire which subsequently invades the stomach and impair the descending function of the stomach, thus resulting in a burning pain in the gastric cavity, acid regurgitation and gastric upset; hyperactivity of fire in the liver and gallbladder is marked by a dry sensation or bitter taste in the mouth, restlessness, irascibility, constipation, red tongue with yellow coating, as well as rapid and taut pulse.

## 3. Insufficiency of stomach yin

Symptoms: Vague stomachache that is aggravated by hunger, a dry mouth and throat, thirst, feverish sensations over the five centers (the palms, the soles and the heart), hunger with no appetite, or poor appetite, frequent retching and dry stools; a red, dry and fissured tongue with scanty or incompletely peeled coating and a thin, rapid pulse.

Analysis of symptoms: Stagnated heat damages yin and malnourishes the stomach collaterals, so there is vague stomachache; deficiency of yin produces internal heat, with such signs as dry mouth and throat, thirst and feverish sensation over the five centers (the palms, the soles and the heart); the stomach qi fails to descend normally, so there is hunger with no appetite, or poor appetite and frequent retching; the large intestine is deficient in fluid, giving rise to dry stools; the red, dry tongue with scanty or incompletely peeled coating and thin, rapid pulse are manifestations of stomachache due to deficiency of yin.

## 4. Deficient cold in the spleen and stomach

Symptoms: Vague stomachache alleviated by pressure and warmth, reduced food intake, vomiting of clear saliva, loose stools, lassitude, listlessness and intolerance of cold with cold limbs; pale enlarged tongue and thin, deep and slow pulse.

Analysis of symptoms: Deficient cold in the spleen and stomach leads to a lack of warmth and nutrition in the collaterals, bringing about vague stomachache; the pain is caused by deficiency and cold, so it can be alleviated by pressure and warmth; dysfunction of the spleen in transportation and transformation results in retention of water and fluid in the stomach, with a result of reduced food intake, vomiting of clear saliva and loose stools; the spleen dominates the muscles and four limbs, so if the spleen yang is inactivated, there will be lassitude, listlessness and intolerance of cold, as well as cold limbs; the pale enlarged tongue and thin, deep and slow pulse are manifestations of inactivated spleen yang with deficient cold in the middle energizer.

## Differential Treatment

### 1. Liver qi invading the stomach

Treatment principle: Soothing the liver and regulating qi.

Prescription and herbs: Supplementary Chaihu Shugan Powder.

Chaihu (Chinese Thorowax Root) 6 g, Zhiqiao (Orange Fruit) 15 g, Xiangfu (Nutgrass Galingale Rhizome) 12 g, Xiangyuan (Citron Fruit) 9 g, Foshou (Finger Citron) 6 g, Luyuemei (Flos Mume) 9 g, Baishao (White Peony Alba) 9 g, Chuanxiong (Szechwan Lovage Rhizome) 6 g, Chenpi (Dried Tangerine Peel) 6 g, Gancao (Liquorice Root) 6 g and Waleng (Calcined Concha Arcae) 30 g.

Modification: If the patient presents with severe pain, Chuanlianzi (Szechwan Chinaberry Fruit) 9 g, Yanhusuo (Corydalis) 9 g and Muxiang (Common Aucklandia Root) 6 g are added to regulate qi and alleviate pain.

### 2. Stagnation of heat in liver and stomach

Treatment principle: Harmonizing the stomach and purging heat.

Prescription and herbs: Supplementary Huagan Decoction.

Chenpi (Dried Tangerine Peel) 9 g, Qingpi (Green Tangerine Peel) 9 g, Yanhusuo (Corydalis) 9 g, Baishao (White Peony Alba) 9 g, Zhizi (Cape Jasmine Fruit) 9 g, Danpi (Cortex Moutan) 9 g, Huanglian (Golden Thread) 3 g, Wuzhuyu (Medicinal Evodia Fruit) 2 g, Dahuang (Rhubarb)

6 g, Duanwaleng (Calcined Concha Arcae) 30 g and Gancao (Liquorice Root) 6 g.

Modification: If the pain is relieved but the liver and stomach still in disorder, modified Danzhi Xiaoyao Powder can be used to dispel heat and relieve stagnation.

### 3. Insufficiency of stomach yin

Treatment principle: Invigorating the stomach and nourishing yin.

Prescription and herbs: Modified Yiguan Decoction and Shaoyao Gancao Decoction.

Beishashen (Coastal Glehnia Root) 12 g, Maidong (Dwarf Lilyturf Tuber) 12 g, Shengdi (Dried Rehmannia Root) 12 g, Shihu (Dendrobium) 9 g, Danggui (Chinese Angelica) 9 g, Chuanlianzi (Szechwan Chinaberry Fruit) 9 g, Yanhusuo (Corydalis) 9 g, Huomaren (Hemp Seed) 15 g, Baishao (White Peony Alba) 30 g and Gancao (Liquorice Root) 6 g.

Modification: For severe stomach pain, Foshou (Finger Citron) 9 g, Bayuezha (Fiveleaf Akebia Fruit) 12 g and Xiangyuanpi (Citron Fruit Peel) 12 g are added to reinforce the action of regulating qi without damaging yin; if there are dry stools, Shengshouwu (Unprepared Fleeceflower Root) 30 g and Yuliren (Chinese Dwarf Cherry Seed) 9 g are used to moisten the intestine and promote defecation.

### 4. Deficient cold in the spleen and stomach

Treatment principle: Invigorating the spleen and warming the interior.

Prescription and herbs: Modified Huangqi Jianzhong Decoction and Liangfu Pill.

Huangqi (Milkvetch Root) 15 g, Dangshen (Radix Codonopsis) 15 g, Baizhu (Largehead Atractylodes Rhizome) 9 g, Guizhi (Cassia Twig) 6 g, Baishao (White Peony Alba) 18 g, Yitang (Cerealose) 30 g, Gaoliangjiang (Lesser Galangal Rhizome) 9 g, Xiangfu (Nutgrass Galingale Rhizome) 12 g and Gancao (Liquorice Root) 6 g.

Modification: For vomiting of profuse clear water, Banxia (Pinellia Tuber) 9 g, Chenpi (Dried Tangerine Peel) 6 g and Fuling (Indian Bread) 12 g can be added to harmonize the stomach, dissolve phlegm and reverse the adverse rising of qi; if there is hemafecia, Huangtu Decoction can be applied to warm the interior and stop bleeding.

## Chinese Patent Medicine

1. Jiangwei Yuyang Tablet: 3~4 tablets for each dose, 3 times a day to treat peptic ulcer with gastric hypersecretion.
2. Hougujun Tablet: 4 tablets for each dose, 3 times a day.

## Simple and Handy Prescriptions

1. Duanwaleng (Calcined Concha Arcae) 150 g, Xiangbeimu (Tendrilleaf Fritillary Bulb) 60 g and Gancao (Liquorice Root) 30 g are ground up into fine powders and swallowed (5 g for each dose) 3 times a day. This prescription is used to treat peptic ulcer with stomach pain and acid regurgitation.
2. Baiji (Common Bletilla Tuber) and Dahuang (Rhubarb) are combined in the ratio of 3:1 and then ground up into fine powders which are sieved before administration. They are taken orally (3 g for each dose) 3~4 times a day for peptic ulcer with bleeding.

## Other Therapies

Dietary therapy:

(1) Cow's milk or soyabean milk 200 ml is boiled and then taken while it is still warm. This is conducted in the morning and evening when the stomach is empty.
(2) Wuzeiyu (Cuttlefish) 500 g is boiled in water and after it is ready, the fish can be taken, but at different times. The bones, or Wuzeigu (Cuttlefish bone), are fried till they are brittle and then cooked in water with Jiangmi (Rice Fruit) 100 g to make porridge.

If there is hematemesis and hemafecia, it is advisable to stop bleeding first; for incessant bleeding, it is appropriate to adopt surgical treatment.

## Cautions and Advice

1. Patients should avoid emotional stimulation, overstrain, irregular lifestyle, tobacco consumption and alcohol abuse.
2. They should consume nutritious yet easily digested food, taking more frequent but smaller meals. They should also cultivate the habit of chewing and swallowing slowly, take meals at fixed times, avoid excessive food intake and avoid coarse, uncooked, cold or hot drinks and foods, as well as spicy, sour and sweet ones. Besides, coffee, strong tea or other stimulating beverages should also be abstained from.

## Daily Exercises

1. Recall the diagnostic key points of peptic ulcer.
2. Explain how peptic ulcer can be treated based on syndrome differentiation.

# Chronic Gastritis

# Week 5: Thursday

Chronic gastritis refers to the long-term inflammation or atrophy of the gastric mucosa due to different etiological factors. It is in essence a restructuring of the gastric mucosa (which is capable of regeneration) due to repeated damages to the gastric epithelium, eventually resulting in an irreversible atrophy or disappearance of the original gastric glands. Clinically this disease is marked by pain in the upper epigastric zone, gastric and abdominal distension, heartburn, nausea, vomiting and poor appetite. As a frequently encountered disease, it generally afflicts men more often than women. In TCM, chronic gastritis is closely associated with the disorders of "stomachache" or "stomach stuffiness".

## Etiology and Pathology

The location of this disease is the stomach and the occurrence of it is closely related to the liver, spleen and stomach, etc. The etiological factors are mainly improper diet and emotional disorder. To be specific, indulgence in alcohol consumption as well as raw, cold and spicy foods can damage the spleen and stomach; excessive worry and contemplation impairs the spleen and uncurbed rage injures the liver (which subsequently causes disharmony between the liver and stomach as well), both of which will lead to this disease; if the disease progresses further, or when the stagnated qi transforms into fire, the stomach yin may be damaged, bringing about dryness in the stomach and dysfunction in descent; moreover, if the spleen yang is deficient, it will fail to warm the body and if some diseases persist, the collaterals or vessels may be obstructed; in either case there may eventually be abnormal ascending and descending of the spleen qi and stomach qi.

## Diagnostic Key Points

1. Chronic gastritis has no pathognomonic symptoms, the severity of which is not consistent with the degree of gastric mucosal lesions.

Most patients present with no symptoms or symptoms of dyspepsia in varying degrees, such as vague pain in the epigastric zone, decreased appetite, gastric or abdominal fullness and distension, heartburn, nausea and vomiting. Patients with atrophic gastritis may also experience anaemia, emaciation, glossitis and diarrhea. There is still a small number of patients experience mucosal erosion, apparent abdominal pain and bleeding.

2. Gastroscopy is the main approach to determining chronic gastritis.
3. Laboratory examination

(1) Gastric acidity determination: Normal or lowered gastric acid level in superficial gastritis and apparent decrease or even absence of gastric acid in the case of atrophic gastritis.

(2) Serum gastrin determination: Normal secretion in antral gastritis, increased production in inflammation of the stomach body and pronounced elevation in the case of malignant anaemia.

(3) Helicobacter pylori examination: Positive result points to a helicobacter pylori infection.

## Syndrome Differentiation

## 1. Mixture of dampness and heat

Symptoms: Burning pain in the gastric cavity, abdominal distension, nausea, retching, thirst, a bitter taste in the mouth and foul breath, yellowish urine, intestinal gurgling sounds, loose stools or constipation; red tongue with crimson tip and margins, yellow, greasy tongue coating and slippery, rapid pulse.

Analysis of symptoms: Internal accumulation of dampness and heat inhibits the smooth functional activity of qi, so there is burning pain in the gastric cavity and abdominal distension; adverse rising of stomach qi results in nausea and retching; internal abundance of dampness and heat blocks the upward flow of body fluid, resulting in thirst, a bitter taste in the mouth and foul breath; damp-heat pours downward and it marked by yellowish urine; damp-heat also impairs the intestinal tract, leading to dysfunction in transportation and transformation, giving rise to intestinal gurgling sounds, loose stools or constipation; the red tongue with crimson tip and margins, yellow, greasy tongue coating and slippery, rapid pulse are manifestations of internal accumulation of dampness and heat.

## 2. Qi stagnation of the liver and stomach

Symptoms: Pain in the gastric cavity involving the hypochondria, distending sensation aggravated by food intake, belching, gastric upset, nausea, vomiting and acid regurgitation; a reddish tongue with white and thin coating and a taut pulse.

Analysis of symptoms: Failure of the liver to promote the free flow of qi impairs the smooth functional activity of qi and is marked by pain in the gastric cavity involving the hypochondria; the liver qi invades the stomach transversely, making the stomach qi fail to descend normally, with distension aggravated by food intake, belching, gastric upset, nausea, vomiting and acid regurgitation; the reddish tongue with white, thin coating and taut pulse are due to qi stagnation of the liver and stomach.

## 3. Deficient cold in the spleen and stomach

Symptoms: Vague stomachache alleviated by warmth and pressure, gastric distension after food intake, vomiting of clear saliva, a reduced appetite, diarrhea, soreness and flaccidity in the four limbs, intolerance of cold with desire for warmth and a lusterless complexion; a reddish tongue with white, thin coating and a thin, feeble pulse or thin, deep pulse.

Analysis of symptoms: Yang deficiency of the spleen and stomach leads to lack of warmth in the collaterals, so there is a vague pain in the stomach; since the pain is deficient in nature, it can be relieved by pressure and because there is the presence of cold, the pain is often alleviated by warmth; owing to the invasion of deficient cold, the spleen becomes deficient and retains water and fluid in the stomach, this is marked by food-triggered distension, vomiting of clear saliva, a reduced appetite and diarrhea; the spleen dominates the four limbs, so if the spleen is deficient, there will be sourness and flaccidity in the four limbs; deficient yang produces internal cold, thus giving rise to an intolerance of cold and desire for warmth; the lusterless complexion, reddish tongue with white, thin coating and thin, feeble pulse or thin, deep pulse are suggestive of cold in the middle energizer with inactivation of spleen yang.

## 4. Insufficiency of stomach yin

Symptoms: Vague stomachache, hunger without appetite, gastric distension after food intake, retching, belching, a dry mouth, a sensation of thirst with preference for cold drinks and dry stools; red, dry and fissured tongue and thin, rapid pulse.

Analysis of symptoms: The stomach yin is damaged and the stomach collaterals are malnourished, resulting in the vague stomachache and sensation of hunger without appetite; the stomach qi fails to descend normally, so there is gastric distension after food intake, accompanied by retching and belching; is deficient and the body fluid is inadequate, resulting in a dry mouth, sensation of thirst and preference for cold drink; the intestines fails to be moistened, presenting as dry stools; the red, dry and fissured tongue and thin, rapid pulse are manifestations of deficient yin.

## 5. Obstruction of stomach collaterals by stasis

Symptoms: Pricking, localized and tender pain in the stomach, bloody black stools; dark red tongue with ecchymosis and thin, unsmooth pulse.

Analysis of symptoms: Stagnation of qi gives rise to blood stasis, causing the pricking, localized and unpressable pain in the stomach; the blood vessels are damaged, as reflected by the bloody black stools; the dark red tongue with ecchymosis and thin, unsmooth pulse are attributable to internal accumulation of blood stasis.

## Differential Treatment

### 1. Mixture of dampness and heat

Treatment principle: Dispelling heat and resolving dampness, harmonizing the middle and alleviating pain.

Prescription and herbs: Modified Banxia Xiexin Decoction.

Banxia (Pinellia Tuber) 9 g, Huangqin (Baical Skullcap Root) 9 g, Huanglian (Golden Thread) 3 g, Pugongying (Dandelion) 30 g, Dangshen (Radix Codonopsis) 12 g, Dazao (Chinese Date) 15 g, Duanwaleng (Calcined Concha Arcae) 30 g and Gancao (Stir-baked Liquorice Root) 6 g.

Modification: If the patient presents with stomach distension, Zhiqiao (Orange Fruit) 15 g is added to regulate qi; if the dampness is relatively severe, Huoxiang (Agastache Rugosa) 9 g and Houpu (Magnolia Bark) 6 g can be added to resolve dampness.

## 2. Qi stagnation of the liver and stomach

Treatment principle: Soothing the liver and regulating qi, harmonizing the stomach and alleviating pain.

Prescription and herbs: Modified Chaihu Shugan Powder and Jinlingzi Powder.

Zhiqiao (Orange Fruit) 15 g, Chaihu (Chinese Thorowax Root) 6 g, Xiangfu (Nutgrass Galingale Rhizome) 9 g, Baishao (White Peony Alba) 9 g, Chuanxiong (Szechwan Lovage Rhizome) 6 g, Chuanlianzi (Szechwan Chinaberry Fruit) 9 g, Yanhusuo (Corydalis) 9 g, Waleng (Concha Arcae) 30 g, Chenpi (Dried Tangerine Peel) 6 g and Gancao (Liquorice Root) 6 g.

Modification: If there is a dry and bitter sensation in the mouth, Zuojin Pill 6 g can be added to disperse stagnant qi and reverse the adverse rising of qi.

## 3. Deficient cold in the spleen and stomach

Treatment principle: Warming the middle energizer and dissipating cold, invigorating the spleen and stomach and promoting digestion.

Prescription and herbs: Modified Xiangsha Liujunzi Decoction and Fuzi Lizhong Pill.

Dangshen (Radix Codonopsis) 15 g, Baizhu (Largehead Atractylodes Rhizome) 12 g, Fuling (Indian Bread) 12 g, Chenpi (Dried Tangerine Peel) 6 g, Banxia (Pinellia Tuber) 9 g, Muxiang (Common Aucklandia Root) 9 g, Sharen (Villous Amomum Fruit) 3 g, Fuzi (Prepared Common Monkshood

Daughter) 6 g, Ganjiang (Dried Ginger) 6 g and Gancao (Liquorice Root) 6 g.

Modification: For listlessness, Huangqi (Milkvetch Root) 15 g can be added to reinforce the effect of nourishing qi; if there is a reduced appetite, Jineijin (Corium Stomachium Galli) 6 g is added to facilitate digestion.

## 4. Insufficiency of stomach yin

Treatment principle: Nourishing yin and invigorating the stomach.

Prescription and herbs: Modified Yeshi Yangwei Decoction.

Beishashen (Coastal Glehnia Root) 9 g, Maidong (Dwarf Lilyturf Tuber) 9 g, Shihu (Dendrobium) 15 g, Baishao (White Peony Alba) 9 g, Biandou (Hyacinth Bean) 9 g, Wumei (Smoked Plum) 3 g, Pugongying (Dandelion) 15 g, Muxiang (Common Aucklandia Root) 6 g, Huomaren (Hemp Seed) 9 g and Gancao (Liquorice Root) 6 g.

Modification: If there is a distending pain in the stomach and belching, Bayuezha (Fiveleaf Akebia Fruit) 12 g, Foshou (Finger Citron) 6 g and Luyuemei (Flos Mume) 9 g are added to reinforce the action of regulating qi without damaging yin.

## 5. Obstruction of stomach collaterals by stasis

Treatment principle: Activating blood and resolving stasis, dredging the collaterals and harmonizing the stomach.

Prescription and herbs: Modified Shixiao Powder and Huoluo Xiaoling Pellet.

Wulingzhi (Faeces Trogopterorum) 9 g (wrapped during decoction), Puhuang (Pollen Typhae) 9 g, Danshen (Radix Salviae Miltiorrhiae) 15 g, Ruxiang (Boswellin) 6 g, Muoyao (Myrrh) 6 g, Yujin (Turmeric Root Tuber) 9 g, Danggui (Chinese Angelica) 9 g and Chenpi (Dried Tangerine Peel) 6 g.

Modification: If there are black stools, Shensanqi (Panax Pseudo-ginseng) 9 g, Huaruishi (Ophicalcite) 15 g and Diyutan (Charred Radix Sanguisorbae)

12 g are added to stop bleeding; for vomiting of blood, Baijifen (Common Bletilla Tuber Powder) 3 g can be added to check bleeding.

## Chinese Patent Medicine

1. Weisu Soluble Granule: 1 small bag for each dose, 3 times a day. It is used to treat chronic gastritis due to disharmony between the liver and stomach.
2. Weifuchun Tablet: 4 tablets for each dose, 3 times a day. It is used to treat chronic gastritis or atrophic gastritis.
3. Yangwei Soluble Granule: 1 small bag for each dose, 3 times a day. It is used to treat chronic gastritis due to weakness of the spleen and stomach.

## Simple and Handy Prescriptions

1. Fresh turnip 200 g is pounded and the juice is extracted. After being warmed in boiling water, the juice can be drunk several times a day to treat chronic gastritis with abdominal distension and poor appetite.
2. Fresh hawthorn fruit is pounded and the juice is extracted. 50 ml of the juice is blended evenly with honey and taken slowly several times a day. It is used for atrophic gastritis.
3. Baihuashecao (Hedyotic Diffusa), Baqia (Bamboo brier), Jiangcan (Stiff Silkworm) and Bihu (House Lizard) are mixed in the ratio of 5:6:1.5:0.1 (120 g in total). The mixed medicinals are boiled in water into a decoction (150 ml), which is taken (50 ml for each dose) 3 times a day. A course of treatment lasts 3 months. It is used for atrophic gastritis with intestinal metaplasia.

## Other Therapies

Dietary therapy:

(1) Cow's milk 200 ml is boiled and taken before sleep for long-term administration. Madzoon 50 ml is warmed in boiling water and taken twice a day when the stomach is empty; a small amount of Yitang

(Cerealose) can be added occasionally. Both liquids can be used to treat atrophic gastritis.

(2) Sugarcane juice 100 ml is taken in the morning and evening, twice a day. It is used to treat atrophic gastritis or chronic gastritis with damage of stomach yin.

## Cautions and Advice

1. Patients should avoid cigarettes and alcohol and take initiative to prevent and treat anaemia.
2. It is advisable for patients to consume easily digestible food and have smaller but more frequent meals in a day. They should also avoid spicy, stomach-irritating foods or drugs, as well as fried, roasted, smoked, milk-based or salt-preserved products. Instead, oranges or hawthorn fruit are recommended to stimulate gastric acid production.
3. Chronic superficial inflammation of the stomach is generally characterized by a favorable prognosis, but in a few cases it may progress into an atrophic one.

## Daily Exercises

1. Recall the diagnostic key points of chronic gastritis.
2. Explain how chronic gastritis can be treated based on syndrome differentiation.

# Gastroptosis

# Week 5: Friday

Gastroptosis is a disease marked by downward displacement of the stomach. In other words, when the patient stands, the location of the stomach is below the normal level, with the lower margin of the stomach reaching the cavity of the pelvis and the perigee of lesser curvature descending below the Tuffier's line. Mild cases of gastroptosis are usually asymptomatic, but the severe ones may cause discomfort and distending pain in the epigastric zone, belching, poor appetite and abnormal defecation. In TCM, gastroptosis is closely associated with "stomach stuffiness" and "abdominal distension".

## Etiology and Pathology

The location of this disease is the stomach and the occurrence of it is related to the spleen and stomach. The spleen, as the postnatal foundation, governs transportation and transformation, manages ascent of the lucid substances and dominates the limbs and muscles. Congenital deficiency of primordial qi or postnatal consumption of qi (due to chronic diseases) can affect the spleen and stomach, which fail to transform water and food properly into qi and blood, resulting in malnourishment of the muscles, qi sinking of the middle energizer and, consequently, gastroptosis; In addition, inactivation of spleen yang may be attributed to a yang-deficient constitution and insufficiency of stomach yin can be caused by a yin-deficient physique.

## Diagnostic Key Points

1. Discomfort and fullness in the epigastric zone that is aggravated by prolonged standing and overstrain, or distending pain in the abdomen, belching, nausea, poor appetite, alternated diarrhea and constipation. In severe cases, there may be palpitations and postural hypotension.
2. Subcostal angle < 90°.
3. X-gastrointestinal barium meal examination is of definitive diagnostic value and may indicate a tension-free stomach and the perigee of the lesser curvature descending below the Tuffier's line.

## Syndrome Differentiation

## 1. Qi sinking of the middle energizer

Symptoms: Distending or sinking sensation in the stomach and abdomen that is aggravated upon exertion, lassitude, poor appetite, frequent belching, a pale complexion and emaciation; pale tongue with white, thin coating and thin, soggy pulse or slow, feeble pulse.

Analysis of symptoms: Deficiency of the spleen leads to qi sinking of the middle energizer, resulting in a distending or sinking sensation in the stomach and abdomen that is aggravated upon exertion; deficiency of the spleen also results in inefficient transformation, marked by lassitude and poor appetite; the failure of spleen qi to ascend and stomach qi to descend is responsible for frequent belching; exhaustion of the source for producing qi and blood causes malnutrition of the muscles, giving rise to the pale complexion and physical emaciation; the pale tongue with white, thin coating and thin, soggy pulse or slow, feeble pulse are manifestations of spleen deficiency.

## 2. Inactivation of spleen yang

Symptoms: Distending sensation and occasional vague pain in the stomach and abdomen that is alleviated by warmth but aggravated by prolonged standing or overstrain, intolerance of cold, preference for warmth, poor appetite, nausea, vomiting and loose stools; pale, enlarged tongue with white, thin coating and thin, slow and feeble pulse.

Analysis of symptoms: Inactivation of the spleen qi and yang leads to insufficient lifting action and morbid sinking tendency, marked by a distending sensation and occasional vague pain in the stomach and abdomen that is aggravated by prolonged standing or overstrain; deficient spleen yang is also responsible for intolerance of cold, preference for warmth and alleviation of distension and pain by warmth; inactivation of spleen yang leads to indigestion of water and food, with such symptoms as poor appetite, nausea, vomiting and loose stools; the pale, enlarged tongue with white, thin coating and thin, slow and feeble pulse are attributable to inactivation of spleen yang.

## 3. Deficiency of stomach yin

Symptoms: Gastric and abdominal distension or fullness, feelings of vexation and malaise that are aggravated by meals or overstrain, thirst and a bitter taste in the mouth with foul breath, or retching, constipation and red, dry mouth and lips; reddish tongue with scanty coating and thin, rapid pulse.

Analysis of symptoms: Deficiency of the spleen causes the sinking of qi, so there is gastric and abdominal distension or fullness, vexation and malaise and aggravation by meals or overstrain; deficiency of stomach yin gives rise to the production of deficient heat, which consumes the yin fluid and presents as thirst and a bitter taste in the mouth with foul breath; the stomach qi fails to descend normally, so there is occasional retching; insufficiency of yin fluid inhibits the moistening of the intestines, which is marked by constipation; the red, dry mouth and lips, reddish tongue with scanty coating and thin, rapid pulse are due to deficiency of the stomach yin.

## Differential Treatment

### 1. Qi sinking of the middle energizer

Treatment principle: Nourishing qi to reinforce the lifting action.

Prescription and herbs: Modified Buzhong Yiqi Decoction.

Huangqi (Milkvetch Root) 15 g, Dangshen (Radix Codonopsis) 12 g, Baizhu (Largehead Atractylodes Rhizome) 9 g, Yiyiren (Coix Seed) 30 g, Danggui (Chinese Angelica) 9 g, Chaihu (Chinese Thorowax Root) 6 g, Shengma (Rhizoma Cimicifugae) 6 g, Gegen (Kudzuvine Root) 15 g, Foshou (Finger Citron) 9 g, Chenpi (Dried Tangerine Peel) 9 g and Gancao (Liquorice Root) 6 g.

Modification: For poor appetite, Jineijin (Corium Stomachium Galli) 6 g, Shenqu (Massa Medicata Fermentata) 9 g and Shanzha (Hawthorn Fruit) 12 g are added to facilitate digestion.

### 2. Inactivation of spleen yang

Treatment principle: Warming yang and lifting qi.

Prescription and herbs: Supplementary Lizhong Pill.

Dangshen (Radix Codonopsis) 12 g, Huangqi (Milkvetch Root) 15 g, Baizhu (Largehead Atractylodes Rhizome) 12 g, Ganjiang (Dried Ginger) 9 g, Rougui (Cassia Bark) 9 g, Chaihu (Chinese Thorowax Root) 6 g, Shengma (Rhizoma Cimicifugae) 6 g, Muxiang (Common Aucklandia Root) 6 g, Foshou (Finger Citron) 6 g and Gancao (Liquorice Root) 6 g.

Modification: For poor appetite, Jineijin (Corium Stomachium Galli) 6 g and Shenqu (Massa Medicata Fermentata) 9 g are added to facilitate digestion; if there are loose stools, Shanyao (Common Yan Rhizome) 15 g and Yiyiren (Coix Seed) 15 g can be added to invigorate the spleen as well as check diarrhea.

### 3. Deficiency of stomach yin

Treatment principle: Nourishing yin and harmonizing the stomach.

Prescription and herbs: Modified Yiwei Decoction.

Beishashen (Coastal Glehnia Root) 12 g, Shihu (Dendrobium) 9 g, Maidong (Dwarf Lilyturf Tuber) 12 g, Shengdi (Dried Rehmannia Root) 12 g, Yuzhu (Fragrant Solomonseal Rhizome) 9 g, Chaihu (Chinese Thorowax Root) 6 g, Shengma (Rhizoma Cimicifugae) 6 g, Lugen (Reed Rhizome) 30 g, Huomaren (Hemp Seed) 15 g, Chenpi (Dried Tangerine Peel) 6 g and Gancao (Liquorice Root) 6 g.

Modification: If there is retching, Shidi (Persimmon Calyx) 9 g and Daodouzi (Jack Bean) 12 g are added to reverse the adverse flow of qi and arrest vomiting.

### Chinese Patent Medicine

Buzhong Yiqi Pill: 4.5 g for each dose, 3 times a day.

### Simple and Handy Prescriptions

1. Taizishen (Heterophylly Falsesatarwort Root) 9 g and Hongzao (Red Date) 10 dates are boiled in a casserole, first over strong fire and then mild fire for 30 minutes. Both the contents and the soup can be consumed.

2. Renshen (Ginseng) 30 g, Huangqi (Milkvetch Root) 50 g and Distillated Spirits 500 ml are sealed in a pot and kept for a month before consumption. 10 ml of the liquid is administered once a day in the morning after breakfast.

## Other Therapies

Dietary therapy: A large, fat pad black rooster is stuffed with 30 g of Huangqi (Unprepared Milkvetch Root), then sutured and stewed in an earthenware cooking pot over both strong fire and mild fire till it is well cooked. The chicken and soup can be taken on an empty stomach, but should not be finished in a single day.

If necessary, a stomach support pad can be worn to facilitate treatment and synthesized proteins can be taken to increase abdominal fat composition and muscular tension.

## Cautions and Advice

1. Patients should perform abdominal muscle strengthening exercises to increase muscular tension.
2. Smaller but more frequent meals are advised but voracious eating or drinking, as well as extreme hunger should be avoided in order to protect the spleen and stomach and prevent gastroptosis. Patients should also control their intake of tea. A little yellow wine may be beneficial because it can drive the flow of qi and blood upward; however, for patients with a history of upper gastrointestinal bleeding, liver disease and alcohol hypersensitiveness, it is strictly forbidden.
3. This disease usually has a favorable prognosis.

## Daily Exercises

1. Recall the different types of gastroptosis based on syndrome differentiation and explain how they can be treated.
2. Recall the cautionary notes for patients with gastroptosis.

# Irritable Bowel Syndrome

# Week 5: Saturday

Irritable bowel syndrome, a common intestinal dynamic disorder, is also known as "functional disorder of the colon", "colonospasm" and "allergic colitis". Clinically, it is marked by abdominal pain and discomfort, diarrhea, constipation or alternated diarrhea and constipation. It generally afflicts people between 20~50 years of age, with females being more susceptible. In TCM, it is closely associated with "abdominal pain", "vomiting" and "precipitation of blood".

## Etiology and Pathology

The location of this disease is the intestine and its occurrence is related to the intestine, spleen, stomach and liver. Specifically, stagnation of liver qi due to emotional depression, co-existence of cold and heat in the body, weakness of the spleen and stomach and deficiency of intestinal yin may all lead to abnormal ascent and descent of the spleen qi and stomach qi, as well as functional disorder of the intestinal qi, creating a predisposition to this disease.

## Diagnostic Key Points

1. Repeated spastic abdominal pain (mainly in the left lower abdomen) for at least 3 months (cumulative time) in a year; sometimes it is accompanied by abdominal distension and discomfort and two of the flowing indications:
2. (a) Relaxation or alleviation of abdominal pain. (b) Abnormal defecation frequency (above 3 times a day or below 3 times a week. (c) Abnormal stools in terms of shape or property (dry or loose). (d) Abnormal defecation process with sensation of incomplete discharge. (e) Stools with mucus.
3. Fecal microscopic examination may show the presence of mucus, but no pus cells nor red blood cells. Except for colonospasm and increased mucus, there are no other positive findings on this examination. Barium

enema test may indicate prominent haustra of the colon, increased tension, or signs of irritation.
4. Exclusion of organic diseases marked by structural or bio-chemical abnormalities.

## Syndrome Differentiation

### 1. Liver qi stagnation with spleen deficiency

Symptoms: Abdominal distension and pain with urge for bowel movements, alleviation after fecal discharge, aggravation by emotional factors, hypochondriac distension, poor appetite, rugitus, flatus, emotional depression or anxiety; thin tongue coating and taut pulse.

Analysis of symptoms: Emotional depression impairs the ability of the liver to promote free flow of qi, resulting in a disorder of qi in ascending and descending, this disorder is marked by melancholia or anxiety, abdominal distension and pain with desire for defecation, alleviation after fecal discharge, hypochondriac distension, poor appetite, rugitus and flatus; disharmony between the spleen and stomach results in poor appetite; the thin tongue coating and taut pulse are attributable to stagnation of liver qi.

### 2. Co-existence of cold and heat

Symptoms: Abdominal pain or rugitus, diarrhea, or alternated diarrhea and constipation, vexation, poor appetite, dry mouth and alleviation of gastric and abdominal discomfort by warmth; slightly red tongue with white greasy coating or yellow greasy coating and taut, slippery pulse.

Analysis of symptoms: Invasion of exogenous pathogenic factors or imbalance of yin and yang create a co-existence of cold and heat and triggers a rebellious flow of qi, marked by abdominal pain, rugitus, diarrhea, or alternated diarrhea and constipation, vexation, poor appetite, a dry mouth and alleviation of gastric and abdominal discomfort by warmth; the slightly red tongue with white greasy coating or yellow greasy coating and taut, slippery pulse are manifestations of mixed cold and heat.

## 3. Weakness of the spleen and stomach

Symptoms: A sallow complexion, poor appetite, lassitude, abdominal distension, loose stools with indigested substances and increased frequency of defecation by cold and oily or stomach-irritating food; a pale tongue with marginal teeth marks and white coating and a slow, soggy pulse.

Analysis of symptoms: Weakness of the spleen and stomach results in exhaustion of the source for producing qi and blood, giving rise to the sallow complexion, poor appetite, lassitude, abdominal distension and loose stools with indigested substances; the pale tongue with marginal teeth marks and white coating and slow, soggy pulse are due to weakness of the spleen and stomach.

## 4. Deficiency of yin with intestinal dryness

Symptoms: Dry stools, difficult defecation, or constipation (several days at a time), chestnut-like stools with mucus, abdominal distension and pain, palpable stools in the lower abdomen and a dry mouth or throat; red tongue with scanty fluid and peeled coating and a thin pulse.

Analysis of symptoms: Dryness in the large intestine impairs smooth transportation, marked by dry stools, difficult defecation, abdominal distension and pain, palpable stools in the lower abdomen and a dry mouth or throat; the red tongue with scanty fluid and peeled coating and thin pulse are manifestations of deficiency of yin.

## Differential Treatment

### 1. Liver qi stagnation with spleen deficiency

Treatment principle: Suppressing the liver and reinforcing the spleen.

Prescription and herbs: Modified Tongxie Yaofang and Sini Powder.

Baizhu (Largehead Atractylodes Rhizome) 12 g, Baishao (White Peony Alba) 30 g, Fangfeng (Divaricate Saposhnikovia Root) 9 g, Chenpi (Dried Tangerine Peel) 6 g, Chaihu (Chinese Thorowax Root) 9 g, Zhishi (Immature Orange Fruit) 15 g and Gancao (Liquorice Root) 6 g.

Modification: If the patient presents with severe abdominal pain, Yanhusuo (Corydalis) 9 g and Chuanlianzi (Szechwan Chinaberry Fruit) 9 g can be added to further help alleviate pain.

## 2. Co-existence of cold and heat

Treatment principle: Regulating heat and cold.

Prescription and herbs: Modified Wumei Pill.

Wumei (Smoked Plum) 9 g, Xixin (Manchurian Wildginger) 6 g, Ganjiang (Dried Ginger) 9 g, Huanglian (Golden Thread) 3 g, Danggui (Chinese Angelica) 9 g, Fuzi (Prepared Common Monkshood Daughter) 3 g, Shujiao (Shichuan Pepper) 9 g, Guizhi (Cassia Twig) 6 g, Dangshen (Radix Codonopsis) 12 g and Huangbai (Amur Cork-tree) 9 g.

Modification: If there is diarrhea, Shanyao (Common Yan Rhizome) 15 g and Yiyiren (Coix Seed) 15 g are added to check diarrhea; for constipation, Huomaren (Hemp Seed) 30 g can be added to moisten the intestine and promote bowel movements.

## 3. Weakness of the spleen and stomach

Treatment principle: Invigorating the spleen and facilitating transformation.

Prescription and herbs: Modified Shenling Baizhu Powder.

Dangshen (Radix Codonopsis) 12 g, Baizhu (Largehead Atractylodes Rhizome) 12 g, Fuling (Indian Bread) 12 g, Shanyao (Common Yan Rhizome) 15 g, Yiyiren (Coix Seed) 15 g, Baibiandou (White Hyacinth Bean) 15 g, Lianzirou (Lotus Seed Kernel) 9 g, Jiegeng (Platycodon Root) 6 g, Sharen (Villous Amomum Fruit) 3 g and Gancao (Liquorice Root) 6 g.

Modification: For severe diarrhea, Yuyuliang (Limonite) 15 g and Chishizhi (Red Halloysite) 15 g are added to invigorate the spleen and stop diarrhea.

## 4. Deficiency of yin with intestinal dryness

Treatment principle: Nourishing yin and moistening the intestine.

Prescription and herbs: Modified Zengye Decoction and Runchang Pill.

Xuanshen (Figwort Root) 9 g, Maidong (Dwarf Lilyturf Tuber) 9 g, Shengdi (Dried Rehmannia Root) 9 g, Danggui (Chinese Angelica) 9 g, Maren (Edestan) 30 g, Taoren (Peach Seed) 9 g and Zhiqiao (Orange Fruit) 6 g.

Modification: For severe abdominal distension, Zhishi (Immature Orange Fruit) 30 g is added to unblock stagnation; if there is constipation, Shengshouwu (Unprepared Fleeceflower Root) 30 g and Wangjiangnan (Cassiae Occidentalis) 30 g can be added to promote defecation.

## Chinese Patent Medicine

1. Runchang Pill (Intestine-Moistening Pill): 4.5 g for each dose, twice a day.
2. Shenling Baizhu Tablet: 4 tablets for each dose, 3 times a day.

## Simple and Handy Prescriptions

1. Laifuzi (Radish Seed) 30 g, Chenpi (Dried Tangerine Peel) 9 g and Zhuru (Bamboo Shavings) 9 g are boiled in water and taken twice a day.
2. Baishao (White Peony Alba) 30 g and Gancao (Stir-baked Liquorice Root) 9 g are boiled in water and taken twice a day.

## Other Therapies

Dietary therapy:

(1) Twenty plums are decocted over a mild then strong fire and after the decoction is ready, a small amount of cerealose is added; this can be taken twice a day.
(2) Shengshouwu (Unprepared Fleeceflower Root) 30 g is simmered into a thick decoction and Jiangmi (Rice Fruit) 100 g and clean water is added. The mixture is made into porridge and taken twice a day.

In addition to herbal therapies, proper psychological regulation is also important, so patients should seek psychological consultation when necessary.

## Cautions and Advice

1. This disease is a functional disorder, so organic diseases of the gastro-intestinal tract should be excluded during the diagnosis. For middle-aged and old patients, the possibility of colon tumors should be ruled out. Unless the patients are physically very weak, there is no need for bedrest. They should develop a regular lifestyle and engage in moderate physical exercise so as to strengthen the constitution and facilitate functional recovery of the nerves.
2. Diet: Patients should consume more soft and easily digestible food and avoid stomach-irritating food or sauces. For those with abdominal distension, consumption of bean products should be restricted; for those with constipation, fiber-rich foods are advisable; for those with loose stools, the amounts of vegetables, fruits, seafood and dairy products should be controlled. In addition, to relieve the symptoms, it is advisable to take more cellulose-rich food.
3. Prognosis: The functional disorder of the gastrointestinal tract may relapse even if it had previously been cured, but generally the disease will not involve the whole body. For severe malnutrition with cachexia, the prognosis is relatively poor, with a 5% death rate.

## Daily Exercises

1. List the diagnostic key points of irritable bowel syndrome.
2. Explain how irritable bowel syndrome can be treated based on syndrome differentiation.

# Intestinal Cancer

# Week 6: Monday

Intestinal cancer, a common malignant tumor in the digestive canal, has the second highest death rate among all the cancers. The main clinical symptoms are change of stools in terms of shape, or stools with pus and blood, abdominal pain and palpable lower abdominal lumps. The ratio of males to females is 1.65:1, with 75% of the patients being between 31~60 years. In TCM, intestinal cancer is closely associated with "masses and accumulations", "visceral toxins", "lesser abdominal mass in women", "anoectal carcinoma", "intestinal accumulation", "intestinal and anal bleeding" and "dysentery".

## Etiology and Pathology

This disease arises from the intestine and its occurrence is closely related to the liver, spleen and intestine. The etiological factors are weakness of the spleen and stomach, insufficiency of healthy qi, improper diet, excessive intake of fatty, sweet or mouldy food (which impairs the spleen and stomach and eventually the kidneys and healthy qi), emotional depression (which causes stagnation of the liver qi), exogenous invasion of virulent damp-heat, chronic dysentery and diarrhea (which leads to disorder of qi and blood in the intestine). The above-mentioned factors can all result in dysfunction of the large intestine in transportation and disorder of the collaterals, which trigger the accumulation of phlegm, dampness and toxic heat, creating a predisposition to this disease.

## Diagnostic Key Points

1. Clinically, it is marked by changes in bowel habits and in fecal shape and texture, such as thinned and flattened stools or bloody and purulent stools, tenesmus, constipation or diarrhea, abdominal distension or pain and lumps in the abdomen or rectum. In the advanced stage, there may be progressive emaciation, low grade fever, cachexia, jaundice and ascites.

2. Definitive diagnosis of the disease requires digital rectal examination, rectal speculum, sigmoidoscopy or fibercolonscopy and biopsy.
3. Imaging tests such as X-ray barium meal examination, especially gas-barium double contrast radiograph, can identify the location and nature of this disease. B ultrasonic test, CT and MRI can determine the character, size and location of the masses, as well as the conditions of celiac lymph nodes and hepatic metastasis.
4. Quantitive and dynamic examination on arcinoembryonic antigen (CEA) is of certain diagnostic value to the evaluation of therapeutic effects.

## Syndrome Differentiation

### 1. Accumulation of dampness and heat

Symptoms: Paroxysmal abdominal pain, tenesmus, a scorching sensation in the anus, possible fever, chest distress, nausea, a bitter taste in the mouth, stools with mucus, pus or blood and yellowish urine; red tongue with yellow, greasy coating and rapid, slippery pulse.

Analysis of symptoms : Internal accumulation of damp-heat leads to stagnation of qi, which is marked by paroxysmal abdominal pain, tenesmus and chest distress; the scorching sensation in the anus, or fever, bitter taste in the mouth and yellowish urine are attributable to abundant damp-heat in the interior; damp-heat damages the blood vessels of the large intestine, giving rise to stools with mucus, pus or blood; the red tongue with yellow, greasy coating and rapid, slippery pulse are due to accumulation of dampness and heat.

### 2. Internal obstruction of stasis and toxins

Symptoms: Abdominal distension and pain at a fixed location, abdominal masses with tenderness, dysentery with dark purple blood, pus and tenesmus; a dark purple tongue with ecchymosis, thin yellow tongue coating and rapid, taut pulse, or thin, unsmooth pulse.

Analysis of symptoms: Blood stasis, in combination with pathogenic toxins, blocks the flow of qi and blood and damages the meridians, causing abdominal distension and pain at a fixed location, unpressable abdominal

---

242     *Introduction to Chinese Internal Medicine*

masses, dysentery with dark purple blood, pus and tenesmus; the dark purple tongue with ecchymosis, thin yellow tongue coating and rapid, taut pulse, or thin, unsmooth pulse are manifestations of severe blood stasis with impairment of pathogenic toxins.

## 3. Deficiency of the spleen with stagnation of qi

**Symptoms:** Abdominal distension, poor appetite, rugitus, scurrying pain, loose or bloody stools, lassitude and a sallow complexion; pale tongue with white-thin or greasy coating and slippery, soggy pulse.

**Analysis of symptoms:** Disharmony between the liver and spleen leads to liver depression and qi stagnation, which is marked by abdominal distension, rugitus and scurrying pain; dysfunction of the spleen in transportation and transformation brings about such symptoms as loose stools and poor appetite; exhaustion of the source for producing qi and blood results in lassitude and a sallow complexion; failure of the kidneys to control blood gives rise to hemafecia; the pale tongue with white-thin or greasy coating and slippery, soggy pulse are manifestations of spleen deficiency.

## 4. Yang deficiency of the spleen and kidneys

**Symptoms:** Vague and lingering pain in the abdomen, intolerance of cold, lack of warmth in the limbs, shortness of qi, weariness, loose stools, diarrhea before dawn or with increased frequency, weakness and soreness of the waist and knees and a pale complexion; a pale, enlarged tongue with white-thin coating or greasy coating and thin, deep pulse or thin, soggy pulse with the chi-region being weak.

**Analysis of symptoms:** Deficiency of spleen yang and kidney yang gives rise to predominance of yin-cold and stagnation of qi, marked by vague and lingering pain in the abdomen, intolerance of cold, lack of warmth in the limbs, shortness of qi, weariness, loose stools, diarrhea before dawn or with increased frequency, weakness and soreness of the waist and knees and a pale complexion; the pale, enlarged tongue with white-thin coating or greasy coating and thin, deep pulse or thin, soggy pulse with the chi-section being weak are signs of yang deficiency.

## 5. Yin deficiency of the liver and kidneys

Symptoms: Dizziness, waist soreness, tinnitus, low grade fever, night sweats, feverish sensations over the five centers (the palms, the soles and the heart), a bitter taste in the mouth and dry throat and dry stools; red tongue with little or no coating and thin, taut pulse or thin, rapid pulse.

Analysis of symptoms: Deficiency of the liver and kidneys is marked by dizziness, waist soreness and tinnitus; deficiency of yin produces internal heat, giving rise to low grade fever, night sweats, feverish sensation over the five centers (the palms, the soles and the heart), mouth bitterness and throat dryness; depletion of intestinal yin-fluid is responsible for dry stools; the red tongue with little or no coating and thin, taut pulse or thin, rapid pulse are manifestations of internal heat due to deficiency of yin.

## Differential Treatment

### 1. Accumulation of dampness and heat

Treatment principle: Dispelling heat, resolving dampness and eliminating toxins.

Prescription and herbs: Modified Huaijiao Diyu Decoction and Baitouweng Decoction.

Huaijiao (Japanese Pagodatree Pod) 9 g, Diyu (Garden Burnet Root) 12 g, Baitouweng (Chinese Pulsatilla Root) 15 g, Qinpi (Ash Bark) 9 g, Huangqin (Baical Skullcap Root) 9 g, Huanglian (Golden Thread) 9 g, Huangbai (Amur Cork-tree) 9 g, Baijiangcao (Dahurian Patrinia Herb) 15 g, Machixian (Purslane Herb) 15 g, Yiyiren (Coix Seed) 15 g and Gancao (Liquorice Root) 6 g.

Modification: If there is presence of abundant toxic heat, Baihuashecao (Hedyotic Diffusa) 30 g, Banbianlian (Chinese Lobelia Herb) 15 g and Banzhilian (Barbated Skullcup Herb) 15 g are added to dispel heat and remove toxins.

## 2. Internal obstruction of stasis and toxins

Treatment principle: Resolving stasis and promoting flow of qi.

Prescription and herbs: Modified Gexia Zhuyu Decoction.

Wulingzhi (Faeces Trogopterorum) 9 g, Guiwei (Carda part of Radix Angelicae Sinensis Root) 9 g, Honghua (Safflower) 9 g, Chuanxiong (Szechwan Lovage Rhizome) 9 g, Taoren (Peach Seed) 9 g, Chishao (Red Peony Root) 9 g, Wuyao (Combined Spicebush Root) 9 g, Yanhusuo (Corydalis) 9 g, Xiangfu (Nutgrass Galingale Rhizome) 12 g, Zhiqiao (Orange Fruit) 6 g, Yiyiren (Unprepared Coix Seed) 15 g amd Gancao (Liquorice Root) 6 g.

Modification: If there is severe blood stasis with pain, Sanleng (Common Burreed Tuber) 9 g and Ezhu (Zedoray Rhizome) 9 g are added to break stasis and alleviate pain.

## 3. Deficiency of the spleen with stagnation of qi

Treatment principle: Invigorating the spleen and regulating qi.

Prescription and herbs: Modified Xiangshao Liujunzi Decoction.

Muxiang (Common Aucklandia Root) 6 g, Sharen (Villous Amomum Fruit) 3 g, Dangshen (Radix Codonopsis) 12 g, Baizhu (Largehead Atractylodes Rhizome) 12 g, Fuling (Indian Bread) 12 g, Banxia (Pinellia Tuber) 9 g, Chenpi (Dried Tangerine Peel) 6 g and Gancao (Liquorice Root) 6 g.

Modification: For hemafecia, Zhaoxintu (Humus Flava Usta) 30 g and Sanqifen (Sanchi) 3 g are used to stop bleeding.

## 4. Yang deficiency of the spleen and kidneys

Treatment principle: Invigorating the spleen and kidneys with warmth.

Prescription and herbs: Modified Shenling Baizhu Powder and Sishen Pill.

Dangshen (Radix Codonopsis) 12 g, Fuling (Indian Bread) 12 g, Baizhu (Largehead Atractylodes Rhizome) 12 g, Jiegeng (Platycodon Root) 6 g,

Shanyao (Common Yan Rhizome) 15 g, Baibiandou (White Hyacinth Bean) 9 g, Yiyiren (Coix Seed) 15 g, Lianzi (Lotus Seed) 9 g, Sharen (Villous Amomum Fruit) 3 g, Buguzhi (Malaytea Scurfpea Fruit) 9 g, Roudoukou (Nutmeg) 6 g, Wuzhuyu (Medicinal Evodia Fruit) 3 g and Gancao (Liquorice Root) 6 g.

Modification: For severe cold in the body and limbs, Fuzi (Prepared Common Monkshood Daughter) 3 g and Ganjiang (Dried Ginger) 9 g are added to warm yang and dissipate cold.

## 5. Yin deficiency of the liver and kidneys

Treatment principle: Nourishing the liver and kidneys.

Prescription and herbs: Modified Zhibai Dihuang Pill.

Zhimu (Common Anemarrhena Rhizome) 9 g, Huangbai (Amur Cork-tree) 9 g, Shudihuang (Prepared Rhizome of Rehmannia) 9 g, Shanzhuyu (Asiatic Cornelian Cherry Fruit) 9 g, Shanyao (Common Yan Rhizome) 12 g, Fuling (Indian Bread) 12 g, Danpi (Cortex Moutan) 9 g and Zexie (Oriental Waterplantain Rhizome) 9 g.

Modification: For constipation, Shengdi (Dried Rehmannia Root) 30 g, Shengshouwu (Unprepared Fleeceflower Root) 30 g and Huomaren (Hemp Seed) 30 g are added to moisten the intestine and promote defecation.

## Chinese Patent Medicine

1. Pingxiao Capsule: 8 capsules for each dose, 3 times a day.
2. Fufang Banmao Capsule: 3 capsules for each dose, twice a day.

## Simple and Handy Prescriptions

1. Baihuashecao (Hedyotic Diffusa) 15 g, Tengligen (Radix Actinidiae) 15 g and Baiying (Bittersweet) 15 g are boiled in water and taken twice a day.

## Other Therapies

Dietary therapy:

(1) Miren (Coix Seed) and Biandou (Hyacinth Bean) are added to Jiangmi (Rice Fruit) and cooked. It can be taken frequently at meals.
(2) Vegetable juice is extracted from Sigua (Fresh Sponge gourd) or Siguanteng (Thick Luffa Stem) for drinking.

Surgical intervention: The main radical cure for intestinal cancer is surgery or radiotherapy and chemotherapy in some cases. TCM therapy can be applied at any stage of this disease.

## Cautions and Advice

1. With the development of intestinal tumors, some patients may present with intestinal obstruction, bleeding or perforation, suppurative peritonitis, pericolic abscess and rectovesical fistula. Once the disease is confirmed, consultation on the follow up treatment necessary should be immediate so that such appropriate treatment can be administered. Periodic checks are also imperative in order for any relapse or metastasis to be promptly identified and addressed accordingly.
2. Patients should develop a regular lifestyle and keep themselves optimistic and in good spirits. For those with praeternaturalis anus, food that may cause flatulence should be avoided; the anal bag should be emptied and changed regularly to keep the skin around the orificium fistulae dry and clean; defecation should also be regular.
3. They should keep to a light diet that is low in fat and high in cellulose. A small amount of animal protein permissable, but they should avoid food that is too oily or food that can trigger tumor growth.
4. Prognosis: The natural course of the disease for those ineffectively treated is 9.5 months on average; the 5-year survival rate for those who received radical surgery of the large intestine is 50% in recent years. Young patients generally have a relatively higher rate of unfavorable prognosis as compared to elderly patients. Howover, the

prognosis of this disease is also influenced by the location of the tumors, the extent of infiltration, the degree of differentiation, the lymphatic or distant metastasis, the promptness of discovery and the appropriateness of treatment.

## Daily Exercises

1. Concisely describe the etiology and pathology of intestinal cancer.
2. Explain how intestinal cancer can be treated based on syndrome differentiation.

# Gastric Cancer
# Week 6: Tuesday

Gastric cancer refers to the malignant cancerization of the gastric epithelium. It is one of the most common types of malignant tumor. Clinically, it is marked by gastric discomfort, abdominal distension and pain, poor appetite, nausea, vomiting, emaciation, abdominal masses and black stools. Gastric cancer generally occurs in the pylorus and sometimes the lesser curvature of the stomach and cardiac region. It mostly afflicts old or middle-aged people, especially males. In TCM, gastric cancer is closely associated with "stomach pain", "regurgitation" and "abdominal mass".

## Etiology and Pathology

This disease stems from the spleen, stomach and liver and mainly afflicts the stomach. Emotional depression often leads to stagnation of qi; dietary impairment generally gives rise to production of phlegm and dampness; and pathogenic toxins tend to damage the stomach collaterals, resulting in qi stagnation, food retention and blood stasis in the stomach. Prolonged affliction may debilitate the body and in some cases, pathogenic heat remains in the stomach and consumes the stomach yin; in other cases, pathogenic factors can exhaust qi and damage yang, creating a predisposition to deficient cold in the spleen and stomach.

## Diagnostic Key Points

1. Emaciation, lassitude, poor appetite, gastric distension or vague pain, aversion to meat, nausea, vomiting and hemafecia of unknown origin at the early stage; abdominal masses, lymphadenectasis and cachexia at the late stage.
2. Gastrointestinal X-ray barium meal examination: Regional filling defect and cancerous niche sign, stenosis or obstruction.
3. Gastroscopy can provide direct visualization of the conditions of carcinomatous change.

4. Biopsy: Identification of the malignant cells is of definitive diagnostic value.

5. Abdominal laparotomy is of definitive diagnostic value.

## Syndrome Differentiation

### 1. Disharmony between the liver and stomach

Symptoms: Gastric distension and discomfort due to emotional depression and occasional distending or vague pain, poor appetite, frequent belching; thin tongue coating and taut pulse.

Analysis of symptoms: Emotional depression impairs the ability of the liver to maintain normal flow of qi, qi invades the stomach and causes functional disorder of qi, resulting in gastric distension and occasional distending or vague pain; the stomach qi fails to descend normally, causing poor appetite and frequent belching; the taut pulse is suggestive of liver diseases and pain.

### 2. Stagnation of phlegm, heat, blood and toxins

Symptoms: Burning pain in the gastric region, nausea, vomiting of sputum and saliva or even blood, occasional fever, mouth dryness with thirst, dry or bloody stools, scanty reddish urine, dry and lusterless skin; purple tongue with ecchymosis and yellow, greasy tongue coating and slippery, rapid pulse.

Analysis of symptoms: Stagnation of phlegm, heat, blood and toxins in the middle energizer inhibits the smooth functional activity of qi, causing burning pain in the gastric region, nausea and vomiting of sputum and saliva; abundance of heat and toxins brings about fever, mouth dryness with thirst, dry stools, scanty reddish urine and dry and lusterless skin; retention of phlegm, heat, blood and toxins damages the collaterals or vessels, resulting in haematemesis and hemafecia; the yellow, greasy coating and slippery, rapid pulse are indicative of phlegm and heat, whereas the purple tongue with ecchymosis is a sign of blood stasis.

### 3. Consumption of yin by stomach heat

Symptoms: Vague pain in the gastric region, dryness in the mouth and throat, nausea, retching, hectic fever, night sweats, dry skin, progressive emaciation, constipation, scanty reddish urine and palpable masses in the abdomen, pelvis and armpit; reddish tongue with scanty coating and thin, rapid pulse.

Analysis of symptoms: Prolonged affliction damages the stomach yin, causing vague pain in the gastric region, dryness in the mouth and throat, nausea and retching; deficiency of yin gives rise to internal heat which is marked by hectic fever, night sweats, dry skin, progressive emaciation, constipation and scanty reddish urine; accumulation of phlegm, heat, toxins and blood stasis in the interior is responsible for the palpable masses in the abdomen, pelvis and armpit; the reddish tongue with scanty coating and thin, rapid pulse are manifestations of internal heat due to deficiency of yin.

### 4. Inactivation of spleen yang

Symptoms: Vague pain in the stomach, lassitude, pale complexion, cold body and limbs, difficult food intake or eating in the morning but vomiting in the evening, loose stools, facial edema and swollen limbs; pale tongue with white coating and a thin, deep and feeble pulse.

Analysis of symptoms: Prolonged affliction debilitates the spleen yang which then fails to warm the stomach collaterals, so there is vague pain in the stomach; deficiency of yang qi produces yin cold, marked by lassitude, pale complexion and cold body and limbs; deficiency of spleen yang leads to poor digestion, resulting in difficult food intake or eating in the morning but vomiting in the evening, as well as loose stools; deficiency of yang brings about internal retention of water and dampness, giving rise to facial edema and swollen limbs; the pale tongue with white coating and thin, deep and feeble pulse are due to inactivation of spleen yang.

### Differential Treatment

### 1. Disharmony between the liver and stomach

Treatment principle: Soothing the liver and regulating qi, harmonizing the stomach and alleviating pain.

Prescription and herbs: Modified Jinlingzi Powder and Xiaoyao Powder.

Chuanlianzi (Szechwan Chinaberry Fruit) 9 g, Yanhusuo (Corydalis) 9 g, Xiangfu (Nutgrass Galingale Rhizome) 9 g, Zhiqiao (Orange Fruit) 15 g, Chaihu (Chinese Thorowax Root) 9 g, Baizhu (Largehead Atractylodes Rhizome) 9 g, Fuling (Indian Bread) 9 g, Gancao (Liquorice Root) 6 g, Danggui (Chinese Angelica) 9 g, Baishao (White Peony Alba) 9 g, Qingpi (Green Tangerine Peel) 6 g and Chenpi (Dried Tangerine Peel) 6 g.

Modification: If there is severe belching, Xuanfuhua (Intussusceer) 12 g and Daizheshi (Red Bole) 30 g can be added to reduce adverseness.

## 2. Stagnation of phlegm, heat, blood and toxins

Treatment principle: Dissolving phlegm and expelling stasis, eliminating toxins and dispelling heat.

Prescription and herbs: Supplementary Xiaoxianxiong Decoction.

Huanglian (Golden Thread) 3 g, Banxia (Pinellia Tuber) 9 g, Quangualou (Snakegourd Fruit) 15 g, Xiakucao (Common Selfheal Fruit-Spike) 9 g, Sanleng (Common Burreed Tuber) 9 g, Ezhu (Zedoray Rhizome) 9 g, Shuyangquan (Bittersweet) 15 g, Shemei (Indian Mockstrawberry Herb) 30 g, Shensanqi (Panax Pseudo-ginseng) 9 g, Shuiniujiao (Buffalo Horn) 30 g and Gancao (Unprepared Liquorice Root) 9 g.

Modification: In cases of haematemesis and hemafecia, Zhaoxintu (Humus Flava Usta) 30 g and Baiji (Common Bletilla Tuber) 9 g are added to stop bleeding; for vomiting of profuse sputum and saliva, Dannanxing (Bile Arisaema) 12 g and Jiangzhuru (Ginger-prepared Bamboo Shavings) 9 g are added to dissolve phlegm and reduce adverseness.

## 3. Consumption of yin by stomach heat

Treatment principle: Nourishing the stomach and replenishing yin, dispelling heat and expelling stasis.

Prescription and herbs: Modified Yangwei Decoction and Shixiao Powder.

Yuzhu (Fragrant Solomonseal Rhizome) 9 g, Shihu (Dendrobium) 12 g, Beishashen (Coastal Glehnia Root) 12 g, Maidong (Dwarf Lilyturf Tuber) 12 g, Gouqizi (Barbary Wolfberry Fruit) 12 g, Biandou (Hyacinth Bean)

12 g, Chuanlianzi (Szechwan Chinaberry Fruit) 9 g, Puhuang (Pollen Typhae) 9 g, Wulingzhi (Faeces Trogopterorum) 9 g (wrapped during decoction) and Xiakucao (Common Selfheal Fruit-Spike) 9 g.

Modification: For dryness in the throat, Lugen (Reed Rhizome) 30 g can be added to promote fluid production; if there is hectic fever and night sweats, Digupi (Chinese Wolfberry Root-Bark) 12 g, Nuodaogen (Glutinous Rice Root) 9 g and Bietaogan (Persicae Immaturus) 9 g are added to nourish yin, dispel heat and stop sweating.

## 4. Inactivation of spleen yang

Treatment principle: Warming yang and supplementing qi, invigorating the spleen and alleviating pain.

Prescription and herbs: Supplementary Shenling Baizhu Powder and Liangfu Pill.

Huangqi (Milkvetch Root) 15 g, Dangshen (Radix Codonopsis) 12 g, Baizhu (Largehead Atractylodes Rhizome) 9 g, Ganjiang (Dried Ginger) 6 g, Fuzi (Prepared Common Monkshood Daughter) 3 g, Biandou (Hyacinth Bean) 12 g, Shanyao (Common Yan Rhizome) 12 g, Yiyiren (Coix Seed) 15 g, Gaoliangjiang (Lesser Galangal Rhizome) 9 g, Xiangfu (Nutgrass Galingale Rhizome) 12 g, Chenpi (Dried Tangerine Peel) 6 g and Gancao (Liquorice Root) 6 g.

Modification: In cases of edema in the face, feet and limbs, Zexie (Oriental Waterplantain Rhizome) 12 g, Cheqianzi (Plantain Seed) 12 g (wrapped during decoction), Zhuling (Polyporus) 12 g and Fuling (Indian Bread) 12 g are added to promote urination and relieve edema.

## Chinese Patent Medicine

Pingxiao Capsule: 8 capsules for each dose, 3 times a day.

## Simple and Handy Prescriptions

1. Shuyangquan (Bittersweet) 30 g, Baihuashecao (Hedyotic Diffusa) 30 g, Banzhilian (Barbated Skullcup Herb) 30 g, Longkui (Solanum

Nigrum) 15 g and Huangmaoercao (Goldhair Hedyotis Herb) 15 g are decocted in water and separated into 3 portions and taken at 3 different times within a day.
2. Lianmiaobiqi (Chinese water chestnut) 30 g, Yiyiren (Unprepared Coix Seed) 30 g and Liligen (Radix Actinidiae) 30 g are boiled in water and taken once a day.

## Other Therapies

Dietary therapy:

(1) Pork 250 g is well cooked and eaten with garlic (and a little soy sauce if preferred). It can be served to patients with gastric cancer for strengthening the constitution or post-operative rehabilitation.
(2) Rice 150 g and Yiyiren (Coix Seed) 50 g are cooked and taken at meals. This is used to treat various types of gastric cancer.

## Cautions and Advice

1. Patients should cultivate a regular, controlled diet and avoid intake of or exposure to possible cancerogenic substances.
2. Patients should have a diet that comprises a higher intake of protein but lower intake of fat, sugar and salt. Fresh vegetables and fruits are also advisable, but pickled food is forbidden.
3. It is important that gastric cancer should be discovered early and treated promptly. If a surgery is deemed suitable, it should be performed as early as possible and radiotherapy, chemotherapy and Chinese herbal treatment should be administered afterwards to ensure a favorable prognosis.

## Daily Exercises

1. Explain how gastric cancer can be treated based on syndrome differentiation.
2. Recall the cautionary notes for patients with gastric cancer.

# Ulcerative Colitis

# Week 6: Wednesday

Ulcerative colitis, also called chronic non-specific ulcerative colitis, is a chronic inflammatory disease marked by ulceration of the mucous membranes of the rectum and colon, with unidentified causes. The main clinical symptoms are chronic and repetitive diarrhea, bloody stools with mucus or pus, tenesmus, abdominal pain and sometimes fever, emaciation, or anaemia. This disease can afflict people of any age, particularly those who are 20~30 years old. Males have a slightly higher incidence rate than females. In TCM, ulcerative colitis is considered to be closely associated with "dysentery", "diarrhea" and "hemafecia".

## Etiology and Pathology

This disease mainly attacks the intestine and is due primarily to disorders of the liver, spleen, stomach and intestine. At the beginning it is generally caused by emotional depression, which leads to stagnation of liver qi and its invasion into the spleen and stomach; improper diet such as excessive intake of fatty and sweet food and a constitution that is dominant in damp-heat, coupled with intake of uncooked, cold food, may damage the spleen and stomach, leading to dysfunction of the spleen in transportation and transformation and confusion of the lucid with the turbid; pathogenic summer-heat, dampness and toxic heat invade the body and impair the intestine, bringing about stagnation of qi and blood and eventually suppuration; chronic bleeding consumes blood and exhausts yin and if the disease persists, the collaterals will be affected, resulting in internal obstruction of blood stasis; prolonged affliction debilitates the spleen yang and kidney yang, causing failure of the lucid yang to ascend and qi sinking of the middle energizer, as well as inefficient warming-transporting and inconsolidation of the stomach gate.

## Diagnostic Key Points

1. Common symptoms: Diarrhea, stools with fresh blood, bloody stools with mucus or pus, tenesmus, abdominal pain, fever, poor appetite, emaciation and anaemia.

2. Sigmfoid colon endoscopy: Diffusive congestion and edema in the intestinal mucosa, increased brittleness of the mucosa with a propensity to bleed, frequent occurrence of erosion or multiple ulcers in different sizes and covered with purulent mucus exudate; in the late stage there are pseudo-polypi, pale mucus membrane, maculae atrophicae, stiffness of the intestinal wall and disappearance of the haustra coli.

3. X-ray barium enema: In the acute phase, there is thickening and derangement of the plica due to edema; when there is ulceration, the mural margin becomes serrated; in the late stage, there are mural fibroplasia, disappearance of the haustra coli, stiffened intestinal wall, shortened intestinal canal and narrowed enteric cavity resembling a water pipe.

4. Laboratory examination: Examination of the excrement and urine shows a large number of red and white blood cells or pus cells; blood routine test may suggest anaemia.

## Syndrome Differentiation

### 1. Production of damp-heat due to spleen deficiency

Symptoms: Diarrhea in varying frequency, tenesmus, or a burning sensation in the anus, bloody stools with mucus or pus and fishy smell, abdominal pain, scanty reddish urine, weariness, emaciation, fever, a bitter taste in the mouth, poor appetite; yellow and greasy tongue coating and thin, rapid and slippery pulse.

Analysis of symptoms: Deficiency of the spleen produces dampness, the stagnation of which generates heat and impairs the intestinal tract, leading to dysfunction in transformation and transportation, with such signs as diarrhea in varying frequency; damp-heat fumigates the intestinal tract and damages the collaterals, leading to stagnation of qi and blood with pus, so there are bloody stools with mucus or pus and a fishy smell; pathogenic damp-heat accumulates in the intestine, hampering the smooth functional activity of qi, this is marked by abdominal pain and tenesmus; damp-heat pours downward, bringing about a burning sensation in the anus and scanty reddish urine; deficiency of spleen qi is responsible for lassitude, poor appetite and emaciation; fever, the bitter taste in the mouth and yellow greasy tongue coating are all due to internal accumulation of damp-heat; the thin pulse is suggestive of spleen deficiency and the slippery, rapid pulse is attributable to damp-heat.

## 2. Hyperactivity of the liver with spleen deficiency

Symptoms: Abdominal pain followed and relieved by fecal discharge, occurrence due to depression, anger, stress or agitation, bloody stools with pus, distension and fullness in the chest and hypochondria, restlessness, irascibility, belching, poor appetite, rugitus, abdominal distension and headache in fits and starts; slightly red tongue and taut, thin pulse.

Analysis of symptoms: Emotional impairment leads to failure of the liver to maintain normal flow of qi, qi invades the spleen and causes indigestion, marked by emotion-induced abdominal pain that is followed and relieved by fecal discharge; stagnation of qi and blood produces pus, so there are purulent bloody stools; hyperactivity of the liver gives rise to distension and fullness in the chest and hypochondria, restlessness, irascibility and headache in fits and starts; stagnation of qi causes belching, rugitus and abdominal distension; deficiency of the spleen is responsible for poor appetite and the slightly red tongue and taut, thin pulse are attributable to hyperactivity of the liver with spleen deficiency.

## 3. Obstruction of blood stasis in the intestinal tract

Symptoms: Abdominal pricking pain aggravated by pressure, stools with purulent blood or dark black blood clots, a dark, lusterless complexion, dark red tongue with ecchymosis and thin, taut pulse.

Analysis of symptoms: Obstruction of blood stasis in the intestinal tract hampers the smooth functional activity of qi, causing lower abdominal pricking pain that is aggravated by pressure; stagnation of qi and blood produces pus, giving rise to stools with purulent blood or dark black blood clots; the dark, lusterless complexion, dark-red tongue with suggillation and thin, taut pulse are all manifestations of qi stagnation and blood stasis.

## 4. Weakness of the spleen and stomach

Symptoms: Loose stools (sometimes with mucus, intestinal filth and puru-lent blood), or even incessant diarrhea triggered by improper diet, lassi-tude, a poor appetite, a pale complexion; pale tongue with white coating and thin, soggy pulse.

Analysis of symptoms: Weakness of the spleen and stomach leads to indi-gestion of water and food and inseparation of the lucid and turbid, marked by loose stools (sometimes with mucus, intestinal filth and purulent blood), or even incessant diarrhea triggered by improper diet; deficiency of the spleen and stomach produces inadequate qi and blood, with such signs as lassitude, a poor appetite and pale complexion; the pale tongue with white coating and thin, soggy pulse are manifestations of weakness of the spleen and stomach.

## 5. Production of internal heat due to deficiency of yin

Symptoms: Diarrhea at times, vague pain in the abdomen, stools with thick and bright-red blood hectic fever in the afternoon, night sweats, vexation and insomnia; reddish tongue with scanty coating and thin, rapid pulse.

Analysis of symptoms: Prolonged diarrhea damages the yin blood, so besides diarrhea, there is vague pain in the abdomen and stools with thick and bright-red blood; deficiency of yin produces internal heat which manifests as hectic fever in the afternoon and night sweats; deficient heat disturbs the heart spirit, leading to vexation and insomnia; the reddish tongue with scanty coating as well as thin, rapid pulse are manifestations of internal heat due to deficiency of yin.

## 6. Yang deficiency of the spleen and kidneys

Symptoms: Abdominal pain, rugitus and diarrhea before dawn, alleviation after fecal discharge, bloody stools with mucus, lack of warmth in the body (especially the limbs), a bland taste in the mouth, reduced food intake, preference for hot drinks, waist soreness, weariness and pale com-plexion; pale tongue with white coating and thin, deep and feeble pulse.

Analysis of symptoms: Prolonged diarrhea leads to deficiency of kidney yang and the subsequent inactivation of spleen yang, as well as dysfunction in transportation and transformation, marked by abdominal pain and diarrhea; the stagnated intestinal qi is unblocked through fecal discharge, so there is alleviation after diarrhea; yin cold congeals qi and blood and damages the intestinal collaterals, bringing about bloody stools with mucus; deficiency of yang gives rise to internal cold, so the disease is often triggered by cold and there is lack of warmth in the body (especially the limbs); insufficiency of kidney yang results in waist soreness and weariness; deficiency of spleen yang is responsible for the bland taste in the mouth, reduced food intake and preference for hot drinks; the pale complexion, pale tongue with white coating and a thin, feeble and deep pulse are all manifestations of deficiency of spleen yang and kidney yang.

## Differential Treatment

### 1. Production of damp-heat due to spleen deficiency

Treatment principle: Dispelling heat and removing toxins, resolving dampness and dissipating stagnation.

Prescription and herbs: Supplementary Lianli Decoction and Baitouweng Decoction.

Dangshen (Radix Codonopsis) 12 g, Chaobaizhu (Fried Largehead Atractylodes Rhizome) 12 g, Baitouweng (Chinese Pulsatilla Root) 30 g, Jinyinhua (Honeysuckle Flower) 9 g, Qinpi (Ash Bark) 9 g, Huanglian (Golden Thread) 3 g, Huangbai (Amur Cork-tree) 9 g, Diyutan (Charred Radix Sanguisorbae) 12 g, Lianzirou (Lotus Seed) 12 g, Paojiangtan (Charred Ginger) 9 g, Muxiang (Common Aucklandia Root) 3 g, Binglang (Areca Seed) 9 g, Zhiqiao (Orange Fruit) 12 , Gegen (Kudzuvine Root) 9 g and Gancao (Liquorice Root) 6 g.

Modification: If there is presence of bloody stools with pus, Baijifen (Common Bletilla Tuber Powder) 3 g and Xianhecao (Hairyvein Agrimonia Herb) 30 g are added to treat hemafecia.

## 2. Hyperactivity of the liver with spleen deficiency

Treatment principle: Suppressing the liver and supporting the spleen, checking diarrhea and stopping pain.

Prescription and herbs: Modified Tongxie Yaofang Prescription and Xiaoyao Powder.

Chaihu (Chinese Thorowax Root) 6 g, Fangfeng (Divaricate Saposhnikovia Root) 9 g, Baizhu (Largehead Atractylodes Rhizome) 9 g, Fuling (Indian Bread) 12 g, Shanyao (Common Yan Rhizome) 15 g, Yiyiren (Coix Seed) 15 g, Weijiang (Roasted Ginger) 6 g, Gancao (Liquorice Root) 6 g, Baishao (White Peony Alba) 9 g, Baijifen (Common Bletilla Tuber Powder) 3 g and Chenpi (Dried Tangerine Peel) 9 g.

Modification: For apparent abdominal distension and belching, Yujin (Turmeric Root Tuber) 9 g, Zhiqiao (Orange Fruit) 12 g and Chenpi (Dried Tangerine Peel) 6 g are added to regulate qi; if there isheadache, restlessness and irascibility, Huangqin (Baical Skullcap Root) 9 g, Zhizi (Cape Jasmine Fruit) 9 g and Longdancao (Radix Gentianae) 6 g are added to dispel heat.

## 3. Obstruction of blood stasis in the intestinal tract

Treatment principle: Regulating qi and activating blood, expelling stasis and checking diarrhea.

Prescription and herbs: Modified Gexia Zhuyu Decoction and Shaoyao Decoction.

Danggui (Chinese Angelica) 9 g, Chishao (Red Peony Root) 9 g, Chuanxiong (Szechwan Lovage Rhizome) 9 g, Honghua (Safflower) 3 g, Wulingzhi (Faeces Trogopterorum) 9 g (wrapped during decoction), Muoyao (Myrrh) 9 g, Yanhusuo (Corydalis) 9 g, Wuyao (Combined Spicebush Root) 9 g, Binglang (Areca Seed) 9 g, Muxiang (Common Aucklandia Root) 6 g, Huangqin (Baical Skullcap Root) 9 g, Huangbai (Amur Cork-tree) 9 g, Baijifen (Common Bletilla Tuber Powder) 3 g, Diyu (Garden Burnet Root) 15 g, Huaihua (Pagodatree Flower) 9 g and Gancao (Liquorice Root) 6 g.

Modification: If the blood stasis is severe, Sanleng (Common Burreed Tuber) 9 g and Ezhu (Zedoray Rhizome) 9 g are added to dissipate blood stasis.

## 4. Weakness of the spleen and stomach

Treatment principle: Nourishing qi and moving up yang, invigorating the spleen and stopping diarrhea.

Prescription and herbs: Supplementary Buzhong Yiqi Decoction.

Huangqi (Milkvetch Root) 15 g, Dangshen (Radix Codonopsis) 12 g, Baizhu (Largehead Atractylodes Rhizome) 12 g, Fuling (Indian Bread) 12 g, Chaihu (Chinese Thorowax Root) 6 g, Shengma (Rhizoma Cimicifugae) 9 g, Shanyao (Common Yan Rhizome) 15 g, Biandou (Hyacinth Bean) 15 g, Lianzirou (Lotus Seed) 9 g, Muxiang (Common Aucklandia Root) 3 g, Sharen (Villous Amomum Fruit) 3 g, Jiegeng (Platycodon Root) 3 g, Danggui (Chinese Angelica) 9 g, Chenpi (Dried Tangerine Peel) 6 g, Dazao (Chinese Date) 15 g and Gancao (Liquorice Root) 6 g.

Modification: For chronic diarrhea with slippage, Hezi (Medicine Terminalia Fruit) 9 g, Yuyuliang (Limonite) 15 g and Chishizhi (Red Halloysite) 15 g are added to astringe the intestine and check diarrhea.

## 5. Production of internal heat due to deficiency of yin

Treatment principle: Nourishing yin blood, dispelling heat and stopping diarrhea.

Prescription and herbs: Supplementary Zhuche Pill.

Shengdi (Dried Rehmannia Root) 12 g, Danggui (Chinese Angelica) 9 g, Baishao (White Peony Alba) 9 g, Ejiao (Donkey-hide Glue) 9 g, Digupi (Chinese Wolfberry Root-Bark)12 g, Baiwei (Blackend Swallowwort Root) 9 g, Huangqin (Baical Skullcap Root) 9 g, Huanglian (Golden Thread) 3 g, Paojiang (Prepared Dried Ginger) 6 g and Gancao (Liquorice Root) 6 g.

Modification: If there is presence of stools with bright red blood, Huaihua (Pagodatree Flower) 9 g, Cebaiye (Chinese Arborvitae Twig and Leaf)

12 g and Diyutan (Charred Radix Sanguisorbae) 12 g are added to cool blood and stop bleeding.

## 6. Yang deficiency of the spleen and kidneys

Treatment principle: Warming and nourishing the spleen and kidneys, astringing the intestine and stopping diarrhea.

Prescription and herbs: Modified Zhenren Yangzang Decoction and Sishen Pill.

Dangshen (Radix Codonopsis) 15 g, Baizhu (Largehead Atractylodes Rhizome) 9 g, Gancao (Liquorice Root) 6 g, Rougui (Cassia Bark) 3 g, Roudoukou (Nutmeg) 9 g, Paojiang (Prepared Dried Ginger) 6 g, Buguzhi (Malaytea Scurfpea Fruit) 9 g, Wuweizi (Chinese Magnolivine Fruit) 3 g, Hezi (Medicine Terminalia Fruit) 9 g, Yingsuke (Poppy Capsule) 6~9 g, Wuzhuyu (Medicinal Evodia Fruit) 3 g, Baishao (White Peony Alba) 9 g, Danggui (Chinese Angelica) 9 g, Muxiang (Common Aucklandia Root) 6 g and Dazao (Chinese Date) 15 dates.

Modification: For waist soreness and cold limbs, Fuzi (Prepared Common Monkshood Daughter) 6 g and Ganjiang (Dried Ginger) 6 g can be added to warm yang and dissipate cold.

## Chinese Patent Medicine

1. Guben Yichang Tablet: 4 tablets for each dose, twice a day.
2. Liushen Pill, Yunnan Baiyao, Xilei Powder can be administered orally at the same time and can also be used to give an enema.

## Simple and Handy Prescriptions

Baitouweng (Chinese Pulsatilla Root) 30 g, Huangqin (Baical Skullcap Root) 9 g, Huanglian (Golden Thread) 6 g, Muxiang (Common Aucklandia Root) 6 g and Binglang (Areca Seed) 9 g are decocted and taken once a day.

## Other Therapies

Dietary therapy:

(1) Jiangmi (Rice Fruit) 100 g and Biandou (Fresh Hyacinth Bean) 30 g are boiled in water until the decoction becomes thick and finally a small amount of spring onion and salt can be added. This porridge can be taken regularly.
(2) Lianzi (Lotus Seed) 15 g (immersed in cold water for 1 hour) and Shanyao (Common Yan Rhizome) 30 g are boiled in water until the decoction becomes thick. This porridge can be taken to treat spleen deficiency.

Chinese medical coloclysis: Baitouweng (Chinese Pulsatilla Root) 30 g, Kushen (Lightyellow Sophora Root) 30 g, Dijincao (Creeping Euphorbia) 15 g, Baijiangcao (Dahurian Patrinia Herb) 15 g, Mingfan (Alum) 15 g, Huaihua (Pagodatree Flower) 15 g, Baiji (Common Bletilla Tuber) 10 g, Cebaitan (Charred Cacumen Platycladi) 10 g and Diyutan (Charred Radix Sanguisorbae) 10 g are boiled into a 250 ml-thick decoction for retention-enema.

If there is profuse bleeding and both Chinese and Western medicines can not stop it, with such complications as intestinal stenosis, obstruction and perforation, or abscess, fistulization and canceration, surgical treatment is advisable.

## Cautions and Advice

1. In the acute phase, or when the disease is severe, patients should rest in bed and avoid emotional stimulation, overstrain, dietary irregularity and secondary infection.
2. Patient should have a light, easily digestible and nutritious diet. Warm porridge is highly recommended for its action in facilitating recovery. Consumption of oily, fatty and sweet food should be controlled, so as to prevent intestinal slippage.

3. Most patients have a favorable prognosis, but in these cases, the risk of canceration is actually increased. If there are complications, the prognosis is usually unfavorable.

## Daily Exercises

1. Recall the etiology and pathology of ulcerative colitis.
2. Explain how ulcerative colitis can be treated based on syndrome differentiation.

# Intestinal Tuberculosis

# Week 6: Thursday

Intestinal tuberculosis refers to a chronic specific infection due to invasion of the tubercle bacillus into the intestinal tract. Intestinal tuberculosis is, under most circumstances, secondary to pulmonary tuberculosis, especially the open pulmonary tuberculosis. It is clinically marked by abdominal pain, loose stools or constipation, right lower abdominal masses, fever and night sweats. This disease usually occurs in young and middle-aged people, with females more susceptible than males. In TCM, intestinal tuberculosis is closely associated with "dysentery", "abdominal pain" and "diarrhea".

## Etiology and Pathology

This disease is located in the intestine and is closely linked to the spleen and kidneys. The occurrence of it is due to insufficiency of healthy qi coupled with infection of "consumptive worms (tubercle bacillus)". For instance, improper sterilization and isolation, dining with patients with pulmonary tuberculosis, or frequent swallowing of sputum containing consumptive worms by patients with pulmonary tuberculosis can all lead to invasion of the consumptive worms into the intestinal tract, marked by a condition in which the root is deficient while the branch is in excess (insufficiency of the spleen and kidneys with qi stagnation and blood stasis).

## Diagnostic Key Points

1. The pre-existence of extra-intestinal tuberculosis in young and middle-aged patients or the manifestation of controlled infection of primary lesion yet with aggravation of tuberculotic virulent blood symptoms.
2. Clinical manifestations: Alimentary canal disorders such as abdominal pain, loose stools or constipation, or alternated constipation and diarrhea, complicated by general symptoms such as fever and night sweats.
3. Masses in the abdomen, particularly the right lower abdomen, with or without tenderness, or presence of unidentified intestinal obstruction.

4. X-ray barium meal test on the gastrointestinal tract: Irritation due to ulcerative inflammation of the ileum, or filling defect and stenosis due to hyperplasia. This method is of significant value to the diagnosis of intestinal tuberculosis.

5. Laboratory auxiliary examination:

(1) Blood test: Possible moderate anaemia, increased level of lymphocytes and marked acceleration of blood sedimentation.

(2) Intestinal discharge test: A small number of pus cells and red blood cells. Presence of tubercle bacillus in condensed stools is indicative of intestinal tuberculosis, but only in the absence of tubercle bacillus in sputum.

6. For suspicion of intestinal tuberculosis but without a definitive diagnosis, antituberculosis drugs can be administered for 2~3 weeks, and then the clinical symptoms are observed and analyzed to ascertain the disease.

## Syndrome Differentiation

### 1. Yang deficiency of the spleen and kidneys

Symptoms: Vague pain in the abdomen with paroxysmal aggravation, loose stools or diarrhea before dawn, lassitude, cold body and limbs, poor appetite, weakness and soreness of the waist and knees and a pale complexion; pale tongue with thin coating and thin, feeble pulse.

Analysis of symptoms: Deficiency of spleen yang and kidney yang fails to warm the body, leading to stagnation of qi and congealing of cold, this is marked by vague pain in the abdomen with aggravated paroxysm; deficiency of the spleen results in indigestion of water and food and deficiency of the kidneys leads to inactivation of the spleen yang, resulting in loose stools or diarrhea before dawn; deficiency of yang produces internal cold, giving rise to lassitude with cold body and limbs; deficiency of the spleen is responsible for poor appetite; deficiency of the kidneys gives rise to weakness and soreness of the waist and knees; a pale complexion, a pale tongue with thin coating and a thin, feeble pulse are all attributable to yang deficiency of the spleen and kidneys.

## 2. Obstruction of blood stasis

Symptoms: Pricking pain with tenderness in the right lower abdomen, fixed abdominal masses and sometimes constipation; dark purple tongue with occasional ecchymosis and thin, unsmooth pulse.

Analysis of symptoms: Owing to obstruction of blood stasis in the vessels, there is pricking pain in the right lower abdomen; since the blood stasis is tangible, the pain is aggravated when pressure is applied and the abdominal masses are fixed in location; obstruction of blood stasis in the intestinal tract results in constipation; the dark purple tongue with occasional ecchymosis and thin, unsmooth pulse are both due to blood stasis.

## 3. Deficiency of healthy qi and excess of pathogenic factors

Symptoms: Lassitude, hectic fever, night sweats, poor appetite, alternated diarrhea and constipation, tender pricking pain in the right lower abdomen and fixed abdominal masses; red tongue with thin coating and thin, feeble pulse or thin, rapid pulse.

Analysis of symptoms: Deficiency of qi brings about lassitude; deficiency of yin results in hectic fever and night sweats; deficiency of the spleen causes poor appetite and loose stools; obstruction of blood stasis in the intestinal tract leads to constipation; and obstruction of blood stasis in the collaterals gives rise to the pricking pain in the right lower abdomen; since the blood stasis is tangible, the pain is aggravated when pressure is applied and the abdominal masses are fixed in location; the red tongue with thin coating and thin, feeble pulse or thin, rapid pulse are caused by deficiency of qi and yin.

## Differential Treatment

## 1. Yang deficiency of the spleen and kidneys

Treatment principle: Nourishing yin and warming yang, invigorating the spleen and tonifying the kidneys.

Prescription and herbs: Fuzi Lizhong Pill and Sishen Pill.

Fuzi (Prepared Common Monkshood Daughter) 6 g, Ganjiang (Dried Ginger) 9 g, Dangshen (Radix Codonopsis) 12 g, Baizhu (Largehead Atractylodes Rhizome) 12 g, Shanyao (Common Yan Rhizome) 15 g, Biandou (Hyacinth Bean) 15 g, Buguzhi (Malaytea Scurfpea Fruit) 9 g, Wuzhuyu (Medicinal Evodia Fruit) 3 g, Roudoukou (Nutmeg) 9 g, Baibu (Stemona Root) 15 g, Chenpi (Dried Tangerine Peel) 6 g and Gancao (Liquorice Root) 6 g.

Modification: For cold-natured constipation, Roucongrong (Desertliving Cistanche) 9 g, Rougui (Cassia Bark) 9 g, Danggui (Chinese Angelica) 9 g and Shengma (Rhizoma Cimicifugae) 6 g are added to warm yang and promote defecation.

## 2. Obstruction of blood stasis

Treatment principle: Resolving stasis and dissipating accumulation, moving qi and resolving stagnation.

Prescription and herbs: Supplementary Shaofu Zhuyu Decoction.

Danggui (Chinese Angelica) 9 g, Chuanxiong (Szechwan Lovage Rhizome) 9 g, Chishao (Red Peony Root) 9 g, Wulingzhi (Faeces Trogopterorum) 9 g, Puhuang (Pollen Typhae) 9 g (wrapped during decoction), Muoyao (Myrrh) 6 g, Zhiqiao (Orange Fruit) 12 g, Yanhusuo (Corydalis) 9 g, Ganjiang (Dried Ginger) 9 g, Xiaohuixiang (Fennel) 6 g, Baibu (Stemona Root) 15 g and Gancao (Liquorice Root) 6 g.

Modification: For apparent masses, Xiangbeimu (Bulbus Fritillariae Thunbergii) 9 g, Sanleng (Common Burreed Tuber) 9 g and Ezhu (Zedoray Rhizome) 9 g are added to soften and dissipate nodules.

## 3. Deficiency of healthy qi and excess of pathogenic factors

Treatment principle: Replenishing qi and nourishing yin, resolving stasis and expelling pathogenic factors.

Prescription and herbs: Modified Yigong Powder and Qinjiao Biejia Powder.

Huangqi (Milkvetch Root) 15 g, Dangshen (Radix Codonopsis) 12 g, Baizhu (Largehead Atractylodes Rhizome) 12 g, Fuling (Indian Bread) 12 g, Biejia (Turtle Shell) 15 g, Zhimu (Common Anemarrhena Rhizome) 9 g, Baishao (White Peony Alba) 9 g, Danggui (Chinese Angelica) 9 g, Qinjiao (Largeleaf Gentian Root) 9 g, Qinghao (Sweet Wormwood Herb) 9 g, Digupi (Chinese Wolfberry Root-Bark) 9 g, Baibu (Stemona Root) 15 g, Ruxiang (Boswellin) 6 g, Muoyao (Myrrh) 6 g, Sanleng (Common Burreed Tuber) 9 g, Ezhu (Zedoray Rhizome) 9 g, Chenpi (Dried Tangerine Peel) 6 g and Gancao (Liquorice Root) 6 g.

Modification: If there are loose stools and poor appetite, Biejia (Turtle Shell) is replaced with Biandou (Hyacinth Bean) 15 g and Yiyiren (Coix Seed) 15 g to invigorate the spleen and stop diarrhea; for constipation, Huomaren (Hemp Seed) 9 g, Shengdi (Dried Rehmannia Root) 30 g and Shouwu (Fleeceflower Root) 30 g are added to moisten the intestine and promote defecation.

## Chinese Patent Medicine

1. Shenling Baizhu Tablet: 4 tablets for each dose, 3 times a day.
2. Qinbudan Tablet: 5 tablets for each dose, twice a day.

## Simple and Handy Prescriptions

1. Baibu (Stemona Root) 20 g is boiled in water and taken 1 dose a day.
2. Shanyao (Common Yan Rhizome) 500 g is steamed, peeled and pounded into paste and then Xianou (Fresh Lotus Root) 500 g is pounded to extract its juice; afterwards, the paste and juice are evenly mixed and taken as food.

## Other Therapies

Dietary therapy:

(1) A tender pulled chicken (preferably silkie), Huangqi (Milkvetch Root) 20 g, Xiyangshen (American Ginseng) 3 g, Baibu (Stemona

Root) 10 g, Dongsun (Winter Bamboo Shoot Slice) 30 g and Shuhuotui (Processed Ham) 3 slices are simmered over slow fire for 2 hours before consumption.

(2) A pulled duck is stuffed with 10 g of Dongchongxiacao (Chinese Caterpillar Fungus) and then steamed for 2 hours after adding seasonings for flavour.

The Western anti-tuberculosis drugs should be properly selected and administered in sufficient amount and duration.

If there is the presence of intestinal obstruction, acute perforation and massive intestinal bleeding, the application of surgical treatment can be taken into consideration.

## Cautions and Advice

1. The patients should take more rest, keep a proper diet and strengthen physical exercises. They should also maintain life cultivation, abstain from alcohol and coitus, regulate daily life and emotions and adapt to weather changes so as to enhance the therapeutic effects.
2. The patients should have sufficient nutrition supply such as vitamins and protein as well as adequate calory intake. For those with weak constitutions and long durations, the tonifying food is highly recommended while fatty, warm or spicy food should be prohibited; consumption of cigarettes and alcohol is also inadvisable.

## Daily Exercises

1. Concisely describe the diagnostic key points of intestinal tuberculosis.
2. Recall the different syndromes classified under intestinal tuberculosis and explain how they can be differentiated prior to treatment.

# Cirrhosis

# Week 6: Friday

Cirrhosis is a systemic wasting disease marked by chronic, progressive and diffusive hepatic disorders due to repeated damages to the liver by various pathogenic factors. Clinically, it is classified into two stages: hepatic functional compensation and decompensation. The compensation stage is characterized by mild symptoms, such as discomfort in the hepatic region, poor appetite, abdominal distension, weariness and splenohepatomegalia. In the decompensation stage, the clinical symptoms are aggravated, complicated by hypohepatia, portal hypertension, splenomegaly, ascites, edema, alimentary tract hemorrhage, anaemia and hepatic coma. Cirrhosis is closely associated with such TCM concepts as "drum belly", "concretions and conglomerations (lower abdominal masses)" and "accumulations and gatherings".

## Etiology and Pathology

The location of this disease is the liver and its occurrence is closely linked to the liver, spleen and kidneys. Emotional depression, improper diet, alcohol abuse, parasitic tympanties and prolonged jaundice can all lead to depression of the liver, stagnation of qi and dysfunction of the spleen; if the condition of liver depression and qi stagnation persists, there will be presence of blood stasis; if deficiency of the spleen with retention of dampness lingers on, the kidney yin and kidney yang can be affected, giving rise to the morbid state marked by deficiency of the primary aspect (deficiency of the liver, spleen and kidneys) and excess of the secondary aspect (qi stagnation, blood stasis and water accumulation) and co-existence of excess and deficiency.

## Diagnostic Key Points

1. The patient has a history of viral hepatitis, schistosomiasis, nutritional disturbance and alcohol abuse.
2. The compensation stage is characterized by mild symptoms, such as discomfort in the hepatic region, weariness, emaciation, poor

appetite, distending pain in the chest and hypochondria, abdominal pain, diarrhea, nausea and vomiting, splenohepatomegalia and a sallow or dark complexion.

3. In the decompensation stage, the clinical symptoms are aggravated, with such manifestations as hardened, enlarged (but contracted thereafter) liver, ascites, pleural fluid, hemorrhagic tendency, anaemia, jaundice, spider telangiectasia, liver palm, mammoplasia in males, varicosis in the abdominal wall, rupture of varicose veins in the esophagus and gastric fundus and hepatic coma.

4. Laboratory examination: Positive result indicated by tests on some hepatic functions and decreased level of white blood cells and platelets (particularly the latter) during hypersplenia.

5. X-ray barium swallowing test on the esophagus shows varicose veins in the esophagus.

6. Ultrasonic examination is of certain diagnostic value.

7. Hepatic CT, MRI and biopsy are conducive to the definitive diagnosis.

## Syndrome Differentiation

### 1. Stagnation of qi with retention of dampness

Symptoms: Enlarged, distending yet non-stiff abdomen, a distending sensation below the costal region with occasional pain, reduced food intake, belching, distention after food intake, scanty urine; white greasy tongue coating and taut pulse.

Analysis of symptoms: Liver depression, qi stagnation and retention of dampness in the middle energizer give rise to the enlarged, distending yet non-stiff abdomen and distending sensation below the costal region with occasional pain; weakness of the spleen and stomach results in dysfunction of transportation and transformation, marked by reduced food intake, belching and distention after food intake; obstruction of the waterways is responsible for scanty urine; the white greasy tongue coating and taut pulse are both manifestations of stagnation of qi with retention of dampness.

## 2. Damp-cold encumbering the spleen

Symptoms: Enlarged, full and distending abdomen like a bag containing water upon palpation, distending and stuffy sensation in the chest and gastric region that is alleviated by warmth, cold body (especially the limbs), lassitude, loose stools, scanty urine; white greasy tongue coating and slow pulse.

Analysis of symptoms: Retention of cold, dampness and water is responsible for the enlarged, full and distending abdomen like a bag containing water upon palpation; cold water encumbers the spleen yang, resulting in the distending and stuffy sensation in the chest and gastric region that is alleviated by warmth; encumbrance of the spleen yang and inactivation of yang qi causes the body and limbs to feel cold and this is accompanied by lassitude; the spleen fails to transform and transport the retained water, resulting in scanty urine; the retained water infiltrates the large intestine, bringing about loose stools; the white greasy tongue coating and slow pulse are due to abundance of dampness with decline of yang.

## 3. Internal accumulation of damp-heat

Symptoms: Enlarged, stiff and distending abdomen, acute pain in the gastric cavity and abdomen, fever with restlessness, a bitter taste in the mouth, reduced food intake, body heaviness, scanty reddish urine, constipation or diarrhea and sometimes yellowish eyes and complexion; red tongue tip or margin, yellow-greasy coating and rapid-taut pulse.

Analysis of symptoms: Dampness and heat combine and turbid water accumulates in the interior, hampering the smooth functional activity of qi, this gives rise to the enlarged, stiff and distending abdomen and acute pain in the gastric cavity and abdomen; damp-heat steams upward leading to feverish dysphoria and dry mouth; retention of damp-heat in the stomach and intestine is responsible for reduced food intake, body heaviness, constipation or diarrhea; damp-heat pours downward, bringing about scanty reddish urine; damp-heat fumigates the upper body, giving rise to jaundice; the red tongue tip or margin, yellow-greasy coating and rapid-taut pulse are manifestations of damp-heat.

## 4. Blood stasis in the liver and spleen

Symptoms: Enlarged, stiff and distending abdomen, scurrying pain in the hypochondriac and abdominal region, palpable and slightly hard masses in the right hypochondria, enlarged veins, dark complexion, thin and silk-like capillary nevus in the face, neck, chest and arms, red marks in the palms, purple-brown lips, thirst, atrophy of the gums, nosebleed and dark stools; dark purple tongue with occasional ecchymosis and thin, unsmooth pulse.

Analysis of symptoms: Retention of blood stasis in the collaterals of the liver and spleen as well as obstruction of the waterways lead to accumulation of water in the interior, marked by the enlarged, stiff and distending abdomen, scurrying pain in the hypochondriac and abdominal region, palpable and slightly hard masses in the right hypochondria and enlarged veins; blood stasis progresses into the kidneys in the long run, bringing about a dark complexion, thin and silk-like capillary nevus in the face, neck, chest and arms, red marks in the palms and purple-brown lips; accumulation of turbid water results in thirst; overflowing of blood in the yin collaterals is responsible for atrophy of the gums, nosebleed and dark stools; the dark-purple tongue with occasional ecchymosis and thin, unsmooth pulse are due to retention of blood stasis.

## 5. Yang deficiency of the spleen and kidneys

Symptoms: Enlarged, full and distending abdomen that is alleviated in the morning and aggravated in the evening, mental and physical lassitude, intolerance of cold with cold limbs, gastric stuffiness, poor appetite, loose stools, yellowish or pale complexion, weakness and soreness of the waist and knees, edema of the lower limbs and scanty urine; pale enlarged tongue and thin, deep pulse.

Analysis of symptoms: Deficiency of spleen yang and kidney yang leads to accumulation of cold water, giving rise to the enlarged, full and distending abdomen that is alleviated in the morning and aggravated in the evening; yang qi fails to flow inside and outside the body, marked by spiritual and physical lassitude, intolerance of cold and cold limbs; spleen yang fails to promote digestion, leading to gastric stuffiness, poor appetite and loose stools; deficiency of kidney yang is responsible for weakness and soreness of the waist and knees; retention of water and dampness in the lower energizer is characterized by scanty urine and pedal edema; deficient yang fails to nourish the upper energizer, resulting in yellowish or pale complexion; the pale and enlarged tongue and thin-deep pulse are manifestations of yang deficiency.

## 6. Yin deficiency of the liver and kidneys

Symptoms: Enlarged, stiff and distending abdomen, hypochondriac pain, waist soreness, emaciated limbs, or even varicose veins, dark complexion and purple lips, dry mouth, vexation, feverish complexion and reddened palms, occasional low grade fever, gingival bleeding, nosebleed and scanty urine; purple-red tongue with little fluid and thin, rapid and taut pulse.

Analysis of symptoms: Deficiency of liver yin and kidney yin leads to retention of fluid, accumulation of water and stasis of blood, marked by the enlarged, stiff and distending abdomen, hypochondriac pain, waist soreness, emaciated limbs, or even protruding bluish veins; stagnation of qi and blood is responsible for the dark complexion and purple lips; deficiency of yin fluid is characterized by dry mouth and scanty urine; exuberance of fire due to yin deficiency is manifested as vexation, feverish complexion, reddened palms and occasional low grade fever; heat drives blood rampant, resulting in gingival and nasal bleeding; the purple-red tongue with little fluid and thin, rapid and taut pulse are manifestations of yin deficiency with blood stasis.

## Differential Treatment

### 1. Stagnation of qi with retention of dampness

Treatment principle: Soothing the liver and promoting flow of qi, removing dampness and relieving fullness.

Prescription and herbs: Modified Chaihu Shugan Powder and Wuling Powder.

Chaihu (Chinese Thorowax Root) 6 g, Foshou (Finger Citron) 6 g, Zhiqiao (Orange Fruit) 12 g, Xiangfu (Nutgrass Galingale Rhizome) 12 g, Baishao (White Peony Alba) 9 g, Chuanxiong (Szechwan Lovage Rhizome) 9 g, Cangzhu (Atractylodes Rhizome) 9 g, Houpu (Magnolia Bark) 9 g, Zhuling (Polyporus) 12 g, Fuling (Indian Bread) 12 g, Zexie (Oriental Waterplantain Rhizome) 12 g, Chenpi (Dried Tangerine Peel) 6 g and Gancao (Liquorice Root) 6 g.

Modification: If there is scanty urine, Cheqianzi (Plantain Seed) 12 g (wrapped during decoction) can be added to promote water discharge.

## 2. Damp-cold encumbering the spleen

Treatment principle: Warming the middle energizer and dissipating cold, resolving dampness and promoting water discharge.

Prescription and herbs: Supplementary Shi Pi Yin (Spleen-Fortifying Potion).

Fuzi (Prepared Common Monkshood Daughter) 6 g, Ganjiang (Dried Ginger) 9 g, Baizhu (Largehead Atractylodes Rhizome) 12 g, Zhuling (Polyporus) 12 g, Fuling (Indian Bread) 12 g, Cheqianzi (Plantain Seed) 15 g (wrapped during decoction), Mugua (Papaya) 9 g, Houpu (Magnolia Bark) 9 g, Muxiang (Common Aucklandia Root) 6 g, Dafupi (Areca Peel) 12 g, Caoguo (Fructus Tsaoko) 9 g and Gancao (Liquorice Root) 6 g.

Modification: For oliguresis, Zexie (Oriental Waterplantain Rhizome) 20 g, Chenhulu (Aged Bottle-gourd) 9 g and Chongsun (Henon Bamboo Dried Shoot) 9 g are added to promote water discharge; if there is severely poor appetite with greasy tongue coating, Jiangbanxia (Ginger-prepared Pinellia Tuber) 9 g and Jineijin (Corium Stomachium Galli) 6 g can be added to resolve dampness and promote appetite.

## 3. Internal accumulation of damp-heat

Treatment principle: Dispelling heat and eliminating dampness, relieving edema and expelling jaundice.

Prescription and herbs: Modified Yinchenhao Decoction and Zhongman Fenxiao Pill.

Yinchen (Virgate Wormwood Herb) 15 g, Huangqin (Baical Skullcap Root) 9 g, Huanglian (Golden Thread) 3 g, Zhizi (Cape Jasmine Fruit) 9 g, Zhimu (Common Anemarrhena Rhizome) 9 g, Houpu (Magnolia Bark) 9 g, Banxia (Pinellia Tuber) 9 g, Zhiqiao (Orange Fruit) 6 g, Chenpi (Dried Tangerine Peel) 6 g, Zhuling (Polyporus) 12 g, Fuling (Indian Bread) 12 g, Zexie (Oriental Waterplantain Rhizome) 15 g, Cheqianzi (Plantain Seed) 15 g (wrapped during decoction) and Gancao (Liquorice Root) 6 g.

Modification: If there is scanty reddish urine, Huangbai (Amur Cork-tree) 9 g and Huashi (Talc) 30 g are added to dispel heat and discharge water.

## 4. Blood stasis in the liver and spleen

Treatment principle: Activating blood and resolving stasis, promoting flow of qi and relieving edema.

Prescription and herbs: Modified Tiaoying Potion.

Chuanxiong (Szechwan Lovage Rhizome) 6 g, Danggui (Chinese Angelica) 9 g, Chishao (Red Peony Root) 9 g, Sanleng (Common Burreed Tuber) 9 g, Ezhu (Zedoray Rhizome) 9 g, Yanhusuo (Corydalis) 9 g, Chenpi (Dried Tangerine Peel) 6 g, Binglang (Areca Seed) 9 g, Dafupi (Areca Peel) 9 g, Tinglizi (Herba Leonuri) 15 g, Chifuling (Indian Bread Pink Epidermis) 12 g, Sangbaipi (White Mulberry Root-Bark) 9 g and Gancao (Liquorice Root) 6 g.

Modification: If there are black stools, Zhaoxintu (Humus Flava Usta) 30 g, Shensanqi (Panax Pseudo-ginseng) 9 g, Baijifen (Common Bletilla Tuber Powder) 3 g and Diyutan (Charred Radix Sanguisorbae) 9 g are added to stop bleeding.

## 5. Yang deficiency of the spleen and kidneys

Treatment principle: Invigorating the spleen and kidneys with warmth, transforming qi and relieving edema.

Prescription and herbs: Modified Fuzi Lizhong Pill and Zhenwu Decoction.

Fuzi (Prepared Common Monkshood Daughter) 9 g, Rougui (Cassia Bark) 3 g, Paojiang (Prepared Dried Ginger) 3 g, Dangshen (Radix Codonopsis)

12 g, Baizhu (Largehead Atractylodes Rhizome) 12 g, Fuling (Indian Bread) 12 g, Chishao (Red Peony Root) 9 g, Danggui (Chinese Angelica) 9 g, Ezhu (Zedoray Rhizome) 9 g, Sanleng (Common Burreed Tuber) 9 g, Dafupi (Areca Peel) 12 g and Cheqianzi (Plantain Seed) 30 g (wrapped during decoction).

Modification: In cases of edema in the lower limbs and oliguresis, Zhuling (Polyporus) 12 g, Zexie (Oriental Waterplantain Rhizome) 15 g, Chenhulu (Aged Bottle-gourd) 9 g, Chongsun (Henon Bamboo Dried Shoot) 9 g and Huashi (Talc) 30 g can be added to promote urination and relieve edema.

## 6. Yin deficiency of the liver and kidneys

Treatment principle: Tonifying the liver and nourishing the kidneys, regulating qi and resolving stasis.

Prescription and herbs: Modified Yiguan Decoction and Gexia Zhuyu Decoction.

Shashen (Root of Straight Ladybell) 12 g, Maidong (Dwarf Lilyturf Tuber) 12 g, Shengdi (Dried Rehmannia Root) 12 g, Shudi (Prepared Rhizome of Rehmannia) 12 g, Gouqizi (Barbary Wolfberry Fruit) 12 g, Guiban (Tortoise Shell) 15 g, Chuanlianzi (Szechwan Chinaberry Fruit) 9 g, Yanhusuo (Corydalis) 9 g, Zhiqiao (Orange Fruit) 15 g, Danggui (Chinese Angelica) 9 g, Chishao (Red Peony Root) 9 g, Honghua (Safflower) 3 g, Wulingzhi (Faeces Trogopterorum) 9 g (wrapped during decoction), Danpi (Cortex Moutan) 9 g and Qiancao (Indian Madder Root) 15 g.

Modification: If there is ascites with scanty urine, Zhuling (Polyporus) 12 g, Fuling (Indian Bread) 12 g, Chenhulu (Aged Bottle-gourd) 9 g and Zexie (Oriental Waterplantain Rhizome) 20 g are added to promote urination and relieve edema; for low grade fever with flushed face, Guiban (Tortoise Shell) 9 g and Biejia (Turtle Shell) 9 g are added to nourish yin and tonify the kidneys.

## Chinese Patent Medicine

Renshen Biejia Jian Pill: 6 g for each dose, 3 times a day.

## Simple and Handy Prescriptions

1. Baimaogen (Lalang Grass Rhizome) 30 g, Chongsun (Henon Bamboo Dried Shoot) 60 g and Chenhulu (Aged Bottle-gourd) 120 g are decocted together and taken once a day.
2. Malantou (Indian Kalimeris Herb) 250 g and Zhushun (Bamboo Shoot) 150 g are boiled together in water. The decoction is taken once a day.

## Other Therapies

Dietary therapy:

(1) A fat, large male duck (aythya baeri) is boiled for a while and then washed with cold boiled water. Afterwards it is stuffed with Dongchongxiacao (Chinese Caterpillar Fungus) 10 g, Gouqizi (Barbary Wolfberry Fruit) 15 g, Chixiaodou (Rice Bean) 60 g and 5 Caoguo (Fructus Tsaoko) and stitched up with a suture line. It is subsequently steamed for 2 hours. Thereafter the Chinese Caterpillar Fungus and Barbary Wolfberry Fruit are taken out and chewed and the dregs are abandoned. The soup is taken for each dose. The duck is sliced and consumed over a few sittings.

(2) Danggui (Chinese Angelica) 9 g, Gouqizi (Barbary Wolfberry Fruit) 9 g, Gandihuang (Adhesive Rehmannia Dried Root) 10 g, Nuzhenzi (Glossy Privet Fruit) 10 g, Maidong (Dwarf Lilyturf Tuber) 10 g, Shanyao (Common Yan Rhizome) 16 g and Chenpi (Dried Tangerine Peel) 6 g are wrapped in a bag made of absorbent gauze, which is subsequently put into the body of a soft-shelled turtle. The stuffed turtle is boiled in an earthenware cooking pot with proper amounts of water, welsh onion and ginger. After it is well decocted over a slow fire, the medicated bag is taken out. Both the turtle and soup can be taken as medicinal food.

If there is coma, massive bleeding, scanty urine or suppression of urine, an integrated Chinese and Western approach can be adopted to address the conditions proactively.

## Cautions and Advice

1. Proper care and regulation are as important as medical treatment, so patients should try to relax and keep themselves calm and in good spirits. If there is hepatic functional decompensation or complications, they should rest in bed, keep warm and take precautions to prevent infection.

2. It is advisable for patients to keep to a diet of easily digested foods that are rich in calories, proteins, carbohydrates and vitamins. When the hepatic functions are markedly reduced, or when there is such presymptom as hepatic coma, the intake of proteins should be strictly restricted. The consumption of animal fat and oil is also restricted. Alcohol is forbidden. The consumption of coarse, hard or roasted foods, as well as birds and fishes with bone chips should be strictly controlled to avoid rupture of varicose veins in the gastric fundus. If there is edema, it is advisable to take a low-salt diet. If there is constipation, it is appropriate to take more sesame oil, honey, sesame and banana to maintain the smoothness of defecation and prevent hepatic coma.

3. When there is presence of upper gastrointestinal bleeding, hepatic coma, primary hepatic carcinoma, hepatorenal syndrome and electrolyte disturbance, the disease begins to exacerbate, pointing to an unfavorable prognosis.

## Daily Exercises

1. Concisely describe the etiology and pathology of cirrhosis.
2. Explain how cirrhosis can be treated based on syndrome differentiation.

# Primary Hepatic Carcinoma

# Week 6: Saturday

Primary hepatic carcinoma refers to the tumors occurring in the hepatic cells or intrahepatic bile duct cells, clinically marked by pain in the hepatic region, weariness, emaciation, reduced appetite and hepatomegalia; in the late stage, there may be such symptoms as jaundice, ascites, cachexia, bleeding, coma and general prostration. In TCM, primary hepatic carcinoma is considered to be associated with "hypochondriac pain", "liver accumulation", "abdominal mass", "drum belly" and "jaundice".

## Etiology and Pathology

This disease is located in the liver and caused by disorders of the liver, spleen, stomach and kidneys. The etiological factors are exogenous damp-heat and pestilent toxins, emotional depression, improper diet and long-term deficiency of the spleen and stomach. These factors can impair the liver, spleen or kidneys in different ways. Abundant heat and toxins fumigate the liver and gallbladder and drive out the bile, resulting in jaundice; qi stagnation and blood stasis creates a predisposition to masses and accumulations; retention of qi, blood and water in the abdomen gives rise to a drum belly; chronic diseases involve the kidneys, leading to deficient consumption with general prostration. This disease is characterized by deficiency of the primary aspect (deficiency of the liver, spleen, stomach and kidneys) and excess of the secondary aspect (toxic heat, qi stagnation, blood stasis and water retention).

## Diagnostic Key Points

1. In the early stage, there are unidentified discomforts or pain in the hepatic region, or exacerbation of the original hepatic symptoms, accompanied by general malaise, weariness, fever, as well as loss of appetite and body weight.
2. In the middle and late stages, there are such signs as pain in the hepatic region, weariness, emaciation, progressive enlargement of the liver

with tenderness and such features as hardness and superficial nodules; in addition, there may also be some symptoms like jaundice, fever, general weakness, splenomegaly, ascites, cachexia, as well as complications such as hepatic coma and upper gastrointestinal bleeding.

3. Laboratory examination: Blood serum AFP determination, positive; hepatic dysfunction in patients in the middle or late stage; increased blood ammonia level in patients with hepatic coma.

4. It is advisable to make a definitive diagnosis by means of hepatic B-ultrasonic wave, CT, MRI and CT-guided cytological or histological examination.

## Syndrome Differentiation

### 1. Stagnation of liver qi

Symptoms: Hypochondriac distending pain (particularly on the right side), chest distress, abdominal fullness and distension, frequent belching, reduced food intake; thin tongue coating and taut pulse.

Analysis of symptoms: The liver fails to promote free flow of qi, so there is hypochondriac distending pain, particularly on the right side; unsmooth functional activity of qi is responsible for chest distress, abdominal fullness and distension; the liver qi invades the stomach and hampers descent of the stomach qi, this is marked by frequent belching and reduced food intake; the thin tongue coating and taut pulse are due to liver depression and qi stagnation.

### 2. Weakness of the spleen and stomach

Symptoms: Weariness, dizziness, gastric and abdominal discomfort, reduced food intake, loose stools, sallow complexion; pale tongue, thin coating and soggy pulse.

Analysis of symptoms: Deficiency of spleen qi and stomach qi leads to abnormal transportation and transformation, as well as disordered ascent and descent, this is marked by weariness, dizziness, gastric and abdominal discomfort, reduced food intake and loose stools; exhaustion of the source for producing qi and blood is manifested in the sallow complexion; the pale tongue with thin coating and soggy pulse are attributable to weakness of the spleen and stomach.

## 3. Accumulation of dampness and heat

Symptoms: Hypochondriac pain, chest distress, yellowish eyes and body, a bitter taste in the mouth, nausea and vomiting in severe cases, abdominal distension and venous prominence, dry stools and scanty reddish urine; yellow-greasy tongue coating and taut-slippery pulse.

Analysis of symptoms: Stagnation of qi in the liver and gallbladder leads to hypochondriac pain and chest distress; damp-heat drives the bile out of the gallbladder, this is marked by yellowish eyes and body; damp-heat fumigates the middle energizer, causing adverse rising of turbid gastric qi and characterized by the bitter taste in the mouth, nausea and vomiting; dampness and heat combine, leading to the accumulation of turbid water, with such signs as bulging belly and varicose veins appearing in the abdominal wall; pathogenic damp-heat obstructs the intestinal tract, so there are dry stools; damp-heat pours into the bladder downwardly, bringing about scanty and reddish urine; the yellow-greasy tongue coating and taut-slippery pulse are both due to accumulation of dampness and heat.

## 4. Exuberance of heat and toxins

Symptoms: High fever with perspiration, thirst with dry lips, abdominal distension, hypochondriac pain, or yellowish eyes and body, nosebleed, gum bleeding and muscular bleeding, or even haematemesis, hemafecia, constipation, scanty reddish urine and skin suggillation; red tongue with extremely dry coating and surging-rapid pulse.

Analysis of symptoms: Abundance of heat and toxins is manifested as high fever with perspiration and thirst with dry lips; the location of this disease is the liver which is affected by stagnation of heat and qi, giving rise to abdominal distension and hypochondriac pain; toxic heat drives out the bile and thiss is marked by the yellowish eyes and body; toxic heat invades the ying phase and drives blood rampant, leading to nosebleeds, gingival and muscular bleeding, or even haematemesis, hemafecia and dermal suggillation; toxic heat obstructs the intestinal tract, resulting in constipation; toxic heat pours into the bladder downwardly, bringing about oliguresis; the red tongue with extremely dry coating and surging-rapid pulse are manifestations of abundance of heat and toxins.

## 5. Retention of blood stasis

Symptoms: Pricking, localized pain in the right hypochondria, enlarged liver with tenderness and such features as hardness in texture and unevenness in surface, dark and lusterless complexion; dark and purple tongue with white and thin coating and thin-unsmooth pulse.

Analysis of symptoms: Prolonged depression of the liver leads to qi stagnation and blood stasis, so there is pricking pain in the right hypochondria; since the blood stasis is tangible, the pain is fixed and the liver is enlarged with tenderness and such features as hardness in texture and unevenness in surface; the dark and lusterless complexion, dark and purple tongue, white and thin coating and thin-unsmooth pulse are all due to internal retention of blood stasis.

## 6. Yin exhaustion of the liver and kidneys

Symptoms: Weariness, emaciation, lusterless face, dry skin and muscles, prominent enlargement of the liver, aggravated pain, bulging and distending abdomen, varicose veins in the abdominal wall, hectic fever in the late afternoon, dry mouth and tongue, vexation, insomnia, dark and withered complexion, nosebleed, gingival bleeding, or even haematemesis and hemafecia; dry, deep-red tongue and thin, rapid pulse.

Analysis of symptoms: The deficiency of yin-blood of the liver and kidneys leads to weariness, emaciation, hectic fever in the late afternoon, dry mouth and tongue, vexation and insomnia; deficient qi and blood fail to nourish the skin and muscles, so there is a lusterless face, dry skin and muscles and a dark, withered complexion; deficiency of healthy qi and excess of pathogenic factors bring about aggravated qi stagnation, blood stasis and water retention, marked by prominent enlargement of the liver, aggravated pain, bulging and distending abdomen and varicose veins in the abdominal wall; internal heat due to deficiency of yin drives the blood rampant, giving rise to nosebleed, gingival bleeding, or even haematemesis and hemafecia; the dry, deep-red tongue and thin, rapid pulse are attributable to internal heat due to deficiency of liver yin and kidney yin.

## Differential Treatment

### 1. Stagnation of liver qi

Treatment principle: Soothing the liver to relieve stagnation, regulating qi to activate blood.

Prescription and herbs: Modified Chaihu Shugan Powder and Jinlingzi Powder.

Chaihu (Chinese Thorowax Root) 6 g, Zhiqiao (Orange Fruit) 15 g, Xiangfu (Nutgrass Galingale Rhizome) 9 g, Yanhusuo (Corydalis) 9 g, Chuanlianzi (Szechwan Chinaberry Fruit) 9 g, Chuanxiong (Szechwan Lovage Rhizome) 6 g, Danshen (Radix Salviae Miltiorrhiae) 15 g, Chishao (Red Peony Root) 9 g, Baishao (White Peony Alba) 9 g and Gancao (Liquorice Root) 6 g.

Modification: If there is presence of thoracic and abdominal distension with white greasy tongue coating, Yiyiren (Coix Seed) 12 g, Cangzhu (Atractylodes Rhizome) 9 g and Houpu (Magnolia Bark) 9 g can be added to dry the dampness.

### 2. Weakness of the spleen and stomach

Treatment principle: Replenishing qi to invigorate the spleen, harmonizing the stomach to relieve the middle energizer.

Prescription and herbs: Supplementary Shenling Baizhu Powder and Danggui Decoction.

Huangqi (Milkvetch Root) 15 g, Dangshen (Radix Codonopsis) 12 g, Baizhu (Largehead Atractylodes Rhizome) 12 g, Fuling (Indian Bread) 12 g, Shanyao (Common Yan Rhizome) 15 g, Yiyiren (Coix Seed) 15 g,

Biandou (Hyacinth Bean) 12 g, Danggui (Chinese Angelica) 9 g, Muxiang (Common Aucklandia Root) 6 g, Sharen (Villous Amomum Fruit) 3 g, Chenpi (Dried Tangerine Peel) 6 g and Gancao (Liquorice Root) 6 g.

Modification: For anal prolapse due to chronic diarrhea with qi sinking of the middle energizer, Shengma (Rhizoma Cimicifugae) 6 g and Chaihu (Chinese Thorowax Root) 6 g are added to move up yang qi.

## 3. Accumulation of dampness and heat

Treatment principle: Dispelling heat and eliminating dampness, promoting flow of qi and relieving stagnation.

Prescription and herbs: Modified Yinchenhao Decoction and Zhishi Daozhi Pill.

Yinchen (Virgate Wormwood Herb) 30 g, Huangqin (Baical Skullcap Root) 9 g, Huanglian (Golden Thread) 6 g, Zhizi (Cape Jasmine Fruit) 9 g, Dahuang (Unprepared Rhubarb) 9 g, Yujin (Turmeric Root Tuber) 9 g, Danshen (Radix Salviae Miltiorrhiae) 15 g, Zhishi (Immature Orange Fruit) 12 g, Zhuling (Polyporus) 12 g, Fuling (Indian Bread) 12 g, Cheqianzi (Plantain Seed) 12 g (wrapped during decoction) and Zexie (Oriental Waterplantain Rhizome) 12 g.

Modification: In cases of nausea and vomiting, Jiangzhuru (Ginger-prepared Bamboo Shavings) 9 g can be added to reverse the adverse flow of qi and arrest vomiting; for abdominal distension, Chenhulu (Aged Bottle-gourd) 9 g and Chongsun (Henon Bamboo Dried Shoot) 9 g are added to promote water discharge.

## 4. Exuberance of heat and toxins

Treatment principle: Dispelling heat and removing toxins, cooling blood and dissipating stasis.

Prescription and herbs: Modified Xijiao Dihuang Decoction and Huanglian Jiedu Decoction.

Shuiniujiao (Buffalo Horn) 30 g, Shengdi (Dried Rehmannia Root) 30 g, Danpi (Cortex Moutan) 9 g, Chishao (Red Peony Root) 9 g, Jinyinhua (Honeysuckle Flower) 12 g, Xianhecao (Hairyvein Agrimonia Herb) 30 g, Huangqin (Baical Skullcap Root) 9 g, Huanglian (Golden Thread) 3 g, Huangbai (Amur Cork-tree) 9 g, Zhizi (Cape Jasmine Fruit) 9 g and Gancao (Liquorice Root) 6 g.

Modification: For high fever with profuse perspiration, Shigao (Gypsum) 30 g and Zhimu (Common Anemarrhena Rhizome) 12 g are added to dispel heat and purge fire; for constipation, Dahuang (Unprepared Rhubarb) 9 g can be added to purge heat and promote defecation.

## 5. Retention of blood stasis

Treatment principle: Promoting flow of qi to activate blood, resolving stasis to stop pain.

Prescription and herbs: Modified Gexia Zhuyu Decoction and Danshen Potion.

Taoren (Peach Seed) 9 g, Honghua (Safflower) 6 g, Chishao (Red Peony Root) 9 g, Danpi (Cortex Moutan) 9 g, Danggui (Chinese Angelica) 9 g, Chuanxiong (Szechwan Lovage Rhizome) 6 g, Danshen (Radix Salviae Miltiorrhiae) 15 g, Wulingzhi (Faeces Trogopterorum) 9 g (wrapped during decoction), Xiangfu (Nutgrass Galingale Rhizome) 12 g, Chuanlianzi (Szechwan Chinaberry Fruit) 9 g, Yanhusuo (Corydalis) 9 g, Zhiqiao (Orange Fruit) 12 g, Tanxiang (Sandalwood) 3 g, Sharen (Villous Amomum Fruit) 3 g and Gancao (Liquorice Root) 6 g.

Modification: If there is enlargement of the liver, Chuanshanjia (Pangolin Scale) 12 g, Sanleng (Common Burreed Tuber) 9 g and Ezhu (Zedoray Rhizome) 9 g are added to eliminate the stasis and resolve the stagnation; for severe pain, Ruxiang (Boswellin) 9g and Muoyao (Myrrh) 9g can be added to eliminate the stasis and alleviate pain.

## 6. Yin deficiency of the liver and kidneys

Treatment principle: Nourishing the liver and kidneys, cooling blood to stop bleeding.

Prescription and herbs: Modified Yiguan Decoction and Qinghao Biejia Decoction.

Gouqizi (Barbary Wolfberry Fruit) 12 g, Shengdi (Dried Rehmannia Root) 30 g, Shudi (Prepared Rhizome Rehmannia) 30 g, Beishashen (Coastal Glehnia Root) 15 g, Maidong (Dwarf Lilyturf Tuber) 12 g, Danggui (Chinese Angelica) 9 g, Chuanlianzi (Szechwan Chinaberry Fruit) 9 g, Qinghao (Sweet Wormwood Herb) 9 g, Biejia (Turtle Shell) 12 g, Zhimu (Common Anemarrhena Rhizome) 9 g, Huangbai (Amur Cork-tree) 9 g, Danpi (Cortex Moutan) 9 g, Ejiao (Donkey-hide Glue) 9 g, Xianhecao (Hairyvein Agrimonia Herb) 30 g and Cebaiye (Chinese Arborvitae Twig and Leaf) 30g.

Modification: If there is scanty urine, Fuling (Indian Bread) 12 g, Zexie (Oriental Waterplantain Rhizome) 12 g and Cheqianzi (Plantain Seed) 12 g can be added to drain dampness and promote water discharge; for presence of low grade fever, Digupi (Chinese Wolfberry Root-Bark) 12 g and Baiwei (Blackend Swallowwort Root) 12 g are added to dispel the deficient heat.

## Chinese Patent Medicine

1. Pingxiao Capsule: 8 capsules for each dose, 3 times a day.
2. Biejiajian Pill: 3 g for each dose, 3 times a day.

## Simple and Handy Prescriptions

1. Chuanshanjia (Pangolin Scale) 15 g, Biejia (Turtle Shell) 15 g, Sanleng (Common Burreed Tuber) 15 g and Ezhu (Zedoray Rhizome) 15 g are boiled together in water.
2. Cheqianzi (Plantain Seed) 30 g (wrapped during decoction), Fulingpi (Indian Bread Peel) 30 g, Dafupi (Areca Peel) 30 g, Xiguapi (Watermelon Peel) 250 g and Donggua (Chinese waxgourd) 500 g are decocted together. The decoction is made into porridge, which is taken at different times each day. It is used to treat hepatic cancer with ascites.

## Other Therapies

Dietary therapy:

(1) A chicken (or spring chicken) is cooked with 250 g of mushroom and just before they are ready, Caotou (california burclover) 100 g is added and the soup is boiled for a while longer before serving.
(2) A green turtle, several slices of ham and a small amount of mushroom are cooked together. in the soup should be consumed within 1~2 days.

For subclinical carcinoma of the liver at the early stage or those confined to the hepatic marginal zone, it is advisable to conduct surgical treatment as early as possible. Intubation interventional chemotherapy is also of certain curative effect.

## Cautions and Advice

1. Patients should rest well and regulate their emotions and lives. Those patients whose conditions are in the early stage or who have undergone surgical treatment should engage in moderate exercise while continuing to receive medical intervention.
2. Patients should avoid consumption of salty, spicy or oily foods, as well as alcohol. They should keep a balanced diet overall but increase their protein intake slightly. Vegetables and fruits rich in vitamin C, as well as garlic and green tea with the function of preventing canceration are highly recommended.
3. The size of tumors, the method of treatment and the bionomics of the carcinoma are key factors determining the prognosis of this disease.

## Daily Exercises

1. Recall the etiology and pathology of primary hepatic carcinoma.
2. Explain how primary hepatic carcinoma can be treated based on syndrome differentiation.

# Acute Pancreatitis
## Week 7: Monday

Acute pancreatitis refers to the chemical inflammation due to autodigestion of pancreatic tissues activated by pancreatic enzyme, clinically marked by sudden abdominal agony and the accompanying symptoms such as nausea, vomiting, fever, jaundice and in severe cases, shock, respiratory failure and peritonitis. The disease can be either mild or severe. The former is characterized by edematous changes of the pancreas and a limited disease course (recovery within a few days). The latter is characterized by hemorrhage and necrosis of the pancreas, a high death rate and such complications as shock, respiratory failure and peritonitis. In TCM, acute pancreatitis is closely associated with "abdominal pain", "stomachache", "precordial pain due to spleen disorder" and "hypochondriac pain".

## Etiology and Pathology

The occurrence of this disease is closely linked to the liver, gallbladder, spleen, stomach and intestine. The etiological factors are emotional depression, which impairs the ability of the liver to promote free flow of qi and leads to the transformation of the stagnated qi into fire and stasis in the long run; voracious eating and drinking as well as alcohol abuse, which impairs the spleen and stomach and results in internal accumulation of dampness and heat due to dysfunction in digestion; parasites and calculus, which obstruct the biliary tract and disturb qi activity. All these factors can contribute to this disease.

## Diagnostic Key Points

1. The patient has engaged in excessive activities, e.g., alcohol abuse or voracious consumption of food and drink, usually 1~2 hours before occurrence of signs and symptoms.
2. For patients with edema, there may be intense, persistent pain in the upper epigastric zone, or paroxysmal aggravation; this may be accompanied by nausea, vomiting, mild fever, or jaundice; there may also be

tenderness in the gastric zone yet without stiffness of the abdominal muscles; meanwhile there is pronounced increase in the serum and/or urinary amylase levels, as well as in the ratio of clearance of amylase (Cam)/creatinine clearance rate (Ccr), with alleviation in 3~5 days and repeated occurrence in a few cases.

3. Patients with hemorrhage and necrosis often present with acute pain in the whole abdomen, stiff abdominal muscles, peritoneal irritation sign, restlessness or peripheral coldness; prominent decrease in blood calcium level; ascites with highly active amylases detected upon abdominal puncturation; sudden decrease in blood urine amylases level which is inconsistent with the disease; marked decrease in bowel sounds, intestinal tympanites or paralytic ileus; hematein albumin(+); fat necrosis in the limbs; massive bleeding in the alimentary canal; hypoxemia; elevated level of peripheral blood WBC, blood urea nitrogen, blood sugar (for those without a history of diabetes); and in severe cases, acute respiratory failure, acute renal failure, circulatory failure, pancreatic encephalopathy, abnormal metabolism and even death.

## Syndrome Differentiation

### 1. Transformation of stagnated liver qi into fire

Symptoms: Sudden abdominal agony (usually in the middle and upper belly and involving the bilateral hypochondria, the waist and the back), fever, dry throat, a bitter taste in the mouth, belching, nausea, vomiting and dry stools; red tongue with yellow coating and rapid-taut pulse.

Analysis of symptoms: Emotional depression hampers the ability of the liver to promote the free flow of qi and leads to the subsequent stagnation of qi, marked by sudden onset of abdominal pain; qi disorder is characterized by qi migration, so the pain involves the bilateral hypochondria, the waist and the back; prolonged stagnation of qi produces fire, with such signs as fever, bitter taste in the mouth and dry throat; liver qi invades the stomach and prevents the stomach qi from descending, resulting in belching, nausea and vomiting; fire and heat obstruct the intestinal tract, bringing about dry stools; red tongue with yellow coating and rapid-taut pulse are due to the transformation of stagnated liver qi into fire.

## 2. Internal accumulation of damp-heat in the liver and gallbladder

Symptoms: Persistent drilling or acute pain in the abdomen and the bilateral hypochondriac region with paroxysmal aggravation, chest distress, nausea, vomiting, fever or alternate chills and fever, a bitter taste in the mouth, yellowish eyes, body and urine; red tongue with yellow-greasy coating and taut-slippery pulse or rapid-taut pulse.

Analysis of symptoms: Accumulation of dampness and heat in the liver and gallbladder leads to disorder of the liver collaterals, marked by persistent drilling or acute pain in the abdomen and the bilateral hypochondriac region with paroxysmal aggravation; internal obstruction of damp-heat is manifested as chest distress, nausea, vomiting and fever; obstruction of the gallbladder is responsible for alternate attacks of chills and fever, the bitter taste in the mouth and hypochondriac pain; dampness and heat steam the interior alternately, driving the bile to flow out of the intestinal tract, with such signs as yellowish eyes, body and urine; the red tongue with yellow-greasy coating and taut-slippery pulse or rapid-taut pulse are attributable to internal accumulation of damp-heat in the liver and gallbladder.

## 3. Retention of heat and stasis in the stomach and intestine

Symptoms: Persistent abdominal cutting pain involving the bilateral hypochondria, the waist and the back, abdominal distension and fullness with tenderness, ardent fever and chills, nausea and vomiting, thirst with restlessness, constipation, or presence of ecchymosis in the belly or around the umbilicus; dark purple tongue with dry yellow coating and surging rapid pulse.

Analysis of symptoms: Prolonged stagnation of qi transforms into heat and produces stasis, marked by persistent abdominal cutting pain involving the bilateral hypochondria, the waist and the back; the blood stasis is tangible, so there is abdominal distension and fullness with tenderness; the struggle between the healthy qi and pathogenic factors is manifested as ardent fever and chills; invasion of liver fire into the stomach is responsible for causing nausea, vomiting and thirst with restlessness; obstruction of heat in the intestinal tract gives rise to constipation; the ecchymosis in the belly or around the umbilicus and the presence of the dark purple tongue is due to internal obstruction of blood stasis whereas the dry yellow coating and surging rapid pulse are attributable to intense heat in the interior.

## Differential Treatment

### 1. Transformation of stagnated liver qi into fire

Treatment principle: Soothing the liver and relieving depression, dispelling heat and purging fire.

Prescription and herbs: Modified Qingyi Decoction.

Chaihu (Chinese Thorowax Root) 6 g, Binglang (Areca Seed) 9 g, Muxiang (Common Aucklandia Root) 6 g, Yanhusuo (Corydalis) 9 g, Zhiqiao (Orange Fruit) 12 g, Chuanlianzi (Szechwan Chinaberry Fruit) 9 g, Huangqin (Baical Skullcap Root) 9 g, Huanglian (Golden Thread) 3 g, Jinyinhua (Honeysuckle Flower) 12 g, Lianqiao (Weeping Forsythia Capsule) 9 g, Dahuang (Unprepared Rhubarb) 9 g and Mangxiao (Sodium Sulfate) 15 g.

Modification: If there is thirst, Lugen (Reed Rhizome) 30 g can be added to promote fluid production and quench thirst.

### 2. Internal accumulation of damp-heat in the liver and gallbladder

Treatment principle: Soothing the liver and dredging the gallbladder, dispelling heat and eliminating dampness.

Prescription and herbs: Modified Longdan Xiegan Decoction and Yinchenhao Decoction.

Chaihu (Chinese Thorowax Root) 6 g, Longdancao (Radix Gentianae) 6 g, Huangqin (Baical Skullcap Root) 9 g, Huanglian (Golden Thread) 3 g, Yinchen (Virgate Wormwood Herb) 15 g, Zhizi (Cape Jasmine Fruit) 9 g, Cheqianzi (Plantain Seed) 30 g, Zexie (Oriental Waterplantain Rhizome) 12 g, Chuanmutong (Armand Clematis Stem) 6 g, Dahuang (Unprepared

Rhubarb) 6 g, Baishao (White Peony Alba) 20 g and Gancao (Liquorice Root) 3 g.

Modification: If the symptoms are triggered by gallstones, Jinqiancao (Christina Loosestrife) 30 g, Haijinshao (Lygodium) 12 g and Yujin (Turmeric Root Tuber) 12 g are added to disperse the liver and dredge the gallbladder; if it is due to roundworms in the biliary tract, Wumei Pill 9 g is used to control the roundworms.

### 3. Retention of heat and stasis in the stomach and intestine

Treatment principle: Expelling stasis and promoting blood circulation, dispelling heat and dredging the intestines.

Prescription and herbs: Modified Taohong Siwu Decoction and Dachengqi Decoction.

Shengdi (Dried Rehmannia Root) 9 g, Danggui (Chinese Angelica) 9 g, Chishao (Red Peony Root) 9 g, Chuanxiong (Szechwan Lovage Rhizome) 6 g, Taoren (Peach Seed) 9 g, Honghua (Safflower) 6 g, Dahuang (Unprepared Rhubarb) 9 g, Mangxiao (Sodium Sulfate) 15 g, Zhishi (Immature Orange Fruit) 12 g, Houpu (Magnolia Bark) 9 g Baijiangcao (Dahurian Patrinia Herb) 30 g, Hongteng (Sargentgloryvine Stem) 30 g and Didingcao (Herba Violae) 12 g.

Modification: In cases of ardent fever, chills and thirst with restlessness, Shigao (Gypsum) 30 g and Zhimu (Common Anemarrhena Rhizome) 9 g can be added to dispel heat and purge fire.

### Chinese Patent Medicine

1. Longdan Xiegan Pill: 4.5 g for each dose, twice a day.
2. Yinzhihuang Powder (preparation for infusion): 1 bag for each dose, 3 times a day.

### Simple and Handy Prescriptions

1. Machixian (Unprepared Purslane Herb) 500 g and Baijiangcao (Dahurian Patrinia Herb) 500 g are decocted together. The decoction is

taken (50 ml for each dose) as needed, for patients whose conditions are severe, the frequency can be once every hour.

2. Dahuangfen (Unprepared Rhubarb Powder) 15 g and Xuanmingfen (Exsiccated Sodium Sulfate) 30 g are infused into 200 ml water and taken orally or nasally once every 2~4 hours and 3 times a day.

## Other Therapies

Dietary therapy:

(1) Chidou (Adzuki Bean) 150 g, Ludou (Mung Bean) 150 g and Yiyiren (Unprepared Coix Seed) 50 g are boiled in a suitable amount of water. The decoction is taken while it is warm (50 ml per hour) in both the day and night.

(2) A Biejia (Turtle Shell) is carbonized (but its effectiveness is retained) and ground up into extremely fine powder, then blended with sesame oil and taken (0.3 g for each dose) 3 times a day after meals.

It is advisable to adopt such measures as food fasting, gastrointestinal decompression, total intravenous nutritional support and enzyme inhibition, so as to reduce pancreatic enzyme secretion, prevent secondary infection and address the primary disorders of the biliary tract.

If jaundice progresses, obstruction of biliary tract and fever persist, blood-urine amylase remains at a high level and abscess occurs, it is advisable to opt for prompt surgical treatment.

## Cautions and Advice

1. Patients should take initiative in treating diseases of the biliary tract so that acute biliary pancreatitis can be prevented; abstinence from alcohol can reduce the likelyhood of alcoholic pancreatitis; external injuries, surgeries, disorders of the region around the carunculae major, severe infection, related drugs, endocrine metabolism and vascular lesions should be avoided; patients should also cultivate a regular lifestyle and avoid voracious eating and drinking, extreme tension and overstrain.

2. The dietary principles of acute pancreatitis: For those with mild edema, a low-fat, liquid diet in frequent (once every 2 hours) but small amounts is recommended. Such food as rice water, arrow root soup, fruit juice, vegetable soup, soyabean milk and low-fat/skimmed milk. For those with severe edema, a fasting diet should be adopted in the initial 2~3 days after occurrence and when the symptoms are improved, liquids can be administered and the volume can be increased gradually. For pancreatitis with hemorrhage and necrosis, a complete fasting diet should be adopted at the same time of proactive treatment so as to reduce gastric acid secretion and the resultant pancreatic secretion. When the disease becomes stable and well controlled, a semi-liquid diet can be adopted, but it should continue to comprise small meals which are enjoyed more frequently.

3. The dietary principles of chronic pancreatitis: For patients with chronic pancreatitis, a low-fat, soft diet in frequent but small amounts is recommended. In the acute relapse period, the dietary principles are consistent with those applied in acute pancreatitis. For biliary diarrhea, the intake of fat should be restricted and for biliary diabetes, the dietary principles are the same with those applied in common diabetes, meanwhile the intake of fat should be properly restricted.

4. Disease course and prognosis: The disease course and prognosis of acute pancreatitis depends on the severity of the disease and the presence of complications. Patients with edema generally recover within a week without lingering effects, but for patients with hemorrhage and necrosis, the conditions are mostly severe and dangerous, with an unfavorable prognosis and a high chance of fatality.

## Daily Exercises

1. Explain how acute pancreatitis can be classified into the different syndromes.
2. Recall the cautionary notes that should be emphasized when treating acute pancreatitis.

# Hepatic Encephalopathy

# Week 7: Tuesday

Hepatic encephalopathy, once called hepatic coma, refers to the functional disorder of the central nervous system on the basis of metabolic disturbance due to severe hepatic diseases. It is clinically marked by conscious disturbance, behavioral disorder and coma. Subclinical or asymptomatic hepatic encephalopathy is so-called because it has no apparent clinical manifestations and biochemical abnormalities and can only be diagnosed by intricate intelligence test and/or electrophysiological examination. In TCM, hepatic encephalopathy is closely associated with "coma", "acute jaundice" and "liver syncope".

## Etiology and Pathology

This disease is located in the liver and brain and its occurrence is linked to the liver, kidneys, brain, spleen and stomach. Generally, prolonged hepatic diseases coupled with invasion of pathogenic heat and pestilent toxins often lead to impairment of the yin fluid. Besides, hyperactive liver (wood) tends to over-restrict the spleen (earth) and weaken the middle energizer, resulting in accumulation of phlegm and dampness; the turbid phlegm moves upward and clouds the clear orifices, bringing about coma or unconsciousness. This disease is often unfavorable in prognosis and normally marked by excess of the pathogenic factors and deficiency of healthy qi, with yin depletion of the liver and kidneys.

## Diagnostic Key Points

1. Hepatic encephalopathy is mostly caused by various types of cirrhosis (usually post-hepatitis cirrhosis); a small number of cerebropathy are seen in the acute or fulminant hepatic failure stage of severe viral hepatitis, toxic hepatitis and drug-induced liver disease; while the less common include primary hepatic carcinoma, acute fatty liver during pregnancy and severe infection of the biliary tract.

2. Clinically it is divided into four stages: stage 1 is marked by slight changes in character and behavioral disorder; stage 2 is marked by

sleeping disturbance, confusion, behavioral abnormalities and flapping tremors; stage 3 is marked by deep slumber and severe mental disorder; stage 4 is marked by aboulia, coma and paroxysmal convulsion, ankle clonus, hepatic odor and, surprisingly, disappearance of flapping tremor.

3. The common inducing factors of hepatic encephalopathy are upper gastrointestinal bleeding, excessive use of kali-uretic drugs, massive discharge of ascites, adoption of protein-rich diet, application of sleeping and tranquilizing drugs or narcotics, constipation, uremia, surgeries and infection.

4. Apparent functional lesion of the liver or elevated level of blood ammonia.

5. Abnormality in electroencephalogram, which is not only of certain diagnostic value to this disease, but also of significance to its prognosis.

## Syndrome Differentiation

## 1. Impairment of the liver by toxic heat and stirring of wind due to deficient yin

Symptoms: General fever, red cheeks, dry mouth with a bitter taste, insomnia, night sweats, restlessness, babbling, nasal and gingival bleeding, dry stools, scanty reddish urine and sometimes flapping tremors; purple red tongue with little or yellowish rough coating and thin, taut and rapid pulse.

Analysis of symptoms: Toxic heat impairs the liver yin and deficiency of yin, in turn, produces internal heat, marked by general fever, red cheeks, dry mouth with bitter taste, insomnia and night sweats; toxic heat disturbs the spirit, so there is restlessness, babbling and insomnia; heat drives blood rampant, so there is nasal and gingival bleeding; toxic heat scorches the intestinal tract and bladder, leading to dry stools and scanty reddish urine; deficiency of yin produces wind, with such signs as flapping tremors; the purple red tongue, little or yellowish rough coating and thin, taut and rapid pulse are due to toxic heat impairing the liver and deficient yin producing wind.

## 2. Obstruction of the clear orifices (upper orifices) by blood stasis and turbid phlegm

Symptoms: Dark and lusterless complexion, chest distress, abdominal distension, wheezy phlegm in the throat, dementia, indifference and gradual progression into unconsciousness, slurred speech and inability to recognize people, or presence of jaundice, vomiting of dark blood, enlarged abdomen with varicose veins and bloody streaks over the skin; dark tongue with ecchymosis, thick and greasy tongue coating and soggy pulse.

Analysis of symptoms: Dysfunction of the spleen in transportation and transformation gives rise to internal abundance of phlegm and dampness and stagnation of yang qi, marked by dark and lusterless complexion, chest distress, abdominal distension and wheezy phlegm in the throat; phlegm clouds the upper orifices, causing dementia, indifference and gradual progression into unconsciousness, slurred speech and inability to recognize people; stagnation of dampness produces heat which fumigates the liver and gallbladder, predisposing the patient to jaundice; prolonged obstruction of qi and dampness brings about retention of blood stasis, so there ais vomiting of dark blood, enlarged abdomen with varicose veins and bloody streaks over the skin; the dark tongue with ecchymosis, thick and greasy coating and soggy pulse are attributable to internal obstruction of turbid phlegm, qi and blood.

## 3. Extreme weakness of the viscera and depletion of liver yin and kidney yin

Symptoms: Prolonged coma, delirium, panting, stiff limbs, spastic hands and feet, special hepatic odor, scanty urine or retention of urine; deep red tongue with sallow coating and faint, thin and rapid pulse.

Analysis of symptoms: Extreme weakness of the viscera and depletion of liver yin and kidney yin leads to uncurbed yang and disquieted spirit, marked by coma and delirium; deficiency of yin brings about a stirring of wind, leading to stiff limbs and spastic hands and feet; deficiency of the viscera gives rise to panting and special hepatic odor; deficiency of the kidneys is responsible for unsmooth opening and closing of the urinary gate, with such signs as scanty urine or retention of urine; deep red tongue with sallow coating and faint, thin and rapid pulse are manifestations of depleted kidney yin and liver yin.

## Differential Treatment

### 1. Impairment of liver by toxic heat and stirring of wind due to deficient yin

Treatment principle: Nourishing yin and extinguishing wind, purging heat and eliminating toxins.

Prescription and herbs: Modified Sanjia Fumai Decoction and Huanglian Jiedu Decoction.

Lingyangjiaofen (Antelope Horn Powder) 0.3 g, Shengdi (Dried Rehmannia Root) 12 g, Baishao (White Peony Alba) 12 g, Maidong (Dwarf Lilyturf Tuber) 12 g, Ejiao (Donkey-hide Glue) 9 g, Guiban (Tortoise Shell) 12 g, Biejia (Turtle Shell) 12 g, Muli (Oyster Shell) 30 g, Maren (Edestan) 9 g, Huangqin (Baical Skullcap Root) 9 g, Huanglian (Golden Thread) 3 g, Zhizi (Cape Jasmine Fruit) 9 g, Dahuang (Unprepared Rhubarb) 9 g and Gancao (Liquorice Root) 6 g.

Modification: If there is flapping tremor, Tianma (Tall Gastrodis Tuber) 6 g and Gouteng (Gambir Plant) 12 g are added to subdue the liver and extinguish wind; for nosebleed and gingival bleeding, Baimaogen (Lalang Grass Rhizome) 30 g, Baiji (Common Bletilla Tuber) 9 g and Cebaiye (Chinese Arborvitae Twig and Leaf) 9 g are added to stop bleeding.

### 2. Obstruction of the clear orifices (upper orifices) by blood stasis and turbid phlegm

Treatment principle: Expelling stasis and removing stagnation, eliminating phlegm for resuscitation.

Prescription and herbs: Modified Ditan Decoction and Suhexiang Pill.

Banxia (Pinellia Tuber) 9 g, Dannanxing (Bile Arisaema) 12 g, Chenpi (Dried Tangerine Peel) 6 g, Zhiqiao (Orange Fruit) 12 g, Fuling (Indian Bread) 9 g, Gancao (Liquorice Root) 6 g, Changpu (Acorus Calamus) 12 g, Taoren (Peach Seed) 9 g, Honghua (Safflower) 6 g, Chishao (Red Peony Root) 9 g, Chuanxiong (Szechwan Lovage Rhizome) 6 g and Suhexiang Wan (Storax Pill) 1 Pill (swallowed).

Modification: If there is haematemesis, Baiji (Common Bletilla Tuber) 9 g, Shensanqi (Panax Pseudo-ginseng Powder) 3 g and Huaruishi (Ophicalcite) 15 g are added to stop bleeding; for enlarged abdomen with varicose veins, Chenhulu (Aged Bottle-gourd) 9 g and Chongsun (Henon Bamboo Dried Shoot) 9 g can be added to promote urination and relieve edema.

### 3. Extreme weakness of the viscera and depletion of liver yin and kidney yin

Treatment principle: Nourishing yin and subduing yang, extinguishing wind for resuscitation.

Prescription and herbs: Modified Dadingfengzhu Decoction and Angong Niuhuang Pill.

Jizihuang (Uncooked Hen Egg Yolk) 2 yolks, Ejiao (Donkey-hide Glue) 9 g, Gouqizi (Barbary Wolfberry Fruit) 12 g, Baishao (White Peony Alba) 9 g, Wuweizi (Chinese Magnolivine Fruit) 6 g, Shengdi (Dried Rehmannia Root) 30 g, Maidong (Dwarf Lilyturf Tuber) 15 g, Maren (Edestan) 9 g, Guiban (Tortoise Shell) 12 g, Biejia (Turtle Shell) 12 g, Muli (Unprepared Oyster Shell) 30 g, Shichangpu (Grassleaf Sweetflag Rhizome) 12 g, Angong Niuhuang Wan (Bezoar Uterus-Calming Pill) 1 pill (swallowed) and Gancao (Liquorice Root) 6 g.

Modification: In cases of stiff limbs and spastic hands or feet, Gegen (Kudzuvine Root) 12 g, Tianma (Tall Gastrodis Tuber) 6 g and Gouteng (Gambir Plant) 12 g can be added to subdue the liver and extinguish wind; for scanty urine Cheqianzi (Plantain Seed) 15 g (wrapped during decoction) and Zexie (Oriental Waterplantain Rhizome) 15 g are added to promote water discharge with their bland flavors.

## Chinese Patent Medicine

1. Angong Niuhuang Wan (Bezoar Uterus-Calming Pill): 1 pill for each dose, 1~2 times a day.
2. Suhexiang Wan (Storax Pill): 0.5 or 1 pill for each dose, 1~2 times a day.

## Simple and Handy Prescriptions

1. Changpu (Acorus Calamus) 9 g, Tianma (Tall Gastrodis Tuber) 6 g and Gouteng (Gambir Plant) 12 g are boiled in water and taken once a day.
2. Guiban (Tortoise Shell) 15 g, Biejia (Turtle Shell) 15 g and Muli (Oyster Shell) 15 g are boiled in water and taken once a day.

## Other Therapies

Elimination of causative factors:

(1) Promptly control infection and upper gastrointestinal bleeding and avoid rapid and massive kali-uresis and paracentesis.
(2) Try to prevent water, electrolyte and acid-base imbalance.
(3) Administer an enema or catharsis so that the intestinal food retention and blood stasis can be removed, bacteria inhibited and ammonia reduced.

Liver transplantation is generally acknowledged to be effective therapy for the chronic hepatic diseases that are irresponsive to other approaches.

## Cautions and Advice

1. In order to actively prevent and treat hepatic diseases, patients must avoid any factors that may lead to hepatic encephalopathy. Patients with liver diseases must be observed closely so that the prodromal and pre-coma symptoms can be discovered promptly and treated properly in time.

2. To protect brain cells, intracranial temperature should be decreased by using ice caps; for patients in deep coma, the respiratory passage should be kept unblocked, with oxygen being administered by incision of trachea; steps must be taking to prevent and treat brain edema, bleeding and shock.

3. Patients should refrain from protein intake and supplement their diets with high-glucose and vitamin-rich foods; for patients with ascites, salt is strictly restricted; for coma patients who are unable to ingest food, it can be administered by nasogastric tube; for patients with negative nitrogen balance, vegetable protein is highly advisable.

4. Cases with clear-cut, easily removed causative factors (such as bleeding and potassium depletion.) have a relatively favorable prognosis. However, patients with portal-systemic encephalopathy due to intake of protein-rich food after shunting will have a relatively poor prognosis. For those with tendency of ascites, jaundice and bleeding, the prognosis is extremely unfavorable because their hepatic functions are poor. Finally, hepatic encephalopathy due to fulminant hepatic failure is the poorest in prognosis.

## Daily Exercises

1. Concisely describe the diagnostic key points of hepatic encephalopathy.
2. Explain how hepatic encephalopathy can be treated based on syndrome differentiation?

# Wednesday
## Cholecystitis and Cholelithiasis
## Week 7: Wednesday

Cholecystitis and cholelithiasis are the relatively common disorders of the biliary tract. The main symptoms during acute onset are paroxysmal colicky pain in the right upper abdomen or below the xiphoid process radiating to the right shoulders and back, pain upon pressure, rebound tenderness or abdominal muscular tension and sometimes fever and jaundice. In the chronic period, the main symptoms are discomfort in the upper belly, vague pain in the right upper abdomen, abdominal distension, belching and aversion to oily food. In TCM, cholecystitis and cholelithiasis are closely associated with "hypochondriac pain", "chest retention" and "jaundice".

## Etiology and Pathology

Cholecystitis and cholelithiasis are both located at the gallbladder and their occurrence is related to the liver, gallbladder, spleen and stomach. Emotional depression, indulgence in fatty and sweet food, parasitic infestation and exogenous pathogenic invasion may all impair the functions of the liver and gallbladder in promoting free flow of qi and that of the stomach and spleen in transportation and transformation. As a result, the liver qi and gallbladder qi are stagnated and the bile is unable to be smoothly discharged. In addition, dysfunction of the spleen in transportation and transformation may bring about internal accumulation of damp-heat, which transforms into stones (calculus) in the long run; stagnation of qi, blockage of the fu-organs and unsmooth circulation of blood give rise to blood stasis and pus accumulation, creating a predisposition to cholecystitis and cholelithiasis in the end.

## Diagnostic Key Points

1. Acute cholecystitis is often characterized by acute, colicky pain in the epigastric, right hypochondriac or xiphoideusal regions that is

accompanied by fever or jaundice; on the other hand, chronic cholecystitis lacks the typical symptoms possible discomfort in the upper belly, vague pain, abdominal distension, belching and aversion to oily food. By contrast, the clinical manifestations of cholelithiasis are determined by the shape, size and location of the gallstone; during its acute onset, there is severe colicky pain in the right upper abdomen (biliary colic), chills, high fever, or jaundice.

2. There is an increase of peripheral blood WBC and neutrophilic granulocyte during acute onset.

3. The confirmation of cholecystitis and cholelithiasis relies on X-ray or B-ultrasonic examination, with such signs as positive calculus or inflammation.

4. Endoscopic Retrograde Cholangiopancreatography (ERCP), Percutaneous Transhepatic Cholangiography (PCT) and CT are of significant diagnostic value to cholelithiasis unidentified by X-ray or B-ultrasonic examination.

## Syndrome Differentiation

### 1. Liver qi stagnation

Symptoms: Paroxysmal colicky pain in the right upper abdomen radiating to the shoulders and back, aggravation by emotional disturbance, reduced food intake, or a bitter taste in the mouth, belching, nausea, vomiting and sometimes fever with intolerance of cold; slightly red tongue with greasy coating and taut-tense pulse.

Analysis of symptoms: Emotional depression leads to stagnation of liver qi and unsmooth discharge of bile, marked by paroxysmal colicky pain in the right upper abdomen radiating to the shoulders and back and aggravation by emotional disturbance; invasion of liver qi into the stomach results in failure of the stomach qi to descend, with such signs of reduced food intake, bitter taste in the mouth, belching, nausea and vomiting; stagnation of liver qi and gallbladder qi produces heat, so there may be mild fever with intolerance of cold; the slightly red tongue with greasy coating and taut-tense pulse are symptomatic of stagnated liver qi and gallbladder qi.

## 2. Steaming and fumigating of damp-heat

Symptoms: Persistent distending pain or colicky pain in the right upper abdomen involving the shoulder and back, fever, intolerance of cold, chest distress, poor appetite, nausea, vomiting, bitter mouth and dry throat; yellow-greasy coating and taut-tense pulse.

Analysis of symptoms: Accumulation of dampness and heat in the liver and gallbladder brings about disorder of the liver collaterals and obstruction of the biliary tract, marked by persistent distending pain or colicky pain in the right upper abdomen; the gallbladder meridian travels through the lateral side of the body, so there is pain involving the shoulder and back; internal accumulation of dampness and heat gives rise to fever and intolerance of cold; internal obstruction of damp-heat encumbers the spleen and stomach, with such signs as chest distress, poor appetite, nausea, vomiting, bitter mouth and dry throat; the yellow-greasy coating and taut-tense pulse are manifestations of damp-heat in the liver and gallbladder.

## 3. Stagnation of qi and accumulation of heat with blood stasis

Symptoms: Persistent stabbing pain in the hypochondriac region, aggravation at night with involvement of the shoulder and back, palpable masses in the aching position, thoracic and abdominal fullness or distension, persistent jaundice, occasional chills and fever, constipation and yellowish urine; dark purple tongue, ecchymosis on the tongue and lips and rapid-taut pulse.

Analysis of symptoms: Prolonged stagnation of qi and accumulation of heat leads to unsmooth blood circulation and retention of blood stasis, marked by persistent stabbing hypochondriac pain aggravated at night; the gallbladder meridian travels through the lateral side of the body, so there is pain involving the shoulder and back; the blood stasis is tangible, so there are palpable masses in the aching position; stagnation of qi brings about thoracic and abdominal fullness and distension; accumulation of heat creates a predisposition to occasional chills and fever; qi stagnation, heat accumulation, blood stasis and unsmooth bile secretion are responsible for the appearance of persistent jaundice; damp-heat pours down into the large intestine and bladder, with such signs as constipation and yellow-ish urine; the dark purple tongue, the ecchymosis on the tongue and lips and the rapid and taut pulse are all symptomatic of blood stasis.

## 4. Retention of damp-heat and purulent toxins in the liver and gallbladder

Symptoms: Tender and persistent colicky pain in the gastric, abdominal or hypochondriac region involving the shoulder and back, thoracic and abdominal fullness or distension, high fever and chills, sweating, jaundice, or even delirium, coma, constipation and yellowish urine; deep-red tongue, yellow-rough coating and thin-rapid pulse.

Analysis of symptoms: Prolonged retention of damp-heat and purulent toxins in the liver and gallbladder leads to stagnation of qi, marked by impalpable and persistent colicky pain in the gastric, abdominal or hypo-chondriac region and thoracic and abdominal fullness or distension; the gallbladder meridian travels through the lateral side of the body, so there is pain involving the shoulder and back; predominance of pathogenic heat and purulent toxins gives rise to high fever, chills and sweating; damp-heat and purulent toxins drive the bile to flow outside, resulting in jaundice; damp-heat and purulent toxins disturb the heart spirit, bringing about delirium and coma; damp-heat pours down into the large intestine and bladder, with such signs as constipation and yellowish urine; the deep-red tongue, yellow-rough coating and thin-rapid pulse are all due to retention of abundant damp-heat and purulent toxins.

## Differential Treatment

### 1. Liver qi stagnation

Treatment principle: Dispersing the liver to dredge the gallbladder, promoting flow of qi to alleviate pain.

Prescription and herbs: Supplementary Dachaihu Decoction and Jinlingzi Powder.

Chaihu (Chinese Thorowax Root) 6 g, Baishao (White Peony Alba) 9 g, Zhiqiao (Orange Fruit) 15 g, Dahuang (Rhubarb) 9 g, Huangqin (Baical

Skullcap Root) 9 g, Banxia (Pinellia Tuber) 9 g, Yujin (Turmeric Root Tuber) 9 g, Jinqiancao (Christina Loosestrife) 30 g, Xiangfu (Nutgrass Galingale Rhizome) 9 g, Chuanlianzi (Szechwan Chinaberry Fruit) 9 g, Yanhusuo (Corydalis) 9 g and Gancao (Liquorice Root) 6 g.

Modification: In cases of bitter taste in the mouth, belching, nausea and vomiting, Zhujin Pill 9 g can be added to relieve the stomach and descending qi with the pungent and bitter flavors of the herbs.

## 2. Steaming and fumigating of damp-heat

Treatment principle: Clearing and dredging the liver and gallbladder, resolving dampness and eliminating the stones.

Prescription and herbs: Modified Sanjin Decoction and Yinchenhao Decoction.

Jinqiancao (Christina Loosestrife) 30 g, Haijinshao (Lygodium) 12 g, Yujin (Turmeric Root Tuber) 9 g, Jineijin (Corium Stomachium Galli) 6 g, Yinchen (Virgate Wormwood Herb) 15 g, Huangqin (Baical Skullcap Root) 9 g, Zhizi (Cape Jasmine Fruit) 9 g, Huzhanggen (Giant Knotweed Rhizome Root) 9 g, Zhiqiao (Orange Fruit) 9 g, Muxiang (Common Aucklandia Root) 9 g, Yanhusuo (Corydalis) 9 g and Gancao (Liquorice Root) 6 g.

Modification: For unsmooth defecation or constipation, Dahuang (Unprepared Rhubarb) 9 g and Mangxiao (Sodium Sulfate) 15 g are added to purge fire and promote defecation.

## 3. Stagnation of qi and accumulation of heat with blood stasis

Treatment principle: Activating blood and resolving stasis, dispelling heat and purging the lower energizer.

Prescription and herbs: Modified Fuyuan Huoxue Decoction and Paishi Decoction.

Taoren (Peach Seed) 9 g, Honghua (Safflower) 6 g, Chuanshanjia (Pangolin Scale) 9 g, Dahuang (Unprepared Rhubarb) 9 g, Mangxiao (Sodium Sulfate) 15 g, Chaihu (Chinese Thorowax Root) 9 g, Yujin (Turmeric Root

Tuber) 9 g, Zhiqiao (Orange Fruit) 15 g, Muxiang (Common Aucklandia Root) 9 g, Yinchen (Virgate Wormwood Herb) 12 g, Huangqin (Baical Skullcap Root) 9 g, Huzhanggen (Giant Knotweed Rhizome Root) 9 g, Jinqiancao (Christina Loosestrife) 30 g and Gancao (Liquorice Root) 6 g.

Modification: If there is severe distending pain in the abdomen, Yanhusuo (Corydalis) 9 g and Chuanlianzi (Szechwan Chinaberry Fruit) 9 g are added to regulate qi and alleviate pain; for presence of fever, Jinyinhua (Honeysuckle Flower) 9 g, Lianqiao (Weeping Forsythia Capsule) 9 g and Pugongying (Dandelion) 30 g are added to reinforce the action of dispelling heat.

## 4. Retention of damp-heat and purulent toxins in the liver and gallbladder

Treatment principle: Dispelling heat and discharging pus, resolving stasis and removing toxins.

Prescription and herbs: Modified Huanglian Jiedu Decoction and Yinchenhao Decoction.

Huangqin (Baical Skullcap Root) 9 g, Huanglian (Golden Thread) 6 g, Huangbai (Amur Cork-tree) 9 g, Yinchen (Virgate Wormwood Herb) 9 g, Zhizi (Cape Jasmine Fruit) 9 g, Dahuang (Rhubarb) 6 g, Chuanshanjia (Pangolin Scale) 15 g, Jinqiancao (Christina Loosestrife) 30 g, Haijinshao (Lygodium) 12 g, Yujin (Turmeric Root Tuber) 9 g, Pugongying (Dandelion) 30 g, Jinyinhua (Honeysuckle Flower) 9 g and Gancao (Liquorice Root) 6 g.

Modification: For sweating with a thin pulse, Taizishen (Heterophylly Falsesatarwort Root) 30 g, Maidong (Dwarf Lilyturf Tuber) 9 g and Wuweizi (Chinese Magnolivine Fruit) 6 g are added to supplement qi, reduce sweat and restore pulsation; in cases of coma and delirium, Angong Niuhuang Wan (Bezoar Uterus-Calming Pill) 1 pill should be swallowed immediately to open the orifices with the aromatic flavor of the herbs.

## Chinese Patent Medicine

1. Danning Pian: 5 tablets for each dose, 3 times a day.
2. Jindan Pian: 4 tablets for each dose, 3 times a day.

## Simple and Handy Prescriptions

1. Huzhanggen (Giant Knotweed Rhizome Root) 15 g, Huangqin (Baical Skullcap Root) 9 g, Muxiang (Common Aucklandia Root) 6 g, Zhiqiao (Orange Fruit) 9 g and Gancao (Liquorice Root) 6 g are boiled in water and taken once a day.
2. Jinqiancao (Christina Loosestrife) 30 g, Haijinshao (Lygodium) 12 g, Yujin (Turmeric Root Tuber) 9 g, Yinchen (Virgate Wormwood Herb), Zhizi (Cape Jasmine Fruit) and Gancao (Liquorice Root) 6 g are boiled in water and taken once a day.

## Other Therapies

Dietary therapy:

The following method is applicable to acute cholecystitis, acute onset of chronic cholecystitis and biliary colic.

(1) Jineijin (Corium Stomachium Galli) 5 (in a dried form, not containing any water) are first cleaned and baked on newly-made earthenware and then ground up into extremely fine powder. The powder is administered with separated milk (preparing method: boil the milk first and when it is cold, remove the upper layer of floating substances) once a day after meals.

The following method is applicable to chronic cholecystitis and cholelithiasis.

(2) A black hen with viscera removed is stuffed with 30 g of fresh endothelium corium stomachium galli and 250 g of white turnip. After it is well boiled in water, the stuffed endothelium corium stomachium galli is removed; the chicken can be eaten at different meals, not necessarily on the same day.

There are also other therapies such as calculus removal under endoscope, extracorporeal shock-wave lithotripsy and surgeries.

## Cautions and Advice

1. Patients should balance work and rest, get rid of unhealthy dietary habits and take steps to prevent the acute onset of the disease.
2. During acute onset, a fasting diet is required and the liquid, semi-liquid and light diets can be gradually introduced when there improvement of the symptoms.
3. For the chronic condition, a light diet is recommended and animal fat or cholesterol is strictly restricted. Fresh vegetables, fruits, mushrooms and jelly fungi are advisable for their functions of absorbing intestinal bile acid, suppressing intestinal cholesterol and alleviating inflammation. A minimum of 1500 ml of water should be drunk each day to prevent calculus formation. As for those with obesity, spicy and fried-foods should be prohibited.
4. Cholecystitis and cholelithiasis are generally favorable in prognosis.

## Daily Exercises

1. Recall the diagnostic key points of cholecystitis and cholelithiasis.
2. Explain how cholecystitis and cholelithiasis can be treated based on syndrome differentiation.

# Viral Hepatitis

# Week 7: Thursday

Viral hepatitis is a common communicable disease caused by a variety of hepatitis viruses. It is clinically marked by weariness, fever, jaundice, nausea, vomiting, decreased appetite, pain in the hypochondriac and hepatic regions and hepatic enlargement with tenderness. In severe cases, it leads to bleeding, hepatatrophia and symptoms of the nervous system, or even death. This disease is classified into several types: Hepatitis A, hepatitis B, hepatitis C, hepatitis D and hepatitis E. According to clinical symptoms, it is also divided into the following types: acute hepatitis (with or without jaundice), chronic hepatitis (persistent and active), serious hepatitis (fulminating type and sub-active type) and cholestatic hepatitis. In TCM, viral hepatitis is closely associated with "hypochondriac pain", "jaundice", "consumptive disease", "acute jaundice", "fulminant jaundice" and "liver accumulation".

## Etiology and Pathology

The location of this disease is in the liver, but its occurrence involves other organs apart from the liver such as the gallbladder, the spleen, the stomach and the kidneys. The exogenous factors are mainly pestilent toxins and damp-heat, whereas the endogenous cause is deficiency of healthy qi. Acute hepatitis is characterized by excessiveness, primarily due to invasion of pestilent toxins and damp-heat (which fumigate the liver and gallbladder and impede activity of qi). Chronic hepatitis is often characterized by co-existence of excess and deficiency; the lingering of exogenous pathogenic factors leads to disharmony between the liver and spleen and deficiency of the liver and kidneys, which subsequently causes obstruction of the collaterals or vessels. Cholestatic hepatitis is also marked by co-existence of excess and deficiency, mainly due to retention of damp-heat which fumigates the liver and gallbladder and blood stasis resulting from spleen deficiency. Serious hepatitis is marked by severe or critical conditions, chiefly due to rampant pestilent toxins transforming into fire and dryness, which sink into the ying-blood phase and lead to internal obstruction of pathogenic heat and extreme prostration of primordial qi.

## Diagnostic Key Points

1. Acute hepatitis is marked by weariness, fever, jaundice, poor appetite, nausea, vomiting, hypochondriac pain, abdominal distension and hepatic pain and enlargement. Chronic hepatitis may also present with symptoms or signs normally found in the acute phase and other symptoms like enlarged spleen, liver palm and spider angioma, as well as extrahepatic lesions such as arthritis and chronic nephritis. Serious hepatitis is characterized by sudden onset, rapid progression of jaundice, obvious bleeding tendency, hepatatrophia, hepatic odor, lethargy, spasms, restlessness, delirium, coma, scanty urine or suppression of urine. Cholestatic hepatitis is manifested as relatively severe jaundice, weariness, itch of the skin, enlargement of the liver, white-grey stools and mild symptoms of the alimentary system.

2. In patients with acute hepatitis, the level of serumal glutamate-pyruvate transaminase (SGPT) elevates constantly and so does the level of serum bilirubin. In patients with chronic hepatitis, the hepatic functions are repeatedly or persistently abnormal. In patients with serious hepatitis, the liver functions are severely damaged, the level of serum bilirubin is markedly elevated, the prothrombin time is significantly prolonged, the level of cholesterol is decreased and there is presence of azotemia. In patients with cholestatic hepatitis, the level of direct bilirubin remains elevated for several months or even a year, while the level of glutamate-pyruvate transaminase is slightly increased or normal.

3. Serumal immunologic test on specific antigen or antibody of hepatitis can be used diagnose and differentiate between different types of hepatitis.

4. The pathological examination of hepatic puncturation is of significant diagnostic value to the different types of hepatitis, i.e., the antigens, etiological factors, severity of inflammation and degree of fibrosis of chronic hepatitis can be accurately determined in this manner.

## Syndrome Differentiation

### 1. Accumulation and steaming of damp-heat

Symptoms: Bright-yellow body and eyes, fever, thirst, poor appetite, aversion to greasiness, nausea, vomiting, hypochondriac pain, abdominal distension, constipation, yellowish or reddish urine and enlarged liver with apparent tenderness; red tongue, yellow and greasy coating and rapid and taut pulse, primarily seen in hepatitis with acute jaundice.

Analysis of symptoms: Damp-heat steams the liver and gallbladder, marked by yellowish body and eyes, hypochondriac pain and enlarged liver with apparent tenderness; heat is a yang pathogen, so there is bright-yellow color; heat scorches the body fluid, leading to fever with thirst; accumulation of dampness and heat in the middle energizer results in dysfunction of transportation and transformation, with such signs as poor appetite and aversion to greasiness; the stomach qi fails to descend, characterized by nausea and vomiting; obstruction of intestinal qi is manifested as abdominal distension and constipation; damp-heat pours downward, impeding qi-transformation of the bladder, so there is yellowish or reddish urine; the red tongue, yellow and greasy coating and rapid and taut pulse are symptomatic of damp-heat steaming the liver and gallbladder.

## 2. Deficiency of the spleen with retention of dampness

Symptoms: Fatigue with weak limbs, vague pain below the costal region, reduced food intake, loose stools and sallow complexion; pale tongue, greasy coating and slow-soft pulse, primarily seen in chronic persistent or active hepatitis.

Analysis of symptoms: Deficiency of the spleen with retention of dampness leads to fatigue with weak limbs; damp-heat impedes the functional activity of qi, so there is vague pain below the costal region; deficiency of the spleen with retention of dampness results in poor digestion, marked by reduced food intake and loose stools; the sallow complexion, pale tongue, greasy coating and slow-soft pulse are due to deficiency of the spleen with retention of dampness.

## 3. Disharmony between the spleen and stomach

Symptoms: Doleful expression, hypochondriac distension or pain, frequent sighing, restlessness, irascibility, gastric stuffiness, abdominal distension, belching, poor appetite, nausea, vomiting and loose stools;

white-thin or white-greasy coating and taut pulse, primarily seen in acute hepatitis without jaundice or the relapse phase of chronic persistent hepatitis.

Analysis of symptoms: Stagnation of liver qi leads to doleful expression, hypochondriac distension or pain and frequent sighing; prolonged stagnation produces fire, marked by restlessness and irascibility; disharmony between the spleen and stomach gives rise to abnormal ascending and descending of the spleen qi and stomach qi, so there are gastric stuffiness, abdominal distension, belching, poor appetite, nausea, vomiting and loose stools; the white-thin or white-greasy coating and taut pulse are manifestations of disharmony between the spleen and stomach.

## 4. Yin depletion of the liver and kidneys

Symptoms: Vague pain in the right hypochondria, emaciation, weakness and soreness of the waist and knees, dizziness, tinnitus, blurred vision, frequent gingival atrophy and nosebleed, dry mouth and lips, feverish sensations in the palms and soles and flushed complexion with hectic fever; reddish tongue with scanty coating and thin and rapid pulse, primarily seen in chronic active hepatitis.

Analysis of symptoms: Prolonged affliction damages the liver yin and leads to malnutrition of the collaterals, marked by vague pain in the right hypochondria, emaciation and blurred vision; the kidneys are involved eventually, so there are weakness and soreness of the waist and knees, dizziness and tinnitus; deficiency of liver yin and kidney yin produces deficient heat in the interior, with such signs as dry mouth and lips, feverish sensation in the palms and soles and flushed complexion with hectic fever; the reddish tongue, scanty coating and thin pulse are attributable to deficiency of liver yin and kidney yin.

## 5. Stagnation of qi and blood

Symptoms: Thoracic and gastric distension, belching, nausea, masses below the costal region, distending or pricking pain in the hypochondria, red palms, red markings resembling the spider's thread on the skin, nasal and gingival bleeding, or dark and lusterless complexion and lips; dark-red tongue and thin-unsmooth pulse, primarily seen in chronic active hepatitis and some cases of persistent hepatitis.

Analysis of symptoms: Stagnation of liver qi brings about failure of the stomach qi to descend, marked by thoracic and gastric distension, belching and nausea; stagnation of qi results in blood stasis in the hypochondriac collaterals, which eventually develops into masses below the costal region with distending or pricking pain in the hypochondria; prolonged retention of blood stasis creates a predisposition to red palms and red markings resembling the spider's thread on the skin; retention of blood stasis hampers the production of fresh blood and causes frequent bleeding, so there are nasal and gingival bleeding; the dark-red tongue and thin-unsmooth pulse are due to stagnation of qi and blood.

## 6. Exuberance of pestilent toxins

Symptoms: Sudden onset, rapid progressing of jaundice with bright golden color, high fever polydipsia, hypochondriac distending pain, reduced food intake, vomiting, lethargy, coma and delirium, extreme fatigue, or sometimes hemorrhinia or hemafecia and deep-yellow urine; red-purple tongue, dry-yellow coating and rapid-taut-slippery or rapid-thin pulse, primarily seen in serious hepatitis.

Analysis of symptoms: Damp-heat with toxins fumigates liver and gallbladder and drives the bile to the skin, marked by sudden onset and rapid progressing of jaundice with bright golden color; internal blazing of toxic heat consumes the body fluid, so there are high fever and polydipsia; obstruction of the liver and gallbladder creates a predisposition to unsmooth flow of qi, with such signs as hypochondriac distending pain, reduced food intake and vomiting; invasion of heat-toxins into the pericardium is characterized by lethargy, coma and delirium; rampancy of blood driven by heat is manifested as hemorrhinia or hemafecia; damp-heat pours into the bladder downwardly, resulting in deep-yellow urine; the red-purple tongue, dry-yellow coating and rapid-taut-slippery or rapid-thin pulse are manifestations of rampancy of pestilent toxins.

## 7. Stagnation of heat in the liver and gallbladder

Symptoms: Prolonged bright-yellow eyes, complexion and body, hypo-chondriac pain involving the back, occasional fever or alternated chills and fever, bitter mouth and dry throat, poor appetite, abdominal distension, nausea and vomiting, constipation and scanty reddish urine; red tongue, yellow-greasy coating and rapid-taut pulse, primarily seen in cholestatic hepatitis.

Analysis of symptoms: Stagnated heat obstructs the biliary tract, leading to leaking of bile with such signs as prolonged bright-yellow eyes, complexion and body; obstruction of the liver and gallbladder creates a predisposition to stagnation of qi which transforms into fire thereafter, so there are bright yellow color and hypochondriac pain involving the back; the gallbladder meridian is in disorder, so there may be fever or alternate attack of chill and fever, bitter mouth and dry throat; stagnated heat in the liver and gallbladder results in abnormal ascending and descending of the spleen qi and stomach qi, characterized by poor appetite, abdominal distension, nausea and vomiting; obstruction of intestinal qi is manifested as constipation; damp-heat pours into the bladder downwardly, with such signs as scanty and reddish urine; the red tongue, yellow-greasy coating and rapid-taut pulse are all symptomatic of stagnated heat in the liver and gallbladder.

## Differential Treatment

### 1. Accumulation and steaming of damp-heat

Treatment principle: Dispelling heat and eliminating dampness, purging fire and removing toxins.

Prescription and herbs: Modified Yinchenhao Decoction and Longdan Xiegan Decoction.

Yinchen (Virgate Wormwood Herb) 18 g, Dahuang (Unprepared Rhubarb) 9 g, Zhizi (Cape Jasmine Fruit) 12 g, Huanglian (Golden Thread) 9 g, Huangqin (Baical Skullcap Root) 9 g, Huangbai (Amur Cork-tree) 9 g, Chuanmutong (Armand Clematis Stem) 6 g, Longdancao (Radix

Gentianae) 6 g, Zexie (Oriental Waterplantain Rhizome) 15 g, Cheqianzi (Plantain Seed) 15 g (wrapped during decoction), Zhuling (Polyporus) 12 g, Fuling (Indian Bread) 12 g, Gancao (Liquorice Root) 6 g.

Modification: In cases of nausea and vomiting, Jiangzhuru (Bamboo Shavings) 9 g and Jiangbanxia (Pinellia Tuber) 9 g are added to harmonize the stomach and relieve vomiting; for severe hepatic heat, Tianjihuang (Hypericum Japonicum Thunb) 30 g and Chuipencao (Strngy Stonecrop Herb) 30 g can be added to clear the liver.

## 2. Deficiency of the spleen with retention of dampness

Treatment principle: Replenishing qi to invigorate the spleen, regulating qi to expel dampness.

Prescription and herbs: Modified Shenling Baizhu Powder and Erchen Decoction.

Dangshen (Radix Codonopsis) 12 g, Baizhu (Largehead Atractylodes Rhizome) 12 g, Fuling (Indian Bread) 12 g, Zhuling (Polyporus) 12 g, Biandou (Hyacinth Bean) 15 g, Shanyao (Common Yan Rhizome) 15 g, Banxia (Pinellia Tuber) 9 g, Houpu (Magnolia Bark) 6 g, Muxiang (Common Aucklandia Root) 6 g, Sharen (Villous Amomum Fruit) 3 g, Chuanlianzi (Szechwan Chinaberry Fruit) 10 g, Chenpi (Dried Tangerine Peel) 6 g, Guya (Milllet sprout) 15 g, Maiya (Malt) 15 g, Gancao (Liquorice Root) 6 g.

Modification: If there are intolerance of cold, cold limbs and diarrhea before dawn, Fuzi (Prepared Common Monkshood Daughter) 6 g and Ganjiang (Dried Ginger) 2 g can be added to warm yang and dissipate coldness.

## 3. Disharmony between the spleen and stomach

Treatment principle: Soothing the liver and regulating qi, invigorating the spleen and harmonizing the middle energizer.

Prescription and herbs: Modified Chaihu Shugan Powder and Sijunzi Decoction.

Chaihu (Chinese Thorowax Root) 6 g, Zhishi (Immature Orange Fruit) 9 g, Xiangfu (Nutgrass Galingale Rhizome) 9 g, Dangshen (Radix Codonopsis) 12 g, Baizhu (Largehead Atractylodes Rhizome) 12 g, Fuling (Indian Bread) 12 g, Yiyiren (Coix Seed) 15 g, Banxia (Pinellia Tuber) 12 g, Houpu (Magnolia Bark) 6 g, Chuanxiong (Szechwan Lovage Rhizome) 6 g, Baishao (White Peony Alba) 9 g, Gancao (Liquorice Root) 6 g.

Modification: In cases of nausea and vomiting, Jiangzhuru (Bamboo Shavings) 9 g can be added to stop vomiting; for loose stools, Shanyao (Common Yan Rhizome) 15 g and Biandou (Hyacinth Bean) 15 g are added to invigorate the spleen and check diarrhea.

## 4. Yin depletion of the liver and kidneys

Treatment principle: Tonifying the kidneys and nourishing deficiency, soothing the liver and replenishing yin.

Prescription and herbs: Modified Yiguan Decoction.

Shengdi (Dried Rehmannia Root) 12 g, Shudi (Prepared Rhizome of Rehmannia) 12 g, Gouqizi (Barbary Wolfberry Fruit) 12 g, Baishao (White Peony Alba) 15 g, Danggui (Chinese Angelica) 9 g, Shashen (Root of Straight Ladybell) 12 g, Maidong (Dwarf Lilyturf Tuber) 12 g, Chuanlianzi (Szechwan Chinaberry Fruit) 9 g, Zhishouwu (Prepared Fleeceflower Root) 12 g, Shanzhuyu (Asiatic Cornelian Cherry Fruit) 12 g, Gancao (Liquorice Root) 6 g.

Modification: If the patient presents with blurred vision, Qingxiangzi (Feather Cockscomb Seed) 9 g and Juemingzi (Cassia Seed) 9 g are added to clear the liver and improve the acuity of vision; in cases of dry mouth and dry lips, Lugen (Fresh Reed Rhizome) 30 g can be added to promote fluid production and quench thirst.

## 5. Stagnation of qi and blood

Treatment principle: Promoting qi flow to dissipate stagnation, activating blood to resolve stasis.

Prescription and herbs: Modified Gexia Zhuyu Decoction.

Wulingzhi (Faeces Trogopterorum) 9 g (wrapped during decoction), Danggui (Chinese Angelica) 9 g, Chuanxiong (Szechwan Lovage Rhizome) 9 g, Taoren (Peach Seed) 9 g, Honghua (Safflower) 6 g, Danshen (Radix Salviae Miltiorrhiae) 15 g, Chishao (Red Peony Root) 9 g, Yanhusuo (Corydalis) 9 g, Xiangfu (Nutgrass Galingale Rhizome) 12 g, Zhiqiao (Orange Fruit) 15 g, Chuanlianzi (Szechwan Chinaberry Fruit) 9 g, Dangshen (Radix Codonopsis) 15 g, Baizhu (Largehead Atractylodes Rhizome) 9 g, Fuling (Indian Bread) 9 g, Gancao (Liquorice Root) 6 g.

Modification: For severe masses below the costal region, Muli (Oyster Shell) 15 g and Chuanshanjia (Pangolin Scale) 15 g are added to soften the hardness and dissipate stagnation.

## 6. Exuberance of pestilent toxins

Treatment principle: Clearing ying and cooling blood, eliminating toxins and draining dampness.

Prescription and herbs: Modified Qingwen Baidu Potion.

Shuiniujiao (Buffalo Horn Slice) 30 g, Dahuang (Rhubarb) 9 g, Zhizi (Cape Jasmine Fruit) 12 g, Huanglian (Golden Thread) 6 g, Yinchen (Virgate Wormwood Herb) 15 g, Huangqin (Baical Skullcap Root) 12 g, Shengdi (Dried Rehmannia Root) 12 g, Xuanshen (Figwort Root) 12 g, Danpi (Cortex Moutan) 12 g, Chishao (Red Peony Root) 12 g, Jinyinhua (Honeysuckle Flower) 9 g, Lianqiao (Weeping Forsythia Capsule) 9 g, Danshen (Radix Salviae Miltiorrhiae) 15 g, Baimaogen (Lalang Grass Rhizome) 30 g, Zicao (Arnebia Root) 12 g, Gancao (Unprepared Liquorice Root) 6 g.

Modification: If there are high fever, mania, coma, delirium and hepatic odor, Angong Niuhuang Wan (Bezoar Uterus-Calming Pill) or Niuhuang Qingxin Pill (Bezoar Sedative Pill) should be administered promptly at 3g a time and 1~3 times a day to dispel heat and open the orifices.

## 7. Stagnation of heat in the liver and gallbladder

Treatment principle: Dispersing the liver and dredging the gallbladder, dispelling heat and removing stagnation.

Prescription and herbs: Modified Sanjin Decoction and Yin-chenhao Decoction.

Jinqiancao (Christina Loosestrife) 30 g, Haijinshao (Lygodium) 12 g, Yujin (Turmeric Root Tuber) 12 g, Jineijin (Corium Stomachium Galli) 6 g, Yinchen (Virgate Wormwood Herb) 30 g, Zhizi (Cape Jasmine Fruit) 9 g, Dahuang (Rhubarb) 9 g, Huangqin (Baical Skullcap Root) 9 g, Fuling (Indian Bread) 12 g, Cheqianzi (Plantain Seed) 15 g (wrapped during decoction), Chuanmutong (Armand Clematis Stem) 6 g, Danshen (Radix Salviae Miltiorrhiae) 15 g, Zhiqiao (Orange Fruit) 15 g, Yanhusuo (Corydalis) 9 g, Gancao (Liquorice Root) 6 g.

Modification: For alternate attack of chill and fever, bitter mouth and dry throat, Chaihu (Chinese Thorowax Root) 6 g can be added to relieve the shaoyang disorder.


## Chinese Patent Medicine

1. Chupencao Power Preparation is infused and administered: 1 bag for each dose and 3 times a day.
2. Yinzhihuang Power Preparation is infused and administered: 1 bag for each dose and 3 times a day.


## Simple and Handy Prescriptions

1. Yinchen (Virgate Wormwood Herb) 10 g, Zhizi (Cape Jasmine Fruit) 6 g, Huangqin (Baical Skullcap Root) 9 g and Chuipencao (Strngy Stonecrop Herb) 30 g are taken 1 dose a day for 15 consecutive days. It is used for hepatitis with acute jaundice.
2. Jigucao (Canton Love-Pea Vine) 9 g, Tianjihuang (Hypericum Japonicum Thunb) 12 g, Danshen (Radix Salviae Miltiorrhiae) 10 g, Baishao (White Peony Alba) 12 g, Longdancao (Radix Gentianae) 4.5 g, Huashi (Talc) 12 g and Chuanmutong (Armand Clematis Stem) 6 g are administered 1 dose a day for 15 consecutive days. It is used for chronic persistent hepatitis and chronic active hepatitis.

## Other Therapies

Dietary therapy:

(1) Water-soaked mushroom (cutting into threads) 50 g and Jingmi (Rice Fruit) 100 g are boiled into thick porridge and taken once day.
(2) Live mudfish 100 g are cooked in a proper amount of water till it is medium-well, then a proper amount of toufu (bean curd), Shanzha (Hawthorn Fruit) 9 g, Jinzhencao (Dwarf Yellow Daylily) 30 g and a small quantity of Shengjiangfen (Fresh Ginger Powder) and salt are added till it is thoroughly cooked. The mudfish should be taken at different meals.

## Cautions and Advice

1. Protection of water source, disinfection of drinking water, sanitation of food and management of excrement and urine should be well conducted. For hepatitis B and C, it is important to prevent dissemination through blood and body fluid. In the active stage of acute or chronic hepatitis, the patients should be isolated for 30 days from the day when it occurs and the patients should also constantly take good rests.
2. The drinks and foods should be fresh, light and easy to digest. They should also be rich in calories, protein and vitamin C. For patients with serious hepatitis, they should take a low-salt, low-fat, high-glucose and calorie-rich diet and refrain from protein until the conditions get better. For those with chronic hepatitis, adequate calories should be guaranteed and the intake of protein can be properly increased. Moreover, alcohol consumption is strictly prohibited for those with hepatitis.
3. Patients with acute hepatitis usually have a favorable prognosis, especially in the case of hepatitis A. Acute hepatitis B is liable to progress into chronic hepatitis and cirrhosis. Hepatitis C and E are apt to become chronic. The prognosis of chronic active hepatitis is poorer than that of chronic persistent hepatitis. The prognosis of serious hepatitis is the most unfavorable, marked by a high case fatality and even for the lucky ones, postnecrotic cirrhosis often ensues. Chronic hepatitis B is closely linked to primary hepatic carcinoma.

## Daily Exercises

1. Recall the various types of viral hepatitis and their diagnostic key points.
2. Explain how viral hepatitis can be treated based on syndrome differentiation.

# Bacillary Dysentery
## Week 7: Friday

Bacillary dysentery is a common acute infection of the intestinal tract by dysentery bacillus, mostly prevalent in summer and autumn. Clinically it is marked by general intoxication, fever, abdominal pain, diarrhea, bloody and purulent stools and tenesmus. It can be divided into two stages: the acute stage (common type, mild type and toxic type) and the chronic stage (chronic persistent type, chronic asymptomatic type and acute attacking type). In TCM, bacillary dysentery is referred to as "Liji" and "Zhixia".

## Etiology and Pathology

The location of this disease is in the intestine, while its occurrence is related to the spleen, stomach and kidneys in addition to the intestine. The causative factors are mainly damp-heat and pestilent toxins, which invade the body and damage the spleen and stomach; besides, damp-heat obstructs the intestine, impeding the flow of qi and hampering the transportation and transformation of food; the stagnation of qi, blood and toxic heat brings about purulent blood, leading to dysentery in the end. If the spleen and stomach are damaged with obstruction of the middle yang, the invasion of dampness will be in combination with cold, leading to damp-cold dysentery; whereas if the spleen and kidneys are already weak, with inability to expel the lingering pathogens, there will be chronic dysentery marked by co-existence of excess and deficiency.

## Diagnostic Key Points

1. This disease is prevalent in summer and autumn.
2. In the acute stage, the patients often present with fever, abdominal pain, diarrhea, purulent and bloody stools and tenesmus. In the chronic stage, repeated occurrence and protraction are common and there are often acute attacks due to certain inductive factors. For the toxic type, the patients may present with high fever, fainting and listlessness, which usually occur prior to abdominal pain and diarrhea.

3. In the acute stage, the patients manifest an increase in the total number of WBC and moderate elevation in neutrophilic granulocyte level.
4. Microscopic examination on feces may show a large quantity of pus cells, red blood cells and macrophages. Pathogenic bacterium obtained from stool culture is decisive in confirming the diagnosis.

## Syndrome Differentiation

### 1. Damp-heat dysentery

Symptoms: Pain in the waist, diarrhea, tenesmus, bloody stools with pus (in red and white colors), a scorching sensation in the anus, scanty and reddish urine and possibly fever, intolerance of cold, headache, or ardent fever with polydipsia; yellow and greasy coating and rapid and slippery pulse; mostly seen in typical acute bacillary dysentery.

Analysis of symptoms: Stagnation of damp-heat in the intestine brings about unsmooth functional activity of qi as well as dysfunction in transportation, marked by abdominal pain, diarrhea and tenesmus; damp-heat fumigates the intestinal tract and impairs the collaterals or vessels, presenting as bloody stools with pus (in red and white colors); damp-heat pours downward, leading to scorching sensation in the anus as well as scanty and reddish urine; exterior-heat syndrome is marked by fever, intolerance of cold, headache, interior heat, or even ardent fever and polydipsia; the yellow and greasy coating as well as the rapid and slippery pulse are both due to steaming of damp-heat.

### 2. Damp-cold dysentery

Symptoms: Dysentery with more pus (in white color) than blood (in red color), accompanied by abdominal pain and spasm, tenesmus, tasteless sensation in the mouth, gastric stuffiness, no thirst, heaviness of the head, weariness of the body and possibly intolerance of cold, mild fever, general ache and absence of sweat; white-greasy coating and slow-soggy pulse; primarily seen in acute bacillary dysentery.

Analysis of symptoms: Stagnation of damp-cold in the intestine leads to unsmooth flow of qi, marked by dysentery, abdominal pain or spasm and tenesmus; damp-cold impairs the qi phase, resulting in dysentery with more pus (in white color) than blood (in red color); damp-cold obstructs the middle energizer, leading to poor digestion, with such signs as tasteless sensation in the mouth, gastric stuffiness, no thirst, heaviness of the head and weariness of the body; since it is accompanied by exterior cold syndrome, there are such symptoms as intolerance of cold, mild fever, general ache and absence of sweat; the white-greasy coating and slow-soggy pulse are both symptomatic of abundant damp-cold in the interior.

## 3. Pestilent toxins dysentery

Symptoms: Sudden onset, severe abdominal pain, aggravated tenesmus, bloody stools with pus in purple red color or like bloody water, ardent fever, thirst, headache, restlessness, chest fullness, poor appetite, vomiting, nausea, or even coma, convulsion, peripheral coldness and bluish or grayish complexion; purple-red tongue, dry-yellow coating and slippery-rapid pulse; mostly seen in acute toxic bacillary dysentery.

Analysis of symptoms : Invasion of pestilent toxins is marked by sudden onset; toxic heat obstructs the intestinal tract, leading to unsmooth functional activity of qi, so there are severe abdominal pain and aggravated tenesmus; toxic heat fumigates the intestinal tract and damages qi and blood, resulting in bloody stools with pus in purple-red color or like bloody water; fluid impairment due to abundant heat is manifested as ardent fever and thirst; heat disturbs the upper part, with such signs as headache; heat harasses the heart spirit, presenting as restlessness; toxic heat obstructs the middle energizer, bringing about malfunction of the spleen in ascending and the stomach in descending, characterized by chest fullness, poor appetite, vomiting and nausea; toxic heat clouds the upper orifices, so there are coma and convulsion; toxic heat consumes yin and in the long run involves yang, giving rise to peripheral coldness and bluish or grayish complexion; the purple-red tongue, dry-yellow coating and slippery-rapid pulse are all manifestations of abundant pestilent toxins.

## 4. Deficient cold dysentery

Symptoms: Chronic dysentery, loose stools with white pus, intermittent onset, vague pain in the abdomen with preference for warmth and pressure, tasteless and thirstless sensation in the mouth, poor appetite and low spirit, intolerance of cold, cold limbs, pale tongue, white and thin coating, deficient pulse or thin and deep pulse; mostly seen in chronic persistent bacillary dysentery .

Analysis of symptoms: Chronic dysentery with deficient cold in the spleen and stomach and damp-cold in the intestine is marked by loose stools with white pus, intermittent onset, vague pain in the abdomen with preference for warmth and pressure, tasteless and thirstless sensation in the mouth, poor appetite and low spirit; inactivation of spleen yang leads to failure of the limbs to warmed, so there are intolerance of cold with cold limbs; the pale tongue, white and thin coating and deficient pulse or thin and deep pulse are manifestations of deficient cold in the spleen and stomach.

## 5. Deficient heat dysentery

Symptoms: Chronic dysentery with thick or sticky red blood and white pus, or discharge of pure blood, vague pain in the abdomen, frequent desire for defecation yet without stools, hectic fever in the afternoon and dry mouth and throat; red tongue with little fluid or coating and thin-rapid pulse; mostly seen in chronic persistent bacillary dysentery.

Analysis of symptoms: Prolonged dysentery impairs the yin blood, marked by thick or sticky blood and pus, or discharge of pure blood and vague pain in the abdomen; consumption of yin-fluid gives rise to deficient heat in the interior, so there are frequent desire for defecation yet without stools, hectic fever in the afternoon and dry mouth and throat; the red tongue with little fluid or coating and the thin-rapid pulse are both symptoms of internal heat due to deficiency of yin.

## 6. Dysentery with vomiting (excess syndrome)

Symptoms: Dysentery with inability to take food, vomiting, chest distress and poor appetite with mouth filthiness; yellow-greasy coating and rapid-slippery pulse; mostly seen in acute toxic bacillary dysentery.

Analysis of symptoms: Accumulation of damp-heat and pestilent toxins in the intestine leads to failure of the stomach qi to descend, so there are inability to take food, vomiting, chest distress and poor appetite with mouth filthiness; the yellow-greasy coating and rapid-slippery pulse are attributable to accumulation of damp-heat and pestilent toxins in the intestine.

## 7. Dysentery with vomiting (deficiency syndrome)

Symptoms: Dysentery with inability to eat food, or with nausea and vomiting, or prompt vomiting after food intake, emaciation, as well as tasteless and thirstless sensation in the mouth; pale tongue and thin-feeble pulse; mostly seen in chronic persistent bacillary dysentery.

Analysis of symptoms: Prolonged dysentery impairs the spleen and stomach, leading to adverse rising of stomach qi, so there are inability to take food, or with nausea and vomiting, or prompt vomiting after food intake; dysfunction of the spleen in transportation and transformation is marked by emaciation as well as tasteless and thirstless sensation in the mouth; the pale tongue and thin-feeble pulse are a result of weakness of the spleen and stomach.

## Differential Treatment

### 1. Damp-heat dysentery

Treatment principle: Dispelling heat, resolving dampness and eliminating toxins; regulating qi, promoting blood circulation and removing stagnation.

Prescription and herbs: Modified Shaoyao Deoction.

Huanglian (Golden Thread) 3 g, Huangqin (Baical Skullcap Root) 9 g, Zhidahuang (Prepared Rhubarb) 9 g, Jinyinhua (Honeysuckle Flower) 12 g, Chishao (Red Peony Root) 9 g, Danggui (Chinese Angelica) 9 g, Gancao (Liquorice Root) 6 g, Muxiang (Common Aucklandia Root) 6 g and Binglang (Areca Seed) 9 g.

Modification: If there is abundant internal heat, Baitouweng (Chinese Pulsatilla Root) 15 g can be added to reinforce the action of dispelling heat; for severe retention of dampness, Zhuling (Polyporus) 12 g and Fuling (Indian Bread) 12 g are added to drain dampness with their bland flavors.

## 2. Damp-cold dysentery

Treatment principle: Warming the interior, resolving dampness and dissipating cold; promoting flow of qi, activating blood and removing stagnation.

Prescription and herbs: Modified Weiling Decoction.

Banxia (Pinellia Tuber) 10 g, Cangzhu (Atractylodes Rhizome) 9 g, Baizhu (Largehead Atractylodes Rhizome) 9 g, Houpu (Magnolia Bark) 6 g, Zhuling (Polyporus) 12 g, Fuling (Indian Bread) 12 g, Zexie (Oriental Waterplantain Rhizome) 12 g, Rougui (Cassia Bark) 3 g, Ganjiang (Dried Ginger) 9 g, Chenpi (Dried Tangerine Peel) 6 g, Zhishi (Immature Orange Fruit) 6 g, Muxiang (Common Aucklandia Root) 6 g, Danggui (Chinese Angelica) 10 g and Gancao (Liquorice Root) 6 g.

Modification: For tasteless sensation in the mouth, Shanzha (Hawthorn Fruit) 15 g and Shenqu (Massa Medicata Fermentata) 9 g are added to promote digestion.

## 3. Pestilent toxins dysentery

Treatment principle: Dispelling heat, cooling blood and eliminating toxins, resolving dampness, opening the orifices and removing stagnation.

Prescription and herbs: Modified Baitouweng Decoction and Zixue Pellet.

Baitouweng (Chinese Pulsatilla Root) 15 g, Huangqin (Baical Skullcap Root) 9 g, Huanglian (Golden Thread) 6 g, Huangbai (Amur Cork-tree) 9 g, Zhidahuang (Prepared Rhubarb) 15 g, Qinpi (Ash Bark) 9 g, Chishao (Red Peony Root) 9 g, Danpi (Cortex Moutan) 9 g, Binglang (Areca Seed) 9 g, Muxiang (Common Aucklandia Root) 6 g, Chenpi (Dried Tangerine Peel) 6 g, Gancao (Liquorice Root) 6 g and 1 ground Zixue Pellet (swallowed).

Modification: In cases of coma and high fever, Shuiniujiao (Buffalo Horn) 60 g, Shengdi (Dried Rehmannia Root) 9 g and 1 Zhibao Pellet (swallowed) are added to dispel heat and open the orifices; for stirring of wind with convulsions, Lingyangjiaofen (Antelope Horn Powder) 0.6 g can be swallowed to dispel heat and extinguish wind; for fulminant dysentery with depletion of yang qi, Renshen (Ginseng) 10 g and Fuzi (Prepared

Common Monkshood Daughter) 10 g should be administered immediately to supplement qi, revive yang and relieve peripheral coldness.

## 4. Deficient cold dysentery

Treatment principle: Warming the middle energizer, invigorating the spleen and tonifying the kidneys; dissipating cold, astringing the intestine and relieving dysentery.

Prescription and herbs: Modified Fuzi Lizhong Decoction and Sishen Pill.

Fuzi (Prepared Common Monkshood Daughter) 6 g, Ganjiang (Dried Ginger) 3 g, Roudoukou (Nutmeg) 6 g, Wuzhuyu (Medicinal Evodia Fruit) 3 g, Dangshen (Radix Codonopsis) 12 g, Gancao (Liquorice Root) 6 g, Baizhu (Largehead Atractylodes Rhizome) 12 g, Danggui (Chinese Angelica) 9 g, Baishao (White Peony Alba) 9 g, Muxiang (Common Aucklandia Root) 6 g, Hezi (Medicine Terminalia Fruit) 3 g, Wuweizi (Chinese Magnolivine Fruit) 6 g and Buguzhi (Malaytea Scurfpea Fruit) 12 g.

Modification: For vague pain in the abdomen with preference for warmth and pressure, Gaoliangjiang (Lesser Galangal Rhizome) 9 g and Paojiang (Prepared Dried Ginger) 9 g can be added to warm the middle energizer and alleviate pain.

## 5. Deficient heat dysentery

Treatment principle: Nourishing yin, supplementing blood and reinforcing the healthy qi; dispelling heat, resolving dampness and relieving dysentery.

Prescription and herbs: Modified Huanglian Ejiao Decoction and Zhuche Pill.

Huanglian (Golden Thread) 3 g, Ejiao (Donkey-hide Glue) 9 g, Huangqin (Baical Skullcap Root) 9 g, Shengdi (Dried Rehmannia Root) 9 g, Baishao (White Peony Alba) 9 g, Danggui (Chinese Angelica) 9 g, Paojiang (Prepared Dried Ginger) 9 g and Gancao (Liquorice Root) 6 g.

Modification: If the patients present with hectic fever in the afternoon, Digupi (Chinese Wolfberry Root-Bark) 12 g and Baiwei (Blackend Swallowwort Root) 9 g are added to subdue the deficient fever.

## 6. Dysentery with vomiting (excess syndrome)

Treatment principle: Bring down qi with bitterness and pungency, harmonizing the stomach and purging heat.

Prescription and herbs: Modified Kaijin Powder.

Huanglian (Golden Thread) 3 g, Shichangpu (Acorus Calamus) 12 g, Banxia (Pinellia Tuber) 9 g, Fuling (Indian Bread) 10 g, Chenpi (Dried Tangerine Peel) 6 g, Heyedi (Lotus Leaf-Base) 9 g, Zhidahuang (Rhubarb) 6 g, Zhuru (Bamboo Shavings) 9 g and Gancao (Liquorice Root) 6 g.

Modification: In cases of vomiting and chest distress, Zhiqiao (Orange Fruit) 12 g can be added to promote the flow of qi.

## 7. Dysentery with vomiting (deficiency syndrome)

Treatment principle: Invigorating the spleen and harmonizing the stomach, reversing the adverse flow of qi and arresting vomiting.

Prescription and herbs: Modified Liujunzi Decoction.

Dangshen (Radix Codonopsis) 12 g, Baizhu (Largehead Atractylodes Rhizome) 12 g, Fuling (Indian Bread) 12 g, Banxia (Pinellia Tuber) 9 g, Shichangpu (Acorus Calamus) 12 g, Lianzirou (Lotus Seed) 9 g, Chenpi (Dried Tangerine Peel) 6 g, Jiangzhuru (Ginger-prepared Bamboo Shavings) 9 g, several drops of Shengjiangzhi (Fresh Ginger Juice), and Gancao (Liquorice Root) 6 g.

Modification: In cases of nausea and vomiting with inability to eat or vomiting induced by food intake, Xuanfuhua (Intussusceer) 12 g and Daizheshi (Red Bole) 30 g can be added to reverse the adverse flow of qi.

## Chinese Patent Medicine

1. Huangliansu Tablet: 2 tablets for each dose, 3 times a day. It is used to treat acute bacillary dysentery.

2. Guben Yichang Pill: 4.5 g for each dose, twice a day. It is used to treat chronic bacillary dysentery.

## Simple and handy prescriptions

1. Baitouweng (Chinese Pulsatilla Root) 30 g, Qinpi (Ash Bark) 30 g, Baijiangcao (Dahurian Patrinia Herb) 15 g, Machixian (Purslane Herb) 15 g, Hongteng (Sargentgloryvine Stem) 15 g and Fengweicao (Huguenot Fern Herb) 15 g, Chishao (Red Peony Root) 9 g and Gancao (Liquorice Root) 6 g are boiled in water to treat acute bacillary dysentery.
2. Machixian (Purslane Herb) 60 g, Biandouhua (Hyacinth Bean Flower) 15 g, Yiyiren (Coix Seed) 15 g, Shanzha (Hawthorn Fruit) 60 g and Qianshi (Gordon Euryale Seed) 15 g are boiled in water to treat chronic bacillary dysentery.

## Other Therapies

Dietary therapy:

(1) Lianzirou (Lotus Seed) 15 g and Nuomi (Glutinous Rice) 30 g (stir-baked till it becomes yellowish) are cleaned and boiled to make porridge.
(2) Shier (Edible Manna Lichen) 10 g is dried and ground up into fine powder. Jiangmi (Rice Fruit) 20 g is boiled in water to make soup. The edible manna lichen powder is added into the rice water when it is boiled. The decoction should be taken at 3 different times within a day.

## Cautions and Advice

1. During the acute stage, isolation and treatment should be prompt and dietary hygiene should always be given special attention.
2. During the acute stage, the consumption of raw, cold, dregs-free, oily, fried or spicy foods should be prohibited. If there is high fever, a light liquid or semi-liquid diet should be adopted. For relatively severe

diarrhea, water should be drunk to replenish the supply in the body; a light, digestible and soft diet can be adopted after the diarrhea ceases.
3. Acute bacillary dysentery has a relatively favorable prognosis.

## Daily Exercises

1. Briefly describe the diagnostic key points of bacillary dysentery.
2. Explain how bacillary dysentery can be treated based on syndrome differentiation.

# CHAPTER 5

# Disorders of the Urinary System

## Acute Glomerulonephritis
## Week 7: Saturday

Acute glomerulonephritis (also called acute nephritis) is mostly caused by an immunological reaction after infection, particularly streptococcal infection. It is marked by diffuse disorders of the glomerulus of both kidneys, with sudden onset of such symptoms as edema, bloody urine, proteinuria and hypertension. It usually afflicts children and young people and it is more common in males than in females. Acute nephritis is closely associated with such TCM concepts as "yang-edema", "wind-edema" and "bloody urine".

### Etiology and Pathology

This disease is related to the lungs, spleen, kidneys and bladder. At the initial stage, the disease is one of "excess", usually due to pathogenic wind that fetters the lungs and impairs their ability to dredge and regulate the waterways, bringing about retention of water in the skin and muscles; it may also be due to improper diet which produces internal water and dampness, this encumbers the spleen and affects its function of ascending the lucid and descending the turbid, resulting in retention of water in the skin and muscles; a third factor is that abundant damp-heat pours into the bladder downwardly and damages the blood vessels, predisposing the patient to bloody urine. At the recovery stage, although the pathogenic factors may decline, the healthy qi also wanes, so this stage is generally characterized by a lingering of pathogenic factors with mild deficiency of healthy qi (primarily deficiency of spleen qi and kidney qi, or consumption of kidney yin).

## Diagnostic Key Points

1. A history of acute streptococcal infection in the tonsillar arch and skin about two weeks before onset of the symptoms mentioned below.
2. Presence of edema, hypertension, bloody scanty turbid urine.
3. Routine urianlysis: Bloody urine and proteinuria in different degrees; elevation of anti-streptolysin O; acceleration of blood sedimentation; decrease of creatinine clearance and dropping of serum CH 5 0 and C 3 level at the initial stage.

## Syndrome Differentiation

### 1. Edema due to wind-heat

Symptoms: Aversion to wind, fever, sore and swollen throat, palpebral edema, or general edema (with the head and face being relatively more severe), scanty and reddish urine and soreness of the bones and joints; red tongue with thin, yellow and greasy coating and floating and rapid pulse.

Analysis of symptoms: External invasion of wind-heat stagnates the defensive qi in the exterior, so there is aversion to wind, fever, as well as a sore and swollen throat; struggle between wind and water leads to overflow of water in the skin and muscles, which is marked by palpebral or general edema; pathogenic heat scorches the lower energizer, resulting in scanty and reddish urine; wind-heat invades the joints, leading to soreness of the bones and joints; the red tongue with thin, yellow and greasy coating and the floating and rapid pulse are symptomatic of overflow of water-dampness due to external invasion of wind-heat.

### 2. Edema due to wind-cold

Symptoms: Intolerance of cold, absence of sweat, mild fever, facial edema, swollen limbs, or general dropsy and oliguresis; white and thin tongue coating and tense and floating pulse.

Analysis of symptoms: Exogenous wind-cold fetters the defensive qi in the exterior, resulting in intolerance of cold, absence of sweat and mild fever; the failure of the lungs to disperse and to dredge and regulate waterways is responsible for the struggle between wind and water and the consequent overflow of water in the skin and muscles, this is marked by facial edema, swollen limbs, or general dropsy and oliguresis; the white and thin tongue coating with tense and floating pulse are manifestations of edema due to wind and cold.

## 3. Spreading of damp-heat

Symptoms: Palpebral and facial edema spreading to the whole body, scanty and reddish urine or bloody urine and pustules on the body surface; red tongue with thin-yellow or greasy-yellow coating and rapid-slippery pulse.

Analysis of symptoms: Stagnation of overflowing water and dampness produces heat, leading to palpebral and facial edema spreading to the whole body; damp-heat pours downward and this is marked by scanty and reddish urine; damp-heat damages the blood vessels, presenting as blood in the urine; damp-heat flows over the skin, leading to pustules on the body surface; the red tongue with thin-yellow or greasy-yellow coating and the rapid-slippery pulse are all attributable to the rampant spreading of damp-heat.

## 4. Retention of cold-dampness

Symptoms: Facial edema with swollen limbs, or general edema, oliguresis, poor appetite, nausea, chest distress, abdominal distension and weariness of the body with a heavy sensation; white-greasy tongue coating and thin-soggy pulse.

Analysis of symptoms: Retained cold-dampness in the interior overflows to the skin and muscles, bringing about facial edema with swollen limbs, or general edema and oliguresis; pathogenic dampness in the interior blocks the flow of qi and impedes the operations of transformation and transportation, resulting in poor appetite, nausea, chest distress and abdominal distension; dampness is characterized by heaviness, so there is weariness of the body with heavy sensation; the white-greasy tongue coating and thin-soggy pulse are both due to internal retention of cold-dampness.

## 5. Qi deficiency of the spleen and kidneys

Symptoms: Subdued edema or mild facial edema in the morning, lassitude, poor appetite and waist soreness; slightly red tongue with, thin coating and thin-soggy pulse.

Analysis of symptoms: Prolonged retention of water and dampness debilitates the spleen qi and kidney qi, resulting in subdued edema with mild facial dropsy in the morning and lassitude; dysfunction of the spleen in transportation and transformation is manifested as poor appetite; deficiency of kidney qi is responsible for soreness in the waist; the slightly red tongue with thin coating and thin-soggy pulse are manifestations of qi deficiency.

## 6. Deficiency of kidney yin

Symptoms: Disappearance of edema, dry mouth with occasional low grade fever, night sweats, waist soreness, yellowish urine and dry stools; reddish tongue with scanty coating and thin and rapid pulse.

Analysis of symptoms: Water and dampness transform into heat which consumes yin in the long run, so there is deficiency of yin fluid despite the disappearance of edema, this is marked by a dry mouth with occasional low grade fever and night sweats; insufficiency of kidney yin is responsible for soreness in the waist; damp-heat pours downward, bringing about yellowish urine; deficient yin fluid fails to moisten the intestine, presenting as dry stools; the reddish tongue with scanty coating and the thin and rapid pulse are symptomatic of yin deficiency with heat.

## Differential Treatment

### 1. Edema due to wind-heat

Treatment principle: Dispersing wind and dispelling heat, promoting urination to relieve edema.

Prescription and herbs: Modified Yinqiao Powder.

Jingjie (Fineleaf Schizonepeta Herb) 9 g, Fangfeng (Divaricate Saposhnikovia Root) 9 g, Jinyinhua (Honeysuckle Flower) 30 g, Lianqiao

(Weeping Forsythia Capsule) 9 g, Cheqianzi (Plantain Seed) 30 g (wrapped during decoction), Zexie (Oriental Waterplantain Rhizome) 15 g, Zhuling (Polyporus) 12 g, Fuling (Indian Bread) 12 g, Xiaoji (Field Thistle Herb) 30 g, Daji (Japanese Thistle Herb) 30 g, Banlange (Isatis Root) 9 g, Fuping (Duckweek) 9 g, Huashi (Talc) 30 g and Gancao (Liquorice Root) 6 g.

Modification: For severe fever, Shengshigao (Gypsum) 30 g and Huangqin (Baical Skullcap Root) 10 g can be added to reinforce the action of dispelling heat.

## 2. Edema due to wind-cold

Treatment principle: Dispersing wind and dissipating cold, promoting urination to relieve edema.

Prescription and herbs: Modified Yuebi Jiazhu Decoction.

Shengmahuang (Unprepared Ephedra) 6 g, Guizhi (Cassia Twig) 6 g, Zisu (Purple Common Perilla) 15 g, Fangfeng (Divaricate Saposhnikovia Root) 9 g, Baizhu (Largehead Atractylodes Rhizome) 9 g, Zexie (Oriental Waterplantain Rhizome) 15 g, Fuling (Indian Bread) 15 g, Zhuling (Polyporus) 15 g, Cheqianzi (Plantain Seed) 30 g (wrapped during decoction), Shengjiangpi (Fresh Ginger Peel) 3 g and Shenggancao (Liquorice Root) 6 g.

Modification: If there is fever, Jingjie (Fineleaf Schizonepeta Herb) 9 g and Douchi (Black Curd Beans) 9 g can be added to disperse wind and dispel heat.

## 3. Spreading of damp-heat

Treatment principle: Dispelling heat and resolving dampness, promoting water discharge and stopping blood.

Prescription and herbs: Modified Mahuang Lianqiao Chixiaodou Decoction and Xiaoji Yinzi.

Mahuang (Ephedra) 9 g, Xingren (Almond) 9 g, Sangbaipi (White Mulberry Root-Bark) 9 g, Lianqiao (Weeping Forsythia Capsule) 12 g, Jinyinhua (Honeysuckle Flower) 9 g, Pugongying (Dandelion) 30 g, Zhizi

(Cape Jasmine Fruit) 10 g, Zihuadiding (Tokyo Violet Herb) 30 g, Daji (Japanese Thistle Herb) 30 g, Xiaoji (Field Thistle Herb) 30 g, Baimaogen (Lalang Grass Rhizome) 30 g, Puhuang (Pollen Typhae) 9 g, Oujie (Lotus Rhizome Node) 9 g, Chixiaodou (Rice Bean) 30 g, Huashi (Talc) 30 g and Gancao (Liquorice Root) 6 g.

Modification: For severe edema, Zexie (Oriental Waterplantain Rhizome) 15 g and Cheqianzi (Plantain Seed) 15 g (wrapped during decoction) are added to promote urination and relieve edema.

## 4. Retention of cold-dampness

Treatment principle: Dissipating cold and drying dampness, promoting urination to relieve edema.

Prescription and herbs: Modified Weiling Powder and Wupi Potion.

Guizhi (Cassia Twig) 9 g, Baizhu (Largehead Atractylodes Rhizome) 9 g, Cangzhu (Atractylodes Rhizome) 15 g, Chuanpu (Sichuan Cortex Magnoliae Officinalis) 6 g, Banxia (Pinellia Tuber) 9 g, Zhuling (Polyporus) 15 g, Fuling (Indian Bread) 15 g, Cheqianzi (Plantain Seed) 30 g (wrapped during decoction), Dafupi (Areca Peel) 12 g, Sangbaipi (White Mulberry Root-Bark) 9 g, Shengjiangpi (Fresh Ginger Peel) 3 g, Chenpi (Dried Tangerine Peel) 6 g and Gancao (Liquorice Root) 6 g.

Modification: For abdominal distension, Zhiqiao (Orange Fruit) 12 g can be added to regulate qi.

## 5. Qi deficiency of the spleen and kidneys

Treatment principle: Invigorating the spleen and tonifying the kidneys, supplementing qi and relieving edema.

Prescription and herbs: Modified Shenling Baizhu Powder.

Huangqi (Milkvetch Root) 15 g, Dangshen (Radix Codonopsis) 12 g, Baizhu (Largehead Atractylodes Rhizome) 12 g, Zhuling (Polyporus) 15 g, Fuling (Indian Bread) 15 g, Shanyao (Common Yan Rhizome) 15 g, Yiyiren (Coix Seed) 15 g, Biandou (Hyacinth Bean) 12 g, Lianzirou (Lotus Seed) 9 g, Sharen (Villous Amomum Fruit) 3 g, Chenpi (Dried Tangerine Peel) 6 g and Gancao (Liquorice Root) 6 g.

Modification: If there is bloody urine, Xianhecao (Hairyvein Agrimonia Herb) 30 g, Qiancao (Indian Madder Root) 12 g and Xueyutan (Carbonized Hair) 9 g can be added to stop bleeding; for proteinuria, Qianshi (Gordon Euryale Seed) 30 g can be added to astringe and consolidate.

## 6. Deficiency of kidney yin

Treatment principle: Nourishing yin and tonifying the kidneys, dispelling heat and discharging water.

Prescription and herbs: Modified Zhibai Dihuang.

Zhimu (Common Anemarrhena Rhizome) 12 g, Huangbai (Amur Cork-tree) 9 g, Shengdi (Dried Rehmannia Root) 15 g, Shanzhuyu (Asiatic Cornelian Cherry Fruit) 9 g, Shanyao (Common Yan Rhizome) 15 g, Zexie (Oriental Waterplantain Rhizome) 15 g, Danpi (Cortex Moutan) 9 g, Fuling (Indian Bread) 15 g, Digupi (Chinese Wolfberry Root-Bark) 15 g, Huanliancao (Ecliptae Herba) 15 g, Xianhecao (Hairyvein Agrimonia Herb) 30 g, Huashi (Talc) 30 g, Cheqianzi (Plantain Herb) 15 g (wrapped during decoction) and Gancao (Liquorice Root) 6 g.

Modification: For persistent low grade fever, Yinchaihu (Starwort Root) 6 g, Qinghao (Sweet Wormwood Herb) 15 g and Baiwei (Blackend Swallowwort Root) 9 g can be added to dispel the deficient heat.

## Chinese Patent Medicine

1. Shenling Baizhu Tablet: 4 tablets for each dose, 3 times a day.
2. Zhibai Dihuang Pill: 4.5 g for each dose, twice a day.

## Simple and Handy Prescriptions

1. Zhuling (Polyporus) 30 g, Fuling (Indian Bread) 30 g, Cheqianzi (Fresh Plantain Herb) 30 g and Yumixu (Stigmata Maydis) 30 g are boiled in water. The decoction is used to treat edema.
2. Daji (Japanese Thistle Herb) 30 g, Xiaoji (Field Thistle Herb) 30 g, Baimaogen (Fresh Lalang Grass Rhizome) 60 g and Xianhecao (Hairyvein Agrimonia Herb) 60 g are boiled in water. The decoction is applicable for the patients with bloody urine.

## Other Therapies

Dietary therapy:

(1) A blackfish, Donggua (Chinese waxgourd) 500 g (cut into slices with peel) and Chixiaodou (Rice Bean) 50 g are boiled together in a cooking pot with clear water. The soup should be made without adding salt. This is used to treat acute nephritis with apparent edema.

(2) 250 g of rice fruit is boiled till it is half cooked, then an egg and 250 g of shepherd's purse are added to make porridge. This is used to treat acute nephritis with bloody urine.

## Cautions and Advice

1. Patients should take caution against catching the common cold and ensure they receive thorough treatment of the repeated tonsillitis and skin ulcers; they should also take good rest in bed and adopt a salt-free diet when they have symptoms of edema and scanty urine.

2. Apart from adopting a low-salt diet, patients with acute nephritis should also restrict their daily intake of protein (less than 1 g of protein / 1000 g of body weight); instead, they should take more carbohydrates; milk and eggs are also preferable; the intake of protein cannot be increased until the recovery phase when the volume of urine begins to pick up. In addition, animal viscera, beans and any foods with these as constituents are inadvisable.

3. Acute nephritis is usually favorable in prognosis and has the tendency of spontaneous recovery. Nevertheless, it should still be treated proactively once diagnosed and the complications should also be prevented and controlled.

## Daily Exercises

1. Concisely describe the diagnostic key points of acute nephritis.
2. Explain how the patterns of acute nephritis can be differentiated.

# Chronic Glomerulonephritis
## Week 8: Monday

Chronic Glomerulonephritis (chronic nephritis) refers to the different types of diffuse or focal inflammation of bilateral glomeruli due to various causes; it is a collective term for the diseases originating from the renal glomerulus with similar clinical manifestations, different pathological changes and varying prognoses. Clinically, it is marked by edema, proteinuria, bloody urine, hypertension and renal inadequacy. Most cases are characterized by a slow onset and a chronic persistent development, while a small number of cases stem from acute nephritis. In TCM, chronic nephritis is considered to be closely associated with "edema", "yin-water", "waist pain" and "deficiency-consumption.

### Etiology and Pathology

This disease is mainly due to the functional disorders of the lungs, spleen, liver and kidneys. Deficiency of the lungs leads to transformation of qi into water instead of essence, deficiency of the spleen results in failure of earth to control water and deficiency of the kidneys brings about uncontrolled circulation of water. If the disease persists, the disorder of yang will involve yin, leading to deficiency of kidney yin and the subsequent deficiency of liver yin (because water fails to nourish wood) and, furthermore, hyperactivity of liver yang (because yin fails to restrict yang). Deficiency of qi and yin gives rise to unsmooth flow of blood, marked by blood stasis. In the end, the result is critical conditions such as deficiency of yin and yang, exhaustion of the spleen and kidneys and internal abundance of turbid yin.

### Diagnostic Key Points

1. This disease is marked by a slow onset and a protracted course, with such clinical manifestations as proteinuria, bloody urine or red blood cells in the urine (under microscopic examination), edema, hypertension and renal inadequacy. Owing to the protracted disease course of chronic nephritis and the gradual destruction of nephrons, renal atrophy and failure are very common in the late stage.

2. According to the clinical manifestations, it can be subdivided into the following five types:

Common type: Mild or medium edema; possible moderate elevation of blood pressure; moderate proteinuria (+ ~ + +) under uroscopy, above 10 RBCs/ high power field from urinary sediment examination and varying degrees of cylindruria; functional lesions of the kidneys to some degrees, decreased endogenous creatinine clearance rate, increased volume of nocturnal urine, decreased function of urinary concentration, dropping of urine osmotic pressure, urine specific gravity (relative density) below 1.015 and azotemia; weariness, poor appetite, waist soreness and anaemia in most patients.

Hypertension type: Similar to the common type, but with its own characteristics of persistent, moderate or marked elevation of blood pressure (particularly diastolic pressure).

Nephrosis type: Moderate or severe edema, marked proteinuria, hypoproteinemia and possibly hyperlipemia. It may also be accompanied by different degrees of hypertension, bloody urine, anaemia and renal inadequacy.

Mixed type: Possessing the characteristics of the above-mentioned types simultaneously.

Acute type: Susceptibility to respiratory tract infection and acute onset; edema, elevation of blood pressure, bloody urine discernable by the naked eye, urine protein (+ ~ + + +) and possibly cylindruria; alleviation by rest or symptomatic treatment, or involuntary relief , but with functional lesions of the kidneys and anaemia in varying degrees.

3. Renal puncturation biopsy is conducive to the definitive diagnosis.

## Syndrome Differentiation

### 1. Retention of water-dampness due to qi deficiency of the lungs and kidneys

Symptoms: Sallow complexion with mild yet persistent edema, lassitude, susceptibility to common cold and soreness in the lumbar vertebrae; pale tongue with white, thin and moist coating with teeth marks, thin and feeble pulse.

Analysis of symptoms: Failure of the lungs in dispersion and purification leads to retention of water and qi, marked by facial edema; the defensive qi fails to consolidate the exterior, resulting in susceptibility to the common cold; the kidneys are in charge of water and fluid with the functions of transforming qi and promoting circulation of water, so if the kidney essence is deficient, there will be such manifestations as sallow complexion, lassitude and soreness in the lumbar vertebrae; the pale tongue, the white, thin and moist coating with teeth marks and the thin and feeble pulse are all symptomatic of retention of water-dampness due to deficiency of lung qi and kidney qi.

## 2. Overflowing of water-dampness due to yang deficiency of the spleen and kidneys

Symptoms: Apparent general edema with pleural fluid, ascites, abdominal distension, scanty urine, whitish complexion, intolerance of cold, cold limbs, listlessness, nocturnal emissions, impotence or menstrual irregularity, soreness in the lumbar vertebrae or weakness of the legs, poor appetite, or loose stools; pale and enlarged tongue with teeth marks, white, thin and greasy coating and thin and deep pulse or deep, slow and feeble pulse.

Analysis of symptoms: Deficient spleen yang and kidney yang fail to distribute the water and dampness properly, leading to retention of which is marked by apparent general edema with pleural fluid, ascites, abdominal distension and scanty urine; deficient spleen yang and kidney yang fail to warm the body and nourish the waist, manifesting in a whitish complexion, intolerance of cold, cold limbs, listlessness, nocturnal emissions, impotence or menstrual irregularity and soreness in the lumbar vertebrae or weakness of the legs; the normal operations of transportation and transformation are hampered, giving rise to poor appetite or loose stools; deficiency of the kidneys leads to insecurity of the essence checkpoint, with such signs as nocturnal emissions, impotence, or menstrual irregularity; the pale and enlarged tongue with teeth marks, the white, thin and greasy tongue coating and the thin and deep pulse or deep, slow and feeble pulse are all manifestations of overflowing of water-dampness due to deficiency of spleen yang and kidney yang.

## 3. Yin exhaustion of the liver and kidneys with floating of deficient yang

Symptoms: Dizziness, headache, feverish sensations over the five centers (the palms, the soles and the heart), flushed and feverish complexion, tinnitus, dry eyes with blurred vision, dry mouth and throat, soreness in the lumbar vertebrae, nocturnal emissions, menstrual irregularity, oliguresis with unsmooth urination, or possibly mild edema and difficult defecation; reddish tongue with scanty coating and thin-taut or thin-rapid pulse.

Analysis of symptoms: Yin deficiency of the liver and kidneys gives rise to hyperactivity of liver yang, this is marked by dizziness, headache, tinnitus and dry eyes with blurred vision; internal heat due to deficiency of yin is manifested as feverish sensation over the five centers (the palms, the soles and the heart), a flushed and feverish complexion and a dry mouth and throat; deficiency of kidney essence is responsible for soreness in the lumbar vertebrae, nocturnal emissions and menstrual irregularity; exhaustion of liver yin and kidney yin brings about oliguresis, unsmooth urination and difficult defecation; deficiency of the kidneys results in functional disorder of qi transformation, so there is mild edema; the reddish tongue with scanty coating and thin-taut or thin-rapid pulse are due to deficiency of liver yin and kidney yin.

## 4. Deficiency of qi and yin with internal obstruction of blood stasis

Symptoms: Lusterless or dark complexion, shortness of qi, weariness, or susceptibility to common cold, post meridiem low grade fever or feverish sensation in the palms and soles, dry mouth and throat or persistent soreness of the throat; slightly red tongue with scanty coating and thin, thin-rapid or thin-unsmooth pulse.

Analysis of symptoms: Prolonged affliction consumes qi as well as yin-blood, leading to unsmooth circulation of blood, marked by lusterless or dark complexion; deficiency of qi results in shortness of qi, weariness, or susceptibility to the common cold; deficiency of yin brings about post meridiem low grade fever or feverish sensation in the palms and soles, dry mouth and throat or persistent soreness of the throat; deficiency of qi and yin gives rise to deficient heat in the interior, with such signs as a slightly red tongue with scanty coating and thin pulse or thin-rapid pulse; the unsmooth flow of blood is responsible for the thin and unsmooth pulse.

## 5. Failure of the spleen and kidneys with internal turbid dampness

Symptoms: Dark, lusterless and swollen complexion, listlessness, emaciation, chest distress, abdominal distension, poor appetite, nausea, vomiting, scanty urine or clear and profuse urine, diarrhea or constipation, or even restlessness, coma and spasms; pale and enlarged tongue, white, thin and greasy or grayish yellow and greasy tongue coating and thin and deep pulse or thin and taut pulse.

Analysis of symptoms: Extreme depletion of primordial qi and exhaustion of the spleen and kidneys lead to internal abundance of turbid dampness, marked by a dark, lusterless and swollen complexion, listlessness and emaciation; failure of turbid yin to descend results in chest distress, abdominal distension, poor appetite, nausea and vomiting; failure of the kidney's controlling function is manifested as scanty or clear and profuse urine; deficiency of the spleen results in poor digestion, with such signs as diarrhea or constipation; turbid dampness disturbs the clear orifices upwardly, predisposing the patient to restlessness, coma and spasms; the pale and enlarged tongue, the white, thin and greasy coating or grayish yellow and greasy coating and the thin and deep pulse or thin and taut pulse are all attributable to failure of the spleen and kidneys with internal turbid dampness.

## Differential Treatment

## 1. Retention of water-dampness due to qi deficiency of the lungs and kidneys

Treatment principle: Simultaneous nourishment of the lungs and kidneys, supplementing qi to relieve edema.

Prescription and herbs: Modified Yupingfeng Powder and Fangji Huangqi Decoction.

Huangqi (Milkvetch Root) 30 g, Baizhu (Largehead Atractylodes Rhizome) 12 g, Fangfeng (Divaricate Saposhnikovia Root) 9 g, Zhuling (Polyporus) 12 g, Fuling (Indian Bread) 12 g, Zexie (Oriental Waterplantain Rhizome) 12 g, Chenhulu (Aged Bottle-gourd) 12 g, Yimucao (Motherwort Herb) 15 g, Zelanye (Herba Lycopi Leaf) 15 g, Baijiangcan (Silkworm Larva) 9 g, Cantui (Cicada Slough) 6 g and Gancao (Liquorice Root) 6 g.

Modification: For severe weariness, Dangshen (Radix Codonopsis) 12 g and Huangjing (Solomonseal Rhizome) 9 g are added to nourish qi.

## 2. Overflowing of water-dampness due to yang deficiency of the spleen and kidneys

Treatment principle: Warming the kidneys and spleen, transforming qi to relieve edema.

Prescription and herbs: Modified Zhenwu Decoction and Shipi Potion.

Ganjiang (Dried Ginger) 9 g, Fuzi (Prepared Common Monkshood Daughter) 6 g, Caoguo (Fructus Tsaoko) 9 g, Baizhu (Largehead Atractylodes Rhizome) 12 g, Fuling (Indian Bread) 15 g, Cheqianzi (Plantain Seed) 30 g (wrapped during decoction), Zexie (Oriental Waterplantain Rhizome) 15 g, Dafupi (Areca Peel) 12 g, Mugua (Papaya) 9 g, Muxiang (Common Aucklandia Root) 6 g, Houpu (Magnolia Bark) 9 g and Gancao (Liquorice Root) 6 g.

Modification: In cases of abdominal distension and scanty urine, Chenhulu (Aged Bottle-gourd) 9 g can be added to promote urination and relieve edema.

## 3. Yin exhaustion of the liver and kidneys with floating of deficient yang

Treatment principle: Nourishing the liver and kidneys, supplementing yin to suppress yang.

Prescription and herbs: Modified Zuogui Potion.

Shengdi (Dried Rehmannia Root) 15 g, Guiban (Tortoise Shell) 9 g, Gouqizi (Barbary Wolfberry Fruit) 9 g, Shanyao (Common Yan Rhizome) 15 g, Shanzhuyu (Asiatic Cornelian Cherry Fruit) 9 g, Fuling (Indian Bread) 12 g, Zexie (Oriental Waterplantain Rhizome) 12 g, Dongkuizi (Malva Verticillata L) 9 g, Zhenzhumu (Nacre) 30 g, Lingcishi (Magnetitum) 30 g and Gancao (Liquorice Root) 6 g.

Modification: If there is waist soreness and nocturnal emissions, Jinyingzi (Cherokee Rose Fruit) 9 g and Qianshi (Gordon Euryale Seed) 9 g can be added to reinforce the kidneys in consolidation; for severe tinnitus, Shichangpu (Acorus Calamus) 12 g can be added to treat the aural disorder.

## 4. Deficiency of qi and yin with internal obstruction of blood stasis

Treatment principle: Replenishing qi and nourishing yin, dispelling heat and activating blood.

Prescription and herbs: Modified Shenqi Dihuang Decoction.

Shenghuangqi (Raw Milkvetch Root) 15 g, Taizishen (Heterophylly Falsesatarwort Root) 15 g, Shengdi (Dried Rehmannia Root) 9 g, Shanzhuyu (Asiatic Cornelian Cherry Fruit) 9 g, Nuzhenzi (Glossy Privet Fruit) 9 g, Danpi (Cortex Moutan) 9 g, Fuling (Indian Bread) 12 g, Shanyao (Common Yan Rhizome) 15 g, Zexie (Oriental Waterplantain Rhizome) 15 g, Danshen (Radix Salviae Miltiorrhiae) 15 g, Yimucao (Motherwort Herb) 15 g, Cantui (Cicada Slough) 6 g, Baijiangcan (Silkworm Larva) 9 g and Gancao (Stir-baked Liquorice Root) 6 g.

Modification: For post meridiem low grade fever or feverish sensation in the palms and soles, Guiban (Tortoise Shell) 9 g and Digupi (Chinese Wolfberry Root-Bark) 12 g are added to nourish yin and dispel heat; if there is obvious internal obstruction of blood stasis, Ezhu (Zedoray Rhizome) 9 g and Shuizhi (Leech) 9 g are added to activate blood and expel stasis.

## 5. Failure of the spleen and kidneys with internal turbid dampness

Treatment principle: Supplementing the primordial qi and reinforcing the healthy qi, eliminating toxins and bringing down turbidity.

Prescription and herbs: Modified Zhenwu Decoction and Liujunzi Decoction.

Dangshen (Radix Codonopsis) 12 g, Baizhu (Largehead Atractylodes Rhizome) 12 g, Fuling (Indian Bread) 12 g, Banxia (Pinellia Tuber) 9 g, Shengjiangpi (Fresh Ginger Peel) 9 g, Chenpi (Dried Tangerine Peel) 6 g, Fuzi (Prepared Common Monkshood Daughter) 6 g, Shengdahuang (Raw Rhubarb) 6~9 g, Huanglian (Golden Thread) 6 g, Cheqianzi (Plantain Seed) 15 g (wrapped during decoction) , Zexie (Oriental Waterplantain Rhizome) 15 g and Gancao (Liquorice Root) 6 g.

Modification: In cases of nausea and vomiting, Zhuru (Bamboo Shavings) 9 g can be added to inhibit the adverse rising of qi; for presence of coma, Suhexiang Pill is administered to open the orifices with aromatic herbs.

## Chinese Patent Medicine

1. Shenyan Siwei Tablet: 4 tablets for each dose, 3 times a day.
2. Bailing Capsule: 4 capsules for each dose, 3 times a day.

## Simple and Handy Prescriptions

Yumixu (Stigmata Maydis) 60 g, Haijinsha (Japanese Climbing Fern Spore) 30 g and Mabiancao (European Verbena Herb) 60 g are boiled in water and consumed.

## Other Therapies

Dietary therapy:

(1) A spring chicken and 120 g of Huangqi (Milkvetch Root) are thoroughly boiled in a casserole. Both the chicken and soup can be consumed.

(2) A blackfish and 500 g of Donggua (Peeled Chinese waxgourd) are cooked together without salt.

## Cautions and Advice

1. Patients should take steps to prevent and treat acute nephritis actively and promptly, avoid strenuous activities, ward off cold and dampness, prevent infection and refrain from drugs detrimental to the kidneys.
2. Chronic nephritis has a slow disease course and symptoms can be alleviated by dietary treatment such as taking nutritious food to recover the renal functions. If there is elevation of blood cholesterol, the intake of fat should be restricted; for edema and hypertension, a low-salt diet can be adopted; for anaemia, it is advisable to consume food rich in iron, vitamins B and C; for patients with hypertension, it is appropriate to adopt a light diet and avoid wind-stirring food, spicy food, stomach-irritating food and seafood; for edema without elevation of blood urea nitrogen, it is advisable to adopt a protein-rich diet; for elevation of blood urea nitrogen, a low-protein diet can be adopted.
3. Most patients can maintain relatively satisfactory renal functions for a very long time with active treatment. If there is presence of azotemia, it should be given due attention and timely treatment; once the condition is aggravatedto the extent of renal failure, the prognosis will be unfavorable.

## Daily Exercises

1. Recall the diagnostic key points of chronic nephritis.
2. Explain how chronic nephritis can be treated based on syndrome differentiation.

# Nephrotic Syndrome
# Week 8: Tuesday

Nephrotic syndrome, a group of clinical symptoms, refers to the disorder of the renal glomerulus due to a variety of etiological factors. The main pathological change is the increased permeability of plasma-albumin through the glomerular filtration membrane. Clinically, it is characterized by the presence of profuse proteins in the urine, albuminaemia, hyperlipemia and edema in varying degrees. Nephrotic syndrome is clinically divided into two types: primary nephrotic syndrome and secondary nephrotic syndrome. The former refers to the disorders caused by primary glomerulopathy, while the latter refers to those secondary to other diseases or resulting from specific pathogenic factors. In addition, primary nephrotic syndrome is subdivided into Type I and Type II. In TCM, nephrotic syndrome is closely associated with "edema", "bloody urine", "lumbago" and "deficiency consumption".

## Etiology and Pathology

The exogenous factors of this disease is wind, dampness, heat, toxins, overstrain and excessive sexual activity. The endogenous factors are mainly functional disorders of the lungs, spleen, kidneys and triple energizer in distributing water and nutrients. If the exogenous pathogenic factors invade the lungs, there will be failure of the lungs in dispersion and purification, as well as its inability to dredge and regulate waterways; if the spleen fails in its functions of transportation and transformation, there can be indigestion of water and food as well as internal retention of water and dampness; if the kidney qi is insufficient, there may be ungoverned opening and closing of the water pass, predisposing the patient to edema; if water and dampness overflow, the yang qi will be stagnated; if the patient has a yang-deficient constitution, there can be deficiency of spleen yang and kidney yang; if the edema persists, the yin-blood will be consumed insidiously, resulting in deficiency of liver yin and kidney yin; if the water disorder involves the blood phase, the collaterals can be injured in the long run, leading to co-existence of edema and blood stasis; if the disease involves too many viscera, there will inevitably be disassociation between yin and yang and such critical conditions as exhaustion of primordial yang, depletion of genuine yin and internal abundance of turbid toxins.

## Diagnostic Key Points

1. Apparent edema.
2. Routine blood test and 24h urine protein+ + + ~ + + + +; quantity >3.5 g/24h; presence of bloody urine or red blood cells under microscopic examination (microscopic urinary sediment >10 red blood cells/highpower field) in Type II nephrotic syndrome.
3. Hypoalbuminemia (which occurs to most of the plasma proteins).
4. Apparent increase in the level of plasma lipids, cholesterol and triglyeride (triacylglycerol); increase in the concentration of low or very low density lipoprotein; normal or slightly decreased concentration of high density lipoprotein.
5. Different degrees of functional lesion of the kidneys in Type II nephrotic syndrome, with such manifestations as reduced creatinine clearance rate, or even increased serum creatinine and urea nitrogen level.
6. The determination of the level of serum complement C3is of diagnostic value to membrane proliferation.
7. The main pathological types during diagnosis are minimal lesions, mesenterium proliferation, membranous or focal segmented sclerosis and membrane proliferation.

## Syndrome Differentiation

### 1. Overflow of wind and water

Symptoms: Palpebral or facial edema rapidly affecting the whole body, soreness and heaviness in the limbs, difficulty in micturition; possible aversion to wind, nasal obstruction and cough; white and thin tongue coating, floating and tense pulse, which may be complicated by redness, swelling and pain in the throat.

Analysis of symptoms: Pathogenic wind invades the body from the exterior and struggles with water and dampness, leading to palpebral or facial edema rapidly spreading to the whole body; dysfunction of the lungs in dispersion and purification impairs it from dredging and regulating the waterways, resulting in soreness and heaviness in the limbs and difficulty in micturition; for predominance of wind-cold, there are symptoms such as aversion to wind-cold, nasal obstruction, cough, white and thin tongue coating, or floating and tense pulse; for predominance of wind-heat, it is manifested as a reddened, swollen and painful pharyngeal, red tongue with yellow coating, as well as floating and rapid pulse.

## 2. Transformation of pathogenic dampness into heat

Symptoms: General edema, shiny and tense skin, thirst, restlessness with fever, thoracic and abdominal stuffiness and fullness, red urine, constipation, or skin sores and ulcers; red tongue with yellow and greasy coating and slippery and rapid pulse.

Analysis of symptoms: Pathogenic water and dampness stagnate in the skin and muscles and turn into heat, resulting in edema all over the body with shiny and tense skin; damp-heat permeates throughout the triple energizers, predisposing the patient to abnormal ascending and descending of qi that is marked by thoracic and abdominal stuffiness and fullness; retention of damp-heat blocks the upward flow of fluid, with such signs as thirst, restlessness and fever; predominance of pathogenic heat is manifested as constipation and red urine; damp-heat transforms into toxins and manifests itself on the skin, leading to dermal sores and ulcers; the red tongue with yellow and greasy coating as well as the slippery and rapid pulse are attributable to an internal accumulation of damp-heat.

## 3. Deficiency of primordial kidney qi

Symptoms: Mild edema, or facial edema in the morning and calf edema in the evening, weakness and soreness of the waist and knees, weariness and drowsiness; slightly red tongue with white and thin or white and greasy coating, as well as thin and deep pulse.

Analysis of symptoms: The deficient kidneys fail to transform the water qi, which accumulates in the interior, this is marked by mild edema or facial edema in the morning and calf edema in the evening; the waist is the "house of the kidneys", so deficiency of the kidneys is manifested as weakness and soreness in the waist and knees; deficiency of kidney essence leads to weariness and drowsiness; the slightly red tongue with white and thin or white and greasy coating, as well as the thin and deep pulse are manifestations of deficiency of kidney qi due to retention of water and dampness.

## 4. Binding of water and stasis

Symptoms: Repeated facial edema and swollen limbs, progressively dry and scaly skin, dark complexion, filiform congestion, petechia and ecchymosis, possibly accompanied by lumbago and red urine; pale or dark-red tongue, petechia on the margin of the tongue, sublingual bruise, thin and yellow or greasy tongue coating, as well as thin and unsmooth pulse.

Analysis of symptoms: Water-dampness and blood stasis bind together and permeate throughout the exterior, leading to facial edema and swollen limbs; blood stasis impedes blood circulation, resulting in dry and scaly skin, dark complexion, filiform congestion, petechia and ecchymosis; retention of blood stasis causes deviation of blood flow and obstruction of channels, marked by lumbago and red urine; pale or dark-red tongue, petechia on the margin of the tongue, sublingual bruise, thin and yellow or greasy tongue coating, as well as thin and unsmooth pulse are all due to binding of water and stasis.

## 5. Yang deficiency of the spleen and kidneys

Symptoms: General edema observed when pressing a submerged finger and ascites in severe cases, shortness of breath, chest distress, loose stools, oliguresis, cold body and limbs and white complexion; obesity, pale tongue, with thin or greasy coating, as well as thin and deep pulse.

Analysis of symptoms: Retained water and dampness and malfunctioning of the entries and exits to the spleen and kidneys lead to retention of water and fluid in the body and overflow to the skin, this is marked by general edema and ascites in severe cases; turbid dampness flows upward, predisposing the patient to shortness of breath and chest distress; a deficient spleen fails to transform the food, resulting in loose stools; yang fails to transform qi, leading to oliguresis; deficient yang qi fails to warm the body, causing a white complexion and cold body and limbs; obesity, the pale tongue with thin or greasy coating, as well as thin and deep pulse are caused by deficiency of spleen yang and kidney yang with internal abundance of water and dampness.

## 6. Yin exhaustion of the liver and kidneys

Symptoms: Repeated occurrences of mild edema, dizziness, restlessness with fever, thirst, sore and swollen throat, irascibility, night sweats, soreness in the waist and red urine; red tongue and thin, rapid and taut pulse.

Analysis of symptoms: Yin deficiency of the liver and kidneys leads to retention of water and dampness, so there are repeated occurrences of mild edema; internal heat due to deficiency of yin is manifested as thirst and a sore and swollen throat; hyperactivity of yang due to deficiency of yin is marked by dizziness; deficient heat disturbs the heart spirit upwardly, leading to irascibility; deficiency of the kidneys is responsible for waist soreness; deficiency of yin produces internal heat, with such signs as night sweat and feverish dysphoria; damp-heat pours downward, resulting in red urine; the red tongue and the thin, rapid and taut pulse are both symptomatic of yin deficiency of the liver and kidneys.

## 7. Exhaustion of yin and yang

Symptoms: Deficient palpebral edema, lassitude, sallow complexion, faint voice, thoracic and abdominal distension and fullness, nausea and vomiting, poor appetite, urinous odor in the mouth, oliguresis or profuse nocturnal urination, or even coma, itching, spasms and melena; pale tongue with greasy and rotten coating, as well as thin, weak and slippery pulse.

Analysis of symptoms: Retained turbid dampness transforms into toxins, which damage the qi and blood and exhaust yin and yang, this is marked by deficient palpebral edema, lassitude, a sallow complexion and faint voice; turbid toxins fail to descend, resulting in unsmooth functional activity of qi, resulting in thoracic and abdominal distension and fullness; turbid dampness flows upward, leading to nausea, vomiting, poor appetite and a urinous odor in the mouth; exhaustion of yin and yang predisposes the patient to oliguresis or profuse nocturnal urination; deficiency of the spirit causes coma; unsmooth flow of blood leads to malnutrition of the tendons, skin and muscles, marked by itching and spasms; the spleen fails to control the blood, leading to extravasation and the presence of melena; the pale tongue with greasy and rotten coating, as well as the thin, weak and slippery pulse are due to exhaustion of yin and yang with internal abundance of turbid toxins.

## Differential Treatment

### 1. Overflow of wind and water

Treatment principle: Soothing wind and dispersing the lung tissue, promoting qi flow and relieving edema.

Prescription and herbs: Modified Yuebi Jiazhu Decoction

Mahuang (Ephedra) 6 g, Shigao (Raw Gypsum) 30 g, Baizhu (Largehead Atractylodes Rhizome) 12 g, Gancao (Liquorice Root) 6 g, Shengjiangpi (Fresh Ginger) 9 g, Fuping (Duckweek) 9 g, Zexie (Oriental Waterplantain Rhizome) 12 g, Fulingpi (Indian Bread Peel) 12 g and Cheqianzi (Plantain Seed) 12 g (wrapped during decoction).

Modification: For relative predominance of wind-cold, Jingjie (Fineleaf Schizonepeta Herb) 9 g, Fangfeng (Divaricate Saposhnikovia Root) 9 g, Suye (Beef-steak Plant Leaf) 9 g and Sangbaipi (White Mulberry Root-Bark) 12 g are added to disperse wind, dissipate cold and drain water; for relative predominance of wind-heat, Baimaogen (Lalang Grass Rhizome) 30 g, Lugen (Reed Rhizome) 30 g, Huangqin (Baical Skullcap Root) 9 g and Lianqiao (Weeping Forsythia Capsule) 9 g can be added to disperse wind, dispel heat and remove water.

### 2. Transformation of pathogenic dampness into heat

Treatment principle: Draining damp-heat, promoting urination and relieving edema.

Prescription and herbs: Modified Shuzao Yinzi.

Qianghuo (Incised Notoptetygium Rhizome or Root) 9 g, Shengdahuang (Unprepared Rhubarb) 9 g, Shanglu (Pokeberry Root) 12 g, Zexie (Oriental

Waterplantain Rhizome) 15 g, Chixiaodou (Rice Bean) 30 g, Chuanjiaomu (Semen Zanthoxli) 3 g, Binglang (Areca Seed) 9 g, Dafupi (Areca Peel) 12 g, Fulingpi (Indian Bread Peel) 12 g and Gancao (Liquorice Root) 6 g.

Modification: For urgent constipation, the dosage of Dahuang (Rhubarb) should be increased to 15 g to reinforce the action of purgation. Furthermore, Hanfangji (Fourstamen Stephania Root) 12 g and Tinglizi (Herba Leonuri) 15 g can be added to promote water discharge.

## 3. Deficiency of primordial kidney qi

Treatment principle: Supplementing primordial qi to nourish the kidneys, promoting urination to relieve edema.

Prescription and herbs: Modified Jisheng Shenqi Pill and Zhuling Powder.

Shudi (Prepared Rhizome of Rehmannia) 9 g, Shanyao (Common Yan Rhizome) 15 g, Shanzhuyu (Asiatic Cornelian Cherry Fruit) 9 g, Zexie (Oriental Waterplantain Rhizome) 15 g, Fuling (Indian Bread) 12 g, Zhuling (Polyporus) 12 g, Yiyiren (Coix Seed) 15 g, Dangshen (Radix Codonopsis) 12 g, Baizhu (Largehead Atractylodes Rhizome) 12 g, Yinyanghuo (Epimedium Herb) 12 g and Gancao (Liquorice Root) 6 g.

Modification: For extreme weariness, Shenghuangqi (Unprepared Milkvetch Root) 30 g and Xianhecao (Hairyvein Agrimonia Herb) 30 g are added to nourish primordial qi; for severe waist soreness, Duzhong (Eucommia Bark) 9 g, Niuxi (Twotoothed Achyranthes Root) 9 g and Sangjisheng (Chinese Taxillus Herb) 9 g are added to nourish the kidneys and strengthen the waist.

## 4. Binding of water and stasis

Treatment principle: Activating blood and resolving stasis, alleviating edema and removing stagnation.

Prescription and herbs: Modified Taohong Siwu Deoction and Zhuling Powder.

Danggui (Chinese Angelica) 9 g, Shengdi (Dried Rehmannia Root) 9 g, Shudi (Prepared Rhizome of Rehmannia) 9 g, Chishao (Red Peony Root) 9 g, Taoren (Peach Seed) 9 g, Chuanxiong (Szechwan Lovage Rhizome)

9 g, Honghua (Safflower) 6 g, Yimucao (Motherwort Herb) 15 g, Zexie (Oriental Waterplantain Rhizome) 15 g, Zhuling (Polyporus) 12 g, Fuling (Indian Bread) 12 g and Gancao (Liquorice Root) 6 g.

Modification: If there is severe blood stasis, Shuizhi (Leech) 9 g can be added to expel the stasis.

## 5. Yang deficiency of the spleen and kidneys

Treatment principle: Nourishing the spleen and tonifying the kidneys, warming yang to relieve edema.

Prescription and herbs: Modified Zhenwu Decoction and Shipi Potion.

Fuzi (Prepared Common Monkshood Daughter) 9 g, Baizhu (Largehead Atractylodes Rhizome) 12 g, Ganjiang (Dried Ginger) 9 g, Dafupi (Areca Peel) 12 g, Zexie (Oriental Waterplantain Rhizome) 15 g, Fuling (Indian Bread) 12 g, Chenhulu (Aged Bottle-gourd) 9 g, Chongsun (Henon Bamboo Dried Shoot) 9 g, Baishao (White Peony Alba) 9 g, Houpu (Magnolia Bark) 9 g, Muxiang (Common Aucklandia Root) 6 g and Gancao (Liquorice Root) 6 g.

Modification: For ascites, Tinglizi (Herba Leonuri) 9 g and Cheqianzi (Plantain Seed) 15 g (wrapped during decoction) are added to relieve edema and expel retained fluid.

## 6. Yin exhaustion of the liver and kidneys

Treatment principle: Tonifying the liver and nourishing the kidneys, dispelling heat and discharging water.

Prescription and herbs: Modified Erzhi Pill, Dabuyin Pill and Zhuling Decoction.

Nuzhenzi (Glossy Privet Fruit) 9 g, Huanliancao (Ecliptae Herba) 9 g, Zhimu (Common Anemarrhena Rhizome) 9 g, Guiban (Tortoise Shell) 15 g, Shengdi (Dried Rehmannia Root) 15 g, Huangbai (Amur Cork-tree) 9 g, Zexie (Oriental Waterplantain Rhizome) 15 g, Fuling (Indian Bread) 15 g, Zhuling (Polyporus) 15 g, Yiyiren (Coix Seed) 15 g, Yimucao (Motherwort Herb) 30 g and Gancao (Liquorice Root) 6 g.

Modification: For relatively severe edema, Cheqianzi (Plantain Seed) 15 g, Chenhulu (Aged Bottle-gourd) 9 g, Chongsun (Henon Bamboo Dried Shoot) 9 g are added to promote urination and relieve edema; for bloody urine, Daji (Japanese Thistle Herb) 12 g and Xiaoji (Field Thistle Herb) 12 g are added to dispel heat, cool blood and stop bleeding.

## 7. Exhaustion of yin and yang

Treatment principle: nourishing yin and yang, tonifying the kidneys and discharging turbidity.

Prescription and herbs: Modified Zuogui Pill and Wenpi Decoction.

Shudi (Prepared Rhizome of Rehmannia) 9 g, Shanyao (Common Yan Rhizome) 15 g, Gouqizi (Barbary Wolfberry Fruit) 9 g, Shanzhuyu (Asiatic Cornelian Cherry Fruit) 9 g, Niuxi (Twotoothed Achyranthes Root) 9 g, Sangjisheng (Chinese Taxillus Herb) 12 g, Tusizi (Dodder Seed) 12 g, Lujiaojiao (Deerhorn Glue) 9 g, Guiban (Tortoise Shell) 9 g, Fuzi (Prepared Common Monkshood Daughter) 9 g, Dahuang (Rhubarb) 9 g, Liuyuexue (Junesnow) 30 g, Danshen (Radix Salviae Miltiorrhiae) 15 g and Gancao (Liquorice Root) 6 g.

Modification: In cases of nausea and vomiting, Zhuru (Bamboo Shavings) 9 g can be added to bring down the adverse flow of qi and arrest vomiting; for unconsciousness or muddled mind, Shichangpu (Acorus Calamus) 12 g is added to dissolve phlegm for resuscitation.

## Chinese Patent Medicine

1. Zuogui Pill: 4.5 g for each dose, twice a day.
2. Jisheng Shenqi Pill: 4.5 g for each dose, twice a day.

## Simple and Handy Prescriptions

1. Huangqi (Milkvetch Root) 45 g, Yiyiren (Coix Seed) 15 g, Dilong (Angle Worm) 15 g, Danshen (Radix Salviae Miltiorrhiae) 15 g, Yimucao (Motherwort Herb) 15 g and Jinyinhua (Honeysuckle Flower) 9 g are boiled in water and then administered.
2. Yumixu (Stigmata Maydis) 15 g, Xiguapi (Watermelon Peel) 15 g, Donggua (Chinese waxgourd) 250 g, Biandou (Hyacinth Bean) 50 g

and Cheqianzi (Plantain Herb) 25 g are boiled in water and administered twice a day.

## Other Therapies

Dietary therapy:

(1) Huangqi (Milkvetch Root) 30 g, Fuling (Indian Bread) 25 g, Sharen (Villous Amomum Fruit) 6 g and Shengjiang (Fresh Ginger) 9 g are boiled in water for 30 minutes and then 250 g of carp is added. Afterwards the ingredients are decocted without salt under mild fire for 40 minutes. Both the fish and soup can be consumed once a day or every other day.
(2) 250 ml milk and an egg can be consumed every morning.
(3) Chinese herbal enema: Dahuang (Rhubarb) 30 g, Diyu (Garden Burnet Root) 15 g, Muxiang (Common Aucklandia Root) 9 g and Liuyuexue (Junesnow) 30 g are boiled into 200 ml of medicated juice, which is consumed for retention-enema.

## Cautions and Advice

1. Patients should take good rest, prevent infection and keep to a salt-free diet during the period of edema.
2. Watermelon, Chinese waxgourd, coix seed and corn are suitable foods to relieve edema; crab, shrimp, cigarettes and alcohol are forbidden. When the edema begins to subside, the patient can switch to a low-salt diet and take small amounts of other previously prohibited food while at the same time consume moderate amounts of protein-rich or vitamin-rich foods such as chicken, duck, crucian and lean meat.
3. A clear understanding about the types of nephrotic syndrome is conducive to the treatment and prognosis of this disease.

## Daily Exercises

1. Concisely describe the diagnostic key points of nephrotic syndrome.
2. Explain how nephrotic syndrome can be treated based on syndrome differentiation.

# Pyelonephritis

# Week 8: Wednesday

Pyelonephritis refers to the inflammation of the renal parenchyma and pelvis, mostly owing to direct bacterial infection. It is usually accompanied by inflammation of the lower urinary tract and clinically it can be divided into the acute stage and chronic stage. The primary symptoms are lumbago, frequent and dripping discharge of urine, urgent urination, or painful urination. It can afflict people of all ages, especially women of child-bearing age. In TCM, pyelonephritis is considered to be closely associated with "pyretic stranguria", "bloody stranguria" and "over-strained stranguria".

## Etiology and Pathology

The onset of acute pyelonephritis, or an acute episode of chronic pyelonephritis, is triggered by excessive intake of spicy, fatty and sweet food or over-consumption of alcohol, breeding damp-heat which pours into the bladder downwardly. It may also be triggered by invasion of foul secretion of the external genitalia into the bladder, which brings about accumulation of damp-heat. Accumulation of damp-heat in the lower energizer will inevitably impede the functional activity of qi and obstruct the lower orifices, giving rise to frequent, dripping discharge of urine, urgent urination and painful urination. Chronic pyelonephritis is caused by prolonged retention of damp-heat which impairs the healthy qi and consumes body fluid, resulting in deficiency of renal qi and yin as well as deficiency of the spleen and kidneys, resulting in deficiency of healthy qi and excess of pathogenic factors with lingering of damp-heat.

## Diagnostic Key Points

1. During the onset of acute pyelonephritis, the patients often present with high fever, chills, lumbago, occasional abdominal colicky pain, frequent, urgent and painful urination, burning sensation in the urethral orifice during urination and unsmooth urination; sometimes there may be headache, nausea and vomiting.

2. More than half of the patients with chronic pyelonephritis have a history of acute pyelonephritis, with unremarkable symptoms such as weariness, low grade fever, waist soreness and lumbago; patients may also have such symptoms of the lower urinary tract as frequent, urgent and painful urination.
3. Uronoscopy may indicate the presence of bacteriuria.
4. Clean catch midstream urine culture finds colony-forming units >105/ml, which is of diagnostic significance.

## Syndrome Differentiation

During the acute phase (onset of acute pyelonephritis, or acute episode of chronic pyelonephritis):

### 1. Damp-heat pouring downward

Symptoms: Frequent, dripping discharge of urine, urgent, painful and unsmooth urination, a burning sensation in the urethral orifice during urination and possibly scanty urine, impalpable lumbago, yellow and greasy tongue coating, soggy and rapid or slippery and rapid pulse.

Analysis of symptoms: Pathogenic dampness and toxic heat pour into the bladder downwardly, impeding the functional activity of qi and obstructing the lower orifices, this brings about frequent and dripping discharge of urine, urgent, painful and unsmooth urination, a burning sensation in the urethral orifice during urination and possibly scanty urine; damp-heat pours downward and impairs the kidneys, leading to impalpable lumbago; the yellow and greasy coating as well as the soggy and rapid or slippery and rapid pulse are manifestations of damp-heat retaining in the interior.

### 2. Heat stagnating in the shaoyang region

Symptoms: Scorching, dripping and turbid urine, urgent and painful urination, distending pain in the lower abdomen, alternated chills and fever, hypochondriac distending pain, vexation, a bitter taste in the mouth, poor appetite with unwillingness to speak; thin and yellow tongue coating and rapid and taut pulse.

Analysis of symptoms: Damp-heat in the liver and gallbladder pours downward, resulting in scorching, dripping and turbid urine, urgent and painful urination and a distending pain in the lower abdomen; failure of the liver to promote free flow of qi causes it to stagnate into heat and attack the shaoyang region upwardly, so there are alternate attacks of the chills and fever, hypochondriac distending pain, vexation, a bitter taste in the mouth and poor appetite with unwillingness to speak; the thin and yellow tongue coating and the rapid and taut pulse are symptomatic of heat stagnating in the shaoyang region.

## 3. Damp-heat obstructing the interior

Symptoms: Chills and high fever aggravated in the afternoon, yellowish red urine, unsmooth and painful urination, a foul odor in the mouth, full and stuffy sensation in gastric and abdominal region, hunger with no desire for drinking, dry or loose stools, pain in the waist and abdomen; yellow and greasy tongue coating and slippery and rapid pulse.

Analysis of symptoms: Internal obstruction of damp-heat is manifested as chills and high fever; dampness, a yin pathogen, can cause fever aggravated in the afternoon; damp-heat pours into the bladder and obstructs the urinary tract, resulting in unsmooth and painful urination with yellowish red urine; damp-heat obstructs the middle energizer and inhibits qi movements, bringing about a foul odor in the mouth, a full and stuffy sensation in the gastric and abdominal region, hunger with no desire for drinking and pain in the abdomen; heat accumulates in the intestine, resulting in constipation; damp-heat invades the intestinal tract, leading to loose stools; damp-heat impairs the kidneys, presenting as lumbago; the yellow and greasy tongue coating and the slippery and rapid pulse are due to internal obstruction of damp-heat in the stomach and intestine.

During the chronic phase (chronic pyelonephritis):

## 1. Deficiency of the spleen and kidneys

Symptoms: Frequent urination with incessant dripping, aggravated upon physical exertion, accompanied by nausea and vomiting, poor appetite, abdominal distension, loose stools, intolerance of cold, cold limbs, facial edema and swollen limbs, weakness and soreness of the waist and knees; pale tongue with white coating or teeth marks, deep and feeble pulse.

Analysis of symptoms: Long-term affliction predisposes a patient to deficiency of yin and yang, as well as deficiency of the spleen and kidneys, resulting in impeded qi-transformation of the bladder, unconsolidated function of kidney qi and unsmooth discharge of urine, all of which is marked by frequent urination with incessant dripping that is aggravated upon physical exertion; deficiency of the spleen leads to retention of dampness and stagnation of qi, with such signs as nausea, vomiting, poor appetite, abdominal distension and loose stools; the simultaneously deficient spleen and kidneys fail to warm and transport water-dampness, which overflows to the skin and muscles, bringing about facial edema and swollen limbs; the deficient kidneys fail to warm yang and the body, causing an intolerance of cold and cold limbs; deficiency of the kidneys is responsible for weakness and soreness of the waist and knees; the pale tongue with white coating and the deep and feeble pulse are due to deficiency of the spleen and kidneys; teeth marks on the tongue are attributable to internal obstruction of turbid dampness.

## 2. Retention of damp-heat due to kidney deficiency

Symptoms: Frequent, urgent and unsmooth urination, aggravated upon physical exertion, accompanied by weariness, profuse sweating, dizziness, tinnitus, weakness and soreness of the waist and knees, feverish sensations in the palms and soles and dry mouth and lips; reddish tongue with scanty or little coating, thin and rapid pulse or thin and deep pulse.

Analysis of symptoms: Prolonged retention of pathogenic heat predisposes the patient to deficiency of renal qi and yin as well as inefficient qi-transformation of the bladder, bringing about a lingering of damp-heat and unsmooth discharge of urine, this results in frequent, urgent and unsmooth urination aggravated upon physical exertion; deficiency of the kidneys is responsible for weariness and secretion of profuse yin fluid, the sweat; deficiency of the kidneys also gives rise to insufficiency of the marrow sea and malnutrition of the brain, characterized by dizziness and tinnitus; inadequacy of kidney qi is manifested as weakness and soreness of the waist and knees; deficiency of yin produces internal heat, with feverish sensation in the palms and soles and a dry mouth and lips; the reddish tongue with scanty or little coating and the thin and rapid or thin and deep pulse are caused by deficiency of kidney qi and kidney yin.

## Differential Treatment

During the acute phase:

### 1. Damp-heat pouring downward

Treatment principle: Dispelling heat, eliminating dampness and relieving stranguria.

Prescription and herbs: Modified Bazheng Powder.

Bianxu (Polygonum Aviculare L.) 9 g Qumai (Lilac Pink Herb) 9 g, Cheqianzi (Plantain Seed) 30 g (wrapped during decoction), Chuanmutong (Armand Clematis Stem) 6 g, Huashi (Talc) 30 g, Zhizi (Cape Jasmine Fruit) 9 g, Dahuang (Rhubarb) 9 g, Dengxincao (Common Rush) 3 g and Gancaoshao (Liquorice Root Tip) 3 g.

Modification: If there is severe heat, Jinyinhua (Honeysuckle Flower) 9 g, Lianqiao (Weeping Forsythia Capsule) 9 g and Pugongying (Dandelion) 30 g can be added to reinforce the action of dispelling heat; if there is scanty urine, Zexie (Oriental Waterplantain Rhizome) 15 g, Zhuling (Polyporus) 12 g and Fuling (Indian Bread) 12 g are added to promote urination and eliminate dampness.

### 2. Heat stagnating in the shaoyang region

Treatment principle: Clearing the liver, promoting bile secretion and relieving stranguria.

Prescription and herbs: Modified Xiaochaihu Decoction and Longdan Xiegan Decoction.

Chaihu (Chinese Thorowax Root) 9 g, Longdancao (Radix Gentianae) 6 g, Huangqin (Baical Skullcap Root) 9 g, Zhizi (Cape Jasmine Fruit) 9 g,

Cheqianzi (Plantain Seed) 30 g (wrapped during decoction), Zexie (Oriental Waterplantain Rhizome) 12 g, Chuanmutong (Armand Clematis Stem) 3 g, Huashi (Talc) 30 g, Shengdi (Dried Rehmannia Root) 15 g, Danggui (Chinese Angelica) 9 g and Gancaoshao (Liquorice Root Tip) 3 g.

Modification: For severe hypochondriac pain, Yanhusuo (Corydalis) 9 g and Chuanlianzi (Szechwan Chinaberry Fruit) 9 g are added to soothe the liver and regulate qi.

## 3. Damp-heat obstructing the interior

Treatment principle: Dispelling heat, resolving dampness and relieving stranguria.

Prescription and herbs: Modified Sanren Decoction and Daochi Chengqi Decoction.

Xingren (Almond) 9 g, Zhuye (Henon Bamboo Leaf) 6 g, Baikouren (Fructus Amomi Rotundus) 6 g, Banxia (Pinellia Tuber) 9 g, Houpu (Magnolia Bark) 9 g, Yiyiren (Coix Seed) 15 g, Huashi (Talc) 30 g, Mutong (Caulis Hocquartiae) 3 g, Baitongcao (Medulla Tetrapanacis) 6 g, Cheqianzi (Plantain Seed) 15 g (wrapped during decoction), Shengdi (Dried Rehmannia Root) 15 g, Huangqin (Baical Skullcap Root) 9 g, Huanglian (Golden Thread) 3 g, Huangbai (Amur Cork-tree) 9 g and Gancaoshao (Liquorice Root Tip) 3 g.

Modification: For loose stools, Shanyao (Common Yan Rhizome) 15 g and Fuling (Indian Bread) 15 g are added to invigorate the spleen and stop diarrhea; for fullness and distension in the stomach and abdomen, Zhishi (Immature Orange Fruit) 12 g and Chenpi (Dried Tangerine Peel) 6 g can be added to regulate qi.

During the chronic phase (chronic pyelonephritis):

## 1. Deficiency of spleen and kidneys

Treatment principle: Invigorating the spleen and nourishing the kidneys, dispelling heat and eliminating dampness.

Prescription and herbs: Modified Shenling Baizhu Powder and Zhibai Dihuang Pill.

Dangshen (Radix Codonopsis) 12 g, Baizhu (Largehead Atractylodes Rhizome) 12 g, Baibiandou (White Hyacinth Bean) 15 g, Yiyiren (Coix Seed) 15 g, Huaishanyao (Huaihe Common Yan Rhizome) 15 g, Zhimu (Common Anemarrhena Rhizome) 9 g, Huangbai (Amur Cork-tree) 9 g, Shengdi (Dried Rehmannia Root) 9 g, Zexie (Oriental Waterplantain Rhizome) 15 g, Fuling (Indian Bread) 12 g, Huashi (Talc) 30 g, Sharen (Villous Amomum Fruit) 3 g and Chenpi (Dried Tangerine Peel) 6 g.

Modification: In cases of nausea, vomiting and poor appetite, Zisu (Purple Common Perilla) 9 g, Banxia (Pinellia Tuber) 9 g and Jineijin (Corium Stomachium Galli) 6 g are added to resolve turbidity, reduce adverseness and promote appetite; for intolerance of cold with cold limbs, Yinyanghuo (Epimedium Herb) 12 g and Xianmao (Common Curculigo Rhizome) 12 g can be added to warm the kidneys and dispel cold; if there is facial edema and swollen limbs, Cheqianzi (Plantain Seed) 15 g (wrapped during decoction) and Dafupi (Areca Peel) 12 g can be used to promote urination and relieve edema.

## 2. Retention of damp-heat due to kidney deficiency

Treatment principle: Nourishing yin, tonifying the kidneys and eliminating dampness.

Prescription and herbs: Supplementary Zuo Gui Pill.

Shengdi (Dried Rehmannia Root) 15 g, Guiban (Tortoise Shell) 9 g, Zhimu (Common Anemarrhena Rhizome) 9 g, Huangbai (Amur Cork-tree) 9 g, Shanzhuyu (Asiatic Cornelian Cherry Fruit) 9 g, Huangqi (Milkvetch Root) 30 g, Dangshen (Radix Codonopsis) 12 g, Shanyao (Common Yan Rhizome) 12 g, Gouqizi (Barbary Wolfberry Fruit) 9 g, Niuxi (Twotoothed Achyranthes Root) 9 g, Tusizi (Dodder Seed) 12 g, Lujiaojiao (Deerhorn Glue) 12 g, Zexie (Oriental Waterplantain Rhizome) 9 g, Fuling (Indian Bread) 12 g and Gancaoshao (Liquorice Root Tip) 6 g.

Modification: For severe problems with urination, Bianxu (Polygonum Aviculare L.) 9 g, Qumai (Lilac Pink Herb) 9 g and Cheqianzi (Plantain Seed) 15 g can be added to dispel damp-heat in the lower energizer.

## Chinese Patent Medicine

Zuo Gui Pill: 4.5 g for each dose, twice a day.

## Simple and Handy Prescriptions

1. Bianxu (Polygonum Aviculare L.) 15 g, Qumai (Lilac Pink Herb) 15 g, Chuanxinlian (Common Andrographis Herb) 15 g, Yazhicao (Common Dayflower Herb) 15 g are boiled in water and taken once a day.
2. Fresh celery 250 g and raw liquorice root 10 g are decocted in water and taken once a day.

## Other Therapies

Dietary therapy:

(1) Fresh lotus root 500 g, cane sugar 500 g and fresh water chestnut 500 g are crushed to make juice. The mixed juice is taken once a day.
(2) A green turtle about 250 g in weight is steamed with desired amounts of spring onion, ginger, yellow wine and salt.

Sodium Bicarbonate is administered (1 g for each dose) 3 times a day. It can alkalify the urine and alleviate the irritation symptoms of the bladder. It is advisable to conduct anti-infection treatment under bacterial culture of urine and drug sensitivity test.

## Cautions and Advice

1. Patients should take initiative in treatment during the acute phase to relieve symptoms and prevent recurrence. They are also encouraged to drink plenty of water (more than two liters per day) so as to promote urinary discharge. The source of inflammation should be identified and treated as early as possible. Gestational, post-partum or menstrual hygiene must be well managed and the smoothness of defecation also maintained.
2. In acute pyelonephritis or an acute episode of chronic pyelonephritis, patients should avoid oily, spicy or stomach-irritating foods, as well as tobacco and alcohol. They are advised to take foods which can dispel

heat and promote urination, such as Chinese waxgourd, green gram sprout, mustard and Indian kalimeris herb.; a light, water-rich diet is also recommended, comprising various vegetables and fruits. Patients with chronic pyelonephritis can aim for moderate nourishment by supplementing yin instead of excessive tonification by warming yang; soft-shelled turtle, tortoise, duck, white fungus gourd, lily bulb and horseshoe are appropriate foods.

3. Acute pyelonephritis, if treated promptly, can have a favorable prognosis. On the other hand, chronic pyelonephritis is refractory and the leading cause for chronic renal insufficiency; once renal insufficiency becomes chronic, the prognosis will become unfavorable.

## Daily Exercises

1. Describe the diagnostic key points of pyelonephritis.
2. Explain how chronic pyelonephritis can be treated based on syndrome differentiation.

# Renal Tuberculosis

# Week 8: Thursday

Renal tuberculosis is caused by tubercle bacillus, which spreads to the kidneys from the lungs or other tubercle foci though hematogenous dissemination, progressively destroying the renal parenchyma and causing cortical or hylic lesions of the kidneys. It may also affect the renal duct, bladder and tract, or even the reproductive system. Being a chronic disease, it is marked by simultaneous destruction and repair. The clinical symptoms are low grade fever, weariness, lumbago, frequent, urgent urination and painful urination of bloody urine. It mostly afflicts young and middle-aged people 20~40 years of age, with males being more susceptible. In TCM, renal tuberculosis is considered to be closely associated with "kidney consumption", "deficiency consumption", "fever due to internal damage", "bloody stranguria" and "lumbago".

## Etiology and Pathology

The location of this disease is in the kidneys and its occurrence is related to the lungs, spleen, liver and bladder in addition to the kidneys. The etiological factor is a consumptive worm (tubercle bacillus), which travels through the lungs or directly to the kidneys. It may lead to simultaneous disorder of the lungs and kidneys and deficiency of qi and yin; the prolonged retention of damp-heat in the bladder exhausts liver yin and kidney yin, producing exuberant fire and, in the late stage, bringing about deficiency of spleen yang and kidney yang with qi stagnation and blood stasis.

## Diagnostic Key Points

1. The clinical symptoms are marked by irregular low grade fever, night sweats, fatigue, listlessness, decreased appetite, vexation and insomnia; if the tubercle bacillus irritates the membrane of the bladder, there may be frequent, urgent and painful urination of bloody urine.; if pyuria irritates the urinary tract, there will be a localized burning pain and dull or colicky pain in the renal region.

2. When there is pyonephrosis or massive fibrous hyperplasia and calcification, lumps can be found in the loins.
3. Urinary test finds tubercle bacillus and bloody urine, which is of critical diagnostic value to this disease. In severe cases, the urine is turbid with broken bits resembling water that has been used to wash meat.
4. Tuberculin test is conducive to the diagnosis.

## Syndrome Differentiation

### 1. Deficiency of kidney yin and lung yin

Symptoms: Cough of short duration, scanty or bloody sputum in a bright-red color, painful urination of bloody urine, lumbago, dry mouth, dry throat, feverish sensation in the palms and soles and night sweats; red tongue with little coating and thin-rapid pulse.

Analysis of symptoms: A deficiency of lung yin leads to abnormal dispersion and descent, marked by cough of short duration and scanty sputum; internal heat due to deficiency of yin damages the lung collaterals, producing sputum with bright-red blood; heat invades the lower energizer and scorches the collaterals, so the urine is bloody and painful to excrete; insufficiency of kidney yin gives rise to internal heat which drives sweat out, this is marked by a dry mouth and throat, feverish sensation in the palms and soles and night sweats; the waist is the "house of the kidneys", so deficiency of the kidneys is manifested as lumbago; the red tongue with scanty coating and the thin and rapid pulse are symptomatic of internal heat due to deficiency of yin.

### 2. Damp-heat pouring downward

Symptoms: Oliguresis, frequent or urgent urination with scorching heat and pricking pain, bloody urine or pyuria, cramping sensation of the lower abdomen and distending pain in the waist; yellow and greasy tongue coating, rapid and soggy pulse or rapid and slippery pulse.

Analysis of symptoms: Damp-heat pours downward, leading to abnormal qi-transformation of the bladder, with such signs as oliguresis, frequent or urgent urination with scorching heat and pricking pain, bloody urine or pyuria, cramping sensation of the lower abdomen and distending pain in the waist; damp-heat damages the blood collaterals, leading to bloody urine; damp-heat and toxins are responsible for pyuria; the yellow and greasy tongue coating and the rapid and soggy pulse or rapid and slippery pulse are due to internal obstruction of damp-heat.

## 3. Deficiency of liver yin and kidney yin

Symptoms: Dizziness, dry eyes, blurred vision, hectic fever in the afternoon, red cheeks, feverish sensations over the five centers (the palms, the soles and the heart), night sweats, scanty reddish urine with blood, emaciation, sore and painful waist and knees, numb limbs, tinnitus, irregular menstruation in women and nocturnal emissions in men; red tongue with little or yellow coating and thin and rapid pulse.

Analysis of symptoms: Deficiency of liver yin results in dizziness, dry eyes and blurred vision; internal heat due to deficiency of yin is manifested as hectic fever, red cheeks, feverish sensation over the five centers and night sweats; heat scorches the lower energizer and damages the blood collaterals, resulting in scanty reddish urine with blood; deficiency of liver yin and kidney yin leads to emaciation, weakness of the waist and knees, numbness in limbs, tinnitus, irregular menstruation in women and nocturnal emissions in men; the red tongue with little or yellow coating and the thin and rapid pulse are caused by insufficiency of the liver and kidneys and exuberance of fire due to yin deficiency.

## 4. Deficiency of spleen yang and kidney yang

Symptoms: Scanty urine, uroschesis or aconuresis, waist soreness or distending pain, abdominal distension after food intake, nausea and vomiting, reduced food intake, loose stools, lassitude, heavy limbs without warmth, urinous odor in the mouth and sallow complexion; pale tongue with white coating and thin and feeble pulse.

Analysis of symptoms: Deficiency of spleen yang and kidney yang results in failure of qi to transform water and abnormal control of the bladder, marked by incontinence or scanty urine due to involuntary suppression; deficiency of kidney yang is responsible for waist soreness or distending pain; dysfunction of the spleen in transportation and transformation predisposes the patient to an accumulation of cold-dampness in the interior and unsmooth functional activity of qi, resulting in lassitude, heavy limbs without warmth, abdominal distension after food intake, nausea and vomiting, reduced food intake and loose stools; deficiency of the kidneys predisposes the patient to dysfunction in qi transformation and accumulation of turbid dampness, so there is a urinous odor in the mouth; the sallow complexion, pale tongue with white coating and thin and feeble pulse are all attributable to deficiency of spleen yang and kidney yang.

## 5. Qi stagnation and blood stasis

Symptoms: Soreness or pricking pain in the waist and back aggravated at night, frequent urination with scanty urine and painful urination with bloody urine; dark mouth, lips and tongue with or without ecchymosis and deep-tense or even unsmooth pulse.

Analysis of symptoms: The disease can spread to the blood phase or the collaterals, so there is soreness or a pricking pain in the waist and back brought about by blood stasis; since both blood and night pertain to yin, the pain is aggravated at night; blood stasis obstructs the kidneys and causes dysfunction of qi transformation, marked by frequent urination with scanty urine; qi stagnation and blood stasis are responsible for painful urination with bloody urine; the dark mouth, lips and tongue with or without ecchymosis and the deep-tense or even unsmooth pulse are manifestations of obstruction of blood stasis.

## Differential Treatment

## 1. Deficiency of kidney yin and lung yin

Treatment principle: Moistening the lungs and kidneys, nourishing yin and stopping bleeding.

Prescription and herbs: Modified Baihe Gujin Pill and Qinghao Biejia Decoction.

Baihe (Lily Bulb) 9 g, Maidong (Dwarf Lilyturf Tuber) 9 g, Xuanshen (Figwort Root) 9 g, Shengdi (Dried Rehmannia Root) 9 g, Baishao (White Peony Alba) 9 g, Jiegeng (Platycodon Root) 6 g, Beimu (Fritillariae Tuber) 9 g, Biejia (Turtle Shell) 9 g, Zhimu (Common Anemarrhena Rhizome) 9 g, Qinghao (Sweet Wormwood Herb) 9 g, Danpi (Cortex Moutan) 12 g, Daji (Japanese Thistle Herb) 12 g, Baimaogen (Lalang Grass Rhizome) 30 g, Baibu (Stemona Root) 9 g and Gancaoshao (Liquorice Root Tip) 6 g.

Modification: For severe coughing with blood and bloody urine, Baiji (Common Bletilla Tuber) 9 g and Xiaoji (Field Thistle Herb) 12 g are added to relieve bloody urine.

## 2. Damp-heat pouring downward

Treatment principle: Clearing and unblocking the bladder, resolving dampness and eliminating toxins.

Prescription and herbs: Supplementary Bazheng Powder and Daochi Powder.

Bianxu (Polygonum Aviculare L.) 9 g, Qumai (Lilac Pink Herb) 9 g, Cheqianzi (Plantain Seed) 15 g (wrapped during decoction), Huashi (Talc) 30 g, Chuanmutong (Armand Clematis Stem) 6 g, Zhuye (Henon Bamboo Leaf) 6 g, Huangbai (Amur Cork-tree) 9 g, Zhimu (Common Anemarrhena Rhizome) 9 g, Shengdi (Dried Rehmannia Root) 15 g, Baibu (Stemona Root) 9 g and Gancaoshao (Liquorice Root Tip) 6 g.

Modification: For bloody urine, Daji (Japanese Thistle Herb) 12 g, Xiaoji (Field Thistle Herb) 12 g and Qiancaotan (Charred Indian Madder Root) 12 g are added to treat bloody urine.

## 3. Deficiency of liver yin and kidney yin

Treatment principle: Supplementing the liver and tonifying the kidneys, nourishing yin and bringing down fire.

Prescription and herbs: Modified Yiguan Decoction and Dabuyin Pill.

Shengdi (Dried Rehmannia Root) 12 g, Shashen (Root of Straight Ladybell) 9 g, Maidong (Dwarf Lilyturf Tuber) 9 g, Gouqizi (Barbary Wolfberry Fruit) 9 g, Guiban (Tortoise Shell) 15 g, Biejia (Turtle Shell)

15 g, Danggui (Chinese Angelica) 9 g, Chuanlianzi (Szechwan Chinaberry Fruit) 9 g, Zhimu (Common Anemarrhena Rhizome) 9 g, Huangbai (Amur Cork-tree) 9 g and Baibu (Stemona Root) 9 g.

Modification: If the patient presents with blurred vision, Juhua (Chrysanthemum Flower) 9 g and Qingxiangzi (Feather Cockscomb Seed) 9 g are added to clear the liver and improve acuity of vision; for tinnitus, Shichangpu (Acorus Calamus) 12 g and Lingcishi (Magnetitum) 30 g are added to nourish the kidneys and open ear orifices.

### 4. Deficiency of spleen yang and kidney yang

Treatment principle: Invigorating the spleen and nourishing qi, warming the kidneys and discharging turbidity.

Prescription and herbs: Modified Buzhong Yiqi Decoction and Jisheng Shenqi Pill.

Rougui (Cassia Bark) 9 g, Fuzi (Prepared Common Monkshood Daughter) 6 g, Huangqi (Milkvetch Root) 30 g, Dangshen (Radix Codonopsis) 12 g, Baizhu (Largehead Atractylodes Rhizome) 12 g, Shanyao (Common Yan Rhizome) 15 g, Shudi (Prepared Rhizome of Rehmannia) 15 g, Niuxi (Twotoothed Achyranthes Root) 9 g, Danggui (Chinese Angelica) 9 g, Cheqianzi (Plantain Seed) 15 g (wrapped during decoction), Zexie (Oriental Waterplantain Rhizome) 15 g, Fuling (Indian Bread) 12 g, Baibu (Stemona Root) 15 g and Chenpi (Dried Tangerine Peel) 6 g.

Modification: If the patient presents with loose stools, Yiyiren (Coix Seed) 15 g and Biandou (White Hyacinth Bean) 9 g are added to invigorate the spleen and stop diarrhea.

### 5. Qi stagnation and blood stasis

Treatment principle: Activating blood and resolving stasis, promoting qi flow and unblocking vessels.

Prescription and herbs: Modified Chenxiang Powder and Didang Pill.

Chenxiang (Chinese eaglewood Wood) 3 g, Chenpi (Dried Tangerine Peel) 6 g, Wuyao (Combined Spicebush Root) 9 g, Zhishi (Immature Orange Fruit) 12 g, Taoren (Peach Seed) 9 g, Honghua (Safflower) 3 g, Chishao

(Red Peony Root) 9 g, Danggui (Chinese Angelica) 9 g, Chuanshanjia (Pangolin Scale) 12 g, Wangbuliuxing (Cowherb Seed) 9 g, Shiwei (Shearer's Pyrrosia Leaf) 9 g, Dongkuizi (Malva Verticillata L) 12 g and Huashi (Talc) 30 g.

Modification: For bloody urine, Sanqifen (Sanchi Powder) 3 g is consumed daily to treat bloody urine.

## Chinese Patent Medicine

1. Qinbudan Tablet: 5 tablets for each dose, twice a day.
2. Liuwei Dihuang Pill: 4.5 g for each dose, twice a day.

## Simple and Handy Prescriptions

1. Baibu (Stemona Root) 12 g, Danpi (Cortex Moutan) 9 g, Shengdi (Dried Rehmannia Root) 18 g, Shudi (Prepared Rhizome of Rehmannia) 18 g, Gouqizi (Barbary Wolfberry Fruit) 15 g, Zhibiejia (Baked Turtle Shell) 30 g and Nuodaogen (Glutinous Rice Root) 30 g are decocted together. The decoction is consumed once a day.
2. Fresh lotus root 500 g is pounded to make juice and Shanyao (Common Yan Rhizome) 500 g is steamed, peeled and pounded into a paste and added to the lotus root for consumption.

## Other Therapies

Dietary therapy:

(1) Dongchongxiacao (Chinese Caterpillar Fungus) 10 g and flavoring are put into a plucked duck and steamed for 2 hours. Both the duck and soup can be eaten.
(2) 300 g of fresh Jicai (Shepherd's Purse) is cut into pieces and then boiled in water with 300 g of Tofu (Beancurd). The soup is thickened by adding starch. For unilateral renal tuberculosis in the advanced stage, surgical treatment is advisable.

## Cautions and Advice

1. Patients with suspected pulmonary tuberculosis or other tuberculoses should take a urinary test so as to diagnose and treat renal tuberculosis as early as possible. They should take adequate rest and regulate their thoughts.
2. Patients with renal tuberculosis are encouraged to consume foods rich in calories, protein, lactose and vitamins A, B, C and D; they also ought to eat more vegetables, fruits and various light and water-containing foods to maintain the smoothness of urination and defecation, as well as reinforce the action of diuresis. For weakness due to prolonged affliction, it is advisable for the patients to take tonics. Warm, hot, aromatic and spicy drinks and foods, as well as cigarettes and alcohols are strictly prohibited.
3. Renal tuberculosis, if diagnosed promptly and treated properly, has a favorable prognosis. However, if it is discovered too late and the kidneys are severely injured or there is presence of ureter stricture, the prognosis is relatively unfavorable and, in this case, a surgery may be needed.

## Daily Exercises

1. Explan how renal tuberculosis can be diagnosed.
2. Concisely describe the etiology and pathology of renal tuberculosis.
3. Explain how renal tuberculosis can be treated based on syndrome differentiation.

# Urinary Calculosis
# Week 8: Friday

Urinary calculosis refers to the abnormal accumulation of crystallized substances or organic matrixes in the urinary tract, including renal calculus, ureter calculus, bladder calculus and urethra calculus. The main symptoms are paroxysmal colicky pain in the waist and lower abdomen, bloody urine, discharge of calculus in different sizes, frequent, urgent, interrupted and difficult urination. This disease is commonly seen in people 20~40 years of age, with the ratio of male to female being 4.5:1. In TCM this disease is considered to be closely associated with "stony stranguria", "bloody stranguria" and "over-strained stranguria".

## Etiology and Pathology

Urinary calculosis is located in the kidneys and bladder yet closely linked to other organs such as the liver and spleen. It is mainly caused by accumulation of damp-heat in the lower energizer, which condenses the urine and turns the impurities in the urine into stones or calculi; or by stagnation of qi and fire in the lower energizer and deficiency of the kidneys, which lead to impeded qi-transformation of the bladder and dysfunction of urinary functions, predisposing the patient to calculus in the end; if the disease is persistent, the heat will consume yin-fluid and the dampness may encumber yang qi, resulting in deficiency of the spleen and kidneys, qi stagnation and blood stasis which is, in essence, a disorder marked by deficiency of healthy qi and excess of pathogenic factors.

## Diagnostic Key Points

1. Pain is the main symptom of urinary calculosis. For renal calculus, the pain is dull and colicky in the renal region or epigastric zone; for ureter calculus, the pain is typically colicky and intolerable, with a sudden onset or sometimes nausea and vomiting; for bladder calculus, the pain is in the pubic or perineal region and occurs at the end of urination.
2. There may be such symptoms as bloody urine, calculus in different sizes, frequent, urgent, interrupted and difficult urination.

3. Urine microscopy indicates the presence of red blood cells.
4. Urinary tract X-ray scan is of significant diagnostic value to this disease.
5. Venous urography and retrograde pyelography can, under most circumstances, display the location, size, shape and number of the calculi, as well as the general conditions of the entire urinary tract.
6. B-ultrasonic test can be a complementary tool to X-ray scan to identify the negative calculus.

## Syndrome Differentiation

### 1. Accumulation of dampness and heat in the lower energizer

Symptoms: Occasional waist soreness, or unbearable colicky pain in the waist and abdomen, unsmooth urination, or sudden disruption of urination, pricking pain or a scorching sensation, calculus in the urine at times, yellowish red urine, or bloody urine, foul breath and a bitter taste in the mouth as well as constipation; red tongue with yellow and greasy coating and slippery and rapid pulse.

Analysis of symptoms: Accumulation of damp-heat in the lower energizer condenses the urine and turns the impurities into stones or calculi, which remain in the interior and impede the kidney qi, manifesting in occasional waist soreness, or unbearable colicky pain in the waist and abdomen; damp-heat pours downward, leading to abnormal qi-transformation of the bladder, this is marked by unsmooth urination; the calculus obstructs the urinary tract, so there is sudden disruption of urination and pricking pain or a scorching sensation; the calculus damages the collaterals, resulting in bloody urine; internal abundance of dampness and heat is responsible for foul breath and the bitter taste in the mouth as well as the yellowish red urine; damp-heat accumulates in the large intestine, bringing about constipation; the yellow and greasy tongue coating and the slippery and rapid pulse are both manifestations of damp-heat.

### 2. Liver qi stagnation transforming into fire

Symptoms: Hypochondriac distension, lumbago which involves the lower abdomen and medial surface of the thigh in severe cases, unsmooth, dripping, or interrupted urination and enlarged lower abdomen with an unbearable sensation; thin and yellow tongue coating and a rapid and taut pulse.

Analysis of symptoms: Persistent depression of liver qi produces fire which, in combination with qi, accumulates in the lower energizer, leading to impeded qi-transformation of the bladder, this is marked by hypochondriac distension and lumbago involving the lower abdomen and medial surface of the thigh; calculus obstructs the urinary tract, so urination is unsmooth, dripping, difficult or interrupted; dysfunction of qi-transformation by the bladder results in retention of urine, causing an enlarged lower abdomen with unbearable sensation; the thin and yellow tongue coating and the rapid and taut pulse are due to stagnation of liver qi transforming into fire.

## 3. Qi deficiency of the spleen and kidneys

Symptoms: After prolonged affliction, there is lassitude, vague pain in the waist and abdomen, preference for kneading and pressing, aggravation upon physical exertion, unsmooth urination coupled with weakness in passing urine, a sinking and distending sensation in the lower abdomen, calculus in urine at times, poor appetite, loose stools and a pale complexion; pale tongue with thin coating and teeth marks, as well as a thin and weak pulse.

Analysis of symptoms: Prolonged existence of calculus consumes the primordial qi and debilitates the spleen and kidneys, resulting in lassitude; insufficiency of kidney qi leads to dysfunction of qi transformation, causing vague pain in the waist and abdomen, preference for palpation, aggravation upon physical exertion and inconspicuous unsmooth urination; deficiency of the spleen results in collapse of qi, leading to a sinking and distending sensation in the lower abdomen and weakness in urinary discharge; the calculi are not fully discharged, so there are stones in the urine; dysfunction of the spleen in transportation and transformation leads to poor appetite and loose stools; the pale complexion, pale tongue with thin coating and teeth marks, as well as thin thin and weak pulse are all attributable to deficiency of the spleen and kidneys, as well as insufficiency of qi and blood.

## 4. Deficiency of kidney qi and yin

Symptoms: Prolonged existence of calculus, persistent lumbago, slightly unsmooth urination with continuous dripping of urine, bloody urine in a bright-red color, hectic fever, night sweats, feverish sensations over the five centers (the palms, the soles and the heart), dry mouth and throat, dizziness and tinnitus; reddish tongue with scanty coating and thin and rapid pulse.

Analysis of symptoms: Prolonged affliction of stony stranguria or overuse of bitter-cold herbs to dispel heat may damage the healthy qi; persistent stagnation of qi and accumulation of damp-heat can generate fire and consume yin, leading to deficiency of the kidneys with insufficient qi and yin, marked by constant lumbago, slightly unsmooth urination and continuous dripping of urine; insufficiency of kidneys yin produces deficient fire in the interior, causing hectic fever, night sweats and feverish sensations over the five centers; deficient heat consumes body fluid, resulting in a dry mouth and throat; deficient fire scorches the yin collaterals and drives the blood out of the vessels, bringing about bloody urine in a bright-red color; deficient kidney qi fails to supplement the marrow sea, giving rise to dizziness and tinnitus; the reddish tongue with scanty coating and the thin and rapid pulse are caused by insufficiency of qi and yin.

## Differential Treatment

## 1. Accumulation of dampness and heat in the lower energizer

Treatment principle: Dispelling heat and eliminating dampness, relieving stranguria and discharging stones.

Prescription and herbs: Modified Shiwei Powder, Bazheng Powder and Sanjin Decoction.

Shiwei (Shearer's Pyrrosia Leaf) 15 g, Dongkuizi (Malva Verticillata L) 15 g, Bianxu (Polygonum Aviculare L.) 12 g, Qumai (Lilac Pink Herb) 12 g, Jinqiancao (Christina Loosestrife) 30 g, Haijinshao (Lygodium) 12 g, Jineijin (Corium Stomachium Galli) 9 g, Zhizi (Cape Jasmine Fruit) 9 g,

Cheqianzi (Plantain Seed) 30 g (wrapped during decoction), Huashi (Talc) 15 g, Chuanmutong (Armand Clematis Stem) 6 g and Gancaoshao (Liquorice Root Tip) 9 g.

Modification: For colicky pain in the waist and abdomen, Baishao (White Peony Alba) 30 g can be added to relieve acuteness and stop pain; if there is bloody urine, Daji (Japanese Thistle Herb) 12 g, Xiaoji (Field Thistle Herb) 12 g and Shengdi (Dried Rehmannia Root) 12 g are added to treat bloody urine.

## 2. Liver qi stagnation transforming into fire

Treatment principle: Clearing the liver and promoting the flow of qi, relieving stranguria and discharging stones.

Prescription and herbs: Modified Chenxiang Powder and Shiwei Powder.

Shiwei (Shearer's Pyrrosia Leaf) 15 g, Dongkuizi (Malva Verticillata L) 15 g, Huashi (Talc) 15 g, Jinqiancao (Christina Loosestrife) 30 g, Haijinshao (Lygodium) 12 g, Chenxiang (Chinese eaglewood Wood) 3 g, Chenpi (Dried Tangerine Peel) 9 g, Wangbuliuxing (Cowherb Seed) 9 g, Danggui (Chinese Angelica) 9 g, Baishao (White Peony Alba) 9 g, Longdancao (Radix Gentianae) 6 g and Gancaoshao (Liquorice Root Tip) 9 g.

Modification: If there is hypochondriac distending pain, Chaihu (Chinese Thorowax Root) 9 g, Yanhusuo (Corydalis) 9 g and Chuanlianzi (Szechwan Chinaberry Fruit) 9 g are added to soothe the liver and regulate qi; for difficult, unsmooth and interrupted urination, Cheqianzi (Plantain Seed) 15 g (wrapped during decoction) and Zexie (Oriental Waterplantain Rhizome) 15 g are added to discharge water and drain dampness.

## 3. Qi deficiency of the spleen and kidneys

Treatment principle: Tonifying the kidneys and invigorating the spleen, nourishing deficiency and discharging stones.

Prescription and herbs: Modified Dabuyuan Decoction and Sanjin Decoction.

Huangqi (Milkvetch Root) 12 g, Dangshen (Radix Codonopsis) 12 g, Shanyao (Common Yan Rhizome) 12 g, Fuling (Indian Bread) 12 g, Zexie (Oriental Waterplantain Rhizome) 12 g, Shudi (Prepared Rhizome of Rehmannia) 15 g, Shanzhuyu (Asiatic Cornelian Cherry Fruit) 6 g, Duzhong (Eucommia Bark) 9 g, Bajitian (Mornda Root) 9 g, Chuanniuxi (Twotoothed Achyranthes Root) 12 g, Tusizi (Dodder Seed) 12 g, Jinqiancao (Christina Loosestrife) 30 g, Haijinshao (Lygodium) 12 g, Huashi (Talc) 12 g and Gancaoshao (Liquorice Root Tip) 9 g.

Modification: For weakness in urinary discharge as well as a sinking and distending sensation in the lower abdomen, Shengma (Rhizoma Cimicifugae) 6 g and Gegen (Kudzuvine Root) 9 g are added to lift yang qi.

### 4. Deficiency of kidney qi and yin

Treatment principle: Supplementing qi and nourishing yin, relieving stranguria and dissolving stones.

Prescription and herbs: Modified Zhibai Dihuang Pill and Shiwei Powder.

Shengdi (Dried Rehmannia Root) 9 g, Shudi (Prepared Rhizome of Rehmannia) 9 g, Zhimu (Common Anemarrhena Rhizome) 12 g, Shanyao (Common Yan Rhizome) 15 g, Shanzhuyu (Asiatic Cornelian Cherry Fruit) 9 g, Danpi (Cortex Moutan) 9 g, Zexie (Oriental Waterplantain Rhizome) 15 g, Fuling (Indian Bread) 15 g, Zhuling (Polyporus) 15 g, Huangbai (Amur Cork-tree) 9 g, Huangqi (Milkvetch Root) 30 g, Shiwei (Shearer's Pyrrosia Leaf) 15 g, Dongkuizi (Malva Verticillata L) 15 g, Huashi (Talc) 15 g and Gancaoshao (Liquorice Root Tip) 9 g.

Modification: If there is bloody urine in a bright-red color, Daji (Japanese Thistle Herb) 15 g, Xiaoji (Field Thistle Herb) 15 g, Ejiao (Donkey-hide Glue) 9 g and Baimaogen (Lalang Grass Rhizome) 30 g can be added to nourish yin, dispel heat and stop bleeding.

### Chinese Patent Medicine

1. Jinqiancao Granule: 1 bag for each dose, 3 times a day.
2. Zhibai Dihuang Pill: 4.5 g for each dose, twice a day.

## Simple and Handy Prescriptions

1. A Jineijin (Corium Stomachium Galli) is soaked in water to make tea and taken in the morning.
2. 20 otolithum sciaenaes in the head of a yellow croaker are taken out, baked and ground into fine powder, which is administered (1~2 g for each dose) twice a day with warm boiled water.

## Other Therapies

Dietary therapy:

(1) Fresh bottle-gourd is pounded for extraction of juice, 1 spoonful is taken twice a day.
(2) Stigmata maydis 30 g, corn root 30 g and corncob 30 g are boiled into thick soup, which can be consumed several times a day.

Extracorporeal shock-wave lithotomy and surgical treatment are also applicable.

## Cautions and Advice

1. Urinary calculosis should be treated proactively to prevent complications. Patients should drink plenty of water, with a daily volume of 1500~3000 ml; the effect will be more significant when 200 ml of water is taken at midnight.
2. Patients with oxal calculus should eat less spinach, tomato, potato, bamboo shoot, cocoa, celery, carrot, apple and pear, so as to promote the discharge of oxalate. Patients with uric acid calculus are advised to have a low-protein diet and eat less meat, fish, chicken, animal viscera, peanuts and chestnut, all of which are rich in purine; fresh fruits, vegetables and milk are highly recommended. Patients with phosphate calculus should consume more sour foods, such as smoked plum, lemon, or vinegar-prepared food. Those with calcium calculus are advised to eat less calcium-rich food, such as milk, beancurd and sesame paste; instead, garden peas and pumpkin are recommended.
3. Urinary calculosis, when treated promptly, results in discharge of the calculus and a favorable prognosis. Patients should beware the

unfavorable conditions: the calculus obstructing the urinary tract and causing retention of the urine as well as accumulation of water in the renal pelvis, calices and ureter, leading to renal atrophy and impaired or even loss of renal function in the end; urinary tract calculus can directly damage the membrane of the tract, bringing about congestive edema, or even ulcerative bleeding; obstruction of urinary tract predisposes the patient to infection and may result in such severe complications as hydronephrosis and perinephritis.

## Daily Exercises

1. Concisely describe the diagnostic key points of urinary calculosis.
2. Explain how urinary calculosis can be treated based on syndrome differentiation.

# Chronic Renal Failure
# Week 8: Saturday

Chronic renal failure refers to the severe damage of the kidneys due to a variety of chronic diseases. It develops slowly until it reaches the final stage of uremia. The symptoms are marked by change from polyuria to scanty urine and to anuria in the end; or by such manifestations as anaemia, bleeding, hemorrhinia, nausea, vomiting, poor appetite, a urinous odor in the mouth, weariness, lethargy, apathy, restlessness, convulsion, coma, hypertension, left ventricular hypertrophy, pericarditis, dermal dryness and peeling with an unbearable itching sensation, deep and long breaths and vulnerability to secondary infection. According to the degree of renal damage, renal failure can be divided into four stages: (1) renal functional compensation, (2) azotemia, (3) early stage renal failure and (4) terminal stage renal failure. In TCM, chronic renal failure is closely associated with "frequent vomiting and dysuria", "retention of urine", "deficiency consumption", "edema" and "lumbago".

## Etiology and Pathology

The location of this disease is the kidneys, but the liver, spleen and stomach are also affected by this disease. Chronic diseases often cause damage of the spleen and kidneys and abnormal qi-transformation, resulting in retention of turbid water and accumulation of turbid toxins in the three energizers, finally leading to the clouding of heart orifices, internal stirring of liver wind and various life-threatening complications.

## Diagnostic Key Points

1. At the stage of renal functional compensation and the stage of azotemia, the volume of urine is increased, with marked polyuria and nocturnal urination; at the stage of uremia, there is oliguria or even anuria and edema.
2. Symptoms of the various systems. Hematopoietic system: anaemia, bleeding and hemorrhinia; digestive system: nausea, vomiting, poor

appetite and a urinous odor in the mouth; cardiovascular system: hypertension, left ventricular hypertrophy, myocarditis, pericarditis and coronary artery disease; nervous system: weariness, dizziness, headache, apathy, lethargy, restlessness, convulsions and coma; respiratory system: deep and long breaths; locomotor system: bone ache, spontaneous bone fracture and arthritis.

3. Renal function test: Decrease in endogenous creatinine clearance rate, increase in serum creatinine and marked decrease in phenol red excretion test and urine concentration dilution test.

4. Blood electrolyte disturbance.

## Syndrome Differentiation

### 1. Deficiency of spleen qi

Symptoms: Nausea, abdominal distension, poor appetite and a sticky, greasy and tasteless sensation in the mouth, or a bitter taste in the mouth, dry mouth, dry stools, withered complexion, listlessness and lassitude; yellow, thick and greasy tongue coating and thin, rapid and slippery pulse.

Analysis of symptoms: Persistent deficiency of the spleen leads to retention of turbid dampness, which stagnates into heat and disturbs the normal ascending and descending functions of qi, this is marked by nausea, abdominal distension and poor appetite; the pathogenic turbidity flows upward, creating a sticky, greasy and tasteless sensation in the mouth; accumulation of heat in the lower energizer is responsible for the presence of dry stools; damp-heat scorches the body fluid, resulting in the bitter taste and dryness in the mouth; deficient spleen qi fails to disperse and move up the lucid yang, with such signs as withered complexion, listlessness and lassitude; the yellow, thick and greasy tongue coating and the thin, rapid and slippery pulse are attributable to internal obstruction of damp-heat.

### 2. Yang deficiency of the spleen and kidneys

Symptoms: Fatigue, lassitude, susceptibility to common cold, poor appetite, vomiting of clear water, a urinous odor in the mouth, loose and filthy stools, clear and profuse urine, intolerance of cold, cold limbs and a white or dark complexion; obesity, slightly pale tongue with teeth marks and a white and moist coating, thin and deep pulse, or soggy and thin pulse.

Analysis of symptoms: The deficiency of the spleen qi and kidney qi leads to malnutrition of the muscles in the four limbs, fatigue, lassitude and susceptibility to common cold; dysfunction of the spleen in transformation results in poor digestion and poor appetite; the disorder in the ascent/ descent of the lucid/turbid results in the vomiting of clear water and urinous odor in the mouth; deficiency of kidney qi causes inefficient qi transformation, it is marked by loose and filthy stools as well as clear and profuse urine; exhaustion of yang qi fails to warm and nourish the body, so there is intolerance of cold, cold limbs and a white or dark complexion; yang deficiency of the spleen and kidneys with internal accumulation of damp-cold is manifested as obesity, a slightly pale tongue with teeth marks, white and moist coating, thin and deep pulse, or soggy and thin pulse.

## 3. Yin deficiency of the spleen and kidneys

Symptoms: Lassitude, weakness and soreness of the waist and knees, shortness of breath upon physical exertion, dry mouth and lips, feverish sensations in the palms and soles, which may be accompanied by hectic fever in the afternoon, dry stools, scanty and yellowish urine and pale complexion; red tongue with thin and yellowish greasy coating and thin, deep and rapid pulse.

Analysis of symptoms: Prolonged retention of damp-heat produces dryness and damages yin fluid, leading to insufficiency of both qi and yin of the spleen and kidneys, marked by lassitude; deficiency of the kidneys is manifested as weakness and soreness of the waist and knees; failure of the kidneys to receive qi results in shortness of breath upon physical exertion; deficiency of spleen yin and kidney yin causes disorder in dispersing the moistening fluid, giving rise to a dry mouth and lips; deficiency of yin creates internal heat, characterized by feverish sensation in the palms and soles as well as hectic fever in the afternoon; intestinal dryness due to depletion of yin is manifested as dry stools; deficiency of the kidneys with damp-heat pouring down is responsible for scanty and yellowish urine; the deficient spleen and kidneys fail to distribute the nutritional essence to the face, so there is paleness of the complexion; the red tongue with thin and yellowish greasy coating and the thin, deep and rapid pulse are all due to deficiency of kidney yin and spleen yin with internal retention of damp-heat.

## 4. Obstruction of orifices by turbid yin

Symptoms: Profuse phlegm and saliva, nausea and vomiting, poor appetite, edema with scanty urine, lethargy, floccitation, progressive loss of consciousness, whitish and lusterless complexion and lack of warmth in the limbs; obesity, pale tongue with whitish greasy coating and slow and deep pulse.

Analysis of symptoms: Dysfunction of the spleen in transportation and transformation produces damp-heat and breeds phlegm, marked by an abundance of phlegm and saliva; abnormal ascent and descent of the spleen qi and stomach qi is manifested as nausea, vomiting and poor appetite; deficiency of the spleen brings about retention of water and dampness in the interior and deficiency of the kidneys leads to dysfunction of qi transformation, with such signs as edema and scanty urine; the turbid yin flows upward and clouds the upper orifices, causing lethargy, floccitation and coma; internal obstruction of turbid dampness results in lucid yang failing to ascend, presenting as a whitish and lusterless complexion; dampness obstructs the yang qi, making it fail to warm the body and manifesting by a lack of warmth in the limbs; obesity, pale tongue with whitish greasy coating and slow and deep pulse are all symptomatic of weakness of yang qi and predominance of turbid yin.

## Differential Treatment

### 1. Deficiency of spleen qi

Treatment principle: Invigorating the spleen and resolving dampness, harmonizing the stomach and dispelling heat.

Prescription and herbs: Modified Xiangsha Liujunzi Decoction and Huanglian Wendan Decoction.

Dangshen (Radix Codonopsis) 12 g, Baizhu (Largehead Atractylodes Rhizome) 12 g, Yiyiren (Coix Seed) 15 g, Shanyao (Common Yan Rhizome) 15 g, Muxiang (Common Aucklandia Root) 6 g, Sharen (Villous Amomum Fruit) 3 g, Huanglian (Golden Thread) 6 g, Fuling (Indian Bread) 12 g, Banxia (Pinellia Tuber) 9 g, Chenpi (Dried Tangerine Peel) 6 g, Zhuru (Bamboo Shavings) 3 g, Zhishi (Immature Orange Fruit) 9 g and Gancao (Liquorice Root) 6 g.

Modification: In cases of listlessness and limb weariness, Huangqi (Milkvetch Root) 15 g can be added to reinforce the action of nourishing qi; for the bitter taste and dryness in the mouth, Huangqin (Baical Skullcap Root) 9 g and Zhizi (Cape Jasmine Fruit) 9 g are added to dispel heat and resolve dampness.

## 2. Yang deficiency of the spleen and kidneys

Treatment principle: Warming and nourishing the spleen and kidneys, resolving dampness and bringing down turbidity.

Prescription and herbs: Modified Wenpi Decoction.

Dangshen (Radix Codonopsis) 12 g, Fuzi (Prepared Common Monkshood Daughter) 6 g, Ganjiang (Dried Ginger) 9 g, Xianlingpi (Herba Epimedii) 9 g, Banxia (Pinellia Tuber) 9 g, Houpu (Magnolia Bark) 9 g, Chenpi (Dried Tangerine Peel) 6 g, Zhishi (Immature Orange Fruit) 12 g, Jiangzhuru (Ginger-prepared Bamboo Shavings) 9 g, Zhidahuang (Specially prepared Rhubarb) 9 g and Gancao (Liquorice Root) 6 g.

Modification: For vomiting of clear water, Guizhi (Cassia Twig) 9 g and Fuling (Indian Bread) 12 g are added to warm and dissolve phlegm and retained fluid.

## 3. Yin deficiency of the spleen and kidneys

Treatment principle: Replenishing qi and nourishing yin, clearing dampness and resolving stagnation.

Prescription and herbs: Modified Zhibai Dihuang Decoction and Huanglian Wendan Decoction.

Zhimu (Common Anemarrhena Rhizome) 12 g, Shudi (Prepared Rhizome of Rehmannia) 9 g, Shengdi (Dried Rehmannia Root) 9 g, Shanzhuyu (Asiatic Cornelian Cherry Fruit) 9 g, Gouqizi (Barbary Wolfberry Fruit) 9 g, Shanyao (Common Yan Rhizome) 15 g, Danpi (Cortex Moutan) 9 g, Huanglian (Golden Thread) 6 g, Huangbai (Amur Cork-tree) 9 g, Fuling (Indian Bread) 12 g, Banxia (Pinellia Tuber) 9 g, Chenpi (Dried Tangerine Peel) 6 g, Zhuru (Bamboo Shavings) 3 g, Zhishi (Immature Orange Fruit) 9 g and Gancao (Liquorice Root) 6 g.

Modification: In cases of feverish sensation in the palms and soles, hectic fever in the afternoon and dry mouth and lips, Xuanshen (Figwort Root) 9 g, Maidong (Dwarf Lilyturf Tuber) 9 g, Shihu (Dendrobium) 9 g, Guiban (Tortoise Shell) 9 g can be added to nourish yin, dispel heat and produce fluid.

### 4. Obstruction of orifices by turbid yin

Treatment principle: Resolving turbidity with pungent and warm herbs and eliminating phlegm for resuscitation.

Prescription and herbs: Modified Ditan Decoction and Suhexiang Pill.

Banxia (Pinellia Tuber) 9 g, Chenpi (Dried Tangerine Peel) 6 g, Zhuru (Bamboo Shavings) 3 g, Zhishi (Immature Orange Fruit) 9 g Dangshen (Radix Codonopsis) 12 g, Fuling (Indian Bread) 12 g, Dannanxing (Bile Arisaema) 6 g, Changpu (Acorus Calamus) 9 g, Yujin (Turmeric Root Tuber) 9 g, Gancao (Liquorice Root) 6 g and Shuhexiang Wan (Storax Pill) 1 pill (administered with warm boiled water).

Modification: If there is nausea and vomiting, Jiangzhuru (Ginger-prepared Bamboo Shavings) 9 g can be added to bring down the adverse flow of qi and arrest vomiting; for edema with scanty urine, Chenhulu (Aged Bottle-gourd) 9 g, Chongsun (Henon Bamboo Dried Shoot) 9 g and Zexie (Oriental Waterplantain Rhizome) 15 g are added to promote urination and relieve edema.

### Chinese Patent Medicine

Bailing Capsule: 4 capsules for each dose, 3 times a day.

## Simple and Handy Prescriptions

Huangqi (Milkvetch Root) 15 g, Shufuzi (Prepared Common Monkshood Daughter) 9 g, Danshen (Radix Salviae Miltiorrhiae) 30 g and Liuyuexue (Junesnow) 30 g are boiled in water and consumed once a day.

## Other Therapies

Dietary therapy:

(1) A Wuguji (Silkie) or Tongziji (Spring Chicken) is stuffed with Huangqi (Milkvetch Root) 30 g and Liuyuexue (Junesnow) 60 g which are wrapped in absorbent gauze and then the chicken is well cooked in water. After it is ready, the medicated bag is taken out and the chicken and soup can be served.

(2) A Jiayu (Green Turtle), Huaishanyao (Huaihe Common Yan Rhizome) 30 g and Gouqizi (Barbary Wolfberry Fruit) 9 g are wrapped in absorbent gauze and boiled in water. After it is ready, the medicated bag is removed and then both the meat and soup can be served.
Coloclysis: Zhidahuang (Prepared Rhubarb) 30 g, Liuyuexue (Junesnow) 30 g, Pugongying (Dandelion) 30 g, Danshen (Radix Salviae Miltiorrhiae) 30 g and Shengmuli (Raw Oyster Shell) 30 g are decocted into 200 ml medicinal liquor for retention-enema.
Peritoneal dialysis or hemodialysis is applicable and renal transplantation can be considered if necessary.

## Cautions and Advice

1. This disease should be treated proactively and patients ought to rest well, prevent and suppress infection and control blood pressure; when there is a urinous odor in the mouth, it is advisable to rinse the mouth regularly.
2. Patients should take semi-fluid and low-protein foods, supplement their diet with adequate calories and vitamins and consume more fruits and vegetables; generally salt and water are not restricted; however, if the urine becomes scanty, the intake of salt must be restricted (1~3 g/day)

and so must the amount of water; seafood, spicy delicacies and alcohol are strictly prohibited.

3. Despite the severity of this disease, it can have a favorable prognosis if treated actively. Nonetheless, if there is presence of uremia, the prognosis will be unfavorable.

## Daily Exercises

1. Recall the diagnostic key points of chronic renal failure.
2. Explain how chronic renal failure can be treated based on syndrome differentiation.

# CHAPTER 6

# Disorders of the Hematological System

## Hypoferric Anaemia
## Week 9: Monday

Hypoferric anaemia refers to the microcytic hypochromic hypemia due to inefficient hemoglobin synthesis caused by inadequate storage or deficiency of iron within the body. This disease can be caused by relative deficiency of iron absorption, as is manifested during the growing stage of infants, adolescent development and menstrual onset in females and the period of pregnancy or lactation in women. It can also be caused by blood loss, such as acute or chronic bleeding of the alimentary canal, hemorrhoid bleeding, hookworm disease and menorrhagia. A third factor is functional disturbance of digestion and absorption, such as functional disorder of the stomach and intestines, iron-absorbing dysfunction of the stomach and intestines and inadequate absorption of iron after surgery. Clinically it is the most common form of anaemia and if diagnosed and treated promptly, can have a favorable prognosis. In TCM, it is believed to be closely associated with "deficiency consumption", "green sickness" and "dizziness".

### Etiology and Pathology

The main causes of hypoferric anaemia are chronic bleeding, such as haematemesis, hemafecia, menorrhagia, hemorrhoid bleeding and parasitic malnutrition (hookworm disease). As a result, the spleen and stomach become weak, and thus the exhaustion of the source for qi and blood predisposes the patient to anaemia.

The pathological change is marked by chronic bleeding and malfunction of the spleen and stomach, which fail to transform water and food into nutrients, thereby resulting in anaemia; besides, if there are worms in the intestine, they will absorb the nutrients and deprive the blood of its source, consequently bringing about anaemia.

## Diagnostic Key Points

1. A history of iron-deficiency, chronic bleeding, increased demand for ˙ iron, or utilization disturbance of iron.
2. Clinical manifestations: Lusterless or yellowish complexion, dizziness, weariness, tinnitus and palpitations.
3. Physical signs: Possibly pale mucous membrane, bluish sclera, or flat, uneven and fragile nails; colonychia, glossitis and stomatitis in some cases.
4. Laboratory examination: Increase in serum iron and the association rate of total iron; blood routine test: Microcytic hypochromic anaemia.
5. Decrease or absence of bone marrow sideroblast and exocellular iron.

## Syndrome Differentiation

### 1. Weakness of the spleen and stomach

Symptoms: Sallow complexion, dizziness, lassitude, poor appetite and loose stools; pale and enlarged tongue with white and thin coating and thin pulse.

Analysis of symptoms: Dysfunction of the spleen and stomach deprives the qi and blood of their source, resulting in sallow complexion and lassitude; blood fails to nourish the head and face, leading to dizziness; the spleen and stomach fail in their functions to transform and transport, with such signs as poor appetite and loose stools; the pale and enlarged tongue, the white and thin coating and the thin pulse are all due to weakness of the spleen and stomach with insufficiency of qi and blood.

## 2. Blood deficiency of the heart and spleen

Symptoms: Lusterless complexion, dizziness, tinnitus, palpitations and insomnia; pale tongue with white and thin coating, thin pulse or thin and rapid pulse.

Analysis of symptoms: The heart and spleen is deficient in blood, thus failing to nourish the heart and tranquilize the spirit, leading to palpitations and insomnia; deficient blood fails to nourish the head and face, resulting in dizziness, tinnitus, pale tongue with white and thin coating; the vessels are insufficiently filled by qi and blood, manifesting in a thin pulse.

## 3. Yang deficiency of the spleen and kidneys

Symptoms: Sallow or lusterless complexion, cold body and limbs, pale lips and nails, general edema, or even ascites, palpitations, shortness of breath, tinnitus, dizziness, listlessness, flaccidity in the limbs, loose stools or diarrhea before dawn, clear and profuse urine, impotence in males and amenia in females; pale tongue, possibly accompanied by teeth marks from self-biting and thin and deep pulse.

Analysis of symptoms: Deficiency of spleen yang and kidney yang leads to malfunction of qi-transformation and retention of pathogenic water, this is marked by general edema or even ascites; the spleen dominates the four limbs and since yang qi is too weak to warm the limbs, there is coldness in the body and limbs; deficiency of spleen yang and kidney yang results in decline of fire from the life gate and retention of water and dampness in the interior, with such signs as impotence, loose stools or diarrhea before dawn and clear and profuse urine; the spleen is the postnatal foundation as well as the source for production of qi and blood; furthermore, the kidneys, as the prenatal foundation, govern the bones, produce marrow and store essence which can transform into blood, so deficiency of spleen yang and kidney yang can lead to deficiency of qi and blood which is marked by sallow or lusterless complexion, pale lips and nails, palpitations, shortness of breath, tinnitus, dizziness, listlessness, flaccidity in the limbs, amenia in females, pale tongue with teeth marks and thin and deep pulse.

## Differential Treatment

### 1. Weakness of the spleen and stomach

Treatment principle: Replenishing qi, invigorating the spleen and producing blood.

Prescription and herbs: Modified Liujunzi Decoction.

Huangqi (Milkvetch Root) 15 g, Dangshen (Radix Codonopsis) 15 g, Baizhu (Largehead Atractylodes Rhizome) 10 g, Fuling (Indian Bread) 10 g, Banxia (Pinellia Tuber) 6 g, Chenpi (Dried Tangerine Peel) 6 g, Dazao (Chinese Date) 7 dates and Gancao (Liquorice Root) 5 g.

Modification: For severe dizziness due to blood deficiency, Danggui (Chinese Angelica) 9 g and Shudi (Prepared Rhizome of Rehmannia) 12 g are added to nourish blood.

### 2. Blood deficiency of the heart and spleen

Treatment principle: Replenishing qi, nourishing the heart and supplementing blood.

Prescription and herbs: Modified Guipi Decoction.

Huangqi (Milkvetch Root) 15 g, Dangshen (Radix Codonopsis) 12 g, Baizhu (Largehead Atractylodes Rhizome) 12 g, Fushen (Indian Bread with Hostwood) 12 g, Baishao (White Peony Alba) 12 g, Shudi (Prepared Rhizome of Rehmannia) 12 g, Danggui (Chinese Angelica) 9 g, Zaoren (Semen Ziziphi Spinosae) 12 g, Zhiyuanzhi (Thinleaf Milkwort Fruit) 6 g. Muxiang (Common Aucklandia Root) 6 g, Dazao (Chinese Date) 7 dates and Zhigancao (Stir-baked Liquorice Root) 5 g.

Modification: If there is constipation, Dazao (Chinese Date) should be replaced with Shengshouwu (Raw Fleeceflower Root) 15 g and Jixueteng (Suberect Spatholobus) 15 g to nourish blood and promote defecation.

### 3. Yang deficiency of the spleen and kidneys

Treatment principle: Warming and nourishing the spleen and kidneys.
Prescription and herbs: Modified Shipi Potion and Sishen Pill.

Huangqi (Milkvetch Root) 15 g, Baizhu (Largehead Atractylodes Rhizome) 12 g, Fuling (Indian Bread) 12 g, Gancao (Liquorice Root) 6 g, Fuzi (Prepared Common Monkshood Daughter) 9 g, Dafupi (Areca Peel) 12 g, Houpu (Magnolia Bark) 9 g, Buguzhi (Malaytea Scurfpea Fruit) 12 g, Tusizi (Dodder Seed) 12 g, Rougui (Cassia Bark) 6 g, Lujiaojiao (Deerhorn Glue) 9 g and Danggui (Chinese Angelica) 12 g.

Modification: For severe diarrhea, Huaishanyao (Huaihe Common Yan Rhizome) 15 g, Chaobiandou (Fried Hyacinth Bean) 15 g and Weirouguo (Sarcocarp) 9 g are added to invigorate the spleen, warm the kidneys and nourish the middle energizer; for apparent edema, Zhuling (Polyporus) 12 g and Zexie (Oriental Waterplantain Rhizome) 15 g are added to promote urination and relieve edema.

## Chinese Patent Medicine

1. Guipi Pill: 12 pills for each dose, 3 times a day.
2. Siwu Heji: 10 ml for each dose, 3 times a day.
3. Zaofan Pill: 3 g for each dose, 2~3 times a day after meals.

## Simple and Handy Prescriptions

Huangqi (Milkvetch Root) 12 g, Danggui (Chinese Angelica) 9 g and Dazao (Chinese Date) 7 dates are boiled in water, separated into 2 portions and taken at 2 different times within a day.

## Other Therapies

Abdominal rubbing exercise: Rub the abdomen by starting from Qihai (RN 6) acupoint, two finger-widths below the umbilicus, then circle around the umbilicus in a clockwise direction with gradual increase in diameter till the whole abdomen has been covered. Repeat several times so as to replenish qi, invigorate the spleen, produce blood and supplement the primordial qi.

Dietary therapy: Bocai Zhugan Decoction: Bocai (Spinach) 250g, Zhuxue (Hog Blood) 250 g, Jixue (Chicken Blood) 250 g, or Yaxue (Duck blood)

250 g and Zhugan (Pork Liver) 150 g. The pork liver is fried and then the coagulated blood and spinach are added to make soup. It can nourish blood and supplement deficiency.

## Cautions and Advice

1. Once a clear diagnosis is made, prompt treatment aiming at the causes should be administered.
2. Patients should regulate their diet and consume more iron-rich foods such as animal viscera, chicken egg yolks, soyabeans and apples.

## Daily Exercises

1. Recall the causes of hypoferric anaemia.
2. Recall the patterns of hypoferric anaemia that can be differentiated clinically. Describe their treatment principles and representative prescriptions.

# Aplastic Anaemia
# Week 9: Tuesday

Aplastic anaemia is a syndrome marked by pancytopenia, resulting from non-function of haematogenesis due to marked decrease in bone marrow hemopoietic tissues. The main clinical symptoms are progressive anaemia, bleeding and infection. The causes of this disease are mostly unclear, with the primary type accounting for about 67% and the secondary type accounting for only a small fraction; some serious infections by bacteria, viruses or toxins of parasites may suppress the haematogenesis of bone marrow, thus creating a predisposition to this disease. According to the differences in occurrence, hemogram and blood marrow image, this disease can be divided into two types: acute and chronic. The former has a poor prognosis, whereas the latter, if treated in time, can have a favorable prognosis. Aplastic anaemia is primarily observed in young and middle-aged people. In TCM, it is considered to be closely associated with "deficiency consumption" and "bleeding syndrome".

## Etiology and Pathology

Aplastic anaemia is caused by internal impairment due to overstrain, contraction of pathogenic factors, or exposure to toxic drugs or substances which damage qi and blood; if the impairment persists, there will be deficiency of the spleen and kidneys and insufficient production of essence and blood, thereby creating a predisposition to this disease.

The pathological changes are discussed as follows: Innate deficiency coupled with contraction of the six abnormal climatic factors, impairment of qi and blood by drugs or toxins, or internal injury due to overstrain may all lead to deficiency of the spleen qi and the subsequent insufficiency of qi and blood; deficiency of the spleen can affect the kidneys, leading to lack of kidney essence, which fails to supplement the bone marrow, essence and blood. Commonly, there are disorders of the five zang-organs: a deficient spleen fails to control blood, a deficient heart fails to govern blood, a deficient liver fails to store blood and deficient kidneys fail to supplement essence and blood, thus resulting in unregulated and disharmonized viscera, malnourished meridians and weakened defensive power with vulnerability to exogenous fever.

## Diagnostic Key Points

1. The main clinical manifestations are progressive anaemia, bleeding and repeated infection.
2. The acute aplastic anaemia is marked by sudden onset and rapid progress and commonly initiated by such manifestations as external or internal bleeding, infection and fever; chronic aplastic anaemia is characterized by slow onset and development, with such manifestations as blood deficiency, bleeding, infection and mild fever.
3. Medical examination: Appearance of anaemia, petechia or ecchymosis on the skin mucosa; for severe anaemia, there is an enlarged heart and audible systolic blowing murmur. Generally there is no enlargement of the liver, spleen or lymph nodes.
4. The number of peripheral complete blood cells (red blood cells, white blood cells and platelets) is decreased and the absolute value of reticulocyte is also reduced.
5. Bone marrow examination indicates that the proliferation of some cells is decreased or seriously decreased; decrease or disappearance of megakaryocyte; increase of non-hematopoietic cells in marrow particles.

## Syndrome Differentiation

### 1. Deficiency of qi and blood

Symptoms: Slow onset, pale complexion, dizziness, shortness of breath, weariness, poor appetite and loose stools; pale tongue with thin coating, deficient and taut pulse; occasional muscular bleeding.

Analysis of symptoms: Deficient spleen fails to transform the water and food into qi and blood, resulting in malnutrition of the head and face, resulting in pale complexion and dizziness; the body is malnourished, manifesting in shortness of breath and weariness; dysfunction of the spleen in transformation and the stomach and intestine in reception and transportation are responsible for poor appetite and loose stools; the pale tongue with thin coating and the deficient and taut pulse are symptomatic of deficient qi and blood.

## 2. Yin deficiency of the liver and kidneys

Symptoms: Pale complexion, dizziness, vexation, insomnia, tinnitus, weakness and soreness of the waist and legs, dry throat and mouth, nasal bleeding and presence of various bleeding manifestations; red tongue tip, thin tongue coating and taut, thin and rapid pulse.

Analysis of symptoms: Deficiency of the liver and kidneys brings about inadequacy of yin blood, which leads to malnutrition of the head and face that is marked by pale complexion and dizziness; deficiency of yin produces internal heat and gives rise to upward disturbance of deficient fire, resulting in vexation and dry throat; the waist is the "house of the kidneys", so deficiency of the kidneys is characterized by weakness and soreness of the waist and legs; deficient kidney yin fails to supplement the marrow sea and nourish the brain, presenting as dizziness and tinnitus; deficiency of liver yin and kidney yin brings about deficient fire which damages the collaterals and causes the bleeding manifestations; the red tongue tip, thin tongue coating and taut, thin and rapid pulse are all attributable to deficiency of liver yin and kidney yin.

## 3. Yang deficiency of the spleen and kidneys

Symptoms: Pale or yellowish and lusterless complexion, pale lips and nails, dizziness, blurred vision, lassitude, tinnitus, palpitations, reduced food intake, loose stools, intolerance of cold and cold limbs; pale and enlarged tongue with white coating and thin and deep pulse.

Analysis of symptoms: Deficiency of spleen yang leads to dysfunction in transforming water and food into qi and blood, this is marked by pale or yellowish and lusterless complexion as well as pale lips and nails; insufficient qi and blood fail to nourish the upper energizer, with such signs as dizziness, blurred vision and tinnitus; deficient kidney yang fails to warm the body, so there is intolerance of cold with cold limbs; deficiency of spleen yang and kidney yang brings about inactivation of lucid yang and failure of fire to generate earth, characterized by inadequate food intake and loose stools; blood fails to nourish the heart, presenting as paroxysmal palpitations; the pale and enlarged tongue with white coating and the thin and deep pulse are due to deficiency of yang qi.

## 4. Invasion of toxic heat into the ying-blood

Symptoms: Pale complexion, dizziness or headache with unclear mind, persistent ardent fever, hemorrhinia or hematemesis, hemafecia and purpura, as well as frequent, incessant and extra-menstrual vaginal bleeding; pale tongue with whitish greasy or yellowish rough coating and large, deficient and rapid pulse.

Analysis of symptoms: Deficiency of qi and yin is manifested as pale complexion, dizziness, pale tongue with yellowish rough coating and large, deficient and rapid pulse; invasion of pathogenic factors into the ying-blood phase is responsible for persistent ardent fever; pathogenic factors sink into the pericardium, bringing about coma and delirium; prolonged lingering of pathogenic heat leads to consumption of genuine yin and extravasation of blood, characterized by hematemesis, hemafecia, suggillation, metrorrhagia and metrostaxis.

## Differential Treatment

### 1. Deficiency of qi and blood

Treatment principle: Invigorating qi and nourishing blood.

Prescription and herbs: Modified Bazhen Decoction.

Renshen (Ginseng) 3 g, Huangqi (Milkvetch Root) 12 g, Baizhu (Largehead Atractylodes Rhizome) 12 g, Baishao (White Peony Alba) 12 g, Danggui (Chinese Angelica) 9 g, Chuanxiong (Szechwan Lovage Rhizome) 6 g, Shudi (Prepared Rhizome of Rehmannia) 15 g, Fuling (Indian Bread) 12 g, Gancao (Liquorice Root) 6 g and Dazao (Chinese Date) 15 g.

Modification: For deficiency of the heart with fright, Wuweizi (Chinese Magnolivine Fruit) 6 g and Longgu (Os Draconis) 30 g are added to calm the heart and tranquilize the mind; if there is muscular bleeding, Xianhecao

(Hairyvein Agrimonia Herb) 15 g and Huanliancao (Ecliptae Herba) 12 g are added to control blood circulation and stop bleeding.

## 2. Yin deficiency of the liver and kidneys

Treatment principle: Nourishing the liver and kidneys.

Prescription and herbs: Modified Dabuyuan Decoction.

Renshen (Ginseng) 3 g, Shudi (Prepared Rhizome of Rehmannia) 12 g, Shanzhuyu (Asiatic Cornelian Cherry Fruit) 9 g, Duzhong (Eucommia Bark) 12 g, Gouqizi (Barbary Wolfberry Fruit) 12 g, Danggui (Chinese Angelica) 9 g, Baishao (White Peony Alba) 12 g, Shouwu (Fleeceflower Root) 9 g, Huaishanyao (Huaihe Common Yan Rhizome) 12 g, Zhiguiban (Baked Tortoise Shell) 9 g and Gancao (Liquorice Root) 6 g.

Modification: If there is presence of bleeding, Danggui (Chinese Angelica) and Duzhong (Eucommia Bark) are removed; in case of peliosis, Huanliancao (Ecliptae Herba) 12 g, Nuzhenzi (Glossy Privet Fruit) 12 g and Xianhecao (Hairyvein Agrimonia Herb) 15 g are added to nourish the kidneys and liver as well as cool blood to stop bleeding; for nosebleed, Baimaogen (Lalang Grass Rhizome) 15 g and Cebaiye (Chinese Arborvitae Twig and Leaf) 12 g are added to cool blood and stop bleeding; for presence of fever, Qinghao (Sweet Wormwood Herb) 9 g, Digupi (Chinese Wolfberry Root-Bark) 12 g and Danpi (Cortex Moutan) 12 g are added to dispel heat and cool blood.

## 3. Yang deficiency of the spleen and kidneys

Treatment principle: Warming the kidneys and nourishing the spleen, invigorating qi and nourishing blood.

Prescription and herbs: Modified Yougui Pill.

Dangshen (Radix Codonopsis) 15 g, Huangqi (Milkvetch Root) 15 g, Baizhu (Largehead Atractylodes Rhizome) 12 g, Fuling (Indian Bread) 12 g, Shudi (Prepared Rhizome of Rehmannia) 12 g, Huaishanyao (Huaihe Common Yan Rhizome) 15 g, Shanzhuyu (Asiatic Cornelian Cherry Fruit) 9 g, Gouqizi (Barbary Wolfberry Fruit) 12 g, Lujiaojiao (Deerhorn Glue) 9 g, Tusizi (Dodder Seed) 12 g, Duzhong (Eucommia Bark) 12 g, Danggui

(Chinese Angelica) 9 g, Shufukuai (Prepared Common Monkshood Daughter Piece) 9 g, Rougui (Cassia Bark) 2 g, Dazao (Chinese Date) 15 g and Gancao (Liquorice Root) 6 g.

Modification: For intolerance of cold and loose stools, Buguzhi (Malaytea Scurfpea Fruit) 9 g and Xianlingpi (Herba Epimedii) 12 g are added to warm the kidneys and activate yang.

## 4. Invasion of toxic heat into the ying-blood

Treatment principle: Eliminating toxins and cooling blood.

Prescription and herbs: Modified Xijiao Dihuang Decoction.

Xiyangshen (American Ginseng) 9 g, Shengdi (Dried Rehmannia Root) 15 g, Xuanshen (Figwort Root) 12 g, Danpi (Cortex Moutan) 15 g, Chishao (Red Peony Root) 9 g, Xijiaofen (Rhinoceros Horn Powder) 2 g (swallowed), Daqingye (Dyers Woad Leaf) 15 g and Lianqiao (Weeping Forsythia Capsule) 9 g.

Modification: For severe bleeding, Shihui Pill 30 g (wrapped during decoction) can be used to cool blood and stop bleeding; if there is coma and delirium, an Angong Niuhuang Pill is administered after being ground with water, or 4 g of Zixue Dan is swallowed to clear the heart and open the orifices.

## Chinese Patent Medicine

1. Fufang Taipan Tablet: 4 tablets for each dose, 3 times a day.
2. Heche Dazao Pill: 4 g for each dose, twice a day.

## Simple and Handy Prescriptions

1. Renshen (Ginseng) 3 g, or Zihechefen (Human Placenta Powder) 6 g is decocted and taken twice a day to supplement the primordial qi, replenish essence and produce marrow.
2. Huangqi (Milkvetch Root) 12 g, Dangshen (Radix Codonopsis) 9 g, Danggui (Chinese Angelica) 9 g and Dazao (Chinese Date) 7 dates are

boiled in water and separated into 2 portions to be taken at 2 different times within a day. It is used to treat anaemia with deficiency of qi and blood.

## Other Therapies

Dietary therapy: Shenqi Yangrou Decoction: Renshen (Ginseng) 30 g, Huangqi (Milkvetch Root) 50 g and Yangrou (Mutton) 500 g are cooked with condiments added for taste. It is used to invigorate the spleen and warm the kidneys, as well as replenish qi and nourish blood.

## Cautions and Advice

1. The causes should be identified and corresponding treatment implemented immediately.
2. The principle of "treating the branch in case of emergency and treating the root in case of chronic disease" should be applied to address the conditions of blood deficiency, bleeding and infection.
3. Patients must pay attention to dietary regulation, avoid spicy and other stomach-irritating foods and consumemore fresh vegetables or fruits.
4. They should also ward off wind-cold and protect themselves from catching thecommon cold, so as to avoid infection.

## Daily Exercises

1. Recall the clinical characteristics of aplastic anaemia.
2. Describe the common patterns, treatment principles and representative prescriptions of aplastic anaemia.

# Leukemia (Chronic Granulocytic Leukemia)
## Week 9: Wednesday

Chronic granulocytic leukemia refers to the cloning or proliferation of pluripotential hemopoietic stem cells in bone marrow, marked by an increase in the total number of white blood cells and significant proliferation of granulocytic juvenile cells and mature cells at different stages (especially the middle and late stages) in bone marrow and blood. Clinically, the symptoms are fever, anaemia, bleeding and enlargement of the liver, spleen and lymph nodes in varying degrees. This disease, usually afflicting adults and old people, has a poor prognosis. In TCM, it is considered to be closely associated with "accumulations and masses", "deficiency consumption" and "bleeding syndrome".

### Etiology and Pathology

It is believed in TCM that chronic granulocytic leukemia is caused by insufficiency of healthy qi or essential qi coupled with contraction of pestilent toxins, which damages ying-yin, affects the kidneys and impairs the bone marrow.

The pathological changes of this disease are discussed as follows: Insufficiency of healthy qi allows invasion of pathogenic toxins from the exterior to the interior, leading to deficiency of healthy qi with abundance of pathogenic factors that damage ying-yin, affect the kidneys, impair the bone marrow and hinder blood production. Consumption of yin-essence creates a predisposition to internal heat which scorches the blood vessels and drives blood rampant. Chronic diseases exhaust qi and blood and the deficient qi fails to control blood, resulting in bleeding syndromes. Since deficiency of healthy qi incurs invasion of exogenous pathogenic factors, or because impairment of yin and blood produces abundant heat in ying-blood, there will be persistent high fever, progressive consumption or stagnation of qi and blood and obstruction of the collaterals or a presence of masses below the costal region. If the pathogenic toxins are not completely expelled, the disease may recur, causing chronic deficiency of qi and yin.

## Diagnostic Key Points

1. The disease is marked by slow onset, absence of subjective symptoms at the early stage and increase in the number of white blood cells or enlargement of the spleen discovered by chance through physical examination.
2. There are also symptoms such as weariness, profuse sweating, intolerance of heat and low fever; or dizziness, palpitations and shortness of breath due to anaemia.
3. Physical examination indicates that there is enlargement of the spleen and lymph nodes, though generally with no pain.
4. The definitive diagnosis necessitates peripheral hemogram and bone marrow image: Chronic Granulocytic Leukemia is marked by significant increase of granulocytic intermediate-type cells and megakaryocytes, or some chromatin-positive cells. Chronic Lymphocytic Leukemia is characterized by proliferation of small lymphocytes.

## Syndrome Differentiation

### 1. Deficiency of qi and yin

Symptoms: Pale complexion, lassitude, dizziness, palpitations, feverish sensations over the five centers, painful masses below the costal region, weakness and soreness of the waist and knees, spontaneous perspiration, night sweats, hectic fever in the afternoon, thin and rapid pulse; white and thin coating on red and tender tongue and obesity; primarily seen in the active stage of chronic leukemia with manifestations of anaemia.

Analysis of symptoms: Deficiency of qi and blood leads to malnutrition of the brain and is marked by dizziness, qi deficiency also causes malnutrition of the heart, marked by palpitations, malnutrition of the limbs and bones, marked by lassitude, weakness and soreness of the waist and knees and malnutrition of the face, marked by pale complexion; deficient qi fails to consolidate the exterior, resulting in spontaneous perspiration; deficiency of yin produces deficient fire in the interior, bringing about night sweats, hectic fever in the afternoon and a feverish sensation over the five centers; deficiency of qi fails to transform body fluid, giving rise to obstruction of phlegm and stasis below the costal region, resulting in the formation of painful hypochondriac masses; the red and tender tongue, with white and thin coating, corpulence and thin and rapid pulse are attributable to deficiency of qi and yin.

## 2.  Stagnation of qi with blood stasis

Symptoms: Abdominal distension, conspicuous masses below the costal region, or painful masses in the limbs, distending pain in the chest and hypochondria, fluctuant low-grade fever, spontaneous perspiration, night sweats, dark and lusterless complexion, reduced appetite and weariness; pale and purple tongue with ecchymosis and taut pulse; primarily seen in the acute or recurrent stage of chronic leukemia.

Analysis of symptoms: Stagnation of qi with blood stasis in the vessels or collaterals predisposes the patient to conspicuous masses below the costal region with both distension and pain, or painful masses in the limbs; accumulation of qi and blood results in imbalance between ying (nutrient phase) and wei (defensive phase), causing tidal low-grade fever, spontaneous perspiration and night sweats; qi stagnation and blood stasis disharmonize the spleen and stomach, presenting as reduced appetite and weariness; the pale and purple tongue with ecchymosis and the taut pulse are symptomatic of blood diseases marked by qi stagnation and blood stasis.

## 3.  Deficiency of healthy qi with blood stasis

Symptoms: Sallow complexion, weariness, low-grade fever, spontaneous perspiration, night sweats, bone ache, general pain, enlarged and hardened masses below the left costal region (enlarged spleen), progressively enlarged superficial nodules, emaciated body, reduced appetite or non-traumatic bleeding; pale and purple tongue with ecchymosis or red and smooth tongue, thin and feeble pulse or thin and taut pulse; primarily seen in the final stage of leukemia.

Analysis of symptoms: Persistent deficiency of healthy qi with blood stasis impedes the production of fresh blood and leads to depletion of ying-qi, marked by a sallow complexion and weariness; imbalance between ying (nutrient phase) and wei (defensive phase) are responsible for spontaneous perspiration, night sweats and low-grade fever; prolonged existence of masses obstructs the blood vessels, characterized by enlarged and hardened masses below the left costal region as well as progressively enlarged superficial nodules; the blood flows outside the vessels, so there is hemorrhinia; insufficiency of middle qi causes dysfunction in transformation and transportation, presenting as reduced appetite and emaciated body; the pale-purple tongue with ecchymosis or red-smooth tongue, as well as the thin-feeble pulse or thin- taut pulse are due to consumption of qi, blood and body fluid with inhibition of qi movements by blood stasis.

## Differential Treatment

### 1. Deficiency of qi and yin

Treatment principle: Replenishing qi, nourishing yin and dispelling heat.

Prescription and herbs: Modified Sancai Fengsui Dan.

Dangshen (Radix Codonopsis) 15 g, Beishashen (Coastal Glehnia Root) 15 g, Shengdi (Rehmannia Dried Rhizome) 15 g, Tiandong (Cochinchinese Asparagus Root) 15 g, Banzhilian (Sun Plant) 15 g, Baihuashecao (Hedyotic Diffusa) 30 g, Qingdai (Natural Indigo) 9 g, Huangbai (Amur Cork-tree) 9 g, Zhiguiban (Baked Tortoise Shell) 15 g, Biejia (Turtle Shell) 15 g and Muli (Oyster Shell) 30 g.

Modification: For hectic fever, Qinghao (Sweet Wormwood Herb) 10 g and Digupi (Chinese Wolfberry Root-Bark) 12 g are added to dispel deficient heat; for presence of masses, Sanleng (Common Burreed Tuber) 9 g, Ezhu (Zedoray Rhizome) 9 g and Taoren (Peach Seed) 9 g are added to activate blood and dissipate the masses.

### 2. Stagnation of qi with blood stasis

Treatment principle: Soothing the liver, regulating qi and resolving stasis.

Prescription and herbs: Modified Gexia Zhuyu Decoction.

Taoren (Peach Seed) 9 g, Honghua (Safflower) 9 g, Chuanxiong (Szechwan Lovage Rhizome) 6 g, Danggui (Chinese Angelica) 9 g, Danpi (Cortex Moutan) 12 g, Chishao (Red Peony Root) 12 g, Zhixiangfu (Nutgrass Galingale Rhizome) 9 g, Zhiqiao (Orange Fruit) 9 g, Yujin (Turmeric Root Tuber) 12 g, Danshen (Radix Salviae Miltiorrhiae) 12 g, Sanleng (Common Burreed Tuber) 15 g, Ezhu (Zedoray Rhizome) 15 g, Banzhilian (Sun Plant) 30 g and Sheshecao (Herba Hedyotis Diffusae) 30 g.

Modification: For constipation, Shengdahuang (Raw Rhubarb) 9 g can be added to dispel heat and dredge the intestines; if there is severe heat, Shengshigao (Raw Gypsum) 30 g and Daqingye (Dyers Woad Leaf) 30 g are added to dispel heat and remove toxins.

### 3. Deficiency of healthy qi with blood stasis

Treatment principle: Invigorating qi, nourishing blood and dissipating stagnation.

Prescription and herbs: Modified Bazhen Decoction and Gexia Zhuyu Decoction.

Dangshen (Radix Codonopsis) 10 g, Huangqi (Milkvetch Root) 15 g, Fuling (Indian Bread) 12 g, Baizhu (Largehead Atractylodes Rhizome) 12 g, Danggui (Chinese Angelica) 9 g, Shengdi (Dried Rehmannia Root) 15 g, Chishao (Red Peony Root) 10 g, Chuanxiong (Szechwan Lovage Rhizome) 10 g, Taoren (Peach Seed) 10 g, Honghua (Safflower) 9 g, Danpi (Cortex Moutan) 10 g, Xiangfu (Nutgrass Galingale Rhizome) 10 g, Sanleng (Common Burreed Tuber) 15 g, Ezhu (Zedoray Rhizome) 15 g, Biejia (Turtle Shell) 15 g and Dibiechong (Eupolyphaga Seu Steleophaga) 15 g.

Modification: If there is bone ache and physical pain, Wulingzhi (Faeces Trogopterorum) 9 g, Ruxiang (Boswellin) 9 g and Muoyao (Myrrh) 9 g are added to activate blood, promote qi flow, dissipate stasis and relieve pain.

### Chinese Patent Medicine

1. Niuhuang Jiedu Tablet: 4 tablets for each dose, 3 times a day after meals.

2. Homoharringtonine Injection: injected intramuscularly, 2 mg for each dose, once a day. A course of treatment lasts a month.

## Simple and Handy Prescriptions

1. Shensanqi (Panax Pseudo-ginseng Powder) 3 g and Baijifen (Common Bletilla Tuber Powder) 6 g are administered twice a day to activate blood and stop bleeding.
2. Qingdai (Natural Indigo) 6~12 g is swallowed twice a day to dispel heat, remove toxins and treat leukemia.

## Other Therapies

Dietary therapy:

(1) Qizao Yiyiren Porridge: Huangqi (Milkvetch Root) 5 g, Dazao (Chinese Date) 10 dates, Shengyiyiren (Raw Coix Seed) 30 g and Jiangmi (Rice Fruit) 50 g are cooked in 1000 ml of water and made into porridge, which is used to invigorate qi, nourish blood and reinforce the healthy qi.
(2) Wuji Tuanyu Decoction: A Wuguji (Silkie) and a Tuanyu (Soft-shelled Turtle) are cut into pieces and cooked in water with seasoning to taste. This is used to supplement qi and nourish the kidneys.

## Cautions and Advice

1. Prompt diagnosis is imperative so as to implement proper treatment, control the progression of the disease and save lives.
2. Mental healing is an important therapy for patients with this disease to conquer negative thoughts and cooperate during the treatment.
3. Patients should rest well and stay in bed during chemotherapy.
4. They must also pay attention to maintain hygiene of the orifices, particularly the mouth, skin, anus and external genitalia, so as to prevent infection.
5. It is advisable to maintain a nutritious and digestible diet, especially vegetables and vitamin-rich food.

## Daily Exercises

1. Recall the main clinical manifestations of chronic granulocytic leukemia.
2. Explain how chronic granulocytic leukemia due to deficiency of qi and yin can be diagnosed and treated.
3. Name the aspects requiring special attention in the treatment of leukemia.

# Leucopenia and Agranulemia
# Week 9: Thursday

Leucopenia and agranulemia refer to the disorders marked by peripheral white blood cell count persistently falling below $4.0 \times 109/$ liter and neutrophilic granulocyte count falling below $2.0 \times 109/$ liter. The clinical symptoms are mainly dizziness, weariness, low-grade fever, palpitations, waist soreness, dental ulcer and infection. They are caused by drugs, chemicals or physical factors and may also be secondary to other diseases, such as hypersplenism and aplastic anaemia. If prompty treated, they can have a favorable prognosis, otherwise, there will be bone marrow depression with an unfavorable prognosis. Leucopenia and agranulemia are believed in TCM to be associated with "deficiency consumption" and "dizziness".

## Etiology and Pathology

From the perspective of TCM, leucopenia and agranulemia are considered to be caused by internal impairment due to overstrain as well as improper care or administration of drugs after the occurrence of disease, which damage the healthy qi and lead to exhaustion of the source for producing qi and blood, deficiency of the spleen and kidneys, decline of ying, wei, qi and blood, as well as imbalance of yin and yang.

The pathological changes are discussed as follows: Innate deficiency and congenital malnourishment cause a weak body, which is then afflicted by internal impairment due to overstrain as well as improper care or administration of drugs after the occurrence of disease, creating a predisposition to deficiency of the spleen and kidneys; deficiency of the spleen gives rise to failure of the nutrients to be dispersed, whereas deficiency of the kidneys is responsible for insufficient genuine qi; thus the source for qi, blood and essence is depleted and the healthy qi becomes deficient.

## Diagnostic Key Points

1. Leucopenia

(1) Clinically, it may be asymptomatic or marked by dizziness, weariness, low-grade fever, decreased appetite, insomnia, dreaminess, intolerance of cold and uneasiness.

(2) It is vulnerable to viral or bacterial infection such as colds.

(3) White cell count below $(2.0{\sim}4.0) \times 109$/liter; differential count may be normal; red cell count and blood platelets count are generally normal.

(4) Bone marrow image: Dysfunctional proliferation or maturation arrest of granulocytic cells.

## 2. Agranulemia

(1) Clinically, it is marked by sudden onset, intolerance of cold, fever, weariness, dental ulcer and infection.

(2) Causative factors are generally identifiable, such as drug reaction or radiation damage.

(3) White cell count below $2.0 \times 109$/liter; significant decrease or absence of granulocytic cells, with an absolute number around $2.0 \times 109$/liter; red cell count and blood platelets count are generally normal.

(4) Bone marrow image: Possible suppression of granulocytic series and decrease or maturity arrest of juvenile cells in the granulocytic series.

## Syndrome Differentiation

## 1. Deficiency of qi and yin

Symptoms: Dizziness, lassitude, spontaneous perspiration, night sweats, dry mouth and throat; slightly red tongue with white and thin coating and deficient large pulse.

Analysis of symptoms: A deficient spleen fails to properly transform water and food into nutrients, qi and blood, resulting in malnutrition of the body which is marked by dizziness and lassitude; deficient qi fails to consolidate the exterior, causing spontaneous perspiration; deficiency of yin produces deficient fire which drives body fluid outside, presenting as night sweats; deficient fire flames up, leading to insufficient fluid in the upper, leading to a dry mouth and throat; the slightly red tongue with white and thin coating and deficient large pulse are due to deficiency of qi and yin.

## 2. Blood deficiency of the heart and spleen

Symptoms: Dizziness, palpitations, insomnia, dreaminess, forgetfulness, lassitude, reduced food intake and loose stools; pale tongue with thin coating, thin or knotted and intermittent pulse.

Analysis of symptoms: A deficient spleen fails to properly transform water and food into nutrients, qi and blood, resulting in malnutrition of the body that is marked by dizziness and lassitude; the dysfunction of the spleen in transformation and the malfunction of the stomach and intestines in reception and transportation are responsible for reduced food intake and loose stools; the deficiency of heart qi, insufficiency of heart blood and malnutrition of the heart spirit are manifested as palpitations, insomnia, dreaminess and forgetfulness; the pale tongue with thin coating and the thin or knotted and intermittent pulse are attributable to deficiency of heart blood and spleen blood.

## 3. Yin deficiency of the liver and kidneys

Symptoms: dizziness, headache, tinnitus, weakness and soreness of the waist and knees, flaccidity of the feet and dryness in the throat; red and dry tongue, with thin and taut pulse.

Analysis of symptoms: A deficiency of liver yin results in hyperactivity of liver yang, which disturbs the clear orifices upwardly and is marked by dizziness, headache and tinnitus; deficient kidney yin fails to nourish the waist where the kidneys dwell, leading to weakness and soreness of the waist and knees and flaccidity of the feet; deficient fire flames upward, giving rise to dryness in the mouth and throat; the red and dry tongue with thin and taut pulse are symptomatic of a hyperactive liver due to deficiency of yin.

## 4. Yang deficiency of the spleen and kidneys

Symptoms: Dizziness, deficient yellow complexion, cold body and limbs, lassitude, reduced food intake, loose stools, rugitus aggravated by cold, waist soreness and profuse urine; pale and enlarged tongue with white coating and weak pulse.

Analysis of symptoms: A deficiency of spleen yang leads to dysfunction in transportation and transformation of water and food into nutrients so as to strengthen the body, this is marked by dizziness, deficient yellow complexion, cold body and limbs as well as lassitude; deficiency of qi results in cold in the middle energizer and inactivation of lucid yang brings about stagnation of cold and qi, with such manifestations as loose stools and rugitus aggravated by cold; deficient yang of the kidneys fails to warm the body, leading to waist soreness, intolerance of cold and cold limbs; inefficient qi-transformation of water is responsible for profuse urine; the pale and enlarged tongue with white coating and weak pulse are manifestations of deficient yang qi.

## Differential Treatment

### 1. Deficiency of qi and yin

Treatment principle: Replenishing qi and nourishing yin.

Prescription and herbs: Modified Sijunzi Decoction and Shengmai Potion.

Dangshen (Radix Codonopsis) 15 g, Baizhu (Largehead Atractylodes Rhizome) 12 g, Fuling (Indian Bread) 12 g, Huangqi (Milkvetch Root) 15 g, Shashen (Root of Straight Ladybell) 12 g, Maidong (Dwarf Lilyturf Tuber) 12 g, Wuweizi (Chinese Magnolivine Fruit) 6 g, Shouwu (Fleeceflower Root) 12 g, Gancao (Liquorice Root) 6 g and Dazao (Chinese Date) 7 dates.

Modification: In cases of severe spontaneous perspiration and night sweats, Nuodaogen (Glutinous Rice Root) 12 g and Bietaogan (Persicae Immaturus) 12 g are added to arrest sweating; for presence of ulcers on the tongue or in the mouth, Huanglian (Golden Thread) 3 g, Mutong (Caulis Hocquartiae) 5 g and Danzhuye (Henon Bamboo Leaf) 9 g are added to clear the heart, purge fire and direct heat downward.

### 2. Blood deficiency of the heart and spleen

Treatment principle: Nourishing the heart and spleen.

Prescription and herbs: Modified Yangxin Decoction.

Dangshen (Radix Codonopsis) 15 g, Huangqi (Milkvetch Root) 15 g, Baizhu (Largehead Atractylodes Rhizome) 12 g, Fuling (Indian Bread) 12 g, Danggui (Chinese Angelica) 9 g, Chuanxiong (Szechwan Lovage Rhizome) 9 g, Wuweizi (Chinese Magnolivine Fruit) 6 g, Baiziren (Chinese Arborvitae Kernel) 12 g, Suanzaoren (Spine Date Seed) 12 g, Rougui (Cassia Bark) 3 g (decocted later), Banxia (Pinellia Tuber) 9 g and Gancao (Liquorice Root) 6 g.

Modification: For gastric distension, vomiting and belching, Chenpi (Dried Tangerine Peel) 6 g can be added to harmonize the stomach and bring down qi; if there is diarrhea after abdominal pain and lack of warmth in the feet and hands, Paojiang (Prepared Dried Ginger) 6 g and Weirouguo (Roasted Sarcocarp) 9 g are added to warm the middle energizer and dissipate cold.

### 3. Yin deficiency of the liver and kidneys

Treatment principle: Nourishing the liver and kidneys.

Prescription and herbs: Modified Zuogui Pill.

Shudi (Prepared Rhizome of Rehmannia) 12 g, Gouqizi (Barbary Wolfberry Fruit) 12 g, Shanyao (Common Yan Rhizome) 12 g, Guiban (Tortoise Shell) 15 g, Niuxi (Twotoothed Achyranthes Root) 9 g, Shanzhuyu (Asiatic Cornelian Cherry Fruit) 9 g, Tusizi (Dodder Seed) 12 g, Huangjing (Solomonseal Rhizome) 12 g and Gancao (Liquorice Root) 6 g.

Modification: If there is relatively severe headache, dizziness and tinnitus, Shijueming (Sea-ear Shell) 30 g, Juhua (Chrysanthemum Flower) 9 g and Gouteng (Gambir Plant) 15 g are used to calm the liver and subdue yang; for relative exuberance of deficient fire with hectic fever and sore throat, Zhimu (Common Anemarrhena Rhizome) 12 g and Digupi (Chinese Wolfberry Root-Bark) 15 g are added to nourish yin and reduce fire.

### 4. Yang deficiency of the spleen and kidneys

Treatment principle: Warming and nourishing the spleen and kidneys.

Prescription and herbs: Modified Huangqi Jianzhong Decoction and Yougui Pill.

Huangqi (Milkvetch Root) 20 g, Guizhi (Cassia Twig) 10 g, Baishao (White Peony Alba) 20 g, Yitang (Cerealose) 30 g, (melted in decoction),

Zhifupian (Prepared Radix Aconitilateralis Preparata) 6 g, Shanyao (Common Yan Rhizome) 12 g, Duzhong (Eucommia Bark) 10 g, Xianlingpi (Herba Epimedii) 12 g, Tusizi (Dodder Seed) 10 g, Danggui (Chinese Angelica) 10 g, Jixueteng (Henry Magnoliavine Stem or Root) 15 g and Zhigancao (Stir-baked Liquorice Root) 6 g.

Modification: If accompanied by diarrhea before dawn, Buguzhi (Malaytea Scurfpea Fruit) 12 g, Roudoukou (Nutmeg) 9 g, Wuzhuyu (Medicinal Evodia Fruit) 3 g and Wuweizi (Chinese Magnolivine Fruit) 6 g are added to warm the spleen and kidneys as well as consolidate the intestine to check diarrhea.

## Chinese Patent Medicine

1. Guipi Pill: 12 pills for each dose, 3 times a day.
2. Liuwei Dihuang Pill: 12 pills for each dose, 3 times a day.
3. Yougui Pill: 6 g for each dose, twice a day.

## Simple and Handy Prescriptions

1. Qiancao (Indian Madder Root) 10 g, Hongzao (Red Date) 15 g and Lianqiao (Weeping Forsythia Capsule) 10 g are boiled in water and separated into 2 portions to be taken at 2 different times within a day. It is used to treat various types of this disease.
2. Taipanfen (Placenta Powder) is administered (1.5 g for each dose) twice a day after being infused in warm boiled water. It is used to treat the defficient spleen and kidneys.
3. Huangqi (Milkvetch Root) 30 g, Jixueteng (Henry Magnoliavine Stem or Root) 30 g, Dazao (Chinese Date) 7 dates and Huangjing (Solomonseal Rhizome) 15 g are boiled in water and separated into 2 portions to be taken at 2 different times within a day. It is used to treat decrease in white blood cell count after chemotherapy.

## Other Therapies

Abdominal self-massage: Rub the abdomen by starting from the Qihai (RN 6) acupoint and circle around the umbilicus in a clockwise direction with gradual increase in diameter till the whole abdomen is covered. Repeat several times so as to replenish qi, produce blood, strengthen the body and supplement the primordial qi.

Exercise therapy: Patients can practice taijiquan (traditional Chinese shadow boxing) when the disease is alleviated so as to strengthen the constitution, regulate qi, blood, yin and yang and consolidate the therapeutic effects.

Dietary therapy: Shuanggu Niurou Porridge: champignon 60 g (cut into threads), mushroom 50 g (sliced), beef 50 g (cut into pieces) and rice fruit 50 g are boiled in 1000 ml of water to make porridge; after adding the seasonings to taste, the porridge can be separated into 2 portions and taken at 2 different times within a day for invigorating the spleen and tonifying the kidneys.

## Cautions and Advice

1. The drugs tending to induce this disease should be strictly controlled and evaluated during clinical administration.
2. Those who have long-term exposure to radioactive substances, X-ray or some special chemicals should take effective precautions and go for periodic blood tests.
3. Interiors should be ventilated to let in fresh air and pathogenic wind-cold must be warded off to prevent catching the common cold.

## Daily Exercises

1. Recall the diagnostic key points of leucopenia and agranulemia.
2. Concisely describe the pathological changes of leucopenia and agranulemia.

# Idiopathic Thrombocytopenic Purpura
# Week 9: Friday

Idiopathic thrombocytopenic purpura, a disease related to autoimmunity, is marked by petechia or ecchymosis of the skin and mucus membrane, or gum bleeding, nosebleed, profuse menstruation and, in severe cases, visceral hemorrhage. Clinically, it is divided into two types: acute and chronic. The former mostly afflicts children and young people, whereas the latter is common in adults, especially females. If promptly treated, it can have a favorable prognosis. It is believed in TCM that this disease is closely associated with "bleeding syndrome" and "deficiency consumption".

## Etiology and Pathology

From the perspective of TCM, this disease is caused by exogenous toxic heat or endogenous production of pathogenic heat, both of which may obstruct the vessels and drive blood to reach the skin; or by improper diet or overstrain, which may damage the heart and spleen and lead to failure of qi to control blood.

The pathological changes are discussed as follows: Exogenous toxic heat hides in the ying-blood phase and damages the vessels, leading to extravasation of blood; pathogenic heat transmits into the interior and fumigates the stomach, or overconsumption of spicy food and alcohol produces heat in the stomach, this heat can disturb the yin-blood and drive it to the skin, manifesting in a sudden onset of extensive bleeding of the skin and mucus membrane; internal damage due to overstrain and repetitive bleeding impairs the heart and spleen and since qi is lost with the consumption of blood, it fails to control blood and results in extravasation; deficiency of yin results not only in malnutrition of the collaterals or vessels, but also in production of exuberant fire which also damages the vessels and drives blood to flow outside, marked by mild bleeding in the skin and mucus membrane without extensive hemorrhage.

## Diagnostic Key Points

1. The acute condition is marked by a sudden onset and severe bleeding symptoms, mainly observed in children. The chronic condition is characterized by a slow onset and obvious bleeding tendency.
2. Blood test: Decreased platelet count, prolonged bleeding time, abnormal blood-clot retraction, positive Leede's test and normal clotting time.
3. Bone marrow image: Increased or normal megakaryocyte count with maturation arrest.
4. Increase in platelet surface IgG, IgM or complement.
5. Exclusion of secondary plate-reduction.

## Syndrome Differentiation

### 1. Rampant flow of blood driven by heat

Symptoms: Purple petechia or ecchymosis on the skin, or with nosebleed, bleeding gums, hemafecia and bloody urine, or fever, dry mouth and constipation; red tongue with yellow coating, as well as rapid and taut pulse; primarily seen in the early stage or acute type of this disease.

Analysis of symptoms: Toxic heat hides in the ying-blood phase, stirs the blood, scorches the vessels and drives blood to flow outside, marked by skin peliosis, or other bleeding symptoms; toxic heat is, in essence, the pathogen of fire-heat, which scorches the interior and causes fever; abundant heat consumes body fluid and this is responsible for dry mouth and constipation; the red tongue with yellow coating as well as the rapid and taut pulse are manifestations of excess heat.

### 2. Exuberance of fire due to yin deficiency

Symptoms: Relatively marked peliosis occurring from time to time, often accompanied by nosebleed, gum bleeding or profuse menstruation, red cheeks, vexation, thirst, feverish sensation in the palms and soles, or hectic fever and night sweats; deep red tongue with scanty coating and thin and rapid pulse; primarily seen in the chronic type of this disease.

Analysis of symptoms: Deficiency of yin produces exuberant deficient fire, which scorches the vessels and drives blood to flow outside, marked by skin peliosis or other bleeding symptoms such as nosebleed, bleeding gums, or profuse menstruation; deficient fire flames up, giving rise to red cheeks and hectic fever; deficient fire disturbs the heart, presenting as vexation; depletion of yin and fluid is responsible for thirst; yin-fire drives the fluid outside, causing night sweats; the deep red tongue with scanty coating and thin and rapid pulse are symptomatic of exuberant fire due to yin deficiency.

### 3. Failure of qi to control blood

Symptoms: Persistent affliction, repetitive occurrence of peliosis, lassitude, dizziness, pale or sallow complexion and poor appetite; pale and enlarged tongue, with thin and feeble pulse; primarily seen in the chronic type of this disease.

Analysis of symptoms: Persistent affliction debilitates the spleen qi, which fails to control the blood, resulting in repetitive occurrence of peliosis; consumption of qi and blood is responsible for lassitude, dizziness and pale or sallow complexion; deficient spleen fails to transport and transform water and food, so the appetite is poor; the pale and enlarged tongue with thin and feeble pulse are both attributable to deficiency of qi and blood.

## Differential Treatment

### 1. Rampant flow of blood driven by heat

Treatment principle: Dispelling heat and removing toxins, cooling blood to stop bleeding.

Prescription and herbs: Modified Qingying Decoction and Shihui Powder.

Xijiaojian (Rhinoceros Horn Tip) 3 g, Shengdi (Dried Rehmannia Root) 30 g, Xuanshen (Figwort Root) 15 g, Zhuyexin (Henon Bamboo Leaf) 12 g, Maidong (Dwarf Lilyturf Tuber) 15 g, Danshen (Radix Salviae

Miltiorrhiae) 30 g, Huanglian (Golden Thread) 6 g, Jinyinhua (Honeysuckle Flower) 15 g, Lianqiao (Weeping Forsythia Capsule) 15 g, Daji (Japanese Thistle Herb) 15 g, Xiaoji (Field Thistle Herb) 15 g, Heye (Lotus Leaf) 6 g, Cebaiye (Chinese Arborvitae Twig and Leaf) 12 g, Baimaogen (Lalang Grass Rhizome) 30 g, Qiancaogen (Indian Madder Root) 15 g, Zonglupi (Fortune windmillpalm sheath-fibre) 12 g and Danpi (Cortex Moutan) 15 g.

Modification: For high fever and severe, extensive bleeding, Shengshigao (Raw Gypsum) 30 g, Longdancao (Radix Gentianae) 9 g and Zicao (Arnebia Root) 9 g are added to purge fire and dispel heat; if there is abdominal pain and hemafecia, Baishao (White Peony Alba) 12 g, Gancao (Liquorice Root) 9 g, Wulingzhi (Faeces Trogopterorum) 9 g (wrapped during decoction), Puhuang (Pollen Typhae) 9 g, Muxiang (Common Aucklandia Root) 6 g and Diyu (Garden Burnet Root) 12 g are used to stop pain, activate blood, regulate qi and stop bleeding.

## 2. Exuberance of fire due to yin deficiency

Treatment principle: Nourishing yin to bring down fire, calming the collaterals to stop bleeding.

Prescription and herbs: (Mainly) Qiangen Powder.

Qiancaogen (Indian Madder Root) 15 g, Huangqin (Baical Skullcap Root) 9 g, Ejiao (Donkey-hide Glue) 9 g, Cebaiye (Chinese Arborvitae Twig and Leaf) 12 g, Shengdi (Dried Rehmannia Root) 15 g and Gancao (Liquorice Root) 6 g.

Modification: If there is apparent hectic fever and night sweats, Xuanshen (Figwort Root) 12 g, Guiban (Tortoise Shell) 9 g, Nuzhenzi (Glossy Privet Fruit) 12 g and Huanliancao (Ecliptae Herba) 12 g are added to reinforce the action of nourishing yin.

## 3. Failure of qi to control blood

Treatment principle: Nourishing qi to arrest bleeding.

Prescription and herbs: Modified Guipi Decoction.

Huangqi (Milkvetch Root) 15 g, Danggui (Chinese Angelica) 10 g, Baizhu (Largehead Atractylodes Rhizome) 10 g, Dangshen (Radix Codonopsis) 12 g, Muxiang (Common Aucklandia Root) 6 g, Yuanzhi (Thinleaf Milkwort Root) 3 g, Suanzaoren (Spine Date Seed) 9 g, Longyanrou (Longan Aril) 9 g, Zhigancao (Stir-baked Liquorice Root) 6 g, Zonglutan (Crinis Trachycarpi) 9 g, Xianhecao (Hairyvein Agrimonia Herb) 30 g and Dazao (Chinese Date) 7 dates.

Modification: If there is kidney deficiency with weakness and soreness of the waist and knees, nocturnal emission, impotence, or irregular menstruation, Shanzhuyu (Asiatic Cornelian Cherry Fruit) 9 g, Tusizi (Dodder Seed) 12 g, Chuanduan (Shichuan Radix Dipsaci) 12 g and Lujiaojiao (Deerhorn Glue) 9 g are added to nourish the kidneys and supplement the essence.

## Chinese Patent Medicine

1. Fufang Taipan Tablet: 4 tablets for each dose, 3 times a day.
2. Guipi Pill: 10 pills for each dose, 3 times a day.

## Simple and Handy Prescriptions

1. Shengshigao (Gypsum) 30 g, Huangbai (Amur Cork-tree) 15 g, Wubeizi (Chinese Gall) 15 g and Ercha (Black Catechu) 6 g are well decocted and then used to rinse the mouth for 5~10 minutes each day. This is used to treat peliosis with relatively severe bleeding gums.
2. Dazao (Chinese Date) 50 dates and Baimaogen (Lalang Grass Rhizome) 30 g are boiled in water, portioned out and taken at 3 different times within a day. This is used to treat the chronic type of this disease.

## Other Therapies

Dietary therapy:

(1) Ouzao Jelly: Dazao (Chinese Date) and Oujie (Lotus Rhizome Node) are mixed in a ratio of 4 to 1 with cane sugar and water into a jelly-like material, which is taken daily to supplement blood as well as arrest bleeding.

(2) Maogen Potion: Baimaogen (Lalang Grass Rhizome) 15 g, Huashengyi (Peanut Coating) 30 g and white sugar are decocted to make tea, with the function of cooling blood to stop bleeding.

## Cautions and Advice

1. This disease should be diagnosed and promptly treated to prevent visceral bleeding or other life-threatening conditions.
2. The acute type of this disease should be addressed with Western medicine, whereas the chronic one can be treated by combining Western medicine with TCM, so as to enhance the therapeutic effects.
3. It is advisable for patients to consume fresh vegetables and fruits, as well as nutritious and easily digestible foods, with the exception of spicy or stomach-irritating ones.

## Daily Exercises

1. Describe the clinical characteristics of idiopathic thrombocytopenic purpura.
2. Recall the treatment principles, methods, prescriptions and herbs for idiopathic thrombocytopenic purpura due to exuberant fire and deficient yin.

# Anaphylactoid Purpura

# Week 9: Friday

Anaphylactoid purpura is an allergic disorder of the blood capillaries, clinically characterized by skin petechia and ecchymosis appearing in crops and distributed symmetrically over the extensor aspect of the limbs and buttocks; abdominal pain or joint swelling and pain are also very common. This disease is caused by the allergic reaction of the body to some irritant substances, which leads to the increase in permeability and friability of the capillary wall. It is commonly observed in children and young people. Clinically there are five types of this disease: skin type (the most common one), abdomen type, joint type, kidney type and mixed type. If properly diagnosed and treated, it can have a favorable prognosis. In TCM, it is believed that anaphylactoid purpura is closely associated with "bleeding syndrome", "macular eruption" and "muscular bleeding".

## Etiology and Pathology

TCM holds that anaphylactoid purpura is mostly caused by abundance of blood heat complicated by invasion of the six abnormal climatic factors, the combat among which drives blood rampant; another cause is pre-existing exuberance of fire and deficiency of yin complicated by invasion of the exogenous pathogenic factors and impairment by some foods or drugs, which results in stagnation of pathogenic heat in the vessels, rampancy of blood circulation and the presence of maculae.

The pathological changes of this disease are discussed as follows: The patient has heat in the blood and then contracts pathogenic wind-fire and damp-toxins, which invade the ying-blood phase and damage the vessels, leading to extravasation; furthermore, if the patient has an improper diet, there will be dysfunction of the spleen and stomach in transportation and transformation, which brings about endogenous production of damp-heat and extravasation of blood; moreover, when deficiency of yin produces exuberant fire, the collaterals, or vessels, may become malnourished and scorched, predisposing the patient to extravasation in the end; finally, deficient spleen qi fails to control the circulation of blood, giving rise to maculae because of the deviated blood.

## Diagnostic Key Points

1. A history of upper respiratory tract infection 1~3 weeks before occurrence.
2. Presence of purpuras in different sizes distributed symmetrically on the lower limbs or buttocks, with occasional paroxysmal abdominal pain, joint swelling and pain, or kidney lesion.
3. Blood test: Normal platelet count and clotting time; positive Leede's test.
4. Routine urianlysis: Possible presence of proteins and red blood cells, or positive result of fecal occult blood test and renal inadequacy.
5. Normal bone marrow image.

## Syndrome Differentiation

### 1. Accumulation of toxic heat

Symptoms: Sudden onset, red complexion, ecchymosis of the skin mucosa which covers large areas in severe cases with bright color and sensation of scorching heat, a bitter taste and dry sensation in the mouth, thirst, constipation, yellowish urine, or nosebleed, gum bleeding and vexation; red and purple tongue with yellow coating and slippery and rapid pulse.

Analysis of symptoms: Abundant toxic heat invades the ying-blood and is marked by a red complexion, feverish body, dry mouth and disturbed mind; pathogenic heat consumes the genuine yin and disturbs the ying-blood, leading to extravasation marked by presence of ecchymosis, or nosebleed and bleeding gums; the deep-red tongue with yellow coating and the slippery and rapid pulse are due to accumulation of toxic heat.

### 2. Deficiency of yin producing heat in the interior

Symptoms: Large area of peliosis in a bright color occurring at times or persistently, commonly with bleeding gums, nosebleed, dizziness, restlessness, slight fever, night sweats, dry and bitter mouth, palpitations, insomnia, feverish sensations over the five centers (the palms, the soles and the heart); red tongue with little coating and thin and rapid pulse.

Analysis of symptoms: Deficiency of yin gives rise to exuberant deficient fire, which damages the vessels and leads to peliosis, or bleeding gums and nosebleed; depleted water fails to coordinate the fire, bringing about disturbance of heart fire, with such signs as vexation, insomnia and feverish sensation over the five centers; deficiency of yin produces exuberant fire, which drives the body fluid outside, presenting as slight fever and night sweats; the reddish tongue with scanty coating and the thin and rapid pulse are symptomatic of exuberant fire with insufficiency of yin-fluid.

### 3. Deficiency of the spleen with oozing blood

Symptoms: Repeated occurrences, long-term chronic skin ecchymosis in slightly dark color, pale complexion, panting with no desire to talk, bland taste in the mouth, poor appetite, occasional presence of loose stools, palpitations and shortness of breath; slightly red and enlarged tongue with white greasy coating and thin and deficient pulse.

Analysis of symptoms: Deficient spleen qi fails to control the blood and is marked by repetitive occurrence of skin ecchymosis that is a slightly dark color and long lasting; deficient qi and blood fail to nourish the bones, leading to pale complexion, panting, reluctance to speak, palpitations and shortness of breath; a deficient spleen fails to transport and transform water and food, resulting in a bland flavor in the mouth, poor appetite and the occasional presence of loose stools; the slightly red and enlarged tongue with white and greasy coating and the thin and deficient pulse are attributable to deficiency of the spleen and blood.

## Differential Treatment

### 1. Accumulation of toxic heat

Treatment principle: Dispelling heat and cooling blood, relieving toxins and resolving macula.

Prescription and herbs: Modified Qingwen Baidu Potion.

Shengshigao (Raw Gypsum) 30 g, Shengdi (Dried Rehmannia Root) 15 g, Xuanshen (Figwort Root) 12 g, Zhuye (Henon Bamboo Leaf) 9 g, Zhimu

(Common Anemarrhena Rhizome) 12 g, Chishao (Red Peony Root) 12 g, Danpi (Cortex Moutan) 15 g, Lianqiao (Weeping Forsythia Capsule) 15 g, Huanglian (Golden Thread) 3 g, Huangqin (Baical Skullcap Root) 15 g, Zicao (Arnebia Root) 15 g and Chaohuaimi (Stir-baked Flos sophorae Immaturus) 12 g.

Modification: If there is gastrointestinal peliosis with vomiting, Banxia (Pinellia Tuber) 9 g can be added to harmonize the stomach and check vomiting; for peliosis with abdominal pain, Baishao (White Peony Alba) 15 g can be added to stop pain; for hemafecia, Chaodiyu (Fried Garden Burnet Root) 15 g is added to cool blood and arrest bleeding.

## 2. Deficiency of yin producing heat in the interior

Treatment principle: Nourishing yin and dispelling heat, cooling blood to stop bleeding.

Prescription and herbs: Modified Qiangen Powder and Erzhi Pill.

Qiancaogen (Indian Madder Root) 10 g, Huangqin (Baical Skullcap Root) 12 g, Cebaiye (Chinese Arborvitae Twig and Leaf) 9 g, Shengdi (Dried Rehmannia Root) 15 g, Ejiao (Donkey-hide Glue) 9 g (melted by heat), Nuzhenzi (Glossy Privet Fruit) 12 g, Huanliancao (Ecliptae Herba) 15 g and Gancao (Liquorice Root) 6 g.

Modification: If there is nosebleed or bloody urine, Jiaoshanzhi (Charred Cape Jasmine Fruit) 9 g, Daji (Japanese Thistle Herb) 9 g and Xiaoji (Field Thistle Herb) 9 g are added to dispel heat and stop bleeding; for severe dryness in the mouth, Shihu (Dendrobium) 15 g and Baimaogen (Lalang Grass Rhizome) 15 g are added to dispel heat and nourish yin.

## 3. Deficiency of the spleen with oozing blood

Treatment principle: Replenishing qi to invigorate the spleen, controlling blood circulation to stop bleeding.

Prescription and herb: Modified Bazhen Decoction.

Dangshen (Radix Codonopsis) 12 g, Huangqi (Milkvetch Root) 15 g, Baizhu (Largehead Atractylodes Rhizome) 12 g, Danggui (Chinese Angelica) 9 g,

Fuling (Indian Bread) 12 g, Shudi (Prepared Rhizome of Rehmannia) 12 g, Baishao (White Peony Alba) 15 g, Chuanxiong (Szechwan Lovage Rhizome) 5 g, Chenpi (Dried Tangerine Peel) 6 g, Xianhecao (Hairyvein Agrimonia Herb) 15 g, Dazao (Chinese Date) 7 dates and Gancao (Liquorice Root) 6 g.

Modification: If there is weakness and soreness of the waist and knees, Shanzhuyu (Asiatic Cornelian Cherry Fruit) 9 g, Tusizi (Dodder Seed) 12 g and Chuanduan (Shichuan Radix Dipsaci) 12 g are added to nourish the kidney qi; if there is a large area of peliosis, it is advisable to add Zicao (Arnebia Root) 12 g, Diyu (Garden Burnet Root) 12 g and Zonglutan (Crinis Trachycarpi) 12 g so as to stop bleeding, resolve stasis and dissipate macula.

## Chinese Patent Medicine

1. Guipi Pill, 12 pills for each dose, 3 times a day.
2. Erzhi Pil, 6 g for each dose, 3 times a day.

## Simple and Handy Prescriptions

1. Zicaogen (Arnebia Root) 20~30 g is boiled in water, separated into 2 portions and taken at 2 different times within a day to cool blood and stop bleeding.
2. Hongzao (Red Date) 20 dates are decocted to make soup. It can be regularly taken to nourish the blood and stop bleeding.

## Other Therapies

External therapy: A proper amount of fetus hair is burned into ashes, which is blown into the nose to arrest bleeding and dissipate macula.

Dietary therapy:

(1) Guizaojian: Hongzao (Red Date) 10 dates and Guirou (Tortoise Meat) 200 g are decocted together. It is administered once a day for nourishing yin and supplementing blood. This is applicable to those with yin deficiency.

(2) Sanxian Potion: Fresh lotus root (with the joints) 100 g, fresh reed rhizome 100 g and fresh imperatae rhizome 100 g are decocted in water. It is served as tea, with the function of cooling blood to stop bleeding.

## Cautions and Advice

1. The key to treating and preventing this disease from recurring is to find and address the causative factors. Re-contact with these substances, such as suspicious drugs or food, must be prohibited.
2. Treatment should eliminate the focus of infection and expel intestinal parasites.
3. Patients are advised to keep a light diet and avoid spicy food or seafood.

## Daily Exercises

1. Describe the clinical characteristics of anaphylactoid purpura.
2. Recall the etiological factors of anaphylactoid purpura.
3. Explain how purpura due to blood heat resulting from deficiency of yin can be treated.

# CHAPTER 7

# Disorders of the Endocrine System

## Hyperthyroidism
## Week 9: Saturday

Hyperthyroidism, or thyroid hyperfunction, is a common endocrine system disease due to excessive secretion of thyroid hormone caused by various etiological factors, clinically marked by hypermetabolism, nervous excitation, diffuse goiter, or protruding eyes. This disease can afflict any age group, but is more common among those who are 20~40 years old, with females being more susceptible. It has a slow onset and an indefinite date of occurrence. Emotional disorder is the most common predisposing factor for this disease. After 2~3 years of persistent treatment, most patients can recover from the disease gradually, but a few of them have a unfavorable prognosis, with such manifestations as hyperthyroid heart disease, thyroid crisis, or endocrine infiltrative exophthalmos. In TCM, hyperthyreosis is believed to be closely associated with "goiter and tumor", "fright" and "liver fire".

### Etiology and Pathology

TCM holds that thyroid hyperfunction is mainly caused by long-term emotional disorder or innate deficiency of the body and closely related to female development or consumption of yin blood in the liver meridian during lactation.

The pathological changes of this disease are discussed as follows: Stagnation of liver qi leads to accumulation of phlegm in the front of the neck, creating a predisposition to goiter. Stagnation of liver qi produces fire which scorches the liver yin and leads to gastric heat, polypepsia, hyperphagia and emaciation. The liver-wood over-restricts the spleen-earth, resulting in dysfunction of the spleen in its functions of transportation and transformation, with the frequent manifestation of diarrhea. Hyperactivity of liver fire causes exuberance of heart fire, marked by palpitations insomnia and irascibility. Abundant fire consumes the yin-fluid, resulting in exhaustion of liver yin and kidney yin, failure of water (the kidneys) to nourish wood (the liver) and internal stirring of deficient wind, marked by tremors of the limbs. When the disease develops into the late stage, the heat manifestations will gradually disappear and be replaced by deficiency of qi and yin.

## Diagnostic Key Points

1. Chief clinical manifestations: Palpitations, intolerance of heat, profuse sweating, bulimia, emaciation, tremors of the fingers, weariness, agitation, diarrhea, scanty menstrual blood volume or even amenorrhea in females and impotence in males; diffusive swelling of the thyroid and protrusion of both eyes to varying degrees; tachycardia, premature beat or atrial fibrillation in some patients.
2. There is an increase in thyroid iodine uptake, blood serum γT3 (reverse triiodothyronine) and FTFT4 (tetraiodothyronine). Serum TGA or TMA is conducive to the identification of etiological factors, while nuclear magnetic resonance can rule out the possibility of thyroid adenoma and other conditions marked by swelling of the thyroid gland.

## Syndrome Differentiation

### 1. Liver qi stagnation transforming into fire

Symptoms: Goiter, protruding eyes with clear and bright vision, polyorexia, dry mouth with thirst, loose stools, irascibility, intolerance of heat, profuse sweating, red face and palpitations; red tongue with thin and yellow coating, rapid and taut pulse. This is a relatively common pattern.

Analysis of symptoms: Emotional disorder leads to the transformation of stagnated liver qi into fire, which accumulates in the liver meridian and combines with phlegm, presenting as goiter and protruding eyes with clear and bright vision; liver fire scorches the stomach yin, bringing about gastric heat, polyorexia and dry mouth with thirst; liver qi over-restricts the spleen, leading to dysfunction in transportation and transformation, as characterized by loose stools; liver fire flames internally, with such manifestations as irascibility, intolerance of heat and profuse sweating; upward disturbance of liver yang with hyperactivity of heart fire and liver fire results in a flushed face and palpitations; the red tongue with thin and yellow coating and the rapid and taut pulse are symptomatic of blazing liver fire.

## 2. Hyperactivity of yang due to yin deficiency

Symptoms: Dizziness, blurred vision, tremors of hands, feverish dysphoria, profuse sweating, dry mouth, polydipsia, hyperphagia, emaciation, palpitations, insomnia, dreaminess, goiter and protruding eyes; red or deep-red tongue with scanty or thin and yellow coating and thin and rapid pulse. This pattern is extremely common.

Analysis of symptoms: Liver fire consumes the liver yin and kidney yin, leading to failure of water to promote wood, and upward disturbance of deficient yang, with such manifestations as dizziness and blurred vision; the deficient wind stirs in the interior, causing tremors of the hands; deficiency of yin produces internal heat, presenting as feverish dysphoria and profuse sweating; deficiency of yin with gastric heat is responsible for hyperphagia and polydipsia; heat consumes the essence and blood, leading to malnutrition of the body, marked by emaciation; heat disturbs the heart spirit, with such signs as palpitations, insomnia and dreaminess; stagnation of liver qi with accumulation of phlegm is manifested as goiter and protruding eyes; the red or deep-red tongue with scanty or thin and yellow coating and thin and rapid pulse are all manifestations of hyperactive yang due to deficiency of yin.

## 3. Deficiency of qi and yin

Symptoms: Uneasy sensation, shortness of breath, severe palpitations, insomnia, dizziness, waist soreness, dry mouth, profuse sweating, listlessness, loose stools and persistent swelling of the neck with goiters; white and thin tongue coating and thin or thin, rapid and feeble pulse. This pattern is seen at the late stage of this disease.

Analysis of symptoms: Prolonged affliction of this disease leads to deficiency of qi and yin, marked by a dry mouth and profuse sweating; deficiency of the lung qi and heart qi is manifested as uneasiness and shortness of breath; deficient heart blood fails to contain the heart spirit, with such signs as severe palpitations and insomnia; deficiency of the liver and kidneys is responsible for dizziness and waist soreness; the deficient spleen is impaired in promoting digestion, presenting as listlessness and loose stools; deficient qi fails to dissipate the phlegmatic accumulation, so there is persistent existence of goiters; the white and thin tongue coating and the thin or thin, rapid and feeble pulse are attributable to deficiency of qi and yin with possible retention of deficient heat.

## Differential Treatment

### 1. Liver qi stagnation transforming into fire

Treatment principle: Clearing the liver and purging the stomach, dissipating the stagnation and resolving goiter.

Prescription and herbs: Modified Longdan Xiegan Decoction.

Longdancao (Radix Gentianae) 6 g, Shanzhizi (Cape Jasmine Fruit) 9 g, Chaihu (Chinese Thorowax Root) 9 g, Huangqin (Baical Skullcap Root) 9 g, Huanglian (Golden Thread) 3 g, Chuanmutong (Armand Clematis Stem) 5 g, Zexie (Oriental Waterplantain Rhizome) 15 g, Danpi (Cortex Moutan) 9 g, Shengdi (Dried Rehmannia Root) 12 g, Xiakucao (Common Selfheal Fruit-Spike) 15 g and Beimu (Fritillariae Tuber) 9 g.

Modification: For dry mouth with thirst, Shihu (Dendrobium) 15 g and Shashen (Root of Straight Ladybell) 15 g can added to nourish the stomach yin; if there are loose stools, Shanyao (Common Yan Rhizome) 15 g and Baibiandou (White Hyacinth Bean) 15 g can be used to invigorate the spleen and check diarrhea.

## 2. Hyperactivity of yang due to yin deficiency

Treatment principle: Nourishing yin to bring down fire, calming the heart to extinguish wind.

Prescription and herbs: Modified Tainwang Buxin Decoction.

Shengdi (Dried Rehmannia Root) 15 g, Xuanshen (Figwort Root) 9 g, Maidong (Dwarf Lilyturf Tuber) 9 g, Zhimu (Common Anemarrhena Rhizome) 9 g, Wuweizi (Chinese Magnolivine Fruit) 6 g, Danshen (Radix Salviae Miltiorrhiae) 15 g, Baiziren (Chinese Arborvitae Kernel) 9 g, Yuanzhi (Thinleaf Milkwort Root) 4.5 g, Longchi (Fossilia Dentis Mastodi) 30 g, Zhenzhumu (Nacre) 30 g, Baishao (White Peony Alba) 15 g and Gouteng (Gambir Plant) 18 g (decocted later).

Modification: For irascibility, Longdancao (Radix Gentianae) 6 g and Chaihu (Chinese Thorowax Root) 9 g can added to clear the liver and purge fire; if there is dizziness and blurred vision, Gouqizi (Barbary Wolfberry Fruit) 15 g, Shihu (Dendrobium) 15 g and Juhua (Chrysanthemum Flower) 9 g are added to clear the liver and improve vision; for obvious tremors of the hands, the amounts of Baishao (White Peony Alba) and Gouteng (Gambir Plant) can be increased and Baijili (Tribulus Terrestris) 12 g and Guiban (Tortoise Shell) 12 g are added to nourish yin and extinguish wind; for persistent swelling of the neck, Beimu (Fritillariae Tuber) 9 g and Muli (Oyster Shell) 30 g can be added to relieve swelling and dissipate stagnation; for protruding eyes with clear and bright vision, Qingxiangzi (Feather Cockscomb Seed) 12 g and Xiakucao (Common Selfheal Fruit-Spike) 12 g can be added to dispel liver fire, dissolve phlegm and dissipate stagnation.

## 3. Deficiency of qi and yin

Treatment principle: Replenishing qi and nourishing yin, dissipating the stagnation and resolving goiter.

Prescription and herbs: Supplementary Shengmai Powder.

Taizishen (Heterophylly Falsesatarwort Root) 15 g, Maidong (Dwarf Lilyturf Tuber) 9 g, Wuweizi (Chinese Magnolivine Fruit) 6 g, Baizhu (Largehead Atractylodes Rhizome) 9 g, Baishao (White Peony Alba) 12 g,

Shanyao (Common Yan Rhizome) 12 g, Baibiandou (White Hyacinth Bean) 12 g, Suanzaoren (Spine Date Seed) 9 g, Banxia (Pinellia Tuber) 9 g, Beimu (Fritillariae Tuber) 9 g, Muli (Oyster Shell) 30 g and Xiakucao (Common Selfheal Fruit-Spike) 12 g.

Modification: If there is shortness of breath and weariness, Huangqi (Milkvetch Root) 15~30 g can be added to supplement qi and nourish deficiency; for obvious dryness in the mouth, Shihu (Dendrobium) 15 g and Beishashen (Coastal Glehnia Root) 15 g can be added to nourish yin and produce fluid; if there arenight sweats, Fuxiaomai (Blighted Wheat) 15 g can be added to nourish the liver and check sweating; for dizziness and waist soreness, Sangjisheng (Chinese Taxillus Herb) 15 g and Duzhong (Eucommia Bark) 9 g are used to nourish the kidneys and strengthen the waist; for persistent existence of goiter, Huangyaozi (Airpotato Yam) 9 g, Danggui (Chinese Angelica) 9 g, Sanleng (Common Burreed Tuber) 9 g and Ezhu (Zedoray Rhizome) 9 g are used to help activate blood and resolve stasis as well as dissipate stagnation and resolve goiters; for retention of deficient heat with thin and rapid pulse, Zhimu (Common Anemarrhena Rhizome) 9 g and Biejia (Turtle Shell) 9 g can be added to dispel the deficient heat.

## Chinese Patent Medicine

1. Xiaoyao Pill: 6 g for each dose, 3 times a day.
2. Jiaokangling Tablet: 3~5 tablets for each dose, 3 times a day.
3. Zhibo Dihuang Pill: 6 g for each dose, 3 times a day.

## Simple and Handy Prescriptions

Danggui (Chinese Angelica) 9 g, Zhebeimu (Zhejiang Fritillariae Tuber) 9 g and Muli (Oyster Shell) 30 g are decocted in water and then separated into 2 portions and administered at 2 different times within a day. The decoction is used to treat diffusive enlargement of the thyroid. If there is deficiency of yin with hyperactivity of yang, Yuanshen (Kakuda Figwort Root) 12 g can be used. To treat deficiency of qi and yin, Huangqi (Milkvetch Root) 30 g can be added to the previous prescription.

## Other Therapies

Frequency spectrum therapy: The thyroid tissues and Zusanli (ST 36) acupoint are treated by direction radiation of WS frequency spectrum; for those with goiters, the Tiantu (RN 22) acupoint is used in combination; for tachycardia, the Neiguan (PC 6) acupoint is combined; and for insomnia, Yongquan (KI 1) acupoint is treated at the same time.

Dietary therapy:

(1) A Jiayu (Green Turtle), Nuzhenzi (Glossy Privet Fruit) 15 g and Gouqizi (Barbary Wolfberry Fruit) 15 g are steamed with seasoning to taste. This is used to treat hyperthyreosis with deficiency of yin and hyperactivity of yang.
(2) Two squabs, Huangqi (Milkvetch Root) 15 g and Gouqizi (Barbary Wolfberry Fruit) 15 g are stewed with seasoning to taste. This is appropriate for patients in the late stage of hyperthyreosis with deficiency of qi and yin.

## Cautions and Advice

1. This disease must be promptly diagnosed and treated. It should be noted that the antithyroid drugs, irradiated iodine and surgical treatment have their toxic or side effects and thus can only be applicable in certain cases. The combined application of Chinese medicine and Western medicine is highly recommended for the unique advantage of this approach. Nevertheless, the traditionally used Haizao (Seaweed) and Kunbu (Kelp or Tangle) for hyperthyreosis should be restricted in dosage because they contain too much iodine.
2. Patients should avoid the inducing factors of the disease, keep themselves in good spirits, prevent infection and adopt a high-protein, high-calorie diet. Oily and iodine-rich food is restricted.

## Daily Exercises

1. Recall the pathological changes of thyroid hyperfunction.
2. Recall the diagnostic key points of thyroid hyperfunction.
3. Explain how hyperthyroidism due to deficiency of yin with hyperactivity of yang and that due to deficiency of qi and yin can be differentiated and treated.

# Hypothyroidism

# Week 10: Monday

Hypothyroidism is a clinical syndrome caused by decreased metabolic activities of the body due to insufficient synthesis or secretion of thyroid hormone, marked by a pale or sallow complexion, listlessness, sleepiness, apathy, edema, intolerance of cold, poor appetite, abdominal distension, constipation and basal metabolic rate. According to the difference in onset age, the disease is divided into three types: cretinism (which occurs in newborns or fetuses), juvenile hypothyroidism (which occurs in childhood) and adulthood hypothyroidism (which begins from adulthood and mostly in middle-aged females). In severe cases, there may be myxedema coma, which points to an unfavorable prognosis. In TCM, hypothyroidism is believed to be associated with "five kinds of tardy growth in infants", "deficiency consumption" and "edema".

## Etiology and Pathology

TCM holds that this disease is mostly caused by innate deficiency or congenital lack of proper care (which lead to deficiency of the spleen and kidneys); or by surgeries and drugs (which result in impairment of primordial yang, or yang qi of the spleen and kidneys).

The pathological changes are discussed as follows: Innate deficiency with weak primordial yang and inadequate kidney essence, or congenital lack of proper care with deficiency of the spleen and dysfunction in reception and transformation, can lead to poor appetite and constipation; a depleted source for the production of qi and blood may result in anaemia, a lusterless complexion and lassitude; insufficient supplement of kidney essence, brain marrow and primordial spirit often brings about apathy and hypophrenia; deficiency of spleen yang and kidney yang is responsible for retention of water in the skin and muscles, or upward attack on the heart and lungs, marked by palpitations and panting and even depletion of the heart yang and kidney yang, which endangers life.

## Diagnostic Key Points

1. Common symptoms are tardy growth in newborns or infants, poor appetite, abdominal distension, constipation, lethargy, dry and rough skin, bradycardia and hypotension. In middle-aged women, symptoms include edema, intolerance of cold, weariness, lethargy, slow reaction, anaemia, loss of hair and decreased appetite with increased body weight.
2. Reduced basal metabolic rate, increased level of blood cholesterols and markedly decreased thyroid iodine uptake.

## Syndrome Differentiation

### 1. Deficiency of qi and blood

Symptoms: Pale and lusterless complexion, listlessness, palpitations, shortness of breath, dizziness, limb flaccidity, poor appetite, abdominal distension, constipation, hypomnesis and intolerance of cold; pale tongue with thin coating and thin pulse.

Analysis of symptoms: Innate deficiency of endowment and lack of proper congenital care can lead to insufficiency of spleen qi, essence and blood, as well as malnourishment of the skin and muscles, with such signs as listlessness, flaccidity in the limbs and pale complexion; the brain is malnourished and there is inadequacy of marrow, marked by dizziness and hypomnesis; insufficient qi and blood fails to nourish the heart and lungs, bringing about palpitations and shortness of breath; deficiency of the spleen with dysfunction in reception and transformation is responsible for poor appetite, abdominal distension and constipation; deficient yang fails to warm the body, characterized by an intolerance of cold; the pale tongue with thin coating and thin pulse are attributable to deficiency of qi and blood.

### 2. Yang deficiency of the spleen and kidneys

Symptoms: Marked general edema, intolerance of cold, cold limbs, sallow complexion, lassitude, poor appetite, body heaviness, indifference, preference for lying down, hypophrenia, rough skin, loss of hair, weakness and soreness of the waist and knees, impotence, infertility, chest distress, palpitations and panting; pale and enlarged tongue with white coating, thin and deep pulse or tardy and deep pulse.

Analysis of symptoms: Yang deficiency of the spleen and kidneys with indigestion of water and food, retention of water and dampness in the skin and muscles, is marked by poor appetite, body heaviness, preference for lying down and general edema; deficiency of the spleen and kidneys with insufficient supplement of primordial qi, essence, blood, marrow and spirit is manifested as indifference, preference for lying down and hypophrenia; the viscera, skin and muscles are malnourished, marked by the sallow complexion, lassitude, rough skin, loss of hair, or weakness and soreness of the waist and knees; water qi attacks the heart, causing palpitations and panting; decline of fire from the life gate is responsible for impotence and infertility, or cold body and limbs; the pale and enlarged tongue with white coating and the thin and deep pulse or tardy and deep pulse are due to deficiency of spleen yang and kidney yang or general decline of yang.

## Differential Treatment

### 1. Deficiency of qi and blood

Treatment principle: Invigorating qi and nourishing blood, nourishing the spleen and warming the kidneys.

Prescription and herbs: Supplementary Bazhen Decoction.

Danggui (Chinese Angelica) 9 g, Chuanxiong (Szechwan Lovage Rhizome) 9 g, Baishao (White Peony Alba) 12 g, Shudi (Prepared Rhizome of Rehmannia) 12 g, Dangshen (Radix Codonopsis) 15 g, Baizhu (Largehead Atractylodes Rhizome) 9 g, Fuling (Indian Bread) 15 g, Zhigancao (Stir-baked Liquorice Root) 3 g, Huangqi (Milkvetch Root) 30 g, Rougui (Cassia Bark) 3 g (decocted later) and Dazao (Chinese Date) 3 dates.

Modification: If there is severe anaemia, Renshen (Ginseng) 6 g, Ejiao (Donkey-hide Glue) 9 g and Shouwu (Fleeceflower Root) 15 g can be added to reinforce the action of invigorating qi and nourishing blood; for abdominal distension with constipation, Binglang (Areca Seed) 9 g and Zhiqiao (Orange Fruit) 9 g are added to regulate qi and promote defecation; in case of edema, Zhuling (Polyporus) 15 g and Zexie (Oriental Waterplantain Rhizome) 15 g can be added to promote urination and relieve edema.

## 2. Yang deficiency of the spleen and kidneys

Treatment principle: Warming yang to relieve edema, nourishing the spleen and kidneys.

Prescription and herbs: Modified Zhenwu Decoction and Jingui Shenqi Pill.

Shufuzi (Prepared Common Monkshood Daughter) 9 g, Ganjiang (Dried Ginger) 3 g, Baizhu (Largehead Atractylodes Rhizome) 9 g, Fuling (Indian Bread) 12 g, Huangqi (Milkvetch Root) 30 g, Fangji (Fourstamen Stephania Root) 9 g, Zexie (Oriental Waterplantain Rhizome) 15 g, Dafupi (Areca Peel) 9 g, Shudi (Prepared Rhizome of Rehmannia) 12 g, Shanyao (Common Yan Rhizome) 12 g, Shanzhuyu (Asiatic Cornelian Cherry Fruit) 9 g and Rougui (Cassia Bark) 3 g (decocted later).

Modification: To promote urination and relieve edema, Zhuling (Polyporus), Cheqianzi (Plantain Seed), Yiyiren (Coix Seed), Dongguapi (Chinese Waxgourd Peel) and Chenhulu (Aged Bottle-gourd) can be adopted; for chest distress, palpitations and panting, Renshen (Ginseng) 6 g ~15 g, Guizhi (Cassia Twig) 9 g, Yimucao (Motherwort Herb) 30 g and Zelan (Herba Lycopi) 15 g are added to nourish the heart qi, warm the chest yang, activate blood circulation and promote water discharge; if there is weakness and soreness of the waist and knees, Duzhong (Eucommia Bark) 9 g, Chuanduan (Shichuan Radix Dipsaci) 9 g, Sangjisheng (Chinese Taxillus Herb) 15 g and Huainiuxi (Twotoothed Achyranthes Root) 9 g can be added to nourish the kidneys and strengthen the waist; for apathy and hypophrenia, Changpu (Acorus Calamus) 9 g and Yuanzhi (Thinleaf Milkwort Root) 4.5 g are used to dissolve phlegm and activate the spirit.

## Chinese Patent Medicine

1. Guipi Pill: 6 g for each dose, 3 times a day.
2. Jisheng Shengqi Pill or Jingui Shenqi Pill: 6 g for each dose, 3 times a day.

## Simple and Handy Prescriptions

Huangqi (Milkvetch Root) 30 g, Dangshen (Radix Codonopsis) 18 g, Baizhu (Largehead Atractylodes Rhizome) 24 g, Fuling (Indian Bread) 30 g, Zhuling (Polyporus) 30 g, Yinyanghuo (Epimedium Herb) 12 g, Danggui (Chinese Angelica) 9 g, Guizhi (Cassia Twig) 9 g and Dafupi (Areca Peel) 9 g are boiled in water and taken once a day. This decoction is used to treat hypothyroidism with long-term edema.

## Other Therapies

External therapy: The medicinal powders of Rougui (Cassia Bark) and Wuzhuyu (Medicinal Evodia Fruit) are blended with fresh ginger juice to make a paste which is applied on the Shenque (RN 8) acupoint every other day. This is used to treat hypothyroidism with edema due to yang deficiency.

Dietary therapy: Huangqi (Milkvetch Root) 50 g and Shouwu (Fleeceflower Root) 15 g are decocted in water and then the decoction (without gruffs) is used to make soup by adding a blackfish, wine, salt and ginger. This is used to treat hypothyroidism with edema and anaemia; dog meat 500 g, common yan rhizome 250 g and desired amounts of fennel, cinnamon bark, ginger, salt and alcohol are well cooked in an earthenware pot. This can be used to treat hypothyroidism with soreness in the waist, cold in the limbs and deep-slow pulse.

## Cautions and Advice

1. This disease, marked by a gradual development, is treated with Western medicine in modern society. However, some patients are intolerant of the therapy, especially the elderly who also have heart diseases. In this

sense, the combined use of Chinese medicine and Western medicine, or the single application of TCM, is highly recommended. For patients with mild symptoms, it is inadvisable to use large doses of warm, dry and yang-invigorating herbs. Myxedema coma, occurring at the most critical stage of this disease, is characterized by a high mortality rate and should be treated primarily with Western medicine.

2. Endemical iodine-deficiency, surgery, radiotherapy and improper application of drugs are common risk factors of this disease and should be avoided.

3. Patients should avoid overstrain, regulate their emotions, supplement their diet with nutrients, refrain from consumption o oily or cold foods and take precautions to prevent themselves from catching the common cold and/or wound infections.

## Daily Exercises

1. Concisely describe the etiology and pathology of hypothyroidism.
2. Explain how hypothyroidism due to yang deficiency of the spleen and kidneys can be diagnosed and treated.

# Benign Thyroid Tumor

# Week 10: Tuesday

Benign thyroid tumor refers to the various types of tumors besides thyroid carcinoma, including thyroid adenoma, thyroid cyst, toxic adenoma and nodular goiter. It is marked by nodules in the neck and, in severe cases, an oppressive sensation in the neck or even unsmooth respiration and hoarse voice. Thyroid adenoma may afflict people of any age, especially females. It has a relatively slow onset and in some cases the thyroid adenoma may retrogress into thyroid cyst, turn into thyroid toxic adenoma, or even progress into malignant tumor. In TCM, benign thyroid tumor is considered to be associated with "goiter and tumor".

## Etiology and Pathology

TCM holds that benign thyroid tumor is caused by internal emotional disorders or exogenous pathogenic factors (such as radiation injury), leading to dysfunction of the liver and spleen, accumulation of qi, phlegm and blood stasis.

The pathological changes of this disease are discussed as follows: The emotional disorders such as excessive worry, contemplation and anger, or invasion of pathogenic factors into the liver meridian, may lead to failure of the liver to promote free flow of qi and the resultant stagnation of qi movements. Liver-wood over-restricts the spleen-earth, bringing about dysfunction of the spleen in transportation and transformation and accumulation of water, dampness, qi and phlegm in the anterior portion of the neck, manifesting as goiters or tumors. In the long run they may disturb the blood phase and become increasingly larger, thereby obstructing the airways, with such signs as unsmooth respiration and hoarse voice.

## Diagnostic Key Points

1. This disease can generally be confirmed if there is a presence of lumps in the thyroid regions with slow growth, distinct margin, smooth surface, relatively soft or hard texture, absence of tenderness, up-down motion during deglutition and no lymphadenectasis.

2. The functions of the thyroid gland are generally normal, with manifestation of cold nodules on radionuclide scanning. Thyroid antibody test, thyroid 131I intake test, thyroid B-ultrasonic test and thyroid biopsy can be conducive to the differentiation between this disease and other types of thyroid enlargement.

## Syndrome Differentiation

### 1. Stagnation of qi with accumulation of phlegm

Symptoms: Soft nodules in the neck without tenderness, a distending sensation in the neck during emotional disturbance, white tongue coating and soggy, taut or slippery pulse.

Analysis of symptoms: The liver promotes free flow of qi, while the spleen governs transportation and transformation, so if there are emotional disorders, or invasion of pathogenic factors into the liver, there will be stagnation of liver qi and over-restriction of liver-wood into the spleen-earth, resulting in dysfunction of the spleen in transportation and transformation; with the malfunction of the spleen, there will be accumulation of water, dampness, phlegm and qi into soft nodules without tenderness; the goiters are present in the anterior portion of the neck, so there is a distending sensation in the neck; the white tongue coating and the soggy, taut or slippery pulse are attributable to stagnation of qi.

### 2. Accumulation of phlegm with blood stasis

Symptoms: Relatively hard nodules in the neck without tenderness, or even unsmooth respiration or deglutition, dark red tongue with occasional ecchymosis, white coating and deep-unsmooth pulse.

Analysis of symptoms: Prolonged stagnation of phlegm and qi brings about blood stasis and the presence of relatively hard goiters in the anterior region of the neck; because the stagnation of qi is the leading cause, there is no pain; accumulation of phlegm and blood stasis obstructs the movements of the lung qi and stomach qi, leading to hoarse voice or even unsmooth respiration or deglutition; the dark red tongue with occasional ecchymosis, the white coating and the deep-unsmooth pulse are all symptomatic of accumulated phlegm and blood.

## Differential Treatment

### 1. Stagnation of qi with accumulation of phlegm

Treatment principle: Regulating qi and relieving depression, dissolving phlegm and dissipating stagnation.

Prescription and herbs: Modified Sihai Shuyu Pill.

Haizao (Seaweed) 30 g, Haidai (Sea Tangle) 30 g, Haigafen (Clam shell Powder) 6 g, Haipiaoxiao (Cuttlebone) 30 g, Kunbu (Kelp or Tangle) 30 g, Beimu (Fritillariae Tuber) 10 g, Muxiang (Common Aucklandia Root) 6 g, Chenpi (Dried Tangerine Peel) 6 g, Qingpi (Green Tangerine Peel) 6 g and Yujin (Turmeric Root Tuber) 12 g.

Modification: If there is vexation and irascibility, Danpi (Cortex Moutan) 9 g and Zhizi (Cape Jasmine Fruit) 9 g can be added to clear the liver and purge fire; for reduced food intake and loose stools, Dangshen (Radix Codonopsis) 12 g, Chaobaizhu (Fried Largehead Atractylodes Rhizome) 12 g and Shanyao (Common Yan Rhizome) 12 g are added to invigorate the spleen and stop diarrhea.

### 2. Accumulation of phlegm with blood stasis

Treatment principle: Dissolving phlegm and regulating qi, dissipating stasis and softening hard nodules.

Prescription and herbs: Modified Haizao Yuhu Decoction.

Haizao (Seaweed) 30 g, Kunbu (Kelp or Tangle) 30 g, Xiakucao (Common Selfheal Fruit-Spike) 15 g, Banxia (Pinellia Tuber) 9 g, Chenpi (Dried Tangerine Peel) 6 g, Qingpi (Green Tangerine Peel) 6 g, Beimu (Fritillariae Tuber) 9 g, Danggui (Chinese Angelica) 9 g, Chuanxiong (Szechwan Lovage Rhizome) 9 g, Sanleng (Common Burreed Tuber) 15 g, Ezhu (Zedoray Rhizome) 15 g and Sheshecao (Herba Hedyotis Diffusae) 30 g.

Modification: For relatively hard nodules, Taoren (Peach Seed) 9 g and Chuanshanjia (Pangolin Scale) 9 g can be added to reinforce the action of breaking stasis and dispersing stagnation.

## Chinese Patent Medicine

1. Xiakucao Paste: 1 spoon for each dose, 3 times a day.
2. Xiaoying Wuhai Pill: 3 g for each dose, 3 times a day.

## Simple and Handy Prescriptions

Xiakucao (Common Selfheal Fruit-Spike) 30 g, Xuanshen (Figwort Root) 10 g, Beimu (Fritillariae Tuber) 10 g and Muli (Oyster Shell) 30 g are boiled in water and then taken twice a day. It is used to treat thyroid adenoma.

## Other Therapies

Dietary therapy:

(1) Sea tangle 50 g and beancurd 250 g are used to make soup with some seasonings.
(2) Acaleph 200 g is dressed with sauces and taken un-warmed.

## Cautions and Advice

1. If there is enlargement of the thyroid, medical diagnosis should be sought at once, regardless of the texture and the age of the patient. If it is confirmed as thyroid tumor, the surgical treatment should be performed as early as possible. As for the benign tumors, proper therapies must be formulated to be consistent with the specific conditions. For thyroid adenoma or cyst, it is advisable to use traditional Chinese medicine.
2. Patients should avoid radiation injury from their childhood, keep themselves in good spirits and refrain from consuming fatty, greasy and sweet foods.
3. They should also go for periodic health checks to ascertain the pathological changes of the disease.

## Daily Exercises

1. Recall the etiological factors of benign thyroid tumor.
2. Recall the diagnostic key points of benign thyroid tumor.
3. Explain how benign thyroid tumor can be treated based on syndrome differentiation.

# Subacute Thyroiditis
# Week 10: Wednesday

There are three types of thyroiditis: acute purulent thyroiditis, subacute thyroiditis and chronic thyroiditis. Clinically, the second and the third one are more common. In this section, we will introduce subacute thyroiditis.

Subacute thyroiditis refers to the inflammation of the thyroid gland due to invasion of viruses or virus-induced allergy, clinically characterized by acute infection of the upper respiratory tract, with diffusive enlargement of the thyroid gland, or the presence of hard nodules only in the thyroid region. There is generally hyperthyroidism in the early stage, transient hypothyroidism in the middle stage and gradual recovery in the late stage. This disease mainly afflicts female patients between 20~30 years of age. It is a self-limiting disease, so there can be a favorable prognosis in most cases despite its recurrent nature. In TCM, subacute thyroiditis is believed to be closely associated with "thyroid swelling" and "heat disorder".

## Etiology and Pathology

TCM holds that subacute thyroiditis is caused by pathogenic fire and heat, or by emotional disorder.

The pathological changes are discussed as follows: pathogenic fire and heat invade the body, leading to accumulation of toxic heat in the anterior portion of the neck; in addition, emotional disorder gives rise to stagnation of liver qi which transforms into fire and scorches the fluid into phlegm, bringing about an accumulation of phlegm and heat in the neck. If the toxic heat or phlegmatic heat further consumes the yin fluid, there will be such syndromes as internal disturbance of deficient heat with deficiency of yin and abundance of fire.

## Diagnostic Key Points

1. Sudden onset, a history of pharyngitis or upper respiratory tract infection, marked swelling and pain in the thyroid region, with fever and hyperthyroidism. In mild cases, there is only the appearance of hard nodules in the thyroid region, without other symptoms.

2. Inefficient thyroid iodine uptake, temporary rising in the level of serum protein-bound iodine, increased basal metabolic rate, accelerated blood sedimentation, elevated level of serum globulin and marked decrease in thyroid 131I intake.

## Syndrome Differentiation

### 1. Abundance of toxic heat

Symptoms: Sudden onset, ardent fever and chills, headache, sore throat, swelling and pain in the neck, slightly red skin; red tongue with thin and yellow coating and floating and rapid pulse.

Analysis of symptoms: Pathogenic fire and heat invade the skin and muscles, leading to intense combat between the healthy qi and pathogenic factors, this is marked by ardent fever and chills, headache and sore throat; toxic heat accumulates in the neck, with such manifestations as swelling, pain and redness of the skin; the red tongue with thin and yellow coating and the floating and rapid pulse are due to accumulation of fire, toxins and heat in the skin and muscles.

### 2. Liver qi stagnation transforming into fire

Symptoms: Swollen and painful neck, palpitations, irascibility, profuse sweating, tremors of hands, a bitter taste in the mouth, thirst and constipation; red tongue with yellow coating or yellow greasy coating and rapid and taut pulse.

Analysis of symptoms: Emotional disorder leads to stagnated liver qi, which transforms into fire and scorches the body fluid into phlegm, bringing about accumulation of phlegm and heat in the neck, with such signs as pain and swelling in the neck; stagnated fire of the liver and gallbladder disturbs the heart spirit, this is marked by palpitations and irascibility; heat consumes the body fluid, bringing about the bitter taste in the mouth, thirst and constipation; rampancy of internal heat is responsible for profuse sweating; liver fire impairs yin, which further gives rise to a stirring of internal wind, characterized by tremors of the hands; the red tongue with yellow coating or yellow greasy coating and the rapid and taut pulse are all attributable to the transformation of stagnated liver qi into fire or mixture of phlegm and heat.

## Differential Treatment

### 1. Abundance of toxic heat

Treatment principle: Dispersing wind and dispelling heat, eliminating toxins and relieving swelling.

Prescription and herbs: Modified Puji Xiaodu Potion.

Huangqin (Baical Skullcap Root) 12 g, Huanglian (Golden Thread) 5 g, Banlange (Isatis Root) 30 g, Lianqiao (Weeping Forsythia Capsule) 12 g, Niubangzi (Great Burdock Achene) 9 g, Xuanshen (Figwort Root) 9 g, Jiegeng (Platycodon Root) 6 g, Shengma (Rhizoma Cimicifugae) 6 g, Chaihu (Chinese Thorowax Root) 9 g, Jiangcan (Stiff Silkworm) 9 g, Xiakucao (Common Selfheal Fruit-Spike) 15 g and Beimu (Fritillariae Tuber) 12 g.

Modification: If there is high fever, Shigao (Gypsum) 30 g (decocted earlier), Zhimu (Common Anemarrhena Rhizome) 9 g and Shanzhi (Cape Jasmine Fruit) 9 g are added to reinforce the action of dispelling heat; for constipation, Quangualou (Snakegourd Fruit) 15 g and Xuanmingfen (Exsiccated Sodium Sulfate) 3 g are added to dispel heat and dredge the intestines.

### 2. Liver qi stagnation transforming into fire

Treatment principle: Soothing the liver and purging heat, dissolving phlegm and dissipating stagnation.

Prescription and herbs: Modified Longdan Xiegan Deoction.

Longdancao (Radix Gentianae) 6 g, Zhizi (Cape Jasmine Fruit) 9 g, Chaihu (Chinese Thorowax Root) 9 g, Huangqin (Baical Skullcap Root) 9 g, Shengdi (Dried Rehmannia Root) 15 g, Chishao (Red Peony Root) 15 g, Danpi (Cortex Moutan) 9 g, Zexie (Oriental Waterplantain Rhizome) 12 g, Zhebeimu (Fritillariae Tuber) 15 g, Huangyaozi (Airpotato Yam) 9 g and Xiakucao (Common Selfheal Fruit-Spike) 15 g.

Modification: If there is distension and fullness in the chest and hypochondria as well as irascibility, Chuanlianzi (Szechwan Chinaberry Fruit) 9 g and Yujin (Turmeric Root Tuber) 9 g are added to reinforce the action of soothing the liver and regulating qi; for palpitations, profuse sweating and apparent tremors of the hands, Chaozaoren (Semen Ziziphi Spinosae) 9 g, Maidong (Dwarf Lilyturf Tuber) 12 g, Duanlongmu (Calcined Fossilia Ossis Mastodi) 30 g and Baishao (White Peony Alba) 15 g are added to nourish the heart and liver, tranquilize the heart and extinguish wind; for feverish dysphoria and night sweats, Huangbai (Amur Cork-tree) 9 g and Zhimu (Common Anemarrhena Rhizome) 9 g can be added to nourish yin and purge fire.

## Chinese Patent Medicine

1. Xiakucao Gao: 1 spoon for each dose, 3 times a day.
2. Jinhuang Gao: External application on the affected area of the thyroid gland.

## Simple and Handy Prescriptions

Pugongying (Dandelion) 30 g and Yejuhua (Wild Chrysanthemum Flower) 15 g are decocted in water and taken as tea several times a day. It is used to treat abundance of toxic heat.

## Other Therapies

External therapy: Yejuhua (Wild Chrysanthemum Flower) and Xianpugongying (Fresh Dandelion) are pounded into a paste, which is thereafter applied on the affected region. In addition, Dahuang (Rhubarb) 12 g, Baifan (Alum) 12 g and Xionghuang (Realgar) 2 g are ground up into powders, blended with vinegar and applied on the affected area.

Dietary therapy:
(1) Mung Bean 50 g is made into porridge with 30 g of candy sugar. It can be served as part of a usual diet.

(2) Indian kalimeris herb 500 g and tonquin beancurd 100 g are immersed in hot water for a while, then sliced, seasoned and blended. It is used to treat subacute thyroiditis in the period of onset.

## Cautions and Advice

1. In the acute stage of this disease, the symptoms can be quickly eliminated by administration of the adrenal cortical hormone, but this treatment cannot prevent the high recurrence rate of the disease. Hence, treatment in combination with TCM therapies based on syndrome differentiation is recommended.
2. In the initial stage of occurrence, patients should take necessary rest in bed and adopt a light diet. For those with high fever, an ice bag can be placed on the thyroid region; while for those whose conditions are complicated by hyperthyroidism, they should avoid emotional stimulation andconsume more nutritious food.
3. Patients should also take precautions against catching the common cold and keep a peaceful mind so as to prevent the disease.

## Daily Exercises

1. Recall the main causes of subacute thyroiditis.
2. Explain how subacute thyroiditis due to accumulation of toxic heat and that due to liver qi stagnation transforming into fire can be differentiated and treated.

# Chronic Lymphocytic Thyroiditis
# Week 10: Wednesday

Chronic lymphocytic thyroiditis, also called Hashimoto thyroiditis, is an autoimmune disease marked by symmetric, diffusive enlargement of the thyroid gland and positive reaction of serum TGA and TMA. This disease is primarily seen in middle-aged females and is also responsible for diffusive goiter in children. It has a slow and asymptomatic onset, with normal thyroid functions and occasional hyperthyroidism in the initial stage. However, when the disease progresses to a certain stage, there will be symptoms of hypothyroidism in most cases. In TCM, chronic lymphocytic thyroiditis is considered to be associated with "qi goiter" and "deficiency consumption".

## Etiology and Pathology

TCM holds that chronic lymphocytic thyroiditis is caused by long-term emotional disorders. The pathological changes of this disease are discussed as follows: Long-term emotional depression results in failure of the liver to promote free flow of qi, resulting in an accumulation of qi and phlegm in the anterior portion of the neck. If the stagnation of qi persists, it will transform into fire and damage yin, bringing about deficient heat in the interior. If the disease protracts, the deficiency of yin will involve yang, marked by deficiency of spleen yang and kidney yang.

## Diagnostic Key Points

1. Clinically, the hardening as well as diffusive and symmetric enlargement of the thyroid gland, regardless of its functional state, may point to this disease.
2. Positive reaction of serum TGA and serum TMA; B-ultrasonic imaging: uneven, low-level echo within the thyroid gland; thyroid gland tissue puncture and cell film preparation: clusters of lymphocytes.

## Syndrome Differentiation

### 1. Stagnation of the liver with retention of phlegm

Symptoms: Diffusive swelling in the front of the neck, or distending sensation in the neck, with chest distress, hypochondriac distension, frequent sighing, aggravation by emotional disturbance; white greasy tongue coating and taut slippery pulse.

Analysis of symptoms: Emotional depression leads to stagnation of liver qi, this is marked by chest distress, hypochondriac distension and frequent sighing; accumulation of qi and phlegm in the anterior portion of the neck is manifested as diffusive swelling in the front of the neck, or distending sensation in the neck; the white and greasy tongue coating and the taut and slippery pulse are due to stagnation of the liver with retention of phlegm.

### 2. Internal heat due to deficiency of yin

Symptoms: Diffusive and painless goiter in the neck, deficient restlessness, insomnia, hectic fever, night sweats, nocturnal emissions, or amenorrhea with scanty menses, or palpitations, uneasiness, tremors of hands and bulging eyes; red tongue, thin and rapid pulse, or thin, rapid and taut pulse.

Analysis of symptoms: Accumulation of phlegm and qi is marked by painless goiter in the neck; stagnant qi transforms into fire which consumes the yin-fluid, causing hectic fever and night sweats; deficiency of kidney yin is responsible for nocturnal emissions in males and amenorrhea or scanty menses in females; deficiency of liver yin brings about hyperactivity of liver yang, causing the hands to tremble and eyes to bulge; liver fire disturbs the heart, with such manifestations as insomnia and palpitations; the red tongue with little fluid and the thin and rapid pulse are symptomatic of internal heat due to deficiency of yin.

### 3. Yang deficiency of the spleen and kidneys

Symptoms: Goiter in the neck, pale complexion, cold body and limbs, weakness and soreness of the waist and knees, dizziness, or facial edema with swollen limbs; pale tongue, white-slippery or greasy coating and thin-deep pulse.

Analysis of symptoms: Prolonged affliction results in deficiency of spleen yang and kidney yang, so there is the persistent existence of goiters; deficiency of spleen qi leads to inadequate production of blood, which fails to nourish the face, causing a pale complexion and dizziness; deficiency of the kidneys in the lower energizer is responsible for the weakness and soreness of the waist and knees; deficiency of yang fails to warm and transport the retained water and dampness, characterized by cold body and limbs, facial edema and swollen limbs; the pale tongue, the white-slippery or greasy coating and the thin-deep pulse are attributable to deficiency of spleen yang and kidney yang.

## Differential Treatment

### 1. Stagnation of the liver with retention of phlegm

Treatment principle: Soothing the liver to relieve depression, regulating qi to dissolve phlegm.

Prescription and herbs: Modified Xiaoyao Powder.

Chaihu (Chinese Thorowax Root) 9 g, Baishao (White Peony Alba) 12 g, Baizhu (Largehead Atractylodes Rhizome) 12 g, Danggui (Chinese Angelica) 9 g, Fuling (Indian Bread) 15 g, Banxia (Pinellia Tuber) 9 g, Bohe (Peppermint) 3 g (decocted later), Xiangfu (Nutgrass Galingale Rhizome) 9 g, Yujin (Turmeric Root Tuber) 9 g, Beimu (Fritillariae Tuber) 12 g, Xiakucao (Common Selfheal Fruit-Spike) 15 g and Chuanlianzi (Szechwan Chinaberry Fruit) 9 g.

Modification: If there is apparent enlargement of the thyroid gland, Taoren (Peach Seed) 9 g and Muli (Oyster Shell) 30 g are added to soften the hard tissue and dissipate stagnation; for emotional depression, worry and insomnia, Chaozaoren (Fried Semen Ziziphi Spinosae) 12 g and Yuanzhi (Thinleaf Milkwort Root) 5 g are added to nourish the heart and tranquilize the mind.

### 2. Internal heat due to deficiency of yin

Treatment principle: Nourishing yin and dispelling heat, softening hardness and dissipating stagnation.

Prescription and herbs: Modified Zhibai Dihuang Pill.

Shengdi (Dried Rehmannia Root) 15 g, Shanyao (Common Yan Rhizome) 15 g, Shanzhuyu (Asiatic Cornelian Cherry Fruit) 9 g, Danpi (Cortex Moutan) 9 g, Digupi (Chinese Wolfberry Root-Bark)15 g, Zexie (Oriental Waterplantain Rhizome) 15 g, Zhimu (Common Anemarrhena Rhizome) 9 g, Huangbai (Amur Cork-tree) 9 g, Xiakucao (Common Selfheal Fruit-Spike) 15 g, Muli (Oyster Shell) 30 g, Guiban (Tortoise Shell) 9 g and Gancao (Liquorice Root) 3 g.

Modification: For palpitations and insomnia, Zhizi (Cape Jasmine Fruit) 9 g, Zhufushen (Indian Bread with Hostwood) 15 g and Chaozaoren (Fried Semen Ziziphi Spinosae) 12 g are added to clear the heart and tranquilize the mind; for frequent nocturnal emissions, Jinyingzi (Cherokee Rose Fruit) 12 g and Fupenzi (Palmleaf Raspberry Pruit) 12 g can be used to nourish the kidneys and secure essence.

## 3. Yang deficiency of the spleen and kidneys

Treatment principle: Warming and nourishing the spleen and kidneys, dissolving phlegm and dissipating stagnation.

Prescription and herbs: Modified Jingui Shenqi Pill and Sijunzi Decoction.

Huangqi (Milkvetch Root) 30 g, Dangshen (Radix Codonopsis) 15 g, Baizhu (Largehead Atractylodes Rhizome) 15 g, Fuling (Indian Bread) 15 g, Shudi (Prepared Rhizome of Rehmannia) 15 g, Shanyao (Common Yan Rhizome) 15 g, Shanzhuyu (Asiatic Cornelian Cherry Fruit) 10 g, Zexie (Oriental Waterplantain Rhizome) 15 g, Fupian (Radix Aconitilateralis Preparata) 9 g, Guizhi (Cassia Twig) 9 g, Haizao (Seaweed) 30 g and Kunbu (Kelp or Tangle) 30 g.

Modification: For weakness and soreness of the waist and knees, Duzhong (Eucommia Bark) 9 g and Chuanduan (Shichuan Radix Dipsaci) 9 g can be added to nourish the kidneys and strengthen the bones; for pale complexion and anaemia, Danggui (Chinese Angelica) 9 g and Jixueteng (Henry Magnoliavine Stem or Root) 30 g can be used to supplement blood.

## Chinese Patent Medicine

1. Xiaoyao Pill: 9 g for each dose, 3 times a day.
2. Xiakucao Paste: 1 spoon for each dose, 3 times a day.

## Simple and Handy Prescriptions

Huangqi (Milkvetch Root) 30 g, Danggui (Chinese Angelica) 9 g, Yinyanghuo (Epimedium Herb) 15 g and Chenpi (Dried Tangerine Peel) 9 g are boiled in water and taken twice a day. It is useful to treat chronic lymphocytic thyroiditis with hypothyroidism.

## Other Therapies

Foot bath therapy: Fuzi (Prepared Common Monkshood Daughter) 30 g, Ganjiang (Dried Ginger) 15 g, Guizhi (Cassia Twig) 15 g and Wuzhuyu (Medicinal Evodia Fruit) 10 g are decocted in water. The decoction is used for foot bath while it is warm or slightly hot for 20 minutes a day. The yongquan acupoint (KI 1) is massaged at the same time. This therapy is used to treat deficiency of spleen yang and kidney yang.

## Cautions and Advice

1. Hypothyroidism is secondary to chronic lymphocytic thyroiditis, which requires long-term administration of thyradin.
2. Patients should keep a peaceful mind, avoid raw and cold food and take precautions to avoid catching the common cold or external infection.

## Daily Exercises

1. List the main clinical characteristics of chronic lymphocytic thyroiditis.
2. Recall the pathological changes of chronic lymphocytic thyroiditis.
3. Explain how chronic lymphocytic thyroiditis due to yang deficiency of the spleen and kidneys can be treated.

# Hypofunction of the Anterior Pituitary

## Week 10: Thursday

Hypofunction of the anterior pituitary, also called Simmonds-Sheehan syndrome, refers to the hypoendocrinism caused by injuries of all or most pituitary glands due to various disorders of the hypothalamus or hypophysis, marked by pale complexion, listlessness, body coldness, waist soreness, hyposexuality, hair loss, atrophy of breasts and amenorrhea. The common causes are ischemic necrosis of the pituitary gland due to postpartum massive bleeding and hypophyseal tumor. In severe cases, there is often hypofunction of the anterior pituitary which, if left untreated, may be life-threatening. In TCM, hypofunction of the anterior pituitary is considered to be closely associated with "postpartum consumption", "dry-blood consumption", "deficiency consumption" and "suppression of menstruation".

## Etiology and Pathology

TCM holds that hypofunction of the anterior pituitary is mostly caused by postpartum massive bleeding, which leads to loss of qi and malnutrition of the kidneys.

The pathological changes are discussed as follows: Childbirth itself is liable to bring on deficiency of the kidneys and the postpartum massive bleeding may render the blood, essence and qi even more inadequate, consequently leading to deficiency of kidney yang, with such signs as feebleness, erotic apathy and sexual atrophy; furthermore, since qi and blood are extremely insufficient, especially the essence and blood in the liver and kidneys as well as qi and blood in the chong-channel and ren-channel, there will be lack of lactation, amenorrhea and hair loss. The kidneys are the prenatal foundation, whereas the spleen is the postnatal foundation, both of which are inter-promoted and inter-dependent, so deficiency of kidney yang will inevitably involve the spleen yang and result in yang deficiency of the spleen and kidneys.

## Diagnostic Key Points

1. Disease history: Massive bleeding during childbirth, ischemic necrosis of the pituitary gland, intracranial vascular lesion, hypophyseal tumor, intracranial trauma, surgery or chemotherapy.
2. Clinical manifestations: Secondary hypofunction of the sex glands, thyroid gland and adrenal gland due to inadequate secretion of trophic hormone by the pituitary gland; pressure symptoms due to hypophyseal tumor; primary symptoms due to other disorders.
3. Inadequate secretion of prolactin, growth hormone, gonadotropic hormone, hormothyrin and adrenocorticotropic hormone; mild or medium normochromic anemia and low level of fasting blood glucose.
4. CT or MRI can reveal hypophyseal tumor in the early stage; electrocardiogram: bradycardia, low-flat T wave, low voltage and protracted P-R interval.

## Syndrome Differentiation

### 1. Deficiency of kidney yang with insufficiency of qi and blood

Symptoms: Pale complexion, lusterless lips, timidity due to deficiency of qi, intolerance of cold, cold limbs, dizziness, withered hair, loss of hair, erotic apathy, lack of lactation, amenorrhea, weakness and soreness of the waist and knees; pale tongue with white coating and deep and feeble pulse.

Analysis of symptoms: Postpartum massive bleeding leads to deficiency of qi, essence and blood, which fail to nourish the upper energizer, this is marked by the pale complexion, lusterless lips, timidity due to deficiency of qi and dizziness; the liver stores blood and the kidneys store essence, so if they are deficient in blood and essence, there will be loss of hair, withered hair and weakness and soreness of the waist and knees; the liver and kidneys are closely linked to the chong-channel and ren-channel, so if the liver and kidneys are deficient, the chong-channel and ren-channel will also be insufficient, marked by a lack of lactation and amenorrhea; since qi and yang as well as yin and yang are interdependent, sudden loss of qi and blood may lead to extreme deficiency of kidney yang, marked by intolerance of cold, cold limbs and erotic apathy; the pale tongue with white coating and the deep and feeble pulse are due to deficiency of kidney yang with insufficiency of qi and blood.

## 2. Yang deficiency of the spleen and kidneys with insufficiency of qi and blood

Symptoms: Sallow complexion, amenorrhea, hypaphrodisia, sexual atrophy, rough skin, intolerance of cold, weariness, swollen limbs, poor appetite, loose stoolss and clear urine; pale and enlarged tongue with white coating, thin and feeble pulse.

Analysis of symptoms: The kidneys are the prenatal foundation, while the spleen is the postnatal foundation, both of which are inter-promoted and inter-dependent, so if the spleen is deficient with inadequacy of qi and blood, there will be sallow complexion and weariness; if the kidneys are malnourished with decline of fire in the life gate, there will be amenorrhea, hypaphrodisia, sexual atrophy, rough skin, intolerance of cold and clear urine; insufficiency of kidney yang may impair the spleen yang, leading to dysfunction in promoting digestion and transportation of water and dampness, with such manifestations as poor appetite and loose stools; the pale and enlarged tongue with white coating and thin and feeble pulse are attributable to yang deficiency of the spleen and kidneys with insufficiency of qi and blood.

## Differential Treatment

### 1. Deficiency of kidney yang with insufficiency of qi and blood

Treatment principle: Nourishing the kidneys and strengthening yang, invigorating qi and replenishing blood.

Prescription and herbs: Modified Erxian Decoction and Bazhen Decoction.

Xianmao (Common Curculigo Rhizome) 9 g, Yinyanghuo (Epimedium Herb) 9 g, Danggui (Chinese Angelica) 9 g, Chuanxiong (Szechwan Lovage Rhizome) 6 g, Baishao (White Peony Alba) 9 g, Shudihuang (Prepared Rhizome of Rehmannia) 12 g, Renshen (Ginseng) 9 g, Baizhu

(Largehead Atractylodes Rhizome) 9 g, Fuling (Indian Bread) 9 g, Zhigancao (Stir-baked Liquorice Root) 3 g, Dazao (Chinese Date) 3 dates and Huangqi (Milkvetch Root) 15 g.

Modification: If there is deficiency of blood and essence, with dizziness, tinnitus, deficient restlessness and constipation, Shouwu (Fleeceflower Root) 15 g, Nuzhenzi (Glossy Privet Fruit) 12 g and Huanliancao (Ecliptae Herba) 12 g are added to nourish the yin-blood of the liver and kidneys; for severe soreness in the waist and loins, Sangjisheng (Chinese Taxillus Herb) 15 g and Duzhong (Eucommia Bark) 9 g can be added to nourish the kidneys and strengthen the bones and loins; for erotic apathy and amenorrhea, Tusizi (Dodder Seed) 9 g and Yimucao (Motherwort Herb) 15 g can be added to warm the kidneys and regulate menstruation; for timidity of qi and intolerance of cold, Zhifuzi (Prepared Common Monkshood Daughter) 9 g and Rougui (Cassia Bark) 2 g (decocted later) can be added to warm the kidneys and activate yang.

## 2. Yang deficiency of the spleen and kidneys with insufficiency of qi and blood

Treatment principle: Invigorating the spleen and warming the kidneys, nourishing deficiency and regulating the chong-channel.

Prescription and herbs: Modified Jingui Shenqi Pill and Danggui Buxue Decoction.

Zhifuzi (Prepared Common Monkshood Daughter) 9 g, Rougui (Cassia Bark) 2 g (decocted later), Shudi (Prepared Rhizome of Rehmannia) 12 g, Shanyao (Common Yan Rhizome) 12 g, Shanzhuyu (Asiatic Cornelian Cherry Fruit) 9 g, Zexie (Oriental Waterplantain Rhizome) 15 g, Fuling (Indian Bread) 15 g, Huangqi (Milkvetch Root) 15 g, Dangshen (Radix Codonopsis) 12 g, Danggui (Chinese Angelica) 9 g, Yinyanghuo (Epimedium Herb) 9 g and Tusizi (Dodder Seed) 9 g.

Modification: If there is lethargy and weariness, Changpu (Acorus Calamus) 6 g and Yujin (Turmeric Root Tuber) 9 g can be added to dissolve phlegm for resuscitation; for apparent edema, Zhuling (Polyporus) 15 g and Mutong (Caulis Hocquartiae) 6 g are added to relieve swelling;

for sexual atrophy with amenorrhea, Xianmao (Common Curculigo Rhizome) 9 g, Bajitian (Mornda Root) 9 g and Yimucao (Motherwort Herb) 15 g can be added to nourish the kidneys and regulate the chong-channel.

## Chinese Patent Medicine

1. Shenrongbu Paste: 10 ml for each dose, twice a day.
2. Jingui Shenqi Pill: 6 g for each dose, 3 times a day.

## Simple and Handy Prescriptions

Gancao (Liquorice Root) 30 g and Renshen (Ginseng) 6 g are prepared and separated into 3 portions and taken at 3 different times within a day. It is used as an alternative treatment for a mild form of this disease.

## Other Therapies

External therapy: Fuzi (Prepared Common Monkshood Daughter), Rougui (Cassia Bark) and Wuzhuyu (Medicinal Evodia Fruit) in equal quantities are ground up into powders, blended with cooking wine and made into paste, which can be applied on the Yongquan acupoint every night.

Dietary therapy:
(1) Shengshaishen (Dried Radix Ginseng) 9 g, or Hongshen (Red Ginseng) 3 g and Hongzao (Red Date) 30 g are steamed and made into soup, which can be consumed every day.
(2) Chinese angelica 10 g, fresh ginger 10 g, mutton 250 g, yellow wine 10 ml and Welsh onion 2 pieces are boiled in water till the mutton is well cooked and then other seasonings can be added for taste before consumption.

## Cautions and Advice

1. This disease has a long duration and patients are often debilitated by it, so they must regulate their diets and consume more high-calorie,

high-protein and high-vitamin foods. Traditional Chinese therapy, relying on syndrome differentiation, is very important to the recovery of body functions, especially when the kidneys are nourished.

2. It is advisable to restrict or prohibit the use of sleeping pills, central nervous depressants and insulin anti-diabetic drugs so as to avoid the aggravation of the illness.

## Daily Exercises

1. Concisely describe the pathological changes of hypofunction of the anterior pituitary.
2. Explain how hypofunction of the anterior pituitary due to yang deficiency of the spleen and kidneys and that due to exhaustion of qi and blood can be differentiated and treated.

# Chronic Adrenocortical Insufficiency

## Week 10: Friday

Chronic hypoadrenia, also called Addison disease, is a chronic clinical syndrome due to destruction of the adrenal gland by autoimmunity, tuberculosis or tumor, which brings about inadequate secretion of the adrenal hormone. It is marked by pigmentation, fatigue, emaciation, hypotension and metabolic disorder of water or salt. Patients are usually between 20~50 years old, with an approximately equal rate of morbidity between males and females. Proactive treatment of this disease can prolong the patients' life span considerably. However, if there is presence of Addisonian crisis, the prognosis will be extremely unfavorable. In TCM, chronic adrenocortical insufficiency is believed to be associated with "deficiency consumption" and "black jaundice".

## Etiology and Pathology

TCM holds that chronic adrenocortical insufficiency is mainly caused by innate deficiency of kidney essence, or postnatal mistreatment or lack of treatment in critical conditions, which severely damages qi, blood, yin and yang, leading to persistent deficiency of the kidneys.

The pathological changes are marked by deficiency of the viscera and weakness of kidney yang. All the etiological factors will ultimately impair the kidneys, the deficiency of which brings on shortness of the visceral qi, characterized by general weakness of the body. Mingmen is located in the renal region, so deficiency of the kidneys is bound to cause decline of mingmen fire, marked by deficiency of kidney yang; the spleen yang relies on the support from kidney yang, so deficiency of the latter is bound to affect the former, characterized by yang deficiency of the spleen and kidneys. The liver and kidneys share the same origin, so insufficiency of kidney essence and primordial yang may also lead to deficiency of liver yin and kidney yin. Furthermore, deficiency of visceral qi leads to inadequacy of blood and hinders smooth circulation, manifesting as symptoms of blood deficiency or blood stasis.

## Diagnostic Key Points

1. Patients may present with pigmentation of the skin in varying degrees from light tan to pitch dark, progressive decrease in body weight, weariness, poor appetite, reduced memory, menstrual disorder, impotence and relatively low blood pressure.
2. Chest scan: relatively small heart shadow; electrocardiogram: low-tension tendency; examination on 24-hour urine and blood: marked decrease in the level of 17; water test and ACTH test: positive.

## Syndrome Differentiation

### 1. Yang deficiency of the spleen and kidneys

Symptoms: Dark skin all over the body, sleepiness, lassitude, facial and pedal edema, poor appetite, loose stools, clear and profuse urine, soreness in the waist and back, intolerance of cold, cold limbs, hyposexuality, dizziness and palpitations; pale, corpulent and tender tongue with white and slippery coating, deep, faint and thin pulse or soggy and feeble pulse.

Analysis of symptoms: Deficiency of kidney yang is manifested as general darkening of the skin; insufficiency of kidney qi leads to decline of mingmen fire, which is marked by soreness in the waist and back, hyposexuality, intolerance of cold, cold limbs, clear and profuse urine; deficiency of spleen yang and kidney yang results in uncontrolled flow of water and dampness, with such signs as facial and pedal edema; deficiency of spleen qi brings about poor digestion with poor appetite and loose stools; deficiency of qi and blood with lucid yang failing to ascend is responsible for sleepiness, lassitude and dizziness; the heart blood is poorly supplemented, causing palpitations; the pale, corpulent and tender tongue with white and slippery coating and the deep, faint and thin pulse or soggy and feeble pulse are all attributable to yang deficiency of the spleen and kidneys.

### 2. Yin deficiency of the liver and kidneys (a rare syndrome)

Symptoms: General darkness of skin, soreness in the waist and knees, dizziness, tinnitus, blurred vision, vexation, insomnia, numbness in the feet and hands, feverish sensations in the palms and soles and menstrual disorder; red tongue with little fluid and thin coating as well as taut and thin pulse.

Analysis of symptoms: The liver and kidneys share the same origin, so insufficiency of yin essence in the liver and kidneys can lead to general darkness of the skin (the color of the kidneys); the tendons, bones and brain marrow are malnourished, so there will be soreness in the waist and knees, numbness in the hands and feet, dizziness, tinnitus and blurred vision; deficiency of yin produces internal heat which disturbs the heart spirit and causes feverish sensation in the palms and soles, vexation and insomnia; deficiency of the liver and kidneys leads to disorders of the thoroughfare vessel and conception vessel, so female patients experience menstrual disorders; the red tongue with little fluid and thin coating and the taut and thin pulse are all due to insufficiency of yin-essence in the liver and kidneys.

## Differential Treatment

### 1. Yang deficiency of the spleen and kidneys

Treatment principle: Warming and invigorating the kidney yang, replenishing qi and invigorating the spleen.

Prescription and herbs: Modified Yougui Pill and Sijunzi Decoction.

Huangqi (Milkvetch Root) 30 g, Dangshen (Radix Codonopsis) 15 g, Baizhu (Largehead Atractylodes Rhizome) 12 g, Fuling (Indian Bread) 12 g, Shudi (Prepared Rhizome of Rehmannia) 12 g, Shanyao (Common Yan Rhizome) 15 g, Shanzhuyu (Asiatic Cornelian Cherry Fruit) 9 g, Tusizi (Dodder Seed) 15 g, Duzhong (Eucommia Bark) 12 g, Buguzhi (Malaytea Scurfpea Fruit) 12 g, Lujiaojiao (Deerhorn Glue) 9 g, melted in decoction, and Fupian (Radix Aconitilateralis Preparata) 9 g.

Modification: If there is severe diarrhea, Muxiang (Common Aucklandia Root) 9 g and Paojiang (Prepared Dried Ginger) 5 g are added to warm the spleen and check diarrhea; for cold body and limbs with apparent listlessness, Xianmao (Common Curculigo Rhizome) 9 g, Yinyanghuo (Epimedium Herb) 6 g and Rougui (Cassia Bark) 3 g (decocted later) can be used to reinforce the action of warming and invigorating the kidney yang; for dark complexion, Honghua (Safflower) 6 g and Danggui (Chinese Angelica) 9 g are added to nourish and activate blood, resolve stasis and remove ecchymosis.

## 2. Yin deficiency of the liver and kidneys

Treatment principle: Tonifying the liver and kidneys, nourishing blood and supplementing essence.

Prescription and herbs: Zuogui Pill and Siwu Decoction.

Shengdi (Dried Rehmannia Root) 12 g, Shanyao (Common Yan Rhizome) 12 g, Shanzhuyu (Asiatic Cornelian Cherry Fruit) 9 g, Gouqizi (Barbary Wolfberry Fruit) 12 g, Tusizi (Dodder Seed) 12 g, Guibanjiao (Tortoise Shell Glue) 9 g (melted in decoction), Danggui (Chinese Angelica) 9 g, Baishao (White Peony Alba) 12 g, Chuanxiong (Szechwan Lovage Rhizome) 9 g and Jixueteng (Henry Magnoliavine Stem or Root) 15 g.

Modification: If there is dizziness and tinnitus with an internal stirring of deficient wind, Juhua (Chrysanthemum Flower) 9 g, Gouteng (Gambir Plant) 15 g (decocted later) and Shijueming (Sea-ear Shell) 30 g (decocted earlier) are used to subdue the liver and extinguish wind; for feverish dysphoria and night sweats, Biejia (Turtle Shell) 9 g and Zhimu (Common Anemarrhena Rhizome) 9 g can be added to nourish yin and dispel heat; for irregular menstruation, Yimucao (Motherwort Herb) 15 g and Taipanfen (Placenta Powder) 3 g (infused in water) are added to nourish the kidneys and regulate the chong-channel.

## Chinese Patent Medicine

1. Jingui Shenqi Pill: 6 g for each dose, 3 times a day.
2. Shenling Baizhu Powder: 6 g for each dose, 3 times a day.

## Simple and Handy Prescriptions

Gancao (Liquorice Root) 15~30 g are decocted and served as tea to treat the condition due to mild yang deficiency of the spleen and kidneys.

## Other Therapies

External therapy: Fuzi (Prepared Common Monkshood Daughter) 15 g, guizhi (Cassia Twig) 15 g, Chuanjiao (Zanthoxyli) 15 g, Danggui

(Chinese Angelica) 15 g, Chuanxiong (Szechwan Lovage Rhizome) 15 g, Honghua (Safflower) 15 g, Sumu (Sappan Wood) 15 g and Shechuangzi (Common Cnidium Fruit) 15 g are decocted in water. The decoction is used for a foot bath (about 30 minutes nightly). It is applicable to treat deficiency of spleen yang and kidney yang.

Dietary therapy: Renshen (Ginseng) 6 g and Danggui (Chinese Angelica) 6 g are decocted for a while before the gruffs are removed. The medicated liquid is afterwards boiled with 500 g of mutton and desired amounts of cinnamon bark, fennel, cooking wine, ginger and onion. After the mutton is well cooked, it can be consumed.

## Cautions and Advice

1. Patients with extremely poor immunity are susceptible to respiratory tract infection, gastrointestinal dysfunction, or even Addisonian crisis. It is advisable to use traditional Chinese therapies since long-term application of the Western treatment method of hormone replacement therapy is likely to incur side-effects.
2. Patients should take good rest and avoid mental as well as physical strain. However, they should engage in appropriate physical exercise to strengthen the body constitution and reduce complications.
3. They should also avoid catching the common cold, trauma, surgical irritation, vomiting, diarrhea, profuse sweating, or excessive stimulation by heat or cold.
4. Foods that are rich in protein, vitamins, carbohydrates and sodium salt (instead of sylvite, so as to maintain the electrolytic balance) are recommended.

## Daily Exercises

1. Recall the main pathological changes of chronic adrenocortical insufficiency.
2. Explain how chronic adrenocortical insufficiency due to yang deficiency of the spleen and kidneys can be diagnosed and treated.

# Diabetes Insipidus
# Week 9: Saturday

Diabetes insipidus is an endocrinal disorder due to the deficiency of the antidiuretic hormone (central or pituitary diabetes insipidus, ADH) or an improper response of the kidneys to ADH) renal diabetes insipidus). It is marked by polydipsia, polyuria and low specific gravity urine. The disease can afflict people of any age, especially youths, with the ratio of male to female patients being 2:1. In TCM, diabetes insipidus is considered to be closely associated with "consumptive thirst" and "consumptive heat".

## Etiology and Pathology

TCM holds that diabetes insipidus is caused by either endogenous or exogenous pathogenic factors. The former refers primarily to an innate deficiency of yin or yang, while the latter to emotional disorder, partiality for a kind of particular food, overstrain or an excessive sexual life and external or surgical trauma. In short, the disease is due to disorder of the distribution of water and fluid resulting from the impairments of the lungs, stomach and kidneys.

The pathological changes are discussed as follows: Innate deficiency of yin, emotional disorder, or preference for spicy and dry food can all lead to internal disturbance of fire-heat originating from the heart, liver and stomach. Fire-heat consumes the lung fluid, resulting in dysfunction of water and fluid in distribution, marked by polydipsia. The kidneys fail to moisten the dry lungs, so there is a strong desire for drinking with inability of the kidneys to concentrate the urine, characterized by excessive drinking with profuse urine. Besides, deficiency cold in the middle energizer causes dysfunction in transporting the water and fluid to the upper energizer, so there are symptoms such as dryness in the mouth, polydipsia and polyuria. Moreover, impairment of kidney yin by overstrain and an excessive sexual life as well as damage of primordial spirit or kidney qi by external or surgical trauma often leads to a failure of body fluid to be transformed, or failure of urine to be condensed, with such signs as polyuria, thirst and polydipsia. Prolonged affliction by this disease debilitates the yin essence, which may further impair yang, resulting in deficiency of qi and yin as well as deficiency of yin and yang.

## Diagnostic Key Points

1. Polyuria, 24 hour urinary output 5~10 L (or more), light-colored or glucose-absent urine, accompanied by thirst, polydipsia, skin dryness and constipation.
2. Specific gravity of urine <1.006 and osmotic pressure of urine <200 mmol/L(mmol/L); ADH-activation test: no marked decrease in the volume of urine; X-ray scan, CT and MRI: intracranial tumor, inflammation and external injury can be found.

## Syndrome Differentiation

### 1. Exuberant heat in the lungs and stomach

Symptoms: Polydipsia, polyuria, polyorexia and constipation; red tongue with yellow-dry coating and surging-rapid or thin-rapid pulse.

Analysis of symptoms: The heart fire and stomach fire consume the lung fluid, leading to dysfunction of water and fluid in distribution, marked by polydipsia; the kidneys fail to moisten the dry lungs, so there is a strong desire for drinking with inability of the kidneys to concentrate the urine, characterized by excessive drinking with profuse urine; abundance of stomach fire is responsible for polyorexia; the lungs are interiorly and exteriorly associated with the large intestine, so deficiency of lung fluid will bring about dryness in the intestine, marked by constipation; the red tongue and yellow-dry coating are signs of fluid damage due to abundant heat and fire; the surging-rapid pulse is present in the initial stage when there is abundant heat, while the thin-rapid pulse is a sign of further damage to the yin-fluid.

### 2. Yang deficiency of the spleen and stomach

Symptoms: Pale and lusterless complexion, drowsiness, weariness, poor appetite, thirst, polydipsia, frequent urination, clear and watery urine; pale tongue with white-greasy coating and thin-feeble pulse.

Analysis of symptoms: "The importance of yang qi is comparable to that of the sky and sun", so yang deficiency of the spleen and stomach is responsible for dysfunction in transforming water and food into qi and blood, this deficiency is marked by poor appetite, pale and lusterless complexion, drowsiness and weariness; unsuccessful qi-transformation of body fluid prevents it from reaching the upper part of the body, leading to dryness in the mouth, polydipsia, frequent urination and clear and watery urine; the pale tongue with white-greasy coating and thin-feeble pulse are due to deficiency of spleen yang and stomach yang.

## 3. Deficiency of kidney yin

Symptoms: Frequent urination with profuse urine, dry mouth and lips, polydipsia, emaciation, lusterless complexion, weakness and soreness in the waist and knees; red tongue with thin coating and thin-deep-rapid pulse.

Analysis of symptoms: The kidneys store essence and governs the opening and closing of the bladder and in this sense, it is deemed the foundation of yin fluid; if the kidneys are deficient and fails to control urination, there will be frequent urination with profuse urine; the loss of yin fluid and deficiency of kidney yin lead to dryness in the mouth and lips as well as polydipsia; deficiency of yin essence results in malnourishment of the body, marked by emaciation and lusterless complexion; the waist is the place where the kidneys dwell and the kidneys control the bones, so deficiency of the kidneys is responsible for weakness and soreness in the waist and knees; red tongue with thin coating and deep-rapid pulse are all attributable to a deficiency of kidney yin, or deficiency of yin with internal heat.

## 4. Deficiency of yin and yang

Symptoms: Dry mouth, polydipsia, dry skin, emaciation, profuse drinking with excessive urination, weakness and soreness in the waist and knees, impotence, premature ejaculation, cold body and limbs and pale complexion; pale tongue with white coating and thin-deep-feeble or deep-weak pulse.

Analysis of symptoms: The yin and yang are interdependent, so deficiency of yin will inevitably affect yang in the long run, leading to deficiency of yin and yang; deficiency of yin in the lungs, stomach and kidneys is manifested as dry mouth, polydipsia, dry skin and emaciation; deficient kidney yang fails to transform or condense the urine, so there is excessive urine; deficiency of the kidneys in the lower energizer, with decline of mingmen fire, is responsible for weakness and soreness of the waist and knees, impotence and premature ejaculation; deficient yang fails to warm the body, so the body and limbs feel cold and the complexion is pale; pale tongue with white coating and thin-deep-feeble or deep-weak pulse are all attributable to deficiency of yin and yang.

## Differential Treatment

### 1. Exuberant heat in the lungs and stomach

Treatment principle: Dispelling stomach fire, nourishing yin and producing fluid.

Prescription and herbs: Modified Baihu Decoction.

Shigao (Gypsum) 30 g (decocted earlier), Zhimu (Common Anemarrhena Rhizome) 9 g, Shashen (Root of Straight Ladybell) 15 g, Maidong (Dwarf Lilyturf Tuber) 15 g, Shihu (Dendrobium) 15 g, Tianhuafen (Trichosanthin) 15 g, Shanyao (Common Yan Rhizome) 15 g, Shanzhuyu (Asiatic Cornelian Cherry Fruit) 9 g and Gancao ( Liquorice Root) 3 g.

Modification: If there is persistent polydipsia and lassitude, Renshen (Ginseng) 6 g can be added to nourish qi and produce fluid; for polyphagia and boulimia, Huanglian (Golden Thread) 3 g and Zhizi (Cape Jasmine Fruit) 6 g are added to dispel stomach fire; for constipation, Shengdi (Dried Rehmannia Root) 15 g and Xuanshen (Figwort Root) 15 g can be used to moisten the intestine and promote defecation; for polyuria, Sangpiaoxiao (Egg Capsule of Mantid) 9 g, Jinyingzi (Cherokee Rose Fruit) 9 g and Fupenzi (Palmleaf Raspberry Pruit) 9 g are added to nourish the kidneys and condense urine.

### 2. Yang deficiency of the spleen and stomach

Treatment principle: Activating yang and transforming qi, invigorating the spleen and producing fluid.

Prescription and herbs: Modified Wuling Powder.

Fuling (Indian Bread) 9 g, Zhuling (Polyporus) 9 g, Baizhu (Largehead Atractylodes Rhizome) 9 g, Zexie (Oriental Waterplantain Rhizome) 9 g, Guizhi (Cassia Twig) 9 g, Dangshen (Radix Codonopsis) 12 g, Shashen (Root of Straight Ladybell) 12 g and Shanyao (Plantain Herb) 12 g.

Modification: If there is apparent lassitude, Renshen (Ginseng) 9 g can be added to replenish qi and invigorate the spleen; for cold limbs and loose stoolss, Fuzi (Prepared Common Monkshood Daughter) 9 g and Ganjiang (Dried Ginger) 3 g are used to warm the middle energizer and invigorate the spleen.

### 3. Deficiency of kidney yin

Treatment principle: Nourishing the kidney yin and promoting fluid production to quench thirst.

Prescription and herbs: Modified Liuwei Dihuang Pill.

Shudi (Prepared Rhizome of Rehmannia) 12 g, Shanyao (Common Yan Rhizome) 12 g, Shanzhuyu (Asiatic Cornelian Cherry Fruit) 10 g, Guiban (Tortoise Shell) 15 g, Tiandong (Cochinchinese Asparagus Root) 15 g, Shashen (Root of Straight Ladybell) 15 g, Maidong (Dwarf Lilyturf Tuber) 15 g and Muli (Oyster Shell) 30 g.

Modification: If there is apparent internal heat, feverish dysphoria and night sweats, Shudi (Prepared Rhizome of Rehmannia) is replaced with Shengdi (Dried Rehmannia Root) 12 g, Huangbai (Amur Cork-tree) 9 g and Zhimu (Common Anemarrhena Rhizome) 9 g are added to nourish the kidneys and dispel heat; for frequent urination with profuse urine, Yizhiren (Bitter-seed Cardamn) 9 g and Sangpiaoxiao (Egg Capsule of Mantid) 12 g can be added to nourish the kidneys and condense urine.

### 4. Deficiency of yin and yang

Treatment principle: Warming the kidneys and replenishing yin, condensing urine and producing fluid.

Prescription and herbs: Modified Jingui Shenqi Pill.

Fuzi (Prepared Common Monkshood Daughter) 9 g, Rouguifen (Cassia Bark Powder) 2 g (infused in water), Shengdi (Dried Rehmannia Root) 9 g, Shudi (Prepared Rhizome of Rehmannia) 9 g, Shanyao (Common Yan Rhizome) 15 g, Shanzhuyu (Asiatic Cornelian Cherry Fruit) 9 g, Fuling (Indian Bread) 9 g, Zexie (Oriental Waterplantain Rhizome) 9 g, Jinyingzi (Cherokee Rose Fruit) 9 g and Fupenzi (Palmleaf Raspberry Pruit) 9 g.

Modification: If there is weariness and shortness of breath, Huangqi (Milkvetch Root) 15 g and Dangshen (Radix Codonopsis) 12 g can be added to supplement qi and nourish deficiency; for impotence and premature ejaculation, Xianmao (Common Curculigo Rhizome) 9 g, Yinyanghuo (Epimedium Herb) 9 g and Tusizi (Dodder Seed) 9 g are used to warm the kidneys and reinforce yang.

## Chinese Patent Medicine

1. Zhibai Dihuang Pill: 6 g for each dose, 3 times a day.
2. Jingui Shenqi Pill: 6 g for each dose, 3 times a day.

## Simple and Handy Prescriptions

Shengshaishen (Dried Radix Ginseng) 9 g, Shihu (Dendrobium) 30 g, Shanyao (Common Yan Rhizome) 15 g and Muli (Oyster Shell) 30 g are decocted and separated into 3 portions to be taken at 3 different times within a day. It is used to treat diabetes insipidus with thirst and polyuria in patients with weak constitution.

## Other Therapies

Dietary therapy:

(1) Live oysters are pounded into paste after the removal of their shells and the meat juice is boiled for warm administration several times a day. It is used to treat diabetes insipidus due to exuberant heat.
(2) Zhishouwu (Fleeceflower Root) 120 g is decocted in water and then the decoction is used to cook Hongzao (Red Date) 120 g, Heizhima (Black Sesame) 100 g, Heizao (Dateplum Persimmon) 60 g,

Huaishanyao (Huaihe Common Yan Rhizome) 60 g and a small black hen (about 500 g) in a earthenware cooking pot. It can be eaten once a day and is used to treat chronic diabetes insipidus in patients with weak constitution.

## Cautions and Advice

1. Patients with diabetes insipidus should take care to prevent severe dehydration and hypernatremia. During treatment, they should consume adequate water but at the same time, prevent water intoxication by refraining from excessive drinking.
2. Patients should increase nutrient intake, restrict salt intake and avoid spicy food.
3. They should also avoid damage to the hypothalamus and pituitary gland by operation or external injury; take initiative in preventing and treating encephalitis and meningitis and address tumors promptly so as to prevent diabetes insipidus.

## Daily Exercises

1. Concisely describe the pathological changes of diabetes insipidus.
2. Explain how diabetes insipidus can be treated based on syndrome differentiation.

# Hypercortisolism
# Week 11: Monday

Hypercortisolism, also called Cushing Syndrome, is caused by a tumor of the adrenal cortex, a tumor of the pituitary gland, or a tumor somewhere other than the pituitary or adrenal glands (ectopic hypercortisolism). The tumor stimulates excessive production of adrenocorticotropic hormone (ACTH), also known as cortisol. Clinically, it is marked by central obesity, moon face, acne, purple striation, hairiness, tendency of diabetes, hypertension, sexual abnormalies or virilism. This disease is primarily seen in females between 20~40 years of age, with the ratio of males to females being 1:2 ~ 1:3. The prognosis may vary with the change in etiological factors, e.g., in cases of adrenal carcinoma, ectopic tumor metastasis, complications of heart failure, cerebrovascular accident, uremia or severe infection, the prognosis can be extremely unfavorable. In TCM, hypercortisolism is associated with "liver-yang" and "phlegm-dampness".

## Etiology and Pathology

TCM holds that hypercortisolism is caused by either endogenous or exogenous pathogenic factors. The former refers to emotional disorder, impairment of the spleen by overstrain, or stagnation of the liver with spleen deficiency, which can bring about generation of damp-heat in the interior. The latter refers to invasion of exogenous damp-heat into the interior, which transforms into fire and consumes yin, ultimately leading to deficiency of yin and yang (for yin and yang are interdependent). In addition, there are other causes such as innate deficiency of yin blood.

The pathological changes are discussed as follows: A sudden emotional change, especially anger, impairs the liver and inhibits it from promoting a free flow of qi, which involves the spleen-earth. In addition, overstrain can also damage the spleen. since the spleen is located in the middle and in charge of transporting and transforming water and dampness, spleen weakness, either due to stagnation of the liver or overstrain, may lead to transformation of dampness into heat and, as a result, internal abundance of dampness and heat, marked by chest-back obesity, a moon face and acne. Dampness and heat transform into fire and scorches the blood and fluid. At the same time, the deficient spleen fails to transport essence and blood to the four limbs, so there can be weakness and atrophy of the limbs. Prolonged stagnation of qi and blood results in blood stasis in the skin, marked by purple striation. If the disease progresses further, there may be exhaustion of liver yin and kidney yin, which leads to hyperactivity of yang and the manifestation of dizziness. In the end there will be deficiency of yin and yang as well as exhaustion of the body and spirit.

## Diagnostic Key Points

1. Central obesity, moon face, acne, purple striation, hairiness, syndrome of hypertension, sexual abnormalies or virilism.
2. Blood eosinopenia, hypopotassemia, impaired glucose tolerance and hyperglycaemia.; increase in blood plasma cortisol and loss of day-night rhythm; positive result of small-dose dexamethasone suppression test.
3. X-ray examination: Enlarged sella, osteoporosis and possibly compressed deformity of the spine.

## Syndrome Differentiation

### 1. Damp-heat in the liver and spleen

Symptoms: Chest-back obesity, moon face, excessive secretion of facial grease, frequent occurrence of acne, purple striation on the skin, atrophy and weakness in the limbs, irascibility, a bitter taste and dry sensation in the mouth, sticky stools and yellowish or reddish urine; red tongue with yellow and greasy coating and taut, slippery and rapid pulse.

Analysis of symptoms: The spleen is located in the middle and in charge of transporting and transforming water and dampness, so invasion of liver qi into the spleen can lead to internal accumulation of phlegm and dampness, marked by chest-back obesity; transformation of dampness into heat results in an internal abundance of dampness and heat, characterized by a moon face, excessive secretion of facial grease and frequent occurrence of acne; damp-heat transforms into fire, which scorches the essence blood, leading to malnutrition of the four limbs and resulting in emaciation and weariness; deficiency of blood increases the likelihood of stasis, so there is purple striation on the skin; upflaming of liver fire is manifested as irascibility and a dry sensation or bitter taste in the mouth; damp-heat pours downward, so there are sticky stools and yellowish or reddish urine; the red tongue with yellow and greasy coating and the taut, slippery and rapid pulse are due to disharmony between the liver and spleen with an internal abundance of dampness and heat.

## 2. Hyperactivity of yang due to deficiency of yin

Symptoms: Headache, dizziness, or even tremors of muscles, restlessness, irascibility, blushing, palpitations, insomnia, dreaminess, nocturnal emissions, weakness and soreness in the waist and knees and menstrual disorder; red tongue with scanty coating and taut, thin and rapid pulse.

Analysis of symptoms: Deficiency of liver yin and kidney yin leads to hyperactivity of liver yang, which disturbs the upper orifices and results in headache or dizziness; internal stirring of deficient wind is responsible for tremors of the muscles; exuberant liver fire flames up, with such manifestations as restlessness, irascibility and flushing; fire disturbs the heart spirit and this ismarked by palpitations, insomnia and dreaminess; fire harasses the semen chamber, presenting as nocturnal emissions; the waist is the "house of the kidneys" and the kidneys control the bones, so deficiency of the kidneys will lead to weakness and soreness in the waist and knees; deficiency of the liver and kidneys brings about dysfunction of the thoroughfare vessel and conception vessel, marked by menstrual disorder; the red tongue with scanty coating and taut, thin and rapid pulse are all symptomatic of hyperactive yang due to deficiency of yin.

## 3. Deficiency of yin and yang

Symptoms: Dizziness, tinnitus, soreness in the waist, weakness in the limbs, tenderness in the bones, a drysensation in the mouth with no thirst, edema in the lower limbs, infertility or cessation of menses in females and impotence or premature ejaculation in males; red and tender or enlarged tongue with white and thin or slightly greasy coating and thin and deep pulse.

Analysis of symptoms: The kidneys store essence and produces marrow to supplement the brain, so prolonged deficiency of kidney yin or essence may lead to dizziness and tinnitus; the waist is the location of the kidneys and the kidneys control the bones, so if the kidneys are deficient, there will be soreness in the waist, weakness in the limbs and tenderness in the bones; the kidneys are in charge of water, when deficiency of yin affects the kidney yang and prevents it from transforming the water and body fluid, there will be be dryness in the mouth with no desire for drinking and edema in the lower limbs; insufficiency of kidney essence leads to a decline of mingmen fire, with such manifestations as infertility or cessation of menses in females and impotence or premature ejaculation in males; the red and tender or enlarged tongue, white and thin or slightly greasy coating and thin and deep pulse are all attributable to deficiency of yin and yang.

## Differential Treatment

### 1. Damp-heat in the liver and spleen

Treatment principle: Soothing the liver and invigorating the spleen, dispelling heat and resolving dampness.

Prescription and herbs: Modified Xiaoyao Powder and Longdan Xiegan Decoction.

Chaihu (Chinese Thorowax Root) 9 g, Danggui (Chinese Angelica) 9 g, Baizhu (Largehead Atractylodes Rhizome) 9 g, Baishao (White Peony Alba) 9 g, Fuling (Indian Bread) 12 g, Shengdi (Dried Rehmannia Root) 12 g, Zexie (Oriental Waterplantain Rhizome) 12 g, Chuanmutong (Armand Clematis Stem) 6 g, Huangqin (Baical Skullcap Root) 9 g, Huanglian (Golden Thread) 3 g, Jiaozhizi (Baked Cape Jasmine Fruit) 9 g and Longdancao (Radix Gentianae) 6 g.

Modification: For insomnia and hyperpragia, Longchi (Fossilia Dentis Mastodi) 30 g (decocted first) and Cishi (Magnetite) 30 g can be added to tranquilize the mind; if there is apparent suggillation, Danshen (Radix

Salviae Miltiorrhiae) 15 g and Zicao (Arnebia Root) 15 g are used to dispel heat and resolve stasis; for acne or agria on the skin, Fuling (Indian Bread) 30 g and Zihuadiding (Tokyo Violet Herb) 30 g can be added to dispel heat and remove toxins.

## 2. Hyperactivity of yang due to deficiency of yin

Treatment principle: Nourishing yin to suppress yang, subduing the liver to extinguish wind.

Prescription and herbs: Modified Tianma Gouteng Potion.

Tianma (Tall Gastrodis Tuber) 9 g, Gouteng (Gambir Plant) 15 g (decocted later), Shijueming (Sea-ear Shell) 15 g, Duzhong (Eucommia Bark) 12 g, Niuxi (Twotoothed Achyranthes Root) 12 g, Sangjisheng (Chinese Taxillus Herb) 12 g, Fushen (Indian Bread with Hostwood) 12 g, Yejiaoteng (Caulis Polygoni Multiflori) 30 g, Longgu (Os Draconis) 30 g, Zhizi (Cape Jasmine Fruit) 9 g, Guiban (Tortoise Shell) 12 g and Shudi (Prepared Rhizome of Rehmannia) 15 g.

Modification: If there is headache, irascibility and relatively high blood pressure, Xiakucao (Common Selfheal Fruit-Spike) 12 g and Lingyangfen (Antelope Horn Powder) 0.3 g (infused in water) can be added to dispel heat, subdue the liver and reduce blood pressure; if there is feverish sensation over the five centers (the palms, the soles and the heart), Zhimu (Common Anemarrhena Rhizome) 9 g, Danpi (Cortex Moutan) 9 g and Biejia (Turtle Shell) 12 g can be used to nourish yin and dispel heat; for disturbance of kidney fire with frequent nocturnal emissions, Huangbai (Amur Cork-tree) 9 g and Tiandong (Cochinchinese Asparagus Root) 15 g are used to nourish yin and bring down fire.

## 3. Deficiency of yin and yang

Treatment principle: Warming the kidneys and nourishing yin.

Prescription and herbs: Supplementary Jisheng Shenqi Pill.

Shudi (Prepared Rhizome of Rehmannia) 15 g, Shanyao (Common Yan Rhizome) 15 g, Shanzhuyu (Asiatic Cornelian Cherry Fruit) 10 g, Zexie (Oriental Waterplantain Rhizome) 10 g, Fuling (Indian Bread) 10 g, Danpi

(Cortex Moutan) 10 g, Rouguifen (Cassia Bark Powder) 2 g (infused in water), Fupian (Radix Aconitilateralis Preparata) 10 g, Niuxi (Twotoothed Achyranthes Root) 10 g, Cheqianzi (Plantain Seed) 15 g (wrapped during decoction), Tusizi (Dodder Seed) 12 g and Yinyanghuo (Epimedium Herb) 12 g.

Modification: If there is weariness, flaccidity in the limbs and susceptibility to common cold, Huangqi (Milkvetch Root) 15 g and Dangshen (Radix Codonopsis) 12 g, or Yupinfeng Powder in combination, can be used to replenish qi and consolidate the superficies; for edema, Zhuling (Polyporus) 15 g, Dongguapi (Chinese Waxgourd Peel) 15 g and Chixiaodou (Rice Bean) 30 g can be added to promote urination and relieve edema; for bone tenderness, Gusuibu (Fortune's Drynaria Rhizome) 12 g and Sangjisheng (Chinese Taxillus Herb) 12 g can be added to nourish the kidneys and strengthen the bones; for impotence, Zihechefen (Human Placenta Powder) 3 g (infused in water) and Xianmao (Common Curculigo Rhizome) 9 g can be used to nourish the kidneys and reinforce yang.

## Chinese Patent Medicine

1. Longdan Xiegan Decoction: 6 g for each dose, 3 times a day.
2. Zhibai Dihuang Pill: 6 g for each dose, 3 times a day.

## Simple and Handy Prescriptions

Shengdi (Dried Rehmannia Root) 30 g, Xuanshen (Figwort Root) 10 g, Zhimu (Common Anemarrhena Rhizome) 10 g and Huangbai (Amur Cork-tree) 10 g are boiled in water and taken twice a day for the treatment of hypercortisolism with hyperactivity of fire and deficiency of yin.

## Other Therapies

External therapy: Zicao (Arnebia Root) 30 g, Fuling (Indian Bread) 30 g and Huanglian (Golden Thread) 10 g are decocted in water, the decoction is cooled and wrapped in antiseptic gauze for application on the acne.

Dietary therapy:

(1) Ludou (Mung Bean) 30 g, Yiyiren (Coix Seed) 50 g and Jiangmi (Rice Fruit) 50 g are made into porridge to address the problem of damp-heat in the liver and spleen, marked by dryness and bitterness in the mouth and greasy tongue coating.

(2) Huangjing (Solomonseal Rhizome) 20 g and Gouqizi (Barbary Wolfberry Fruit) 20 g are cooked together with lean meat 150 g and desired amounts of yellow wine, salt and onion to address the problem of hyperactivity of fire and deficiency of yin, marked by dry mouth, polydipsia, dizziness and waist soreness.

## Cautions and Advice

1. Patients with hypercortisolism, the most common type of hyperadreno-corticism, have greater susceptibility to diabetes and electrolyte distur-bance. If there is adrenal insufficiency after removal of the adrenal gland due to carcinoma or hyperplasia in the organ, it should be prop-erly treated.
2. Patients should avoid overstrain, cold and take precautions against catching the common cold.
3. They should also adopt a low-fat, low-glucose, high-protein and vita-min-rich diet, which is easy to digest.

## Daily Exercises

1. List the clinical characteristics of hypercortisolism.
2. Concisely describe the different patterns of hypercortisolism based on syndrome differentiation.
3. Explain how hypercortisolism due to damp-heat in the liver and spleen and that due to yin deficiency causing hyperactivity of yang can be differentiated and treated.

# Idiopathic Edema
# Week 11: Tuesday

Idiopathic edema, also called "water-retention obesity", "uncomplicated water-sodium retention" and "periodical edema", is a syndrome of water-electrolyte metabolic disturbance due to disorders of the endocrine, vascular and nervous systems. This disease usually afflicts obese women 20~50 years of age during the child-bearing period. Clinically, it is marked by edema and closed linked with the menstrual cycle and weight gain. In TCM, this disease is considered to be closely associated with "edema".

## Etiology and Pathology

TCM holds that idiopathic edema is caused by emotional disorder, which brings about failure of the liver to promote free flow of qi; or by innate deficiency of the kidney qi; or by postnatal mistreatment, which damages the spleen and kidneys and causes retention of water in the skin and muscles.

The pathological changes are characterized by impairment and dysfunction of the liver, spleen and kidneys. The liver functions to promote free flow of qiwhich ensures the normal circulation of water, blood and body fluid. However, if the liver qi is stagnated, there will be blood stasis and retention of water in the skin and muscles (edema). The spleen governs transportation and transformation, and this is affected by improper diet or postnatal nourishment. When the spleen is impaired, there will be retention of phlegm and dampness in the skin and muscles, creating a predisposition to edema. The kidneys are in charge of controlling water, which can be affected by innate deficiency, chronic diseases and excessive sexual activities; during a woman's menstrual period, the nourishment of the chong-channel and ren-channel by kidney essence is imperative, if the kidney essence is lost with menstrual discharge, the kidney yang will be debilitated and fail to promote circulation of water, leading to aggravation of edema during the menstrual period. In addition, edema can also be caused by accumulation of dampness and heat (transformed from dampness).

## Diagnostic Key Points

1. This disease, mostly afflicting people with obesity, can be aggravated when the patient stands, but is alleviated when he or she is in a lying position.
2. Patients with edema during the period of child-bearing can present with aggravation of the symptoms before each menstrual phase, gain in body weight may also aggravate the edema.
3. The various conditions of edema due to other factors should be excluded.
4. Upright vs. supine position water load test is conducive to the diagnosis.

## Syndrome Differentiation

### 1. Qi stagnation and blood stasis

Symptoms: Swelling of limbs during the premenstrual or menstrual period, delayed period or menstrual colic, emotional depression, chest and hypochondriac distension or pricking pain; deep-red tongue or ecchymosis and taut or unsmooth pulse.

Analysis of symptoms: The liver promotes the free flow of qi and regulates emotions. When anger impairs the liver, there will be stagnation of liver qi, emotional depression and chest and hypochondriac distension; the stagnation of liver qi may further lead to the obstruction of the chong-channel and ren-channel, marked by a delayed period or menstrual colic; qi stagnation and blood stasis in the liver meridian are responsible for chest and hypochondriac distension or pricking pain; retention of water in the skin and muscles is characterized by swelling of the limbs during the premenstrual or menstrual period; the deep-red tongue with occasional ecchymosis and the taut or unsmooth pulse are manifestations of qi stagnation and blood stasis.

### 2. Obstruction of phlegm and dampness

Symptoms: Obesity, edema unrelated to menstrual period, general swelling due to deficiency, lethargy, a heavy sensation of the whole body, gastric distension, poor appetite and oliguresis; pale and enlarged tongue with white and greasy coating and slow pulse.

Analysis of symptoms: Deficiency of the spleen results in accumulation of phlegm and dampness in the body, marked by obesity; deficiency of the spleen is also responsible for an overflowing of water and dampness, so there is frequent swelling of the whole body; dampness obstructs the movements of qi and the ascent of lucid yang, bringing about lethargy and general heaviness; obstruction of phlegm and dampness in the middle energizer leads to a poor reception and digestion of food, characterized by gastric distension and poor appetite; retention of phlegm and dampness in the lower energizer is manifested as oliguresis; pale and enlarged tongue with white and greasy coating and slow pulse are manifestations of abundant dampness due to deficiency of the spleen.

## 3. Yang deficiency of the spleen and kidneys

Symptoms: Facial and blepharal edema in the menstrual period, swelling of the head or face in the morning, delayed arrival of menses in a small volume and light color, intolerance of cold, cold limbs, oliguresis, weakness and soreness in the waist and knees, lassitude, gastric distension, poor appetite, abdominal distension and loose stools; pale tongue with white coating, slow and deep pulse or slow and feeble pulse.

Analysis of symptoms: Deficiency of spleen yang and kidney yang, essence and blood, or the chong-channel and ren-channel are responsible for the delayed arrival of menses in a small volume and light color; the loss of qi as well as blood in the menstrual period leads to a failure of yang qi to warm the body, this is marked by intolerance of cold and cold limbs; deficient yang fails to warm and transport water-dampness, so there is facial and blepharal edema during the menstrual period and oliguresis; yang qi begins to decline in the evening, resulting in swelling of the head or face in the morning; deficiency of the spleen and stagnation of qi are manifested as lassitude, gastric distension, poor appetite, abdominal distension and loose stools; deficiency of the kidneys is responsible for weakness and soreness in the waist and knees; the pale tongue with white coating, slow and deep or slow and feeble pulse are all due to deficiency of spleen yang and kidney yang.

## Differential Treatment

### 1. Qi stagnation and blood stasis

Treatment principle: Promoting qi flow and activating blood circulation, inducing urination to relieve edema.

Prescription and herbs: Modified Xuefu Zhuyu Decoction and Wupi Potion.

Chaihu (Chinese Thorowax Root) 9 g, Danggui (Chinese Angelica) 9 g, Chuanxiong (Szechwan Lovage Rhizome) 9 g, Chishao (Red Peony Root) 12 g, Zhiqiao (Orange Fruit) 9 g, Niuxi (Twotoothed Achyranthes Root) 9 g, Yimucao (Motherwort Herb) 15 g, Sangbaipi (White Mulberry Root-Bark) 9 g, Fulingpi (Indian Bread Peel) 15 g, Dafupi (Areca Peel) 9 g, Chenpi (Dried Tangerine Peel) 9 g and Xiangfu (Nutgrass Galingale Rhizome) 9 g.

Modification: If there is apparent menstrual colic or pricking pain in the chest and hypochondria, Chuanlianzi (Szechwan Chinaberry Fruit) 9 g and Yanhusuo (Corydalis) 9 g can be added to soothe the liver and regulate qi, as well as to resolve stasis and stop pain; for severe swelling before menstruation, Wangbuliuxing (Cowherb Seed) 12 g and Zelan (Herba Lycopi) 12 g can be added to activate blood and promote urination.

### 2. Obstruction of phlegm and dampness

Treatment principle: Dissolving phlegm and expelling dampness, promoting urination to relieve edema.

Prescription and herbs: Modified Wuling Powder and Erchen Decoction.

Baizhu (Largehead Atractylodes Rhizome) 15 g, Fuling (Indian Bread) 15 g, Zhuling (Polyporus) 15 g, Guizhi (Cassia Twig) 9 g, Chenpi (Dried Tangerine Peel) 6 g, Banxia (Pinellia Tuber) 12 g, Dafupi (Areca Peel) 9 g, Houpu (Magnolia Bark) 6 g, Zexie (Oriental Waterplantain Rhizome) 12 g and Cheqianzi (Plantain Seed) 12 g (wrapped during decoction).

Modification: For lassitude, Huangqi (Milkvetch Root) 30 g can be added to supplement qi and promote water circulation; if there are loose stools, Yiyiren (Fried Coix Seed) 30 g and Sharen (Villous Amomum Fruit) 3 g (decocted later) can be added to invigorate the spleen and check diarrhea; if phlegm and dampness transforms into heat and dryness, the fluid will be impaired, marked by feverish dysphoria, thirst, constipation, yellow and greasy tongue coating and slippery and rapid pulse. In this case, it can be treated by nourishing yin, promoting urination and purging heat with Supplementary Zhuling Decoction: Zhuling (Polyporus) 15 g, Chifuling (Indian Bread Pink Epidermis) 15 g, Zexie (Oriental Waterplantain Rhizome) 30 g, Huashi (Talc) 20 g (wrapped during decoction), Tinglizi (Herba Leonuri) 15 g (wrapped during decoction), Dahuang (Rhubarb) 3 g (decocted later) and Ejiao (Donkey-hide Glue) 9 g (melted in decoction).

### 3. Yang deficiency of the spleen and kidneys

Treatment principle: Warming yang to relieve edema.

Prescription and herbs: Modified Linggui Zhugan Decoction and Zhenwu Decoction.

Fupian (Radix Aconitilateralis Preparata) 9 g, Guizhi (Cassia Twig) 9 g, Baizhu (Largehead Atractylodes Rhizome) 15 g, Fuling (Indian Bread) 15 g, Ganjiang (Dried Ginger) 6 g, Zexie (Oriental Waterplantain Rhizome) 15 g, Muxiang (Common Aucklandia Root) 9 g, Chenpi (Dried Tangerine Peel) 9 g, Houpu (Magnolia Bark) 9 g and Baishao (White Peony Alba) 15 g.

Modification: If there is lassitude, reduced food intake and loose stools, Huangqi (Milkvetch Root) 15 g, Dangshen (Radix Codonopsis) 12 g and Shanyao (Common Yan Rhizome) 12 g can be added to replenish qi and invigorate the spleen; for delayed arrival of menses in a small volume, Danggui (Chinese Angelica) 9 g, Yimucao (Motherwort Herb) 15 g and Tusizi (Dodder Seed) 15 g can be added to nourish blood and regulate the chong-channel; for severe swelling of the head or face, Mahuang (Ephedra) 9 g and Chixiaodou (Rice Bean) 30 g are used to move up yang, disperse the exterior and promote urination for alleviation of the edema.

### Chinese Patent Medicine

1. Jisheng Shenqi Pill: 6 g for each dose, 3 times a day.
2. Xiaoyao Pill: 6 g for each dose, 3 times a day.

## Simple and Handy Prescriptions

Dongguapi (Chinese Waxgourd Peel) 9 g, Shengjiangpi (Fresh Ginger Peel) 6 g, Dafupi (Areca Peel) 9 g and Chenpi (Dried Tangerine Peel) 6 g are boiled in water and consumed several times a day. It is used to treat frequent edema.

## Other Therapies

External therapy: 4 river-snails (without shells), 5 onions and Cheqianzi (Plantain Herb) 15 g are pounded and made into medicinal paste for application on the umbilical region.

Dietary therapy: Chixiaodou (Rice Bean) 30 g, Yiyiren (Coix Seed) 30 g and Jiangmi (Rice Fruit) 50 g are boiled in water and made into porridge, which is taken in the morning and evening. It is used to treat obese patients with scanty urine and edema.

## Cautions and Advice

1. Generally, idiopathic edema has a favorable prognosis, so it is unnecessary for the patients to be worried; instead, they should maintain a positive and peaceful frame of mind.
2. It is advisable for the patients to control their intake of carbohydrates, animal lipids and salt.

## Daily Exercises

1. Concisely describe the pathological changes of idiopathic edema.
2. Explain how idiopathic edema due to qi stagnation and blood stasis and that due to deficiency of spleen and kidneys can be differentiated and treated.

# Female Climacteric Syndrome
# Week 11: Wednesday

Female climacteric syndrome refers to the systemic pathological changes due to the disorder of the hypothalamus-hypophysis-gonad axis, which results from the retrogressive changes of sexual glands in females when they progress from the prime of their lives into old age. Clinically. it is often characterized by a propensity for anger and crying, baking fever, sweating, feverish sensation over the five centers, dizziness, tinnitus, forgetfulness, palpitations, insomnia, menstrual disorder and anthralgia. It afflicts females around 45~55 years old. Regarded as a disorder occurring at a certain lifestage, climacteric syndrome usually has a favorable prognosis. In TCM, this disease is believed to be closely associated with "lily disease", "visceral agitation", "syndrome of depression", "palpitations", "insomnia", "dizziness", "headache", "massive or incessant extramenstral vaginal bleeding" and "irregular menstruation".

## Etiology and Pathology

TCM holds that female climacteric syndrome is due to deficiency of kidney qi and essence, termination of tiangui (menstruation) and malnutrition of the viscera and meridians when the patients are over 49 years old (the menopause period), which further progresses into disorder of qi and blood, imbalance between yin and yang and pathological changes of the heart, liver and kidneys.

The pathological changes are marked by deficiency of the kidney primordial qi and dysfunction of the visceral qi when the patients are over 49 years old. Stagnation of the liver with deficiency of the gallbladder is manifested as distending pain in the chest and breast, timorousness and a tendency to cry easily. Deficiency of the spleen and stomach with exhaustion of both qi and blood is manifested as uncontrolled primordial spirit, absentmindedness and forgetfulness. Yin-blood is essential to females, so deficiency of the kidneys, blood, chong-channel, ren-channel and meridians is manifested as menstrual disorders, or weakness and soreness in the waist and knees. Deficiency may lead to blood stasis, which is manifested as bone soreness. Deficiency of kidney yin results in hyperactivity of liver yang, presenting as dizziness, headache and tinnitus. Liver fire flames up, bringing about irascibility. Fire-heat scorches the body, resulting in baking fever with sweating; kidney water fails to coordinate the heart fire, leading to hyperactivity of heart fire marked by palpitations and insomnia. In the end, there will be deficiency of kidney yin and kidney yang.

## Diagnostic Key Points

1. This disease usually occurs in females around 45~55 years old, who have removed bilateral ovaries, or experienced artificial menopause due to radiotherapy.
2. The common symptoms are emotional change, propensity for anger and crying, paroxysmal baking fever, sweating, insomnia, dizziness, tinnitus, forgetfulness, palpitations, chest distress, soreness in waist and knees and menstrual disorder. Other internal or women's diseases should be excluded.
3. Laboratory examination: Increase in blood gonadotropic hormone, decrease in estrogen and slight decrease in vaginal smear hormone.

## Syndrome Differentiation

### 1. Stagnation of the liver with deficiency of the gallbladder

Symptoms: Emotional depression, crying and sighing for no apparent reason, palpitations, timorousness, restlessness, distending pain in the chest, hypochondria and breast and menstrual disorder; red tongue with thin coating and taut-thin pulse.

Analysis of symptoms: The liver is the prenatal foundation of women, so when they are over 49 years old, the stagnation of liver qi may lead to emotional depression and propensity for tears and sighing; deficiency of heart qi and gallbladder qi is responsible for palpitations, timorousness and restlessness; stagnation of the liver meridian can result in disorders of the thoroughfare vessel and conception vessel, marked by distending pain in the chest, hypochondria and breast, as well as menstrual disorder; the red tongue, thin coating and taut-thin pulse are all attributable to depression of liver with deficiency of the gallbladder.

## 2. Deficiency of the kidneys with hyperactivity of the liver

Symptoms: Dizziness, headache, tinnitus, feverish sensations over the five centers, baking fever, sweating, irascibility, palpitations, insomnia, menstrual disorder, weakness and soreness in the waist and legs; red tongue with thin and yellow coating and thin, taut and rapid pulse.

Analysis of symptoms: Deficiency of kidney yin leads to hyperactivity of liver yang (due to water failing to nourish the wood), it is marked by dizziness, headache and tinnitus; deficiency of yin results in hyperactivity of yang and abundance of liver fire, characterized by feverish sensation over the five centers, baking fever and sweating; the liver fire flames upward, leading to irascibility; the kidney water fails to curb the heart fire, resulting in palpitations and insomnia; the waist is the "house of the kidneys" and the kidneys control the bones, so deficiency of the kidneys can bring about weakness and soreness in the waist and knees; the deficiency of kidney yin may also cause insufficiency of the liver blood as well as dysfunction of the thoroughfare vessel and conception vessel, marked by menstrual disorders; deficiency of yin produces internal heat, which consumes the body fluid, with such signs as scanty reddish urine and dry stools; the red tongue with thin and yellow coating and thin, taut and rapid pulse are due to deficiency of the kidneys with hyperactivity of the liver.

## 3. Deficiency of the spleen and stomach

Symptoms: Palpitations, insomnia, absentmindedness, forgetfulness, apathy, lassitude, poor appetite, or continual menses; pale tongue with white coating and thin pulse.

Analysis of symptoms: The patient is weak in constitution and has entered into the climacteric period, marked by deficiency of the spleen and stomach, as well as insufficiency of qi and blood; insufficiency of heart blood leads to a malnourished heart spirit and ungoverned primordial spirit, characterized by palpitations, insomnia, absentmindedness, forgetfulness and apathy; deficiency of spleen qi results in poor digestion, leading to lassitude and poor appetite; the deficient spleen fails to arrest bleeding, so there is continual menses; the pale tongue with white coating and thin pulse are all caused by deficiency of the spleen and stomach, as well as simultaneous depletion of qi and blood.

## 4. Deficiency of kidney yin and kidney yang

Symptoms: Dizziness, blurred vision, tinnitus, forgetfulness, soreness or pain in the waist and knees, cold body, aversion to heat, suppression of menses and hyposexuality; slightly red tongue, thin coating and thin, deep and weak pulse.

Analysis of symptoms: Deficiency of kidney essence brings on malnutrition of the brain, marked by dizziness, blurred vision, tinnitus and forgetfulness; since tiangui disappears, menstruation also ceases; deficiency of the kidneys leads to obstruction in the collaterals, so there is soreness or pain in the waist and knees; prolonged deficiency of yin involves the kidney yang, giving rise to deficiency of yin and yang, with such signs as cold body, aversion to heat and hyposexuality; the slightly red tongue with thin coating and thin, deep and weak pulse are attributable to deficiency of kidney yin and kidney yang.

## Differential Treatment

### 1. Stagnation of the liver with deficiency of the gallbladder

Treatment principle: Soothing the liver and relieving stagnation, tranquilizing the spirit andcalming the mind.

Prescription and herbs: Modified Chaihu Shugan Powder and Anshen Dingzhi Pill.

Chaihu (Chinese Thorowax Root) 9 g, Zhiqiao (Orange Fruit) 9 g, Xiangfu (Nutgrass Galingale Rhizome) 9 g, Baishao (White Peony Alba) 12 g, Chuanxiong (Szechwan Lovage Rhizome) 9 g, Zhigancao ( Liquorice Root) 9 g, Fushen (Indian Bread with Hostwood) 15 g, Yuanzhi (Thinleaf Milkwort Root) 5 g, Changpu (Acorus Calamus) 6 g and Longchi (Fossilia Dentis Mastodi) 30 g (decocted first).

Modification: For timorousness, Huaixiaomai (Wheat) 30 g and Cishi (Magnetite) 30 g (decocted first) can be used to tranquilize the spirit and calm the mind; for irregular menstruation, Danggui (Chinese Angelica) 9 g, Yimucao (Motherwort Herb) 15 g and Tusizi (Dodder Seed) 15 g are added to nourish blood and regulate the chong-channel.

## 2. Deficiency of the kidneys with hyperactivity of the liver

Treatment principle: Nourishing yin and tonifying the kidneys, calming the liver and subduing yang.

Prescription and herbs: Modified Zhibai Dihuang Pill and Tianma Gouteng Potion.

Zhimu (Common Anemarrhena Rhizome) 9 g, Huangbai (Amur Cork-tree) 9 g, Shengdi (Dried Rehmannia Root) 15 g, Shanzhuyu (Asiatic Cornelian Cherry Fruit) 9 g, Danpi (Cortex Moutan) 9 g Zexie (Oriental Waterplantain Rhizome) 12 g, Tianma (Tall Gastrodis Tuber) 9 g, Gouteng (Gambir Plant) 15 g (decocted later), Shijueming (Sea-ear Shell) 30 g (decocted first), Zhenzhumu (Nacre) 30 g, Sangjisheng (Chinese Taxillus Herb) 12 g and Duzhong (Eucommia Bark) 12 g.

Modification: If there are menstrual disorders with profuse, continual menses, Tiandong (Cochinchinese Asparagus Root) 15 g and Ejiao (Donkey-hide Glue) 9 g (melted in decoction) can be added to nourish the kidneys and arrest bleeding; for incoordination between the heart and kidneys with restlessness and insomnia, Tianma (Tall Gastrodis Tuber), Gouteng (Gambir Plant) and Shijueming (Sea-ear Shell) can be replaced with Huanglian (Golden Thread) 5 g and Rouguifen (Cassia Bark Powder) 2 g (infused in water) to coordinate the heart and kidneys.

## 3. Deficiency of the spleen and stomach

Treatment principle: Invigorating qi and nourishing blood, nourishing the heart and calming the spirit.

Prescription and herbs: Modified Guipi Decoction.

Dangshen (Radix Codonopsis) 15 g, Huangqi (Milkvetch Root) 20 g, Baizhu (Largehead Atractylodes Rhizome) 12 g, Zhigancao (Liquorice

Root) 6 g, Danggui (Chinese Angelica) 9 g, Longyanrou (Longan Aril) 9 g, Suanzaoren (Spine Date Seed) 12 g, Fushen (Indian Bread with Hostwood) 12 g, Yuanzhi (Thinleaf Milkwort Root) 6 g and Muxiang (Common Aucklandia Root) 6 g.

Modification: If there is continuous menses, Xianhecao (Hairyvein Agrimonia Herb) 15 g and Duan Wuzeigu (Calcined Cuttebone) 15 g can be added to stop bleeding and regulate menstrual discharge; for palpitations with knotted or intermittent pulse, Zhigancao (Stir-baked Liquorice Root) 9 g is replaced with Guizhi (Cassia Twig) 9 g, Shengdi (Dried Rehmannia Root) 12 g and Maidong (Dwarf Lilyturf Tuber) 12 g to warm and activate the heart yang, as well as to nourish the heart yin.

## 4. Deficiency of kidney yin and kidney yang

Treatment principle: Warming the kidneys, supplementing essence and regulating yin and yang.

Prescription and herbs: Supplementary Erxian Decoction.

Xianmao (Common Curculigo Rhizome) 9 g, Xianlingpi (Herba Epimedii) 9 g, Bajitian (Mornda Root) 9 g, Zhimu (Common Anemarrhena Rhizome) 9 g, Huangbai (Amur Cork-tree) 9 g, Danggui (Chinese Angelica) 9 g, Tusizi (Dodder Seed) 15 g, Shudi (Prepared Rhizome of Rehmannia) 15 g, Shanyao (Common Yan Rhizome) 15 g, Shanzhuyu (Asiatic Cornelian Cherry Fruit) 9 g, Gouqizi (Barbary Wolfberry Fruit) 12 g and Sangjisheng (Chinese Taxillus Herb) 15 g.

Modification: If there is lassitude, Huangqi (Milkvetch Root) 15 g and Dangshen (Radix Codonopsis) 12 g can be added to invigorate the spleen and supplement qi; for intolerance of cold with cold limbs, Rouguifen (Cassia Bark Powder) 2 g (infused in water) and Lujiaojiao (Deerhorn Glue) 9 g (melted in decoction) can be used to warm and activate yang; for swollen limbs, Fuling (Indian Bread) 15 g, Zhuling (Polyporus) 15 g, Baizhu (Largehead Atractylodes Rhizome) 15 g and Guizhi (Cassia Twig) 9 g can be used to activate yang and promote water discharge; for sore and painful waist and knees, Buguzhi (Malaytea Scurfpea Fruit) 15 g and Niuxi (Twotoothed Achyranthes Root) 15 g are used to nourish the kidneys and strengthen the bones.

## Chinese Patent Medicine

1. Zhibai Dihuang Pill: 6 g for each dose, 3 times a day.
2. Yougui Pill: 6 g for each dose, 3 times a day.
3. Gengnian An Tablet: 4 tablets for each dose, 3 times a day.

## Simple and Handy Prescriptions

1. Baihe (Lily Bulb) 30 g and Shengdi (Dried Rehmannia Root) 15 g are boiled in water and administered twice a day to address emotional disturbance and propensity for anger and crying.
2. Huaixiaomai (Wheat) 50 g, Zhigancao (Stir-baked Liquorice Root) 9 g and Dazao (Chinese Date) 9 g are boiled in water and administered twice a day to address palpitations and insomnia.
3. Renshenfen (Ginseng Powder) 30 g and Zihechefen (Human Placenta Powder) 30 g are mixed evenly and then capsulized. The capsules are administered 2 g for each dose, 3 times a day. This is used address the deficiency of kidney yin and kidney yang.

## Other Therapies

Dietary therapy:

(1) Gouqizi (Barbary Wolfberry Fruit) 9 g, Juhua (Chrysanthemum Flower) 6 g and Maidong (Dwarf Lilyturf Tuber) 12 g are boiled in water. The decoction is frequently served as tea for the treatment of this disease with exuberance of fire due to deficiency of yin.

(2) Huangqi (Milkvetch Root) 20 g, Shengdi (Dried Rehmannia Root) 10 g, Wuguji (Silkie) 500 g, Hongzao (Red Date) 15 dates and Shengjiang (Fresh Ginger) 3 g are thoroughly boiled in a steam boiler with the decoction of Huangqi (Milkvetch Root) and Shengdi (Dried Rehmannia Root). It is used to treat this disease with deficiency of yin and yang.

## Cautions and Advice

1. In the climacteric period, females are susceptible to hypertension, coronary artery disease, diabetes, metabolic disturbance of lipids, as well as

mental disorders such as anxiety and depression. For this reason, a comprehensive therapy plan is needed.
2. Patients should consume adequate nutrients, calcium and vitamins so as to prevent such disorders as osteoporosis.
3. They should also be actively involved in physical exercise in order to strengthen the constitution and prevent pre-senility.

## Daily Exercises

1. Recall the etiological factors and pathological characteristics of female climacteric syndrome.
2. Explain the different patterns and treatment principles of female climacteric syndrome.

# CHAPTER 8

# Neuropsychic Diseases

## Myasthenia Gravis
## Week 11: Thursday

Myasthenia gravis refers to an autoimmune disease due to sensitization of the auto-acetylcholine receptors (AchR). In other words, it is a chronic disease marked by disorders of muscle contraction resulting from transmission dysfunction in the neuromuscular junction. It is divided into three types according to the different regions involved: ocular myasthenia, bulbar myasthenia and general myasthenia. Some patients may present with mixed types. The symptoms vary, but the main one is fatigability of the affected striated muscles which may temporarily recover or improve after rest or treatment. In severe cases, it can be life-threatening due to dyspnea. The disease is more commonly seen in females than in males at the age ranging from 20 to 35 years old. In TCM, myasthenia gravis is considered to be associated with "flaccidity syndrome" and "deficiency consumption".

### Etiology and Pathology

TCM holds that the occurrence of this disease is closely linked to the spleen, stomach, liver and kidneys. The spleen, being the source of qi and blood and the postnatal foundation, governs transportation and transformation and dominates the muscles and four limbs. The kidneys store essence, governs bones and produces marrow. As such, weakness of the spleen and stomach will lead to qi sinking of the middle energizer, insufficiency of cereal nutrients and malnutrition of muscles; in the long run, the primordial qi may become extremely deficient and the tendons and vessels can be malnourished due to deficiency of liver blood; furthermore, there will not be postnatal supplement to the kidney essence, bringing about withered bones and depleted marrows.

## Diagnostic Key Points

1. The hallmark of myasthenia gravis is fatigability of the skeletal muscle group and emotional fluctuation. In 90% of the cases, the first noticeable symptom is ptosis. Within 1~2 years, it may involve the bulbar muscles, facial muscles, cervical muscles and limb muscles. Symptoms of the ocular type are ptosis, anopsia and diplopia; the bulbar type is marked by low and faint nasal voice, hiccups during food intake, dysarthria, dysphagia, flowing of drinking water out of the nostrils and weakness of the masticatory muscles and facial muscles of expression; the general type is marked by impairment of the striated muscles all over the body in varying degrees, accompanied by myasthenia of the four limbs, aptness to tumbling down, difficulty in going upstairs and dyspnea in severe and life-threatening cases.
2. In some cases there are abnormalities of T3 and T4 and 63%~95% of the patients have increase of AchR antibodies in blood serum. For uncomplicated ocular type, the positive rate is 30%.
3. Thoracic gland CT, MRI and mediastinum aerography may find abnormalities of the thoracic gland in over 90% patients.
4. For those who are suspected to have this disease, fatigue test and drug examination may help make it clear.
5. If it is still unconfirmed, GMG and repeated electric stimulation can be performed (attenuation rate is over 10%).

## Syndrome Differentiation

### 1. Weakness of the spleen and stomach

Symptoms: Ptosis, flaccidity of the limbs aggravating gradually, exacerbation upon physical exertion, alleviation after rests, lassitude, reduced appetite, hiccups during food intake, or even with dysphagia, loose stools, swollen and lusterless complexion; white and thin tongue coating, thin and feeble pulse.

Analysis of symptoms: Weakness of the spleen and stomach leads to qi sinking of the middle energizer, marked by ptosis and swollen, lusterless complexion; weakness of the spleen and stomach also results in deficiency of qi and blood, marked by flaccidity of the limbs aggravating gradually, with exacerbation upon physical exertion and alleviation after rests; insufficiency of middle qi brings about failure of lucid yang to ascend, characterized by lassitude and loose stools; deficiency of the spleen creates a predisposition to abnormal ascending and descending of qi, characterized by reduced appetite, hiccups during food intake, or even dysphagia; the white and thin tongue coating as well as thin and feeble pulse are attributable to weakness of the spleen and stomach.

## 2. Yin deficiency of the liver and kidneys

Symptoms: Ptosis, flaccidity in the lower limbs with inability to stand for a long time, or even restricted movements, soreness and weakness in the lumbar vertebrae, tinnitus, blurred vision, irregular menstruation, nocturnal emissions and impotence, hectic fever and night sweats; reddish tongue with scanty coating and thin and rapid pulse.

Analysis of symptoms: Yin deficiency of the liver and kidneys brings on malnutrition of the tendons, marked by ptosis, flaccidity in the lower limbs with inability to stand for a long time, or even restricted movements; the waist is the "house of the kidneys", so deficiency of the kidneys will result in soreness and weakness in the lumbar vertebrae; the liver opens into the eyes, while the kidneys open into the ears, so insufficiency of the liver and kidneys will give rise to blurred vision and tinnitus; the kidneys store essence, whereas the liver stores blood, thus deficiency of the liver and kidneys can bring about deficiency of essence and blood, with such manifestations as irregular menstruation in females as well as nocturnal emissions and impotence in males; internal heat due to deficiency of yin is responsible for hectic fever and night sweats; the red tongue with scanty coating, as well as the thin and rapid pulse are due to deficiency of liver yin and kidney yin.

## Differential Treatment

### 1. Weakness of the spleen and stomach

Treatment principle: Nourishing qi for ascending, invigorating the spleen and stomach.

Prescription and herbs: Modified Buzhong Yiqi Decoction.

Huangqi (Milkvetch Root) 30 g, Dangshen (Radix Codonopsis) 12 g, Shengma (Rhizoma Cimicifugae) 9 g, Chaihu (Chinese Thorowax Root) 9 g, Baizhu (Largehead Atractylodes Rhizome) 12 g, Shanyao (Plantain Herb) 15 g, Biandou (Hyacinth Bean) 15 g, Yiyiren (Coix Seed) 30 g, Danggui (Chinese Angelica) 9 g, Chenpi (Dried Tangerine Peel) 6 g and Gancao (Liquorice Root) 6 g.

Modification: If there is severe lassitude, Huangjing (Solomonseal Rhizome) 9 g can be added to reinforce the action of nourishing qi.

### 2. Yin deficiency of the liver and kidneys

Treatment principle: Tonifying the liver and kidneys, nourishing yin and dispelling heat.

Prescription and herbs: Modified Huqian Pill.

Niuxi (Twotoothed Achyranthes Root) 9 g, Duzhong (Eucommia Bark) 9 g, Sangjisheng (Chinese Taxillus Herb) 12 g, Suoyang (Songaria Cynomorium Herb) 9 g, Danggui (Chinese Angelica) 9 g, Baishao (White Peony Alba) 9 g, Zhimu (Common Anemarrhena Rhizome) 9 g, Huangbai (Amur Cork-tree) 9 g, Shengdi (Dried Rehmannia Root) 9 g, Shudi (Prepared Rhizome of Rehmannia) 9 g, Guiban (Tortoise Shell) 15 g and Gancao ( Liquorice Root) 6 g.

Modification: For tinnitus, hichangpu (Acorus Calamus) 12 g and Lingcishi (Magnetitum) 30 g can be added to open the ear orifices; for blurred vision, Gouqizi (Barbary Wolfberry Fruit) 9 g and Juhua (Chrysanthemum Flower) 9 g can be used to nourish yin, clear the liver and improve vision.

## Chinese Patent Medicine

1. Buzhong Yiqi Pill: 3 g for each dose, 3 times a day.
2. Zuogui Pill: 3 g for each dose, twice a day.
3. Yougui Pill: 3 g for each dose, 3 times a day.

## Simple and Handy Prescriptions

1. Huangqi (Milkvetch Root) 9 g, Renshen (Ginseng) 3 g, Shengma (Rhizoma Cimicifugae) 6 g and Gouqizi (Barbary Wolfberry Fruit) 3 g are decocted in water and frequently taken as tea.
2. Shenglizi (Chestnuts) 200 g and Shanyao (Common Yan Rhizome) 500 g are decocted in a proper amount of water and then a small quantity of Yitang (Cerealose) is added. This decoction should be frequently taken.

## Other Therapies

Dietary therapy: A female silkie and a male silkie are stuffed with Renshen (Ginseng) 9 g, Shenghuangqi (Raw Milkvetch Root) 60 g and Shengjiang (Fresh Ginger) 6 g and then sutured with thread. Then the silkies are boiled in an earthenware cooking pot with cooking wine and water in equal amounts. At first they are boiled with strong fire and then mild fire till the decoction is condensed. Seasonings can be added according to taste. Both the decoction and chicken meat can be consumed frequently at different times and on different days.

## Cautions and Advice

1. This disease is marked by slow onset, long duration, tendency for alleviation, aptness to relapse and alternated relief and aggravation. Overstrain, emotional disturbance, infection, external injury, childbirth and improper use of drugs can all trigger off this disease. Patients should balance their work and rest, maintain a regular lifestyle, avoid dramatic emotional fluctuations or mental traumas, strengthen the body constitution, be aware of the climatic changes, prevent common cold and promptly treat various infections.
2. Patients should consume nutritious foods such as chicken, beef, mutton, dog meat, eel, oyster and shrimp. Because the patients are very weak in the spleen and stomach, they should take easily digestible food in a small quantity but have more frequent meals. The food should be well cooked or contain certain Chinese herbs with the function of promoting digestion so as to invigorate the stomach qi.

3. The ocular type and bulbar type of myasthenia gravis, if treated actively and properly, can have a relatively favorable prognosis. If the respiratory muscles are involved, critical conditions such as dyspnea may appear (myasthenia crisis, pointing to an unfavorable prognosis).

## Daily Exercises

1. Concisely describe the diagnostic key points of myasthenia gravis.
2. Explain the patterns that myasthenia gravis can be clinically differentiated into, as well as how to treat these variations.

# Progressive Muscular Dystrophy

## Week 11: Friday

Progressive muscular dystrophy is a genetic disease characterized by atrophy or degeneration of the muscle fibers due mostly to long-term ischemia or lack of voluntary contraction of the muscles. This disease can be divided into five types: false hypertrophic type, face-shoulder-brachium type, limb girdle type, ocular type and distal type. The main symptoms are muscular atrophy or decrease in muscular force, which initially occurs at the proximal end of the limbs (shoulder girdle, pelvic girdle), this is marked by symmetrical and progressive myatrophy, or even general muscular atrophy and flaccidity of the limbs in the long run. This disease is often secondary to disorders of the nervous system, or muscular injuries, hyperostosis, bone fracture, muscular spasms and malnutrition. In TCM, progressive muscular dystrophy is considered to be associated with "flaccidity syndrome" and "paralysis and bi-syndrome".

## Etiology and Pathology

TCM holds that the syndrome of flaccidity is closely linked to the lungs, spleen, stomach, liver and kidneys. It is primarily due to emotional impairment, exogenous invasion of damp-heat, overstrain and an excessive sexual life, all of which result in deficiency of the internal organs, essence qi, muscles and tendons. In some cases, invasion of heat into the lungs brings about failure of the five zang-organs to be moistened by the fluid and the resultant malnutrition of the four limbs and tendons. In other cases, invasion of damp-heat into the channels causes unsmooth circulation of nutrient qi and defensive qi, eventually leading to inhibited flow of qi and blood and flaccidity of the tendons and muscles due to malnutrition. In addition, weakness of the spleen and stomach can lead to functional disorders of reception, transformation and distribution, so there will be inadequate qi, blood and body fluid for the nourishment of the five zang-organs, marked by limited range of movements and muscular wasting. Furthermore, deficiency of the liver and kidneys may also deprive the muscles and tendons of nutrients, predisposing them to muscular atrophy and flaccidity.

## Diagnostic Key Points

1. This disease is marked by latent onset, difficulty in walking with frequent falls, a waddling gait and winged scapula and even an inability to walk, progressive muscle wasting and bone deformity. There may also be false hypertrophy of the muscles and supine rising.
2. For patients with prominent, extensive muscles, the excretion of urine creatine is increased whereas that of creatinine is decreased; the creatine phosphokinase level in blood serum is 10~100 times as high as the normal one, which is the result of reduced activity in the late stage due to lack of exercise and wasting of muscles.
3. Electromyogram and muscular biopsy can be helpful to the diagnosis.

## Syndrome Differentiation

### 1. Scorching heat in the lungs with impaired lobes

Symptoms: Sudden onset, fever at first, then flaccidity in the limbs, thirst, vexation, dry throat and skin, choking cough with little sputum, yellowish urine and dry stools; red tongue with yellow coating and thin and rapid pulse.

Analysis of symptoms: Pathogenic heat invades the lungs and damages the qi and yin, leading to failure of the body fluid to moisten the muscles, this is marked by fever and subsequent flaccidity in the limbs; the lung fluid fails to nourish the pulmonary system, resulting in a dry throat, choking cough and scanty sputum; pathogenic heat consumes fluid, so there is thirst; heat disturbs the heart spirit, so there is vexation; consumption of yin-fluid is marked by dry skin; heat in the bladder is manifested as yellowish urine; heat accumulating in the intestine is responsible for the dry stools; the red tongue with yellow coating and thin and rapid pulse are manifestations of impaired qi, yin and body fluid, which is due to exuberance of deficient heat in the interior.

### 2. Immersion of damp-heat

Symptoms: Flaccidity, a heavy sensation, numbness and mild edema in the four limbs (especially the lower ones) and sometimes fever, thoracic and epigastric fullness and distress, reddish urine with burning pain; yellow and greasy tongue coating, thin and rapid pulse.

Analysis of symptoms: Immersion of damp-heat in the skin and muscles leads to stagnation of qi and blood in the meridians, this is marked by flaccidity, a heavy sensation and mild edema in the four limbs; retention of damp-heat results in unsmooth circulation of qi and blood, characterized by numbness; obstruction of damp-heat brings about unsmooth functional activity of qi, presenting as fever as well as thoracic and epigastric fullness and distress; damp-heat pours downward, so there is reddish urine with burning pain; the yellow and greasy tongue coating and the thin and rapid pulse are attributable to immersion of damp-heat in the skin and muscles.

## 3. Weakness of the spleen and stomach

Symptoms: Flaccidity in the limb muscles which aggravates gradually, lassitude, shortness of breath upon exertion, reduced appetite, gastric and abdominal distension after food intake, loosestools and sallow or swollen complexion; pale tongue with white, thin and greasy coating and soggy and thin pulse.

Analysis of symptoms: Deficient spleen and stomach fail to transform water and food into qi and blood, which fail to nourish the muscles and tendons, so there is a lusterless complexion and flaccidity in the limb muscles which aggravates gradually; deficiency of qi is manifested as lassitude and shortness of breath upon physical exertion; dysfunction of the spleen in transportation and transformation results in failure of the stomach qi to descend normally, this is marked by a reduced appetite with gastric and abdominal distension after food intake; deficiency of the spleen is responsible for the failure of lucid yang to ascend, resulting in loose stools; a deficient spleen cannot transport and transform the water and dampness properly, giving rise to facial edema and greasy coating; the pale tongue with white, thin and greasy coating and the soggy and thin pulse are due to weakness of the spleen and stomach being unable to transform food into essence.

## 4. Deficiency of the liver and kidneys

Symptoms: Slow onset, flaccidity in the lower limbs with inability to stand for long periods or even walk, gradual loss of muscle mass in the leg or shin, soreness in the lumbar vertebrae, dry throat, loosened teeth, dizziness, loss of hair, tinnitus and incontinence of urine; reddish tongue with scanty coating and thin, rapid and deficient pulse.

Analysis of symptoms: Deficient liver and kidneys produce inadequate essence and blood to nourish the bones, tendons and muscles, gradually leading to the slow onset of flaccidity syndrome, particularly in the lower limbs with inability to stand for long or even walk; in the long run the muscles and tendons start to waste away, manifested by a shrinking in muscle mass of the legs and shins; a deficient kidney produces insufficient essence and marrow, so there is soreness in the lumbar vertebrae, dryness in the throat, looseness of the teeth and tinnitus; deficiency of liver blood is responsible for dryness in the throat, dizziness and loss of hair; a deficient kidney fails to store the essence, so there are nocturnal emissions, premature ejaculation and enuresis; the reddish tongue with scanty coating and thin, rapid and deficient pulse are all caused by exhaustion of liver yin and kidney yin with heat in the interior.

## Differential Treatment

### 1. Scorching heat in the lungs with impaired lobes

Treatment principle: Dispelling heat and moistening the lungs, nourishing yin to produce fluid.

Prescription and herbs: Modified Qingzao Jiufei Decoction.

Sangye (Mulberry Leaf) 12 g, Shigao (Gypsum) 30 g, Maidong (Dwarf Lilyturf Tuber) 9 g, Xingren (Almond) 9 g, Maren (Edestan) 9 g, Ejiao (Donkey-hide Glue) 9 g, Pipaye (Loquat Leaf) 12 g, Sangbaipi (White Mulberry Root-Bark) 9 g, Dangshen (Radix Codonopsis) 12 g and Gancao (Liquorice Root) 6 g.

Modification: If there is the presence of thirst, Huangfen (Radix Trichosanthis) 12 g, Yuzhu (Fragrant Solomonseal Rhizome) 9 g, Baihe (Lily Bulb) 9 g and Lugen (Reed Rhizome) 30 g are added to nourish yin and produce fluid.

### 2. Immersion of damp-heat

Treatment principle: Dispelling heat, eliminating dampness and promoting smooth flow of qi and blood.

Prescription and herbs: Modified Supplementary Ermiao Powder.

Huangbai (Amur Cork-tree) 9 g, Cangzhu (Atractylodes Rhizome) 9 g, Bixie (Rhizoma Dioscoreae Hypoglaucae) 9 g, Fangji (Fourstamen Stephania Root) 12 g, Chuanmutong (Armand Clematis Stem) 6 g, Yiyiren (Coix Seed) 15 g, Niuxi (Twotoothed Achyranthes Root) 9 g, Danggui (Chinese Angelica) 9 g, Shengdi (Dried Rehmannia Root) 9 g, Shudi (Prepared Rhizome of Rehmannia) 9 g, Chishao (Red Peony Root) 9 g, Danshen (Radix Salviae Miltiorrhiae) 15 g, Taoren (Peach Seed) 9 g, Honghua (Safflower) 3 g and Zhiqiao (Orange Fruit) 12 g.

Modification: If there is fever, QingshuiDoujuan (Semen Sojae Germinatum) 12 g, Jinyinhua (Honeysuckle Flower) 9 g and Lianqiao (Weeping Forsythia Capsule) 9 g can be added to dispel heat.

### 3. Weakness of the spleen and stomach

Treatment principle: Invigorating the spleen and stomach, nourishing qi and moving up the lucid.

Prescription and herbs: Modified Buzhong Yiqi Decoction.

Huangqi (Milkvetch Root) 30 g, Dangshen (Radix Codonopsis) 12 g, Baizhu (Largehead Atractylodes Rhizome) 12 g, Shanyao (Common Yan Rhizome) 15 g, Biandou (Hyacinth Bean) 12 g, Yiyiren (Coix Seed) 15 g, Chenpi (Dried Tangerine Peel) 9 g, Sharen (Villous Amomum Fruit) 3 g, Danggui (Chinese Angelica) 9 g, Chaihu (Chinese Thorowax Root) 9 g, Shengma (Rhizoma Cimicifugae) 6 g and Zhigancao (Stir-baked Liquorice Root) 6 g.

Modification: For reduced appetite, Shenqu (Massa Medicata Fermentata) 9 g and Maiya (Malt) 12 g can be added to promote digestion.

### 4. Deficiency of the liver and kidneys

Treatment principle: Supplementing the liver and tonifying the kidneys, nourishing yin and dispelling heat.

Prescription and herbs: Modified Heche Dazao Pill and Huqian Pill.

Dangshen (Radix Codonopsis) 12 g, Zihechefen (Human Placenta Powder) 12 g, Duzhong (Eucommia Bark) 9 g, Niuxi (Twotoothed Achyranthes Root) 9 g, Maidong (Dwarf Lilyturf Tuber) 9 g, Huangbai

(Amur Cork-tree) 9 g, Zhimu (Common Anemarrhena Rhizome) 9 g, Shudi (Prepared Rhizome of Rehmannia) 9 g, Guiban (Tortoise Shell) 9 g, Suoyang (Songaria Cynomorium Herb) 9 g, Danggui (Chinese Angelica) 9 g, Baishao (White Peony Alba) 9 g and Gancao ( Liquorice Root) 6 g.

Modification: If there is intense heat, Suoyang (Songaria Cynomorium Herb) 9 g can be replaced by Gouqizi (Barbary Wolfberry Fruit) 9 g and Juhua (Chrysanthemum Flower) 9 g so as to dispel liver heat.

## Chinese Patent Medicine

1. Buzhong Yiqi Pill: 3 g for each dose, 3 times a day.
2. Zuogui Pill: 3 g for each dose, twice a day.
3. Yougui Pill: 3 g for each dose, twice a day.

## Simple and Handy Prescriptions

Rice 60 g is made into porridge and then Shanyao (Common Yan Rhizome) 30 g is pounded into a paste with a small quantity of water; the porridge and paste are mixed evenly before adding Baibiandou (White Hyacinth Bean) 15 g; the mixture is boiled until the beans are well cooked. It is consumed twice a day, 1 bowl for each dose.

## Other Therapies

Dietary therapy:

(1) Huangqi (Milkvetch Root) 30 g is extracted to make juice and beef 50 g is cut into small pieces. Afterwards they are boiled with a proper amount of clear water. Before the mixture is completely cooked, 100 g of rice is added to make porridge. This porridge can be taken twice a day.
(2) A pig's knuckle and 50 g of pork tendon are cooked in the decoction made by boiling Duzhong (Eucommia Bark) 30 g and Niuxi (Twotoothed Achyranthes Root) 30 g. Proper amounts of salt and gourmet power are added before it is served.

Proper physical exercise, massage and Achilles tendon lengthening are still the first choice of treatment for patients with muscular dystrophy.

## Cautions and Advice

1. In the development of this disease, patients should perform frequent light exercises and massages. For those confined to bed, they should take active measures to prevent the occurrence of bedsores and pulmonary infection.
2. It is advisable for atients to adopt a protein-rich diet. In the initial stage, the disease, mostly due to excess by nature, should be addressed by taking predominantly cold foods as well as vegetables and fruits instead of oily ones. When the disease progresses into the late stage, it will become deficient in nature, so it is advisable to take more fish, eggs, chicken, lean pork, beef and mutton so as to nourish the blood and muscles. However, this cannot be overdone lest the spleen and stomach be damaged. Since the patients' organs are too deficient to be nourished, the spleen and stomach must be invigorated first before the tonics are applied. Shanzha (Hawthorn Fruit), Yiyiren (Coix Seed), Jidun (corium stomachium galli) and Chenpi (Dried Tangerine Peel) are highly recommended to regulate the spleen and stomach.
3. Family medical history, blood serum CPK and genes should be analyzed so as to discover the carrier as early as possible. Such knowledge about marriage, heredity and eugenics should be made available to the public.

## Daily Exercises

1. Concisely describe the diagnostic key points of progressive muscular dystrophy.
2. Explain how progressive muscular dystrophy can be treated based on syndrome differentiation.

# Trembling Palsy
# Week 11: Saturday

Trembling palsy, also called Parkinson's disease, is a degenerative disease of the central nervous system occurring in middle-aged and old people. The chief degenerative change takes place in the substantia nigra and nigrostriatal passage, leading to a decrease in dopamine-generating cells. The main symptoms are progressive slowness in movement and muscular stiffness and tremors. It mostly afflicts people above the age 50, especially the males. It has a slow onset and a long duration (possibly decades). In TCM, trembling palsy belongs to the category of "tremors", "dizziness" and "liver wind".

## Etiology and Pathology

TCM holds that this disease is caused by deficiency of the liver and kidneys with insufficiency of qi and blood. Deficiency of kidney yin leads to hyperactivity of liver yang (water fails to nourish wood) and subsequently brings about malnutrition, stiffness or spasm of muscles and tendons. Hyperactivity of yang gives rise to a stirring of wind, marked by tremors of the limb extremities; insufficient qi and blood fail to nourish the muscles and tendons all over the body, characterized by tremors and stiffness of the muscles.

## Diagnostic Key Points

1. The disease is characterized by a slow onset, gradual development, progressive slowness in movement, muscular stiffness and tremors and disappearance of postural reflexes.
2. Reduced movement is firstly seen in the fingers and then the homolateral lower limbs and heterolateral upper and lower limbs and sometimes there are "pill-rolling movements", a "mask-like face", "micrographia" and "festinating gait", slurred speech with monotonous tone and dysphagia in severe cases.
3. Special postures may appear: anteversion of head, hunched back, slight flexion or adduction of the four limbs.

## Syndrome Differentiation

## 1. Stirring of wind due to yin deficiency

Symptoms: Dizziness, tinnitus, involuntary twitching of the head, incessant shaking of upper limbs with inability to hold things, tremors of muscles, restlessness, irascibility, insomnia, spasm of muscles and tendons, apathy with inability to smile and pale complexion; red tongue with thin coating and rapid-taut or rapid-thin pulse.

Analysis of symptoms: Deficiency of liver yin and kidney yin is manifested as dizziness and tinnitus; deficiency of yin brings about hyperactivity of yang, which stirs wind and causes involuntary twitching of the head, incessant shaking of upper limbs with inability to hold things and muscle tremors; deficiency of yin brings about hyperactivity of yang, which produces fire and disturbs the heart spirit, this is marked by restlessness, irascibility and insomnia; the liver and kidneys are insufficient, leading to malnutrition of the muscles and tendons, with such signs as spasm of muscles and tendons, apathy with inability to smile and pale complexion; the red tongue with thin coating and rapid-taut or rapid-thin pulse are all attributable to deficiency of the liver and kidneys.

## 2. Stirring of wind due to blood deficiency

Symptoms: Weariness, listlessness, weakness and soreness in the waist and knees, spontaneous perspiration, shortness of breath, dizziness, tremors and spasms of the four limbs, incessant twitching of the head, stiffness of the limbs, unsteady gait with frequent falls; enlarged and slightly red tongue with teeth marks, as well as a thin and deficient pulse.

Analysis of symptoms: Deficiency of primordial qi gives rise to weariness, listlessness and weakness and soreness in the waist and knees; deficiency of lung qi brings about spontaneous perspiration and short breath; blood deficiency is responsible for dizziness; exhaustion of both qi and blood triggers an internal stirring of deficient wind, marked by tremors and spasms of the four limbs and incessant twitching of the head; deficient qi and blood fail to nourish the muscles and tendons, resulting in stiffness of the limbs and an unsteady gait with frequent falls; the corpulent and slightly red tongue with teeth marks, as well as the thin and deficient pulse, are symptomatic of deficient qi and blood.

## Differential Treatment

### 1. Stirring of wind due to yin deficiency

Treatment principle: Tonifying the liver and nourishing the kidneys, subduing yang and extinguishing wind.

Prescription and herbs: Qiju Dihuang Decoction and Zhengan Xifeng Decoction.

Gouqizi (Barbary Wolfberry Fruit) 9 g, Shudi (Prepared Rhizome of Rehmannia) 12 g, Shanzhuyu (Asiatic Cornelian Cherry Fruit) 9 g, Maidong (Dwarf Lilyturf Tuber) 9 g, Baishao (White Peony Alba) 30 g, Xuanshen (Figwort Root) 12 g, Guiban (Tortoise Shell) 12 g, Tianma (Tall Gastrodis Tuber) 12 g, Gouteng (Gambir Plant) 15 g, Shenglonggu (Os Draconis) 30 g, Shengshijueming (Raw Sea-ear Shell) 30 g, Juhua (Chrysanthemum Flower) 9 g, Danpi (Cortex Moutan) 9 g, Niuxi (Twotoothed Achyranthes Root) 15 g, Fuling (Indian Bread) 12 g and Gancao ( Liquorice Root) 6 g.

Modification: If are severe tremors, Quanxie (Scorpion) 6 g and Wugong (Centipede) 3 can be added to subdue the liver and extinguish wind; for tinnitus, Shichangpu (Acorus Calamus) 12 g and Lingcishi (Magnetitum) 30 g can be added to open the ear orifice.

### 2. Stirring of wind due to blood deficiency

Treatment principle: Regulating qi and blood, nourishing deficiency and extinguishing wind.

Prescription and herbs: Modified Bazhen Decoction and Dadingfengzhu Decoction.

Dangshen (Radix Codonopsis) 12 g, Baizhu (Largehead Atractylodes Rhizome) 12 g, Fuling (Indian Bread) l2 g, Shengdi (Dried Rehmannia Root) 12 g, Shudi (Prepared Rhizome of Rehmannia) 12 g, Danggui (Chinese Angelica) 9 g, Baishao (White Peony Alba) 9 g, Chuanxiong

(Szechwan Lovage Rhizome) 9 g, Dazao (Chinese Date) 15 g, Wuweizi (Chinese Magnolivine Fruit) 9 g, Maidong (Dwarf Lilyturf Tuber) 15 g, Guiban (Tortoise Shell) 30 g, Biejia (Turtle Shell) 30 g, Ejiao (Donkeyhide Glue) 9 g, Tianma (Tall Gastrodis Tuber) 9 g, Shengmuli (Oyster Shell) 30 g and Gancao ( Liquorice Root) 6 g.

Modification: If there is severe weariness and listlessness, Huangqi (Milkvetch Root) 30 g and Huangjing (Solomonseal Rhizome) 9 g can be added to nourish qi; for tremors and spasms of the four limbs with incessant twitching of the head, Quanxie (Scorpion) 6 g and Wugong (Centipede) 3 can be added to subdue the liver and extinguish wind.

## Chinese Patent Medicine

1. Quantianma Capsule: 4 capsules for each dose, 3 times a day.
2. Xiewu Tablet: 4 tablets for each dose, 3 times a day.

## Simple and Handy Prescriptions

1. Tianma (Tall Gastrodis Tuber) 60 g, Quanxie (Scorpion) 15 g and Wugong (Centipede) 15 g are ground up into fine powders, which are infused into green tea and taken (4.5 g for each dose)twice a day.
2. Huangqi (Milkvetch Root) 6 g, Renshen (Ginseng) 3 g, Gouqizi (Barbary Wolfberry Fruit) 3 g and Juhua (Chrysanthemum Flower) 3 g are infused into hot water to be drunk as tea.

## Other Therapies

Dietary therapy:

(1) A Jiayu (Green Turtle), Gouqizi (Barbary Wolfberry Fruit) 15 g, Tianma (Tall Gastrodis Tuber) 6 g and Chenpi (Dried Tangerine Peel) 6 g are well decocted in water and then taken at different meals. This should be administered twice a month.
(2) A hen is stuffed with Renshen (Ginseng) 3 g, Huangqi (Milkvetch Root) 9 g, Tianma (Tall Gastrodis Tuber) 6 g, Danggui (Chinese

Angelica) 6 g and Shanyao (Plantain Herb) 15 g, then sutured, seasoned (such as with onion and ginger) and well cooked over a mild fire. Both the chicken and soup can be consumed after the removal of the herbs.

## Cautions and Advice

1. Patients should be actively involved in physical work, keep themselves employed and cultivate vocations. A physical trainer can assist patients in walking and eating in everyday life. In severe cases, the patients should be accompanied when going outside to prevent accidents.
2. Patients' diets should be nutritious, soft and easy to digest; for those with swallowing difficulty, semi-fluid or fluid food such as milk and chicken soup are highly recommended.
3. Drug treatment can temporarily alleviate symptoms, but will fail to stop the progress of this disease fundamentally; if there is dysphagia and dementia, the prognosis will be unfavorable.

## Daily Exercises

1. Concisely describe the diagnostic key points of trembling palsy.
2. Explain how trembling palsy can be treated based on syndrome differentiation.

# Bell's Paralysis
# Week 12: Monday

Bell's paralysis refers to the peripheral facial paralysis (abbreviated as facial paralysis) due to facial neuritis, clinically marked by facial distortion that is mostly unilateral rather than bilateral. This disease is a frequently encountered disease that can afflict at any age, especially between 20~40 years. Mild facial paralysis, if treated promptly, can have a favorable prognosis; the longer the duration before treatment is sought, the poorer the prognosis. In TCM, Bell's paralysis is called "facial paralysis" or "mouth distortion" and closely associated with "stroke".

## Etiology and Pathology

TCM holds that Bell's paralysis is mainly caused by deficiency of healthy qi in the interior and invasion of wind-cold into the head and face from the exterior, bringing on malnutrition of tendons and the occurrence of this disease.

Under the circumstances of fatigue with reduced physical force, the patient is deficient in internal healthy qi, which allows the invasion of pathogenic wind-cold into the head and face, causing stagnation of qi and blood in the meridians, as well as malnutrition of the tendons, marked by facial distortion.

## Diagnostic Key Points

1. The age of onset ranges from 20 to 40 years old and males are more susceptible, mostly when their face is exposed to cold or wind over the long term.
2. Sudden onset, with slight pain behind the ear, inside the ear and in the mastoid process or face on the affected side, drooling spotted when rinsing in the morning, loss of control over facial movements and distortion of the angle of the mouth; retention of food residue in the teeth-cheek space found during food intake, with saliva drooping down along the corner of the mouth.

3. Paralysis of facial muscles, apraxia of lid-closure or hypophasis and reduced lacrimal secretion on the affected side; absence of corneal reflex, flattening of nasolabial fold, ptosis of labial angle on the affected side; inability to close the eye, knit the brow, crease the forehead, puff up the cheek and expose the teeth on the affected side.

## Syndrome Differentiation

### 1. Invasion of pathogenic wind into collaterals

Symptoms: Facial paralysis or distortion due to contraction of wind-cold and dampness at night, or headache; white and thin tongue coating and floating pulse.

Analysis of symptoms: Insufficiency of healthy qi allows the invasion of pathogenic wind-cold into the poorly defended collaterals of the head and face, leading to facial paralysis and distortion; pathogenic wind-cold fetters the exterior, bringing about headache, white and thin tongue coating and floating pulse.

### 2. Deficiency of qi and blood

Symptoms: Chronic distortion of eyes and mouth, dizziness, weariness, poor appetite, palpitations, blurred vision; thin tongue coating and thin pulse.

Analysis of symptoms: Insufficiency of healthy qi creates a predisposition to invasion of wind-cold, which stagnates the qi and blood in the collaterals and causes malnutrition of the tendons, marked by chronic facial distortion; prolonged affliction debilitates the qi and blood simultaneously, with such signs as dizziness, weariness and blurred vision; blood fails to nourish the heart, so there are frequent palpitations; the spleen cannot transform the food properly, so there is poor appetite; the thin tongue coating and thin pulse are both symptomatic of insufficient qi and blood.

### 3. Obstruction by binding phlegm and stasis

Symptoms: Facial distortion, headache, numbness in the limbs, dizziness, lassitude and poor appetite; dark tongue with thin and greasy coating and thin and slippery or thin and unsmooth pulse.

Analysis of symptoms: Insufficiency of healthy qi creates a predisposition to invasion of wind-cold, which obstructs the collaterals in combination with phlegm and stasis, leading to facial paralysis marked by distorted eye and mouth; blood stasis obstructs the collaterals and covers the upper orifices, with such signs as headache and numb limbs; insufficiency of qi and blood is manifested as dizziness and lassitude; the spleen cannot transform the food properly, so there is poor appetite; the dark tongue with thin and greasy coating and thin and slippery or thin and unsmooth pulse are all attributable to deficiency of qi, stagnation of blood and obstruction of binding phlegm and stasis.

## Differential Treatment

### 1. Invasion of pathogenic wind into the collaterals

Treatment principle: Expelling wind and activating blood, harmonizing ying and dredging the collaterals.

Prescription and herbs: Modified Qianzheng Powder.

Baifuzi (Giant Typhonium Rhizome) 9 g, Jiangcan (Stiff Silkworm) 9 g, Quanxiefen (Scorpion Powder) 1.5 g (Swallowed), Danggui (Chinese Angelica) 9 g, Fangfeng (Divaricate Saposhnikovia Root) 9 g, Baizhi (Dahurian Angelica Root) 12 g, Baishao (White Peony Alba) 12 g, Chuanxiong (Szechwan Lovage Rhizome) 6 g, Gouteng (Gambir Plant) 12 g and Tianma (Tall Gastrodis Tuber) 12 g.

Modification: If there is excessive phlegm, Tianzhuhuang (Tabasheer) 12 g and Zhinanxing (Prepaired Rhizoma Arisaematis) 12 g can be added to dissolve phlegm; for dry mouth and throat, Huangqin (Baical Skullcap Root) 12 g and Shengshigao (Gypsum) 30 g are added to dispel heat and purge fire.

### 2. Deficiency of qi and blood

Treatment principle: Nourishing qi and blood, expelling wind and dredging the collaterals.

Prescription and herbs: Modified Bazhen Decoction.

Dangshen (Radix Codonopsis) 9 g, Baizhu (Largehead Atractylodes Rhizome) 12 g, Fuling (Indian Bread) 12 g, Zhigancao (Liquorice Root)

6 g, Danggui (Chinese Angelica) 9 g, Chishao (Red Peony Root) 12 g, Chuanxiong (Szechwan Lovage Rhizome) 6 g, Dilong (Angle Worm) 12 g, Wugong (Centipede) 2, Quanxiefen (Scorpion Powder) 1.5 g (swallowed) and Guizhi (Cassia Twig) 9 g.

Modification: If there is listlessness and shortness of breath, Huangqi (Milkvetch Root) 15 g can be added to nourish the middle qi; for dizziness with blurred vision, Gouqizi (Barbary Wolfberry Fruit) 12 g and Juhua (Chrysanthemum Flower) 9 g are used to nourish the liver and dispel heat in the head and eyes.

## 3. Obstruction by binding phlegm and stasis

Treatment principle: Nourishing qi and activating blood, expelling phlegm and dredging the collaterals.

Prescription and herbs: Modified Buyang Huanwu Decoction and Qianzheng Powder.

Shenghuangqi (Raw Milkvetch Root) 15 g, Danggui (Chinese Angelica) 9 g, Chuanxiong (Szechwan Lovage Rhizome) 6 g, Chishao (Red Peony Root) 9 g, Dilong (Angle Worm) 12 g, Baifuzi (Giant Typhonium Rhizome) 9 g, Taoren (Peach Seed) 9 g, Honghua (Safflower) 9 g and Quanxiefen (Scorpion Powder) 1.5 g (swallowed).

Modification: If there are manifestations of cold, Guizhi (Cassia Twig) 9 g and Qianghuo (Incised Notoptetygium Rhizome or Root) 9 g can be added to warm the meridians and dissipate the cold; for manifestations of heat, Huangqin (Baical Skullcap Root) 12 g and Shengshigao (Raw Gypsum) 30 g are used to dispel heat in the gallbladder and stomach; for apparent phlegmatic dampness, Chenpi (Dried Tangerine Peel) 6 g and Banxia (Pinellia Tuber) 9 g are added to remove dampness and dissolve phlegm; if accompanied by facial convulsion, the amount of Quanxiefen (Scorpion Powder) can be increased and Baishao (White Peony Alba) 15 g, Gancao (Liquorice Root) 6 g and Jixueteng (Suberect Spatholobus) 15 g can be used to relieve convulsions and dredge the collaterals.

## Chinese Patent Medicine

1. Dahuoluo Pill: 1 pill for each dose, 2~3 times a day, when there are manifestations of cold.
2. Niuhuang Qingxin Pill: 1 pill for each dose, 2~3 times a day, when there are manifestations of heat.

## Simple and Handy Prescriptions

1. Wugong (Centipede), Quanxie (Scorpion) and Jiangcan (Stiff Silkworm), in the ratio of 1:2:3, are baked, ground up into powders and administered (2 g for each dose) 3 times a day.
2. Seven castor beans are shelled, pounded into paste and applied at the Qianzheng acupoint on the opposite side of the affected area, that is, if the left side is distorted, the right side will be treated and if the right side is distorted, the left side will be treated.

## Other Therapies

Acupuncture therapy: 2~4 acupoints among Fengchi (GB 20), Yifeng (SJ 17), Yangbai (GB 14), Dicang (ST 4), Xiaguan (ST 7), Hegu (LI 4) and Yingxiang (LI 20) are selected to treat facial paralysis every day in the acute stage and every other day in the chronic stage. Besides, acupoint-penetrating therapy can also be applied, i.e., to puncture Yangbai (GB 14) towards Yuyao (EX-HN 4), to puncture Yingxiang (LI 20) towards Sibai (ST 2) and to puncture Dicang (ST 4) towards Jiache (ST 6). Apart from Hegu (LI 4), other acupoints are all selected on the affected side. For localized needling, the stimulating intensity should be well controlled so as not to stiffen the local muscle; otherwise, the recovery of facial paralysis will be impaired, leading to facial spasm.

Massage therapy: This method can help in the improvement of local numbness, the recovery of facial paralysis, as well as the prevention of facial spasms. The main technique is point-kneading and the selection of points is based on the principles of acupuncture.

Physical therapy: In the acute phase, hot compress, infrared radiation, or short-wave radiation can be applied to the region of stylomastoid foramen behind the ears so as to improve local blood circulation, reduce edema and alleviate local pain.

Functional exercise: Early-stage functional exercise of the facial muscles can significantly shorten the course of treatment. Patients should practise frowning, raising the frontal muscles, closing the eyes, exposing the teeth, puffing up the cheeks and whistling several times a day, a few minutes each time.

## Cautions and Advice

1. At the period of onset, the invasion of pathogenic wind-cold into the local region must be prevented and the affected area should be protected and warmed with a mouth-muffle.
2. In the acute phase, prompt measures must be adopted to improve the blood circulation in the local region and promote the subduing of local inflammation and edema, so that the facial nerve will not be further impaired.
3. The local affected area should be frequently massaged and functional exercises of the facial muscles must be performed as early as possible to facilitate recovery.

## Daily Exercises

1. Concisely describe the etiology and pathology of Bell's paralysis.
2. Explain how facial paralysis due to invasion of pathogenic wind into the collaterals can be diagnosed and treated.

# Ischemic Stroke
# Week 12: Tuesday

Ischemic stroke is a cerebrovascular disorder resulting from a lack of blood supply to the brain, which brings about ischemia, hypoxia, necrosis and infarction of the brain tissues. Clinically, it is manifested as hemiplegia and conscious disturbance. The most common clinical types are cerebral thrombosis and cerebral embolism. This disease can occur regardless of the seasons, but may have seasonal variations. The neurologic defect symptoms, if promptly addressed, can be quickly improved within half a year. However, if there are complications of hypertension, cardiac diseases and diabetes, the recovery will be inhibited. In TCM, this disease belongs to the categories of "stroke", "channel-involved apoplexy", "unilateral paralysis" and "pianfeng (hemiplegia)".

## Etiology and Pathology

TCM holds that ischemic stroke is caused mainly by endogenous factors, such as emotional depression and anger (which stirs internal wind and creates a predisposition to stroke); or improper diet (which brings about dysfunction of the spleen in transportation and transformation of food, change of stagnated phlegm into heat and internal stirring of wind); or overstrain (which insidiously consumes the ying-blood and disturbs the internal wind). In addition, this disease is also influenced by changes in weather.

For those with existing deficiency of qi and blood, the yin and yang lose their balance in the heart, liver, kidneys and spleen, which brings on endogenous production of wind, phlegm, dampness and fire; emotional disorders such as excessive worry, contemplation and anger, or excessive alcohol and food intake, or sexual overstrain, or invasion of exogenous pathogenic factors, can all lead to unsmooth flow of qi and blood, malnutrition of muscles and tendons, hyperactivity of liver yang, internal stirring of wind and rampancy of qi, blood, phlegm and fire in the channels and upper orifices, causing excess in the upper and deficiency in the lower body with separation between yin and yang.

## Diagnostic Key Points

1. For middle and old aged patients, this disease may be secondary to hypertension, atherosclerosis, diabetes and coronary artery disease.
2. This disease usually occurs when the patients are in a resting state, with a clear mind and generally no headache, vomiting or signs of meningeal irritation, or with only mild manifestations of the symptoms mentioned.
3. It has a relatively slow onset, or staged progress.
4. There are also symptoms of hemiplegia, hemianopsia, aphasia, aphasia and damage to the cranial nerve.
5. Examination of cerebrospinal fluid: Normal pressure and other indexes.
6. Brain CT, MRI: Foci of cerebral infarction due to ischemia.

## Syndrome Differentiation

## 1. Invasion of pathogenic wind into channels

Symptoms: Numbness in the skin and muscles, especially those of the hands and feet, sudden distortion of eyes and mouth, slurred speech, angular salivation and even hemiparalysis, or intolerance of cold, fever, spasms of limbs and soreness in the joints; dark and pale tongue with white and thin coating and floating and rapid pulse.

Analysis of symptoms: Insufficiency of healthy qi and deficiency of qi and blood are responsible for numbness in the skin and muscles, especially those of the hands and feet; inadequate defense of the collaterals and exterior allows invasion of pathogenic wind, which obstructs the flow of qi and blood, leading to sudden distortion of the eyes and mouth, slurred speech, angular salivation and even hemiparalysis; pathogenic wind invades the body from the exterior, causing imbalance between ying (nutrient phase) and wei (defensive phase) as well as struggle between pathogenic factors and healthy qi, accompanied by intolerance of cold, fever, spasms of the limbs, soreness in the joints, dark and pale tongue with white and thin coating and floating and rapid pulse.

## 2. Upward harassment of wind-yang

Symptoms: Usually dizziness, headache, tinnitus, insomnia and dreaminess, or sudden distortion of the eyes and mouth, stiffness of the tongue, slurred speech, heaviness in the hands and feet and even hemiparalysis; red tongue with thin and greasy coating and taut, thin and rapid pulse or taut and slippery pulse.

Analysis of symptoms: The kidney yin is usually too deficient to nourish the liver wood, bringing on hyperactivity of liver yang, which is marked by dizziness, headache and tinnitus in usual times; insufficiency of kidney yin leads to dysfunction in communication between the heart and kidneys, causing insomnia and dreaminess; the wind-yang stirs in the interior, mixes with phlegm in the channels and collaterals and impedes the flow of meridian qi, with such signs as sudden distortion of the eyes and mouth, stiffness of the tongue, slurred speech, heaviness in the hands and feet and even hemiparalysis; the taut pulse is a sign of liver wind; the taut, thin and rapid pulse with red tongue are symptoms due to deficiency of liver yin and kidney yin with internal heat; the greasy tongue coating and slippery pulse are attributable to phlegm and dampness.

## 3. Deficiency of qi with blood stasis

Symptoms: Hemiparalysis, awry mouth and tongue, slurred speech or speechlessness, unilateral numbness, pale complexion, shortness of breath, weariness, angular salivation, spontaneous perspiration, palpitations, loose stools, swollen hands and feet; dark tongue with white and thin or white and greasy coating and thin and deep, thin and slow, or thin and taut pulse.

Analysis of symptoms: Deficiency of qi leads to unsmooth flow of blood and obstruction of the collaterals, with such signs as hemiparalysis, awry mouth and tongue, slurred speech or speechlessness and unilateral numbness; deficiency of qi is also responsible for shortness of breath, angular salivation and spontaneous perspiration; deficiency of heart qi is manifested as palpitations, while deficiency of spleen qi is marked by edema in the feet and hands and loose stools; the dark tongue, white and thin or white and greasy tongue coating and the thin and deep, thin and slow, or thin and taut pulse are all symptomatic of blood stasis due to deficiency of qi.

## 4. Stirring of wind due to deficiency of yin

Symptoms: Hemiparalysis, awry mouth and tongue, stiff tongue with speechlessness, unilateral numbness, restlessness, insomnia, dizziness, tinnitus and feverish sensations in the palms and soles; purple red or dark red tongue with little or no coating, as well as thin and taut or thin, taut and rapid pulse.

Analysis of symptoms: Exhaustion of liver yin and kidney yin brings about hyperactivity of yang, internal stirring of deficient wind and obstruction of the collaterals, marked by hemiparalysis, awry mouth and tongue, stiff tongue with slurred speech or speechlessness and unilateral numbness; insufficient kidney yin fails to communicate with the heart, thus the deficient fire will disturb the heart spirit, causing restlessness and insomnia; deficiency of kidney essence and brain marrow are manifested as dizziness and tinnitus; the feverish sensation in the palms and soles, purple red or dark red tongue with little or no coating, as well as the thin and taut or thin, taut and rapid pulse are all due to deficiency of yin with exuberance of fire and stirring of wind in the interior.

## Differential Treatment

## 1. Invasion of pathogenic wind into channels

Treatment principle: Expelling wind and nourishing blood, activating blood and dredging the collaterals.

Prescription and herbs: Modified Daqijiao Deocotion.

Qinjiao (Largeleaf Gentian Root) 9 g, Qianghuo (Incised Notoptetygium Rhizome or Root) 9 g, Fangfeng (Divaricate Saposhnikovia Root) 9 g, Baizhi (Dahurian Angelica Root) 9 g, Danggui (Chinese Angelica) 9 g, Shudi (Prepared Rhizome of Rehmannia) 12 g, Baishao (White Peony Alba) 12 g, Chuanxiong (Szechwan Lovage Rhizome) 9 g, Baizhu (Largehead Atractylodes Rhizome) 12 g, Fuling (Indian Bread) 12 g,

Huangqin (Baical Skullcap Root) 15 g, Shigao (Gypsum) 30 g, Shengdi (Dried Rehmannia Root) 15 g and Xixin (Manchurian Wildginger) 3 g.

Modification: If the patient is old with a weak constitution, Huangqi (Milkvetch Root) 15 g can be added to invigorate qi and reinforce the healthy qi; for vomiting with profuse phlegm, greasy tongue coating and slippery pulse, Dihuang (Rehmannia Root) can be replaced with Banxia (Pinellia Tuber) 9 g, Baifuzi (Giant Typhonium Rhizome) 9 g and Quanxie (Scorpion) 5 g so as to expel wind phlegm and dredge the channels and collaterals.

## 2. Upward harassment of wind-yang

Treatment principle: Nourishing yin and suppressing yang, extinguishing wind and dredging the collaterals.

Prescription and herbs: Modified Zhengan Xifeng Decoction.

Niuxi (Twotoothed Achyranthes Root) 20 g, Baishao (White Peony Alba) 15 g, Tiandong (Cochinchinese Asparagus Root) 12 g, Xuanshen (Figwort Root) 12 g, Longgu (Os Draconis) 30 g, Daizheshi (Red Bole) 15 g, Muli (Oyster Shell) 30g, Guiban (Tortoise Shell) 9 g, Shengmaiya (Raw Malt) 15 g, Chuanlianzi (Szechwan Chinaberry Fruit) 9 g, Yinchen (Virgate Wormwood Herb) 9 g and Gancao ( Liquorice Root) 6 g.

Modification: If there is severe hyperactivity of liver yang, Tianma (Tall Gastrodis Tuber) 12 g, Gouteng (Gambir Plant) 15 g and Juhua (Chrysanthemum Flower) 9 g can be added to subdue the liver and extinguish wind; for restlessness with feverish sensation in the heart, Zhizi (Cape Jasmine Fruit) 9 g and Huangqin (Baical Skullcap Root) 12 g can be added to dispel heat and relieve vexation; for relatively severe headache, Lingyangjiaofen (Antelope Horn Powder 0.6 g (swallowed), Shijueming (Sea-ear Shell) 30 g and Xiakucao (Common Selfheal Fruit-Spike) 12 g can be used to extinguish wind and subdue yang.

## 3. Deficiency of qi with blood stasis

Treatment principle: Nourishing qi, activating blood and dredging the collaterals.

Prescription and herbs: Modified Buyang Huanwu Decoction.

Huangqi (Milkvetch Root) 30 g, Danggui (Chinese Angelica) 9 g, Chuanxiong (Szechwan Lovage Rhizome) 9 g, Chishao (Red Peony Root) 12 g, Taoren (Peach Seed) 12 g, Honghua (Safflower) 9 g, Dilong (Angle Worm) 12 g, Quanxie (Scorpion) 5 g and Chuanniuxi (Twotoothed Achyranthes Root) 12 g.

Modification: If there is relatively severe hemiparalysis, Sangzhi (Mulberry Twig) 12 g, Chuanshanjia (Pangolin Scale) 9 g and Shuizhi (Leech) 9 g can be added to activate blood and dredge the collaterals as well asexpel stasis and produce new tissues; for slurred speech, Shichangpu (Acorus Calamus) 12 g and Yuanzhi (Thinleaf Milkwort Root) 6 g can be added to dissolve phlegm; for loose stools, Taoren (Peach Seed) can be replaced with Baizhu (Largehead Atractylodes Rhizome) 15 g and Shanyao (Common Yan Rhizome) 15 g to invigorate the spleen.

### 4. Stirring of wind due to deficiency of yin

Treatment principle: Nourishing yin and extinguishing wind.

Prescription and herbs: Modified Dadingfengzhu Decoction.

Shengdi (Dried Rehmannia Root) 15 g, Maidong (Dwarf Lilyturf Tuber) 12 g, Baishao (White Peony Alba) 12 g, Wuweizi (Chinese Magnolivine Fruit) 9 g, Shengguiban (Unbaked Tortoise Shell) 12 g, Shengbiejia (Raw Turtle Shell) 12 g, Ejiao (Donkey-hide Glue) 9 g, Shengmuli (Unbaked Oyster Shell) 30 g, Zhigancao (Stir-baked Liquorice Root) 6 g.

Modification: If there is relatively severe hemiplegia, Niuxi (Twotoothed Achyranthes Root) 12 g, Dilong (Angle Worm) 12 g, Wugong (Centipede) 2 pieces and Sangzhi (Mulberry Twig) 9 g can be added to dredge the channels and activate the collaterals; for slurred speech, Shichangpu (Acorus Calamus) 12 g, Yujin (Turmeric Root Tuber) 12 g and Yuanzhi (Thinleaf Milkwort Root) 6 g are used to restore the voice and alleviate discomfort in the throat.

### Chinese Patent Medicine

1. Huoxue Tongmai Capsule: 2~4 capsules, 3 times a day.
2. Naoxueshuan Tablet: 3~4 tablets, 3 times a day.

3. Huatuo Zaizao Pill: 8 g for each dose, 3 times a day.
4. Danshen Injection: 20 ml of the injection is added into 500 ml of 10% glucose for intravenous dripping once a day.

## Simple and Handy Prescriptions

1. Huangqi (Milkvetch Root) 30 g, Chuanxiong (Szechwan Lovage Rhizome) 9 g, Danshen (Radix Salviae Miltiorrhiae) 15 g and Chishao (Red Peony Root) 12 g are boiled in water and separated into 2 portions to be taken at 2 different times within a day, for nourishing qi and activating blood.
2. Shuizhi (Leech), Yujin (Turmeric Root Tuber) and Chuanxiong (Szechwan Lovage Rhizome) are mixed in the ratio of 1.5:2:3 and ground into fine powders before being administered (1.5~2 g for each dose) 3 times a day.

## Other Therapies

Acupuncture and moxibustion treatment: For acupoints on the upper limbs, Jianyu (LI 15), Quchi (LI 11), Waiguan (TE 5) and Hegu (LI 4) can be selected and Jianliao (TE 14), Jianzhen (SI 9), Binao (LI 14) and Yangchi (TE 4) can also be applied in turn; for acupoints on the lower limbs, Huangtiao (GB 30), Yanglingquan (B 34), Zusanli (ST 36) and Kunlun (BL 60) can be selected and Fengshi (GB 20), Juegu (GB 39) and Yaoyangguan (DU 3) can also be applied in turn. This is used to treat hemiparalysis by regulating the channels and promoting the flow of qi and blood. For slurred speech, Jinjing (EX-HN 12) and Yuye (EX-HN 13) can be pricked to let out a certain amount of blood and Neiguan (PC 6), Tongli (HT 5), Lianquan (RN 23) and Sanyijiao (SP 6) can be needled to expel wind, remove phlegm and dredge the orifices and collaterals.

Massage therapy: This is used to treat stroke in the acute phase or recovery phase with unilateral paralysis. Fengchi (GB 20), Jianjing (GB 21), Tianzong (SI 11), Jianyu (LI 15), Quchi (LI 11), Shousanli (LI 10), Hegu (LI 4), Huantiao (GB 30), Yaolingquan (GB 34), Weizhong (BL 40) and Chengshan (BL 57), selected on the affected side, are pushed, pressed, twisted, kneaded, grabbed and scraped so as to promote the circulation of qi and blood and enable the functions of the affected limbs to be recovered.

Medicated pillow therapy: Xiakucao (Common Selfheal Fruit-Spike) 1000 g, Juhua (Chrysanthemum Flower) 1000 g, Danpi (Cortex Moutan) 200 g, Chuanxiong (Szechwan Lovage Rhizome) 400 g and Baizhi (Dahurian Angelica Root) 200 g are crushed into fine pieces and stuffed into a pillow, which is used by the patient every night. This therapy is used to treat ischemic stroke in the acute phase.

Dietary therapy: Tianma Yutou Soup is made by steaming Tianma (sliced) 20 g, a spotted silver carp head 250 g and seasonings such as onion, ginger, alcohol and salt for taste. This therapy is used to subdue the liver and extinguish wind as well as nourish blood and supplement the brain.

## Cautions and Advice

1. Patients should take initiative to prevent and treat hypertension, athero-sclerosis and diabetes so as to reduce the attack rate of ischemic stroke.
2. They should also regulate their lives, avoid wind-cold, balance warmth and cold, adopt a light diet and refrain from cigarettes and alcohol.

## Daily Exercises

1. Concisely describe the etiology and pathology of ischemic stroke.
2. Explain how stroke due to upward disturbance of wind yang resulting from yin deficiency of the liver and kidneys can be diagnosed and treated.

# Hemorrhagic Stroke
# Week 12: Tuesday

Hemorrhagic stroke refers to the primary or spontaneous bleeding of the brain. Clinically, bleeding is manifested as headache and vomiting (due to intracranial hypertension), hemiplegia and disturbances of speech and consciousness (due to disorders of the nervous system). According to the changes in pathology, this disease can be divided into two categories of cerebral hemorrhage and subarachnoid hemorrhage. About 80% of the cases of hemorrhagic stroke occur in the cerebral hemisphere, whilethe remaining 20% of them occur in the brain stem and cerebellum. The common causative factors are agitation, climatic changes and increase in intra-abdominal pressure (due to the effect of promoting defecation). This disease is poor in prognosis and high in mortality and even if the patients survive, there may still be some serious lingering effects. In TCM, hemorrhagic stroke is closely associated with "wind-strike", "unilateral paralysis" and "syndrome of blood stasis".

## Etiology and Pathology

TCM holds that this disease is caused by either endogenous or exogenous factors. The former refers to the functional disorder of the viscera, deficiency of qi and blood and production of pathogenic wind, fire, phlegm and stasis; hyperactivity of the five emotions, improper diet, overstrains and climatic changes are the exogenous factors of this disease. The combination of endogenous and exogenous factors leads to disorders of qi and blood, with bleeding in the brain.

The pathological changes are discussed as follows: When people get old, the qi and blood will become deficient and there will be imbalance of yin, yang, qi and blood. If complicated by excessive worry, contemplation and anger, or improper diet, unbalanced warmth and cold and overstrain, there may be yin deficiency of the liver and kidneys, which creates a predisposition to hyperactivity of liver yang and stirring of liver wind, marked by disordered qi and blood. The internal wind and the disordered qi and blood attack the brain and cause bleeding and impairment of the marrow, with such signs as stiff tongue, slurred speech, hemiplegia, or unclear mind. Disorder in the ascent and descent of qi and blood is the main mechanism for hemorrhagic stroke and the main pathogenesis is that qi, blood, phlegm and fire flow upward with wind, break the blood vessels and obstruct the primordial spirit.

## Diagnostic Key Points

1. This disease occurs mostly in patients above 50 years old, with a history of hypertension or arteriosclerosis.
2. It often occurs when the patients are agitated or doing physical work, commonly being accompanied by headache, vomiting and hemiplegia.
3. The disease can develop rapidly and the patient may progress into a state of unconsciousness and coma within a short time.
4. The examination of cerebrospinal fluid shows that the blood is even while the pressure is high.
5. Brain CT or MRI indicates foci of bleeding.
6. Patients with subarachnoid hemorrhage may present with mental symptoms such as meningeal irritation (deep yet unmarked coma), optic nervous edema and retina bleeding on examination of ocular fundus.

## Syndrome Differentiation

### 1. Acute phase

(1) Blockage (excess) syndrome of stroke

Yang blockage (excess): Sudden hyperactivity of liver yang with stirring of wind.

Symptoms: Abrupt coma and fall, locked jaw, clenched hands and stiff limbs, hemiparalysis, constipation and anuresis, red complexion, fever, wheezy phlegm in the throat and agitation; red tongue with yellow and greasy coating and taut, rapid and slippery pulse or surging and large pulse.

Analysis of symptoms: Sudden hyperactivity of liver yang with stirring of wind and upward attack of qi, blood, phlegm and fire is marked by sudden coma and fall; obstruction of the channels by wind, fire, phlegm and heat is responsible for locked jaw, clenched hands, stiff limbs, hemiparalysis, constipation, anuresis, red complexion, fever, wheezy phlegm in the throat and agitation; the red tongue with yellow and greasy coating and the taut, rapid and slippery pulse or surging and large pulse are manifestations of internal blockage of phlegm and heat.

Yin blockage (excess): Obstruction of turbid phlegm in the collaterals with clouding of the upper orifices

Symptoms: Sudden coma and fall, locked jaw, clenched hands and stiff limbs, white complexion with dark lips, lying in bed without restlessness, lack of warmth in the limbs and abundance of phlegm and saliva; dark tongue with white and greasy coating and slow, deep and slippery pulse.

Analysis of symptoms: Abundant phlegm and dampness obstruct the channels and collaterals, leading to sudden coma and fall, locked jaw, clenched hands and stiff limbs; phlegm and dampness are yin in nature, so the patient may lie quietly; phlegm and dampness block the flow of yang qi, marked by lack of warmth in the limbs, white complexion and dark lips and tongue; the dark tongue with white and greasy coating and slow, deep and slippery pulse are attributable to internal abundance of phlegm and dampness.

## (2) Collapse (deficiency) syndrome: Loss of primordial essence with deficiency of yang and collapse of qi.

Symptoms: Sudden fall with coma, or transformation of blockage syndrome into collapse syndrome; unconsciousness, pale complexion, closed eyes, open mouth, stertor with weak breathing, unclenched hands with cold limbs, profuse sweating, incontinence of urine and feces and flaccid paralysis of limbs; flaccid tongue, thin and feeble pulse or extremely feeble and faint pulse.

Analysis of symptoms: Exhaustion of healthy qi with an impaired heart spirit is caused by extreme deficiency of yin, yang, qi and blood; the depletion syndrome, secondary to the blockage one, is due to upward flaming of wind and fire coupled with phlegm and heat, which scorch the genuine yin and primordial qi; the exhaustion of essence qi of the five zang-organs is responsible for the sudden fall with coma, unconsciousness, closed eyes, open mouth, snoring, unclenched hands, flaccid tongue and incontinence of urine and feces; the weak breathing, profuse and incessant sweating, peripheral coldness and thin and feeble pulse are all due to depletion of yin essence with sudden loss of yang qi.

## 2. Recovery phase

### (1) Deficiency of qi with blood stasis

Symptoms: Hemiparalysis, facial distortion, slurred speech, lassitude, dark and lusterless complexion; dark tongue perhaps with ecchymosis, white and thin tongue coating and thin, weak and unsmooth pulse.

Analysis of symptoms: Deficient qi fails to control blood, which deviates from its normal course and turns into blood stasis; the healthy qi is seriously damaged after disease, so the blood flow within the clear orifices will be unsmooth due to deficiency of qi, this is marked by hemiparalysis, slurred speech and distorted eyes and mouth; deficient qi fails to distribute the blood to the face, so the complexion is dark and lusterless; the dark tongue with possible ecchymosis, white and thin coating and thin, weak and unsmooth pulse are attributable to deficiency of qi with blood stasis.

### (2) Deficiency of the liver and kidneys

Symptoms: Unilateral paralysis of the limbs, numbness, distorted eyes and mouth, hoarseness of voice or aphasia, wheezy phlegm in the throat, dementia, headache and dizziness; reddish tongue with scanty coating and thin and taut pulse.

Analysis of symptoms: Exhaustion of liver yin and kidney yin involves the essence and blood, leading to malnutrition of the channels which is marked by unilateral paralysis of the limbs, numbness and distorted eyes and mouth; the kidney essence fails to nourish the throat, so there is hoarseness of voice or aphasia; damp phlegm obstructs the interior, marked by wheezy phlegm in the throat and dementia; hyperactivity of liver yang is manifested as headache and dizziness; the reddish tongue with scanty coating and the taut and thin pulse are both due to exhaustion of liver yin and kidney yin.

## Differential Treatment

### 1. Acute phase

(1) Blockage (excess) syndrome of stroke

Yang blockage (excess): Sudden hyperactivity of liver yang with stirring of wind.

Treatment principle: Clearing the liver, extinguishing wind and opening the orifices (with pungent and cool herbs).

Prescription and herbs: Angong Niuhuang Pill or Jufang Zhibao Pill can be administered by intragastrical gavage or nasal feeding to open the orifices; afterwards, modified Lingyangjiao Decoction can be used to clear the liver and extinguish wind, as well as nurture yin and subdue yang. Lingyangjiaofen (Antelope Horn Powder) 0.6 g (infused in water), Guiban (Tortoise Shell) 20 g, Shengdi (Dried Rehmannia Root) 15 g, Danpi (Cortex Moutan) 15 g, Baishao (White Peony Alba) 15 g, Bohe (Peppermint) 6 g, Chanyi (Cicada Shell) 3 g, Juhua (Chrysanthemum Flower) 9 g, Xiakucao (Common Selfheal Fruit-Spike) 15 g, Shijueming (Sea-ear Shell) 30 g, Shengdahuang (Raw Rhubarb) 9 g (decocted later).

Modification: If there are spasms, Quanxie (Scorpion) 3 g, Wugong (Centipede) 2 and Jiangcan (Stiff Silkworm) 12 g can be used to extinguish wind and relieve convulsions; for excessive phlegm, Tianzhuhuang (Tabasheer)12 g and Dannanxing (Bile Arisaema) 12 g can be used to dispel heat and dissolve phlegm; for excessive phlegm with deep slumber, Yujin (Turmeric Root Tuber) 9 g and Shichangpu (Acorus Calamus) 12 g are added to reinforce the action of eliminating phlegm and unblocking the orifices.

Yin blockage (excess): Obstruction of turbid phlegm in the collaterals with clouding of the upper orifices.

Treatment principle: Eliminating phlegm, extinguishing wind and opening the orifices (with pungent and warm herbs).

Prescription and herbs: Suhexiang Pill can be immediately used (dissolved in warm boiled water and fed intragastrically or nasally) and then modified Ditan Decoction can be applied.

Banxia (Pinellia Tuber) 9 g, Chenpi (Dried Tangerine Peel) 9 g, Fuling (Indian Bread) 12 g, Zhuru (Bamboo Shavings) 9 g, Changpu (Acorus Calamus) 15 g, Dannanxing (Bile Arisaema) 12 g, Zhishi (Immature Orange Fruit) 9 g, Tianma (Tall Gastrodis Tuber) 12 g, Gouteng (Gambir Plant) 15 g, Chishao (Red Peony Root) 12 g and Shuizhi (Leech) 6 g.

Modification: If there is a marked deficiency of yang such as pale complexion and cold limbs, Huangqi (Milkvetch Root) 15 g and Chuanxiong (Szechwan Lovage Rhizome) 9 g can be added to nourish qi and activate blood.

## (2) Collapse (deficiency) syndrome: Loss of primordial essence with deficiency of yang and collapse of qi.

Treatment principle: Nourishing qi and restoring yang, saving yin and treating collapse.

Prescription and herbs: Modified Shenfu Decoction and Shengmai Powder.

Renshen (Ginseng) 10 g, Fuzi (Prepared Common Monkshood Daughter) 10 g (decocted first), Maidong (Dwarf Lilyturf Tuber) 15 g and Wuweizi (Chinese Magnolivine Fruit) 10 g.

Modification: If there is incessant sweating, Huangqi (Milkvetch Root) 30 g, Longgu (Os Draconis) 30 g, Muli (Oyster Shell) 30 g and Shanzhuyu (Asiatic Cornelian Cherry Fruit) 12 g can be added to reduce sweating and treat collapse.

## 2. Recovery phase

### (1) Deficiency of qi with blood stasis

Treatment principle: Nourishing qi and activating blood, resolving stasis and dredging the collaterals.

Prescription and herbs: Modified Buyang Huangwu Decoction.

Huangqi (Milkvetch Root) 60 g, Danggui (Chinese Angelica) 12 g, Chuanxiong (Szechwan Lovage Rhizome) 9 g, Taoren (Peach Seed) 12 g,

Honghua (Safflower) 9 g, Chishao (Red Peony Root) 12 g, Dilong (Angle Worm) 12 g, Quanxie (Scorpion) 3 g, Dibiechong (Eupolyphaga Seu Steleophaga) 9 g, Chuanniuxi (Twotoothed Achyranthes Root) 12 g and Sangzhi (Mulberry Twig) 12 g.

Modification: If there is flaccidity of the lower limbs, Sangjisheng (Chinese Taxillus Herb) 12 g can be added to nourish the kidneys and strengthen the tendons; for paralysis of a certain limb, Guizhi (Cassia Twig) 9 g can be used to dredge the collaterals; for slurred speech, Yujin (Turmeric Root Tuber) 9 g, Shichangpu (Acorus Calamus) 12 g and Yuanzhi (Thinleaf Milkwort Root) 6 g can be added to remove phlegm and unblock the orifices.

## (2) Deficiency of the liver and kidneys

Treatment principle: Tonifying the liver and kidneys, Nourishing the channels and tendons.

Prescription and herbs: Modified Dihuang Yinzi.

Shengdi (Dried Rehmannia Root) 20 g, Shanzhuyu (Asiatic Cornelian Cherry Fruit) 9 g, Bajitian (Mornda Root) 12 g, Shihu (Dendrobium) 15 g, Roucongrong (Desertliving Cistanche) 12 g, Wuweizi (Chinese Magnolivine Fruit) 9 g, Maidong (Dwarf Lilyturf Tuber) 12 g, Shichangpu (Acorus Calamus) 12 g, Yuanzhi (Thinleaf Milkwort Root) 6 g, Chishao (Red Peony Root) 12 g, Danggui (Chinese Angelica) 9 g and Gancao (Liquorice Root) 6 g.

Modification: For hyperactivity of liver yang, Shijueming (Sea-ear Shell) 30 g and Zhenzhumu (Nacre) 30 g can be used to calm the liver and subdue yang; for spasm of tendons, Baishao (White Peony Alba) 12 g and Mugua (Papaya)15 g can be used to relieve spasms and dredge the collaterals.

## Chinese Patent Medicine

1. Angong Niuhuang Pill: 1 pill for each dose taken twice a day to open the orifices with pungent and cool herbs in the case of stroke with blockage of yang.

2. Suhexiang Pill: 1 pill for each dose taken once a day to open the orifices with pungent and warm herbs in the case of stroke with blockage of yin.
3. Huoxue Tongmai Capsule: 2~4 capsules for each dose taken 3 times a day for stroke with lingering effects.

## Simple and Handy Prescriptions

1. Tianma (Tall Gastrodis Tuber) 9 g, Banxia (Pinellia Tuber) 12 g, Shichangpu (Acorus Calamus) 6 g, Sangjisheng (Chinese Taxillus Herb) 12 g and Longchi (Fossilia Dentis Mastodi) 30 g are boiled in water. This therapy is applied to treat stroke with unconsciousness.
2. Dangshen (Radix Codonopsis) 12 g, Shuizhi (Leech) 10 g and Danpi (Cortex Moutan) 10 g are ground up into powders and made into capsules, with 3 of crude drug in each capsule. Three capsules are taken for each dose and 3 times a day. This therapy is used to treat stroke with bleeding in the recovery phase.

## Other Therapies

Acupuncture therapy:

(1) For blockage syndrome in the acute phase, Renzhong (DU 26), Yongquan (K 1), Baihui (DU 20), Dazhui (DU 14), Hegu (LI 4) and Neiguan (PC 6) can be needled and Shixuan (EX-UE 11) can be pricked for blood-letting. If there is excessive phlegm, Fenglong (ST 40) and Tiantu (RN 22) can be added. For depletion syndrome, Shenque (RN 8), Guanyuan (RN 4) and Qihai (RN 6) can be cauterized with moxa.
(2) Recovery phase: For acupoints on the upper limbs, Jianyu (LI 15), Quchi (LI 11), Waiguan (SJ 5) and Shoushanli (LI 10) can be selected; for acupoints on the lower limbs, Huantiao (GB 30), Weizhong (BL 40), Fengshi (GB 31), Yanglingquan (GB 34), Zusanli (ST 36) and Kunlun (BL 60) can be selected. If there is slurred speech, Jinjin (EX-HN 12) and Yuye (EX-HN 13) can be pricked rapidly to let out blood; for distorted eyes and mouth, Jiache (ST 6), Dicang (ST 4) and Xiaguan (ST 7) can be added.

Medicated pillow therapy: Shengshigao (Gypsum) in a proper amount is broken into pieces to fill the pillow. This therapy is used to treat cerebral bleeding in the acute phase.

Dietary therapy: Celery 250 g and sea tangle 100 g are cut into threads, immersed in hot water for a while and seasoned with sesame oil and salt. This therapy is used to dispel heat and subdue the liver, as well as soften and dissolve phlegm.

## Cautions and Advice

1. Patients often present with the presymptom of stroke such as frequent headache, dizziness and numbness in the limbs, or occasional slurred speech, which must be addressed promptly.
2. When stroke occurs, patients should remain quiet and avoid making unnecessary movements in order to prevent bleeding.
3. It is advisable for patients to adopt a low-salt, low-fat and low-cholesterol diet and consume more vegetables, fruits and bean products. At the same time, they must refrain from cigarettes and alcohol.

## Daily Exercises

1. Explain the differences between hemorrhagic stroke and ischemic stroke in terms of the clinical symptoms, etiology and pathology.
2. Concisely describe the pathogeneses of yin blockage versus yang blockage of hemorrhagic stroke in the acute phase and explain the treatement differences.

# Epilepsy

# Week 12: Wednesday

Epilepsy is a disorder of the brain that is marked by seizures. Clinically, there are symptoms such as transient sensory disability, spasms, loss of consciousness, behavioral disturbance or dysautonomia. Most cases of epilepsy (seizures, called secondary epilepsy, arise from various diseases inside or outside of the brain, while those with unknown causes are called primary epilepsy. Primary epilepsy is mostly seen in children around the age of 5 or adolescents. The prognosis of this disease depends on its etiological factors. Generally speaking, primary epilepsy, if treated promptly and regularly, can be favorable in prognosis and will not lead to death; delay and/or inconsistency in treatment may lead to recurrent and refractory seizures. In TCM, this disease is classified under "epileptic syndrome".

## Etiology and Pathology

The etiological factors of epilepsy are either congenital or postnatal. The former refers to improper nursing during pregnancy (sudden terror of the mother) and fetal hypoplasia. The latter refers to emotional disorder, brain injury, invasion of the six abnormal climatic factors, or improper diet, overstrain and other diseases involving the viscera and creating a predisposition to epilepsy.

    The pathological changes are discussed as follows: If the pregnant mother is suddenly frightened, there will be disorder of qi activity, consumption of essence and deficiency of the kidneys; for this reason the fetal development will be impaired, resulting in epileptic syndrome after birth. Unlike the congenital factors, the postnatal factors are mainly fright and improper diet, both of which can lead to functional disorders of the viscera: sudden fright can disturb the activity of qi, which may further impair the viscera, e.g., damage to the liver and kidneys (marked by deficiency of yin, production of heat and stirring of wind), damage to the spleen and stomach (marked by poor digestion and accumulation of turbid phlegm, which may combine with wind, fire and heat to harass the brain spirit and cloud the heart spirit, creating a predisposition to epilepsy). Furthermore, emotional depression and overstrain can stagnate the liver qi and stir the liver wind which, when combined with phlegm, may obstruct the heart orifices and the channels, thus bringing on epilepsy. Moreover, injuries to the brain may create a predisposition to disturbance of the mind, stagnation of qi and blood and disorder of the collaterals, thereby resulting in epilepsy. It is thus evident that the occurrence of epilepsy is most closely related to the kidneys, liver and spleen and the pathological changes are linked with wind, stasis and phlegm especially.

## Diagnostic Key Points

1. The symptoms are varied, but in most cases, a detailed history of disease, a clear description of clinical characteristics and a thorough health examination combined with electroencephalography (EEG) findings can give a definite diagnosis.
2. Grand mal, or generalized seizure, is marked by loss of consciousness and general spasms. There are two types: primary and secondary. Most cases are considered secondary ones. There are primarily three stages: pre-symptomatic, tonic and clonic.
3. Petit mal is marked by absence of general spasms and conscious disturbance. The simple type is only manifested as loss of consciousness, while the complex type is accompanied by transient stiffness, spasms, or automatism and autonomic nervous symptoms.
4. Partial seizure includes simple partial seizure and complex partial seizure; the former is caused by local lesion of the cerebral cortex; the latter is also called psychomotor seizure.
5. EEG is a most common and important diagnostic method. The EEG findings during intermission and onset, plus various inducing methods, can have a positive detection rate of 80%~85% for all types of epilepsy. If the tracings are conducted during the period of onset, the diagnostic result will be more reliable.

## Syndrome Differentiation

## 1. Obstruction of wind phlegm

Symptoms: Dizziness, chest distress, weariness and local spasms (in some cases there are no presymptoms) before onset; during onset, there are sudden falls, an unclear mind, convulsions, salivation, or possible screaming, urinary and fecal incontinence, or transient unconsciousness and absent-mindedness without spasms; white and greasy tongue coating and taut and slippery pulse.

Analysis of symptoms: Dizziness, chest distress, weariness and local spasms are all presymptoms of wind phlegm flowing up; the liver wind stirs in the interior and, in combination with phlegm, covers the heart spirit, bringing on mental derangement and seizure; the stagnated liver qi impairs the transforming function of the spleen, producing turbid phlegm in the interior, which flows upward with wind, marked by salivation; if the turbid phlegm is not abundant but the wind is predominant, the patient may present with transient unconsciousness and absent-mindedness without spasms; the white and greasy tongue coating as well as the taut and slippery pulse are manifestations of turbid phlegm with wind.

## 2. Internal exuberance of phlegm and fire

Symptoms: During the period of onset, there is a sudden fall andsubsequent unconsciousness, convulsions, salivation, locked jaw, crying or screaming, while typical everyday symptoms include irascibility, vexation, insomnia and the coughing up of sticky phlegm; there is also a bitter taste in the mouth with dryness, constipation, red tongue with yellow and greasy coating and taut, rapid and slippery pulse.

Analysis of symptoms: Relative exuberance of liver fire produces wind and scorches body fluid into phlegm, giving rise to expectoration of sticky phlegm and a bitter taste in the mouth with dryness; the phlegm moves up with the rising of wind, obstructing the heart orifices and disturbing the mind, marked by the sudden fall with unconsciousness, convulsions, salivation and locked jaw; stagnation of liver qi is responsible for irascibility;

fire disturbs the heart spirit, bringing about insomnia and vexation; the red tongue with yellow and greasy coating and the taut, rapid and slippery pulse are attributable to predominance of liver fire and phlegmatic heat.

## 3. Deficiency of the spleen with phlegm and dampness

Symptoms: During the period of intermission, there is lassitude, chest distress and dizziness; while during onset the complexion is dark, luster-less or white and there is peripheral coldness, unconsciousness, curled body with spasms, vomiting, salivation, or low and faint crying; pale and enlarged tongue with white and greasy coating and thin and slippery pulse.

Analysis of symptoms: Deficiency of the spleen yang and kidneys brings about dampness and phlegm, marked by lassitude and chest distress; insufficiency of yang qi leads to coldness in the body, characterized by a dark and lusterless complexion, peripheral coldness and faint crying; dampness and phlegm obstruct the clear orifices, giving rise to an unclear mind, spasms or convulsions; the pale and enlarged tongue with white and greasy coating and the thin and slippery pulse are all manifestations of abundant phlegm and dampness due to insufficiency of spleen yang.

## 4. Deficiency of brain marrow

Symptoms: Long-term epilepsy leads to absent-mindedness, a dark and lusterless complexion, insomnia, forgetfulness, palpitations, dizziness, weakness and soreness of the waist and knees and lassitude; thin and greasy tongue coating and thin and feeble pulse.

Analysis of symptoms: Repeated seizures create a predisposition to deficiency of heart blood and brain marrow as well as insufficiency of liver and kidneys, with consumption of essence and blood, resulting in absent-mindedness, forgetfulness, insomnia, palpitations, dizziness, weakness and soreness of the waist and knees and lassitude; the thin and greasy tongue coating and the thin and feeble pulse are both symptomatic of the deficient heart, liver and kidneys.

## 5. Obstruction of collaterals by blood stasis

Symptoms: This syndrome is mostly seen in chronic epilepsy with a history of brain trauma; during the period of intermission, there is headache, emotional depression andnumbness in the limbs, head or face. During the period of onset, there are fixed symptoms such as local or general spasms, with headache as a lingering effect after onset. Patients with this pattern may have dark and purple tongue with petechia, white and thin tongue coating and unsmooth or taut and tense pulse.

Analysis of symptoms: The head is injured by external force, with blood stasis in the interior, which obstructs the brain vessels, leading to localized pain in the head; obstruction of the vessels is responsible for numbness in the limbs, head or face, fixed spasms during occurrence and marked headache after onset; the dark and purple tongue with petechia, white and thin tongue coating and the unsmooth or taut and tense pulse are all manifestations of blood stasis.

## Differential Treatment

## 1. Obstruction of wind phlegm

Treatment principle: Eliminating phlegm and extinguishing wind, opening the orifices and calming epilepsy.

Prescription and herbs: Mainly Dingxian Pill.

Zhuli (Succus Bambusae) 30 g, Banxia (Pinellia Tuber) 9 g, Shichangpu (Acorus Calamus) 12 g, Dannanxing (Bile Arisaema)12 g, Chuanbei (Tendrilleaf Fritillary Bulb) 9 g, Tianma (Tall Gastrodis Tuber) 12 g, Gouteng (Gambir Plant) 12 g, Quanxiefen (Scorpion Powder) 2 g (swallowed), Jiangcan (Stiff Silkworm) 12 g, Zhiyuanzhi (Prepared Thinleaf Milkwort Root) 6 g, Longchi (Fossilia Dentis Mastodi) 30 g and Fushen (Indian Bread with Hostwood) 9 g.

Modification: If the patient presents with an unclear mind with predominance of phlegm, Tianzhuhuang (Tabasheer) 12 g and Baifuzi (Giant Typhonium Rhizome) 9 g can be added to eliminate phlegm, open the orifices and calm epilepsy.

## 2. Internal exuberance of phlegm and fire

Treatment principle: Clearing the liver and purging fire, dissolving phlegm and opening the orifices.

Prescription and herbs: Modified Longdan Xiegan Decoction and Ditan Decoction.

Longdancao (Radix Gentianae) 6 g, Zhizi (Cape Jasmine Fruit) 9 g, Chuanmutong (Armand Clematis Stem) 5 g, Shengdi (Dried Rehmannia Root) 12 g, Banxia (Pinellia Tuber) 9 g, Zhishi (Immature Orange Fruit) 9 g, Changpu (Acorus Calamus) 12 g, Nanxing (Rhizoma Arisaematis) 9 g, Tianma (Tall Gastrodis Tuber) 12 g, Gouteng (Gambir Plant) 12 g, Dilong (Angle Worm) 12 g and Quanxiefen (Scorpion Powder) 2 g (swallowed).

Modification: For constipation, Shengdahuang (Unprepared Rhubarb) 9 g (decocted later than other herbs) can be added to purge fire and promote defecation; for insomnia, Zaoren (Semen Ziziphi Spinosae) 12 g and Yejiaoteng (Caulis Polygoni Multiflori) 30 g can be added to calm the heart and tranquilize the mind.

## 3. Deficiency of the spleen with phlegm and dampness

Treatment principle: Invigorating the spleen and expelling dampness, dissolving phlegm and calming epilepsy.

Prescription and herbs: Modified Liujunzi Decoction.

Dangshen (Radix Codonopsis) 9 g, Baizhu (Largehead Atractylodes Rhizome) 12 g, Fuling (Indian Bread) 12 g, Chenpi (Dried Tangerine Peel) 6 g, Banxia (Pinellia Tuber) 9 g, Dannanxing (Bile Arisaema) 9 g, Changpu (Acorus Calamus) 12 g, Dilong (Angle Worm) 12 g, Zhiyuanzhi (Prepared Thinleaf Milkwort Root) 6 g, Wugong (Centipede) 2 and Gancao (Liquorice Root) 6 g.

Modification: In cases of cold body and limbs with a predominant deficiency of yang, Fuzi (Prepared Common Monkshood Daughter) 9 g and Ganjiang (Dried Ginger) 6 g can be added to warm yang and resolve dampness.

## 4. Deficiency of brain marrow

Treatment principle: Nourishing essence and blood, supplementing the liver and kidneys.

Prescription and herbs: Modified Dabuyuan Decoction.

Dangshen (Radix Codonopsis) 12 g, Shudi (Prepared Rhizome of Rehmannia) 12 g, Shanyao (Common Yan Rhizome) 15 g, Duzhong (Eucommia Bark) 12 g, Gouqizi (Barbary Wolfberry Fruit) 12 g, Shanzhuyu (Asiatic Cornelian Cherry Fruit) 9 g, Danggui (Chinese Angelica) 9 g, Zhigancao (Stir-baked Liquorice Root) 6 g, Shichangpu (Acorus Calamus) 12g, Yuanzhi (Thinleaf Milkwort Root) 6 g, Tianma (Tall Gastrodis Tuber) 12 g and Gouteng (Gambir Plant) 15 g.

Modification: If there is predominance of kidney deficiency, Guiban (Tortoise Shell) 12 g and Zihechefen (Human Placenta Powder) 6 g (swallowed) can be added to supplement essence and nourish the kidneys.

## 5. Obstruction of collaterals by blood stasis

Treatment principle: Activating blood and resolving stasis, dredging the collaterals and calming epilepsy.

Prescription and herbs: Supplementary Xuefu Zhuyu Decoction.

Taoren (Peach Seed) 9 g, Honghua (Safflower) 9 g, Danggui (Chinese Angelica) 9 g, Chuanxiong (Szechwan Lovage Rhizome) 9 g, Shengdi (Dried Rehmannia Root) 9 g, Chishao (Red Peony Root) 12 g, Baishao (White Peony Alba) 12g, Chaihu (Chinese Thorowax Root) 9 g, Zhiqiao (Orange Fruit) 9 g, Jiegeng (Platycodon Root) 6 g, Niuxi (Twotoothed Achyranthes Root) 12 g, Jiangcan (Stiff Silkworm) 12 g, Dilong (Angle Worm) 12 g and Gancao ( Liquorice Root) 6 g.

Modification: For severe headache, Tianma (Tall Gastrodis Tuber) 12 g and Gegen (Kudzuvine Root) 30 g can be used to subdue the liver and activate blood.

## Chinese Patent Medicine

1. Baijin Pill: 3 g for each dose, 3 times a day for long-term administration.

2. Qingdai Powder: 3 g for each dose, 3 times a day after meals. Once there is no occurrence for half a year, it can be administered twice a day and subsequently reduced to just 1 dose daily if there is no occurrence for a year.

## Simple and Handy Prescriptions

Equal quantities of Quanxie (Scorpion), Wugong (Centipede), Jiangcan (Stiff Silkworm) and Dibiechong (Eupolyphaga Seu Steleophaga) are ground up into powders and then capsulized. Five capsules are taken for each dose, twice a day (in the morning and evening). This medicine is used to extinguish wind and calm epilepsy.

## Other Therapies

Exercise therapy: Proper physical exercises, such as taijiquan and body-building exercise, are beneficial to the body and can reduce the occurrences of this disease.

## Cautions and Advice

1. Patients must not abruptly reduce the amount of anti-epileptic drugs or suddenly discontinue them lest there be epileptic relapse.
2. They must conquer their sense of inferiority and fear and avoid physical or emotional overstrain leading to fatigue or tension.
3. Patients should strengthen their constitution, develop a regular lifestyle and refrain from cigarettes and alcohol.
4. Driving, swimming and going outside alone at night are prohibited. If there are presymptoms, patients should lie down immediately to avoid possible injuries from falling.

## Daily Exercises

1. Recall the main etiological factors of epilepsy. To which viscera it is most closely related in terms of occurrence?
2. Explain how epilepsy due to obstruction of wind and phlegm and epilepsy due to internal exuberance of phlegm and fire can be differentiated.

# Schizophrenia

# Week 12: Thursday

Schizophrenia is a most common type of mental disorder. It is marked by mental, emotional, volitional and behavioral disturbances with no pathological changes of the brain. The most conspicuous symptom is incoordination of emotional activities. It can be classified into different types based on symptoms: paranoiac, adolescent, catatonic, simple and others. It mostly strikes in late adolescence and early adulthood. Spring is the season when this disease takes place most frequently. The prognosis is poor, especially for the simple and adolescent types. In TCM, schizophrenia belongs to the category of "depressive psychosis".

## Etiology and Pathology

TCM holds that schizophrenia is caused by emotional disorders, which impair the liver and spleen and by excessive contemplation, which harms the heart spirit. In addition, the occurrence of this disease is also considered to be closely associated with innate endowment or body constitution.

The pathological changes are discussed as follows: Excessive contemplation damages the heart and spleen with a failure of blood to nourish the heart spirit, this is marked by insomnia, impaired concentration, absent-mindedness, palpitations, propensity for anger and crying and lassitude. Excessive melancholy damages the liver and causes stagnation of live qi and impairment of the spleen and stomach; the spleen fails to transform water properly, thus creating dampness and phlegm which flow upward, obstructing the heart vessels and clouding the spirit, with such manifestations as dementia, disorganized speech, emotional fluctuations and sloppiness of dress and hygiene. Moreover, excessive phlegm and stasis may impede the flow of qi and blood, preventing the visceral qi from communicating with the brain qi and consequently triggering off this disease.

## Diagnostic Key Points

1. The disease is marked by slow onset and symptoms of nervous exhaustion in the initial and acute stages, such as headache and insomnia.

2. This disease can be confirmed if there are at least two of the following aspects, without conscious disturbance and emotional fluctuations: (1) association disturbance; (2) delusion; (3) affective disorder; (4) auditory hallucination; (5) behavioral disturbance; (6) hypobulia; (7) passive experience (8) disorganized thinking or forced thinking.
3. The duration of mental disorder is at least three months.
4. The mental disorders should be discounted if they are associated with brain diseases, somatic diseases, psychoactive substances and non-dependent substances.

## Syndrome Differentiation

### 1. Stagnation of phlegm and qi

Symptoms: Emotional depression, apathy, dementia, incoherent speech or murmuring to oneself, emotional fluctuations and poor appetite; greasy tongue coating and taut and slippery pulse.

Analysis of symptoms: Excessive contemplation and unrealized desire lead to stagnation of liver qi, failure of spleen qi to ascend and clouding of the spirit by stagnated phlegm and qi, with such manifestations as apathy and dementia; turbid phlegm impedes the transforming function of the spleen, giving rise to a poor appetite, greasy tongue coating and taut and slippery pulse.

### 2. Disturbance of the heart by phlegm and fire

Symptoms: Insomnia, timorousness, restlessness, incoherent speech, reddened eyes and complexion, emotional instability and good appetite; red tongue with yellow and greasy coating and slippery and rapid pulse.

Analysis of symptoms: Disharmony between the spleen and stomach brings about the transformation of stagnated qi and phlegm into fire, which disturbs the heart spirit upwardly, with such signs as insomnia, timorousness, restlessness and incoherent speech; phlegmatic fire disturbs the upper energizer, marked by reddened eyes and complexion; phlegmatic fire scorches the interior, giving rise to a good appetite, red tongue with yellow and greasy coating and slippery and rapid pulse.

## 3. Deficiency of the spleen and stomach

Symptoms: Absent-mindedness, delusions, palpitations, timorousness, sentimentality, sorrowfulness, weariness, poor appetite, pale tongue with thin coating and thin and weak pulse.

Analysis of symptoms: Long-term affliction of depressed psychosis leads to insufficiency of the heart and blood and malnutrition of the heart spirit, this is marked by palpitations, timorousness, absent-mindedness, sentimentality, sorrowfulness and delusions; since the qi and blood is declined, the spleen may fail to work properly to transform food, resulting in poor appetite and weariness; the pale tongue with thin coating and thin and weak pulse are all attributable to deficiency of the spleen and stomach as well as qi and blood.

## Differential Treatment

### 1. Stagnation of phlegm and qi

Treatment principle: Regulating qi and relieving stagnation, dissolving phlegm and opening the orifices.

Prescription and herbs: Modified Shunqi Daotan Decoction.

Chenpi (Dried Tangerine Peel) 9 g, Banxia (Pinellia Tuber) 9 g, Dannanxing (Bile Arisaema) 12 g, Fuling (Indian Bread) 12 g, Zhixiangfu (Prepared Nutgrass Galingale Rhizome) 9 g, Yujin (Turmeric Root Tuber) 9 g, Shichangpu (Acorus Calamus) 12 g, Muxiang (Common Aucklandia Root) 6 g and Gancao (Liquorice Root) 6 g.

Modification: If there is absent-mindedness with a dull expression, disorganized speech, widened eyes without blinking and white greasy tongue coating, this is a case of mental confusion due to phlegm obstructing the heart orifices, which can be treated by Suhexiang Pill to open the orifices with aromatic herbs.

### 2. Disturbance of the heart by phlegm and fire

Treatment principle: Dispelling heat and dissolving phlegm, calming the heart and tranquilizing the mind.

Prescription and herbs: Modified Huanglian Wendan Decoction.

Huangqin (Baical Skullcap Root) 12 g, Huanglian (Golden Thread) 6 g, Banxia (Pinellia Tuber) 9 g, Chenpi (Dried Tangerine Peel) 9 g, Fuling (Indian Bread) 12 g, Zhuru (Bamboo Shavings) 9 g, Qingmengshi (Chlorite Schist) 15 g, Shichangpu (Acorus Calamus) 15 g, Tianzhuhuang (Tabasheer)12 g, Gancao (Liquorice Root) 6 g and Dazao (Chinese Date) 7 dates.

Modification: If there is exuberant phlegm and fire with constipation, Shengdahuang (Unprepared Rhubarb) 9 g (decocted later) and Mangxiao (Sodium Sulfate) 9 g (infused) can be added to remove phlegm and reduce fire.

### 3. Deficiency of the spleen and stomach

Treatment principle: Invigorating the spleen and nourishing the heart, supplementing blood and calming the spirit.

Prescription and herbs: Modified Yangxin Decoction and Ganmai Dazao Decoction.

Dangshen (Radix Codonopsis) 9 g, Huangqi (Milkvetch Root) 15 g, Fuling (Indian Bread) 9 g, Danshen (Radix Salviae Miltiorrhiae) 12 g, Chuanxiong (Szechwan Lovage Rhizome) 9 g, Danggui (Chinese Angelica) 9 g, Yuanzhi (Thinleaf Milkwort Root) 6 g, Baiziren (Chinese Arborvitae Kernel) 12 g, Wuweizi (Chinese Magnolivine Fruit) 6 g, Chaozaoren (Fried Semen Ziziphi Spinosae) 12 g, Xiaomai (Wheat) 30 g, Rougui (Cassia Bark) 3 g, Gancao (Liquorice Root) 6 g and Dazao (Chinese Date) 15 g.

Modification: For palpitations and insomnia, Shenglonggu (Raw Os Draconis) 30 g, Hehuanpi (Silktree Albizia Bark) 15 g and Yejiaoteng (Caulis Polygoni Multiflori) 30 g can be added to calm the heart and tranquilize the mind.

### Chinese Patent Medicine

1. Zhusha Anshen Pill: 10 pills for each dose, 3 times a day.
2. Mengshi Guentan Pill: 10 pills for each dose, 3 times a day.
3. Cizhu Pill: 10 pills for each dose, 3 times a day.

## Simple and Handy Prescriptions

Huaixiaomai (Wheat) 30 g, Dazao (Chinese Date) 15 g and Gancao (Liquorice Root) 6 g are boiled in water and take 1 dose a day at 2 different times for nourishing the heart, calming the spirit and moistening dryness.

## Other Therapies

Family therapy: Family members should provide care, kindness and support, as well as communicate openly with the patient. Doing so will help reduce the patient's psychological burden, build self-esteem and conquer the sense of inferiority that plagues him or her. All of these can be helpful for the recovery of the patient.

Dietary therapy: A pig's heart and 10 batches of Indian bread with hostwood and with seasonings for taste are boiled together to nourish the heart and calm the spirit.

Exercise therapy: In the recovery phase, patients can take exercises such as taijiquan, baduanjin and wuqinxi so as to restore the higher nervous activity.

## Cautions and Advice

1. Patients should receive guidance to properly deal with their conditions.
2. Prompt and consistent treatment should be administered to prevent relapse.
3. Patients should adopt a regular lifestyle, stick to a light yet nutritious diet and engage in exercise such as taijiquan, walking and jogging, so as to speed up the recovery of this disease.

## Daily Exercises

1. List the different clinical types of schizophrenia and recall their treatment principles and representative prescriptions.
2. Describe the main clinical characteristics of schizophrenia with stagnation of phlegm and qi.

# Neurastheria
# Week 12: Friday

Neurastheria, also called neurosis, is a functional disorder of the nerves due to long-term overstress or psychic trauma, resulting in dysfunction of the brain with various clinical symptoms, namely agitation, fatigue, mood swings, pain due to tension, sleeping disturbance and dysfunction of the autonomic nerve. These symptoms, however, are not secondary to the diseases of the brain, the body, or other mental disorders. This disease mostly afflicts young and middle-aged people, with females and those who do more mental rather than physical work being more susceptible. In TCM, neurastheria is closely associated with "syndrome of depression", "insomnia" and "palpitations".

## Etiology and Pathology

This disease is mostly caused by emotional disorders, especially long-term depression, excessive contemplation and mental strain, all of which bring about imbalance of yin, yang, qi and blood of the viscera, with a series of clinical symptoms.

## Diagnostic Key Points

1. Agitation, moodiness, disorganized thinking and memory and intolerance of sound and light with hyperesthesia.
2. Fatigue, complaint of low work-efficiency, impaired concentration, reduced memory, weariness, distension in the head with mental confusion and listlessness.
3. Emotional instability, melancholy, anxiety, irascibility, nervousness, excessive self-consciousness of various changes with suspicions or doubts and various corresponding clinical symptoms.
4. Pain due to tension, with distension in the head, stiffness in the neck, soreness in the waist and back and pain in the muscles of the four limbs.
5. Difficulty in falling asleep, disturbed sleeping rhythms, dreaminess, tinnitus, blurred vision, palpitations, shortness of breath, chest distress,

menstrual irregularity, nocturnal emissions, flushed complexion, cold in the feet and hands or even cyanosis.

6. Physical and laboratory examination: No corresponding organic changes.

## Syndrome Differentiation

### 1. Liver-qi stagnation

Symptoms: Emotional depression, mental uneasiness, chest and hypochondriac distension and pain without fixed locations, frequent sighing, abdominal distension, gastric stuffiness, belching, vomiting, reduced appetite, abnormal defecation and menstrual irregularity; thin and greasy coating and taut pulse.

Analysis of symptoms: Emotional disorder leads to failure of the liver to promote the free flow of qi, causing emotional depression and mental uneasiness; stagnation of liver qi and disorder of the liver collaterals are responsible for chest and hypochondriac distension and pain without fixed location, as well as frequent sighing; if the liver qi invades the stomach, the stomach qi will fail to descend normally, giving rise to abdominal distension, gastric stuffiness, belching and vomiting; the liver qi over-restricts the spleen, bringing about a reduced appetite and abnormal defecation; stagnation of liver qi and disorder of the thoroughfare vessel and conception vessel are responsible for menstrual irregularity; the thin and greasy coating and the taut pulse are both manifestations of liver depression and qi stagnation.

### 2. Transformation of stagnated qi into fire

Symptoms: Chest distress, hypochondriac distension, headache, dizziness, reddened eyes, tinnitus, irascibility, dry and bitter mouth, gastric upset with acid regurgitation and dry stools; red tongue with yellow coating and rapid and taut pulse.

Analysis of symptoms: Stagnation of liver qi is marked by chest distress and hypochondriac distension; prolonged stagnation produces fire, marked by headache, dizziness, reddened eyes and tinnitus; the liver fire invades the stomach, bringing about heat in the stomach and intestine, with the symptoms of dry and bitter mouth, gastric upset with acid regurgitation and dry stools; irascibility, red tongue with yellow coating, as well as rapid and taut pulse are all symptomatic of excessive liver fire.

### 3. Stagnation of qi with accumulation of phlegm

Symptoms: Sensation of a foreign body stuck in the throat, chest fullness and stuffiness, bilateral distension and pain in the hypochondria; white and greasy tongue coating and taut and slippery pulse.

Analysis of symptoms: Over-restriction of liver qi in the spleen causes dysfunction of the spleen in transportation and transformation, thus resulting in the accumulation of dampness into phlegm which, combined with qi, obstructs the throat. This manifests as self-consciousness of throat obstruction with a fixed location that poses no difficulty in swallowing in actuality, known as "globus hysteritis"; stagnation of liver qi uninhibits the smooth functional activity of qi, leading to chest fullness and stuffiness, as well as bilateral distension and pain in the hypochondria; the white and greasy tongue coating and taut and slippery pulse are both attributable to stagnation of qi with accumulation of phlegm.

### 4. Malnutrition of the heart spirit

Symptoms: Mental uneasiness, absent-mindedness, involuntary sorrowfulness, vexation, insomnia and frequent yawning, or even disorganized speech; pale tongue with white and thin coating and taut and thin pulse.

Analysis of symptoms: Prolonged stagnation of qi consumes the heart qi and ying-blood, leading to malnutrition of the heart spirit, marked by mental derangement, uneasiness, absent-mindedness, involuntary sorrowfulness, vexation, insomnia and frequent yawning, or even disorder of speech, known as "visceral agitation"; the pale tongue with white and thin coating and the taut and thin pulse are all manifestations of qi stagnation and blood deficiency.

## 5.  Deficiency of the heart and spleen

Symptoms: palpitations, timorousness, excessive contemplation, forget-fulness, dreaminess with frequent startles, dizziness, listlessness, reduced food intake, loose stools and lusterless complexion; pale tongue with teeth imprints, thin coating and thin and feeble pulse or slow and soggy pulse.

Analysis of symptoms: Stagnation of qi and deficiency of blood leads to malnourishment of the heart; excessive contemplation damages the spleen and stomach, bringing on deficiency of the spleen and stomach, with mental uneasiness, palpitations, timorousness, excessive contemplation, palpitations, forgetfulness and dreaminess with frequent startles; dysfunction of the spleen in transportation and transformation is responsible for reduced food intake and loose stools; insufficient qi and blood is manifested as dizziness, listlessness and lusterless complexion; the pale tongue with teeth imprints and thin coating and the thin and feeble pulse or slow and soggy pulse are all attributable to deficiency of qi and blood.

## 6.  Exuberance of fire due to deficiency of yin

Symptoms: Dizziness, head distension, irascibility, palpitations, vexation, insomnia, waist soreness, tinnitus, nocturnal emissions and irregular menstruation; red tongue and taut, thin and rapid pulse.

Analysis of symptoms: The deficiency of visceral yin and ying-blood leads to floating of deficient yang, marked by dizziness, distension of the head and irascibility; consumption of yin-blood and malnutrition of the heart spirit may produce deficient heat which disturbs the heart spirit, giving rise to palpitations, vexation and insomnia; insufficiency of kidney yin creates a predisposition to malnutrition of the waist and disorder of the ear, marked by waist soreness and tinnitus; deficiency of yin produces exuberant fire which disturbs the semen chamber and causes nocturnal emissions in males; malnutrition of the liver and kidneys with disorder of the thoroughfare and conception vessels is responsible for irregular menstruation in females; the red tongue and the taut, thin and rapid pulse are both caused by deficiency of yin with exuberance of fire.

## Differential Treatment

### 1. Liver-qi stagnation

Treatment principle: Soothing the liver and regulating qi, removing stagnation and relieving depression.

Prescription and herbs: Modified Chaihu Shugan Powder and Yueju Pill.

Chaihu (Chinese Thorowax Root) 9 g, Zhiqiao (Orange Fruit) 12 g, Xiangfu (Nutgrass Galingale Rhizome) 12 g, Yujin (Turmeric Root Tuber) 9 g, Qingpi (Green Tangerine Peel) 6 g, Chenpi (Dried Tangerine Peel) 6 g, Chuanxiong (Szechwan Lovage Rhizome) 6 g, Baishao (White Peony Alba) 9 g, Cangzhu (Atractylodes Rhizome) 9 g, Zhizi (Cape Jasmine Fruit) 9 g, Shenqu (Massa Medicata Fermentata) 9 g and Gancao ( Liquorice Root) 6 g.

Modification: For belching and vomiting, Xuanfuhua (Intussusceer) 12 g, Daizheshi (Red Bole) 30 g and Jiangzhuru (Ginger-prepared Bamboo Shavings) 9 g can be added to reverse the adverse flow of qi and arrest vomiting; for suppression of menses, Danggui (Chinese Angelica) 9 g, Taoren (Peach Seed) 9 g and Honghua (Safflower) 9 g can be added to nourish blood, activate blood and regulate menstruation; for profuse menses, Nuzhenzi (Glossy Privet Fruit) 9 g, Huanliancao (Ecliptae Herba) 9 g and Xianhecao (Hairyvein Agrimonia Herb) 30 g can be added to nourish the kidneys, stop bleeding and regulate menstruation; for loose stools, Yiyiren (Coix Seed) 15 g and Shanyao (Common Yan Rhizome) 15 g can be added to invigorate the spleen and check diarrhea; for constipation, Huomaren (Hemp Seed) 9 g and Dahuang (Rhubarb) 9 g can be added to promote defecation.

### 2. Transformation of stagnated qi into fire

Treatment principle: Promoting flow of qi to relieve depression, dispelling heat in the liver.

Prescription and herbs: Modified Danzhi Xiaoyao Powder and Zuojin Pill.

Danpi (Cortex Moutan) 9 g, Zhizi (Cape Jasmine Fruit) 9 g, Chaihu (Chinese Thorowax Root) 9 g, Bohe (Peppermint) 3 g, Danggui (Chinese Angelica) 9 g, Baishao (White Peony Alba) 9 g, Baizhu (Largehead

Atractylodes Rhizome) 12 g, Fuling (Indian Bread) 12 g, Huanglian (Golden Thread) 6 g, Wuzhuyu (Medicinal Evodia Fruit) 3 g and Gancao (Liquorice Root) 6 g.

Modification: For chest distress with hypochondriac distension, Yanhusuo (Corydalis) 9 g and Chuanlianzi (Szechwan Chinaberry Fruit) 9 g can be added to soothe the liver and regulate qi; for headache, Chuanxiong (Szechwan Lovage Rhizome) 6 g can be added to expel wind and stop pain; for tinnitus, Shichangpu (Acorus Calamus) 12 g and Lingcishi (Magnetitum) 30 g are added to treat the ear disorder; for the bitter taste in the mouth, reddened eyes, irascibility and dry stools, Longdancao (Radix Gentianae) 6 g and Dahuang (Rhubarb) 6 g can added to dispel liver heat.

## 3. Stagnation of qi with accumulation of phlegm

Treatment principle: Promoting flow of qi and dissolving phlegm, relieving depression and dissipating stagnation.

Prescription and herbs: Modified Banxia Houpu Decoction.

Banxia (Pinellia Tuber) 9 g, Houpu (Magnolia Bark) 9 g, Fuling (Indian Bread) 12 g, Zisu (Purple Common Perilla) 9 g, Zhixiangfu (Nutgrass Galingale Rhizome) 12 g, Zhiqiao (Orange Fruit) 12 g, Foshou (Finger Citron) 8 g, Bayuezha (Fiveleaf Akebia Fruit) 9 g, Luyuemei (Flos Mume) 9 g, Chenpi (Dried Tangerine Peel) 6 g, Shengjiang (Fresh Ginger) 3 slices and Gancao (Liquorice Root) 6 g.

Modification: If there is chest distress and hypochondriac pain, Yujin (Turmeric Root Tuber) 12 g and Gualou (Snakegourd Fruit) 15 g can be added to relieve the chest; for nausea, vomiting and the bitter taste in the mouth, Huangqin (Baical Skullcap Root) 9 g, Xuanfuhua (Intussusceer) 12 g and Daizheshi (Red Bole) 30 g are added to dispel stomach heat and bring down qi.

## 4. Malnutrition of the heart spirit

Treatment principle: Supplementing qi and nourishing the heart, tranquilizing the spirit and calming the mind.

Prescription and herbs: Modified Ganmai Dazao Decoction and Anshen Dingzhi Pill.

Gancao (Liquorice Root) 9 g, Taizishen (Heterophylly Falsesatarwort Root) 30 g, Xiaomai (Wheat) 30 g, Dazao (Chinese Date) 15 g, Longgu (Calcined Os Draconis) 30 g, Fuling (Indian Bread) 12 g, Fushen (Indian Bread with Hostwood) 9 g, Shichangpu (Acorus Calamus) 12 g, Baiziren (Chinese Arborvitae Kernel) 9 g, Suanzaoren (Spine Date Seed) 9 g, Yejiaoteng (Caulis Polygoni Multiflori) 30 g and Hehuanhua (Albizia Flower) 9 g.

Modification: If there is vexation and insomnia, Muli (Calcined Oyster Shell) 30 g, Lingcishi (Magnetitum) 30 g and Guiban (Tortoise Shell) 9 g can be added to tranquilize the mind with their heavy properties

## 5. Deficiency of the heart and spleen

Treatment principle: Supplementing qi and tranquilizing the mind, invigorating the spleen and nourishing the heart.

Prescription and herbs: Modified Guipi Decoction and Suanzaoren Decoction.

Huangqi (Milkvetch Root) 15 g, Dangshen (Radix Codonopsis) 12 g, Baizhu (Largehead Atractylodes Rhizome) 12 g, Zhigancao (Stir-baked Liquorice Root) 6 g, Fushen (Indian Bread with Hostwood) 12 g, Longyanrou (Longan Aril) 3 g, Suanzaoren (Spine Date Seed) 9 g, Zhiyuanzhi (Prepared Thinleaf Milkwort Root) 6 g, Danggui (Chinese Angelica) 9 g, Zhimu (Common Anemarrhena Rhizome) 9 g, Chuanxiong (Szechwan Lovage Rhizome) 6 g and Muxiang (Common Aucklandia Root) 6 g.

Modification: For severe palpitations, Maidong (Dwarf Lilyturf Tuber) 9 g and Wuweizi (Chinese Magnolivine Fruit) 6 g can be added to astringe yin and revive pulsation; for dreaminess and restless sleep, Yujin (Turmeric Root Tuber) 9 g, Hehuanhua (Albizia Flower) 9 g, Baiziren (Chinese Arborvitae Kernel) 9 g and Yejiaoteng (Caulis Polygoni Multiflori) 30 g can be added to tranquilize the mind.

## 6. Exuberance of fire due to deficiency of yin

Treatment principle: Nourishing yin to purge fire, tranquilizing the mind by subjugation.

Prescription and herbs: Modified Zishui Qinggan Potion and Zhusha Anshen Pill.

Shengdi (Dried Rehmannia Root) 12 g, Shanzhuyu (Asiatic Cornelian Cherry Fruit) 9 g, Fuling (Indian Bread) 12 g, Shanyao (Common Yan Rhizome) 15 g, Zexie (Oriental Waterplantain Rhizome) 12 g, Chaihu (Chinese Thorowax Root) 6 g, Danpi (Cortex Moutan) 9 g, Zhizi (Cape Jasmine Fruit) 9 g, Huanglian (Golden Thread) 3 g, Suanzaoren (Spine Date Seed) 9 g, Danggui (Chinese Angelica) 9 g and Gancao (Liquorice Root) 6 g.

Modification: For dizziness and distension in the head, Tianma (Tall Gastrodis Tuber) 6 g and Gouteng (Gambir Plant) 12 g can be added to calm the liver and subdue yang; for severe insomnia, Zhenzhumu (Nacre) 30 g, Lingcishi (Magnetitum) 30 g and Shengtieluo (Raw Pulvis Ferri) 30 g can be added to tranquilize the mind with their heavy properties; for waist soreness and nocturnal emissions, Zhimu (Common Anemarrhena Rhizome) 9 g, Guiban (Tortoise Shell) 9 g, Buguzhi (Malaytea Scurfpea Fruit) 12 g and Wuweizi (Chinese Magnolivine Fruit) 6 g are used to tonify the kidneys, nourish yin and reduce emissions; for irregular menstruation, Xiangfu (Nutgrass Galingale Rhizome) 12 g, Nuzhenzi (Glossy Privet Fruit) 9 g and Huanliancao (Ecliptae Herba) 9 g can be added to regulate menstruation.

## Chinese Patent Medicine

1. Zhenheling Tablet: 4 tablets for each dose, 3 times a day.
2. Zaoren Anshen Capsule: 2 capsules for each dose before sleep at night.
3. Tianwang Buxin Dan: 3 g for each dose, 3 times a day.

## Simple and Handy Prescriptions

1. Lianzirou (Lotus Seed Pulp) 30 g, Longgu (Os Draconis) 15 g, Longyanrou (Longan Aril) 30 g, Shanyao (Common Yan Rhizome) 20 g and Dazao (Chinese Date) 6 dates (enucleated) are decocted in water for an hour and then Baihe (Lily Bulb) 30 g is added for further decoction. The soup and its ingredients Baihe (Lily Bulb), Longyanrou

(Longan Aril) and Dazao (Chinese Date) can be consumed once a day-with 1 bowl constituting 1 dose.

2. Sangshenzi (Mulberry Seed) 30 g, Zhenzhumu (Nacre) 30 g and Maidong (Dwarf Lilyturf Tuber) 15 g are boiled in water and 1 bowl (constituting 1 dose) is consumed before sleep at night.

3. 12~25 spine date seeds are fired till they are half cooked and then pounded and ground up into powder. The draft of powder is taken before sleep at night.

## Other Therapies

Dietary therapy:

(1) 250 g of lean pork is sliced, mixed with 50 g of lotus pulp and then boiled in water. Seasoning can be added for taste before eating.

(2) Baizhu (Largehead Atractylodes Rhizome) 10 g, Suanzaoren (Spine Date Seed) 10 g, Longyanrou (Longan) 15 longans, Heshouwu (Fleeceflower Root) 15 g, Lingzhi (Mythic Fungus) 15 g and Dazao (Chinese Date) 7 dates are decocted in water. The condensed decoction is then used to cook rice fruit (50 g), with seasoning added for taste once it is cooked. This can be consumed twice a day with 1 bowl constituting 1 dose.

(3) Heizhima (Black Sesame) 50 g and Hutaorou (Walnut) 50 g are fried, ground up into powders and then blended with 15 g of refined sugar. A single spoonful is administered once a day.

## Cautions and Advice

1. Apart from drug treatment, emotional regulation is also very important. Patients should relieve themselves of psychological burdens, avoid various irritations and balance work and rest. It is also advisable for them to avoid emotional fluctuation before sleep, as well as refrain from drinking strong tea, coffee and too much water.

2. Lily bulb, lotus seed, longan and Chinese date can be frequently consumed so as to nourish the heart and calm the spirit. The diet of patients should be composed of light, easily digested foods instead of spicy, oily ones.

3. If patients can exercise self-regulation as mentioned above while simultaneously receiving drug treatment, the disease can be completely cured; otherwise, it may be aggravated and have an unfavorable prognosis.

## Daily Exercises

1. Describe the etiology and pathology of neurastheria.
2. Explain how neurastheria can be treated based on syndrome differentiation.

# Senile Dementia
# Week 12: Saturday

Senile dementia is an acquired overall impairment of the sophisticated functions of the cerebral cortex, clinically marked by forgetfulness, change in personality and exhibition of abnormal thinking and behavior in more severe cases, or even inability to provide self-care, difficulty in walking and death in the late stage. Senile dementia can be classified into three types according to etiological factors: primary retrograde dementia (or Alzheimer's disease), vascular dementia and dementia due to other brain diseases (a relatively rare type). This disease, if promptly diagnosed, treated and controlled, can have a favorable prognosis; however, once it progresses into the stage of severe mental confusion, the prognosis will be unfavorable. In TCM, senile dementia is closely associated with "cognitive dysfunction", "forgetfulness", "idiocy" and "syndrome of depression".

## Etiology and Pathology

TCM holds that senile dementia is caused by deficiency of visceral qi and blood due to senility and impairment of liver and kidney essence due to excessive sexual activities; or by heat consumption of qi, blood and body fluid due to chronic diseases, mental disorders or stroke; or by damage to the liver and spleen due to emotional disorders such as excessive worry, contemplation and anger, as well as improper diet such as excessive intake of alcohol and food; or by stagnation of qi and blood due to prolonged worry and contemplation; or by injury to the brain due to trauma and intoxication.

The pathological changes are discussed as follows: Senility and chronic disease can lead to deficiency of the viscera and brain marrow, imbalance between yin and yang, abnormal transformation of qi, blood and essence, disordered ascent and descent of qi and obstruction of phlegm and blood, all of which are responsible for the dysfunction of brain and the exhibition of various symptoms. Since the qi, blood, yin and yang of the viscera are deficient, the essence qi will be unable to reach the head and nourish the brain marrow as well as the spirit, which then fails to govern the body, especially the five sense organs and nine orifices, thereby presenting as dementia. The location of this disease is in the brain (marrow), but the condition of the heart, kidneys, liver and spleen are also closely linked to it.

## Diagnostic Key Points

1. The disease often occurs in the old age (above 65 years of age in males and over 55 in females).
2. Clinically, there are changes in intelligence, mental state, behavior and the physical body.
3. Primary retrograde dementia usually demonstrates no marked focal neurological signs, while vascular dementia presents with focal neurological signs of stroke.
4. EEG findings: Diffusive rhythm disturbance and diffusive short wave. CT and MRI findings: Brain atrophy and brain ventricle enlargement.

## Syndrome Differentiation

### 1. Deficiency of essence qi

Symptoms: Dull expression, slow movements, poor memory, slurred and disorganized speech, naïve behavior, withdrawal from society, depression, emotional instability, or tremors of the head or limbs, dizziness, blurred vision, poor hearing, weakness and soreness in the waist and knees, hair loss, loosening of teeth, shortness of breath and feebleness of the body; slightly dark tongue with white and thin coating and thin and feeble pulse, especially in the chi region.

Analysis of symptoms: Senility is marked by a weak body with deficiency of essence and marrow, which leads to malnutrition and dysfunction of the primordial spirit, with such signs as silliness or dementia. Insufficiency of kidney essence and brain marrow are responsible for dizziness, soreness in the waist and knees, hair loss and loosening of teeth; insufficiency of essence qi is manifested as deafness, blurred vision and shortness of breath; the slightly dark tongue with white and thin coating and the thin and feeble pulse (especially in the chi region) are attributable to insufficiency of kidney qi.

## 2. Deficiency of the spleen and stomach

Symptoms: Dull expression, melancholy, reluctance to talk, pale complexion, lassitude with a tendency to lie, palpitations, shortness of breath and poor appetite; pale tongue with white and thin coating and thin and feeble pulse.

Analysis of symptoms: Excessive contemplation impairs the heart and spleen, resulting in insufficient blood to nourish the heart and brain and giving rise to mental derangement and dementia; deficiency of qi and blood is responsible for lassitude with a tendency to lie, palpitations, shortness of breath and pale complexion; dysfunction of the spleen in transportation and transformation is manifested as poor appetite; the pale tongue with white and thin coating and thin and feeble pulse are due to deficiency of the spleen and stomach as well as qi and blood.

## 3. Obstruction of the orifices by turbid phlegm

Symptoms: Emotional depression, dull expression, quietness, reluctance to talk or murmuring to oneself, withdrawal from society, emotional instability, unwillingness to communicate with people, heaviness of the head as if it was being wrapped up, poor appetite, gastric and abdominal distension, profuse sputum and saliva in the mouth, pale or lusterless complexion, shortness of breath and weariness; pale and enlarged tongue with white and greasy coating and deep and slippery pulse.

Analysis of symptoms: Stagnated liver qi over-restricts the spleen and stomach, preventing them from transforming the turbid phlegm which accumulates in the chest and clouds the spirit, giving rise to the heaviness of the head and dementia; pale complexion, shortness of breath and weariness may point to deficiency of middle qi; poor appetite, gastric and abdominal distension and profuse sputum and saliva in the mouth are attributable to the malfunctioned spleen; the pale and enlarged tongue with white and greasy coating and the deep and slippery pulse are symptomatic of abundant phlegm and dampness in the interior.

## 4. Stagnation of qi with blood stasis

Symptoms: Dull expression, slow reaction, reluctance to talk, forgetfulness, irascibility, liability to wake up with a start, delirium, insomnia and steady fixation of eyes; dark purple tongue with ecchymosis or petechia, white and thin tongue coating and unsmooth, thin and weak, or deep and slow pulse.

Analysis of symptoms: This syndrome is usually caused by trauma. The brain is the place where the primordial spirit resides and if there is stagnation of qi with blood stasis in the brain, the primordial spirit will be malnourished, presenting as dementia; the dark purple tongue and tardy and unsmooth pulse are manifestations of blood stasis.

## Differential Treatment

### 1. Deficiency of essence qi

Treatment principle: Supplementing essence qi, nourishing the brain and tranquilizing the spirit.

Prescription and herbs: Modified Huanshao Dan.

Shudi (Prepared Rhizome of Rehmannia) 12 g, Gouqizi (Barbary Wolfberry Fruit) 12 g, Shanzhuyu (Asiatic Cornelian Cherry Fruit) 9 g, Chushizi (Papermulberry Fruit) 12 g, Roucongrong (Desertliving Cistanche) 12 g, Duzhong (Eucommia Bark) 12 g, Niuxi (Twotoothed Achyranthes Root) 9 g, Bajitian (Mornda Root) 12 g, Yizhiren (Bitter-seed Cardamn) 15 g, Fuling (Indian Bread) 12 g, Yuanzhi (Thinleaf Milkwort Root) 6 g, Shanyao (Common Yan Rhizome) 15 g, Shichangpu (Acorus Calamus) 12 g, Yujin (Turmeric Root Tuber) 12 g and Dazao (Chinese Date) 7 dates.

Modification: If there isweariness, shortness of breath and unwillingness to speak and walk, Huangqi (Milkvetch Root) 15 g and Dangshen (Radix

Codonopsis) 9 g can be added to replenish qi and invigorate the spleen; for poor appetite with yellow and greasy tongue coating and phlegmatic heat in the middle energizer, the removal of phlegmatic heat should be addressed before the application of nourishing therapy.

## 2. Deficiency of the spleen and stomach

Treatment principle: Invigorating the spleen and supplementing blood, nourishing the heart and improving intelligence.

Prescription and herbs: Modified Guipi Decoction and Dingzhi Pill.

Dangshen (Radix Codonopsis) 12 g, Huangqi (Milkvetch Root) 15 g, Baizhu (Largehead Atractylodes Rhizome) 12 g, Fushen (Indian Bread with Hostwood) 9 g, Suanzaoren (Spine Date Seed) 12 g, Yuanzhi (Thinleaf Milkwort Root) 6 g, Danggui (Chinese Angelica) 9 g, Muxiang (Common Aucklandia Root) 6 g, Shichangpu (Acorus Calamus) 12 g, Yizhiren (Bitter-seed Cardamon) 15 g, Gancao (Liquorice Root) 6 g, Dazao (Chinese Date) 7 dates.

Modification: If there is chest distress and poor appetite, Zhiqiao (Orange Fruit) 9 g and Yujin (Turmeric Root Tuber) 12 g can be added to regulate and relieve the chest discomfort; for incessant sweating, Longgu (Os Draconis) 30 g, Muli (Oyster Shell) 30 g and Fuxiaomai (Blighted Wheat) 15 g can be added to reduce sweating.

## 3. Obstruction of the orifices by turbid phlegm

Treatment principle: Removing phlegm and resolving turbidity, opening the orifices and activating the spirit.

Prescription and herbs: Modified Xixin Decoction.

Dangshen (Radix Codonopsis) 12 g, Baizhu (Largehead Atractylodes Rhizome) 12 g, Fuling (Indian Bread) 12 g, Chenpi (Dried Tangerine Peel) 6 g, Banxia (Pinellia Tuber) 9 g, Zaoren (Semen Ziziphi Spinosae) 12 g, Shichangpu (Acorus Calamus) 12 g, Yujin (Turmeric Root Tuber) 12 g, Yuanzhi (Thinleaf Milkwort Root) 6 g, Gancao (Liquorice Root) 6 g, Fuzi (Prepared Common Monkshood Daughter) 9 g, Shenqu (Massa Medicata Fermentata) 9 g and Roudoukou (Nutmeg) 3 g.

Modification: For apparent stagnation of liver qi, Chaihu (Chinese Thorowax Root) 9 g and Baishao (White Peony Alba) 12 g can be added to soothe the liver and relieve stagnation; for insomnia, Baiziren (Chinese Arborvitae Kernel) 12 g, Yejiaoteng (Caulis Polygoni Multiflori) 30 g and Hehuanpi (Silktree Albizia Bark) 15 g are used to nourish the heart and calm the spirit.

## 4. Stagnation of qi with blood stasis

Treatment principle: Promoting flow of qi and activating blood, unblocking the orifices and refreshing the brain.

Prescription and herbs: Modified Tongqiao Huoxue Decoction.

Taoren (Peach Seed) 9 g, Honghua (Safflower) 9 g, Chishao (Red Peony Root) 12 g, Chuanxiong (Szechwan Lovage Rhizome) 9 g, Shichangpu (Acorus Calamus) 12 g, Yujin (Turmeric Root Tuber) 9 g, Laocong (Dried Spring Onion) 6 g, Shengjiang (Fresh Ginger) 3 slices and Dilong (Angle Worm) 12 g.

Modification: If the disease persists with insufficiency of qi and blood, Danggui (Chinese Angelica) 9 g, Shengdi (Dried Rehmannia Root) 12 g, Dangshen (Radix Codonopsis) 12 g and Huangqi (Milkvetch Root) 15 g can be added to invigorate qi and nourish blood; if there is stagnation of liver qi, Chaihu (Chinese Thorowax Root) 9 g, Zhishi (Immature Orange Fruit) 9 g and Xiangfu (Nutgrass Galingale Rhizome) 12 g are used to soothe the liver, regulate qi and promote circulation of blood.

## Chinese Patent Medicine

1. Naofukang: 3 tablets for each dose, 3 times a day.
2. Huanjingjian Oral Liquid: 10 ml for each dose, 3 times a day.

## Simple and Handy Prescriptions

1. Renshen (Ginseng) 6 g, Baizhu (Largehead Atractylodes Rhizome) 12 g, Fushen (Indian Bread with Hostwood) 9 g and Chenpi (Dried Tangerine Peel) 6 g are boiled in water and then separated into 2 portions to be taken at 2 different times within a day. It is used to treat dementia with deficiency of the spleen and stomach.

2. Danshen (Radix Salviae Miltiorrhiae) 15 g, Chuanxiong (Szechwan Lovage Rhizome) 9 g and Danggui (Chinese Angelica) 9 g are boiled in water and then separated into 2 portions to be taken at 2 different times within a day. It is used to treat dementia with qi stagnation and blood stasis.

## Other Therapies

Dietary therapy:

(1) Fresh Dove Soup: A dove is boiled in water with a small amount of yellow wine. The soup, the meat and the dove's brain can be consumed to nourish the brain and improve intelligence.
(2) Medlar and Pig Brain Soup: A pig brain and 15 g of barbary wolfberry fruit are boiled in water with salt, wine and ginger. It is used to supplement the liver, nourish the brain and improve intelligence.

## Cautions and Advice

1. Senile dementia is hardly treatable, so the prevention of it is of paramount importance. Diseases which may be detrimental to the brain should be promptly treated so as to reduce the damage to the brain.
2. Patients should engage in physical and mental exercises, keep themselves in good spirits and balance work and rest.
3. They are advised to have a light, yet nutritious diet with more fruits and vegetables rather than oily food. They should also refrain from cigarettes and alcohol.

## Daily Exercises

1. Concisely describe the pathological changes of senile dementia.
2. Recall the treatment principle and representative prescription of senile dementia due to depletion of essence qi.
3. List any other points that need to be noted during the treatment of dementia.

# CHAPTER 9

# Connective Tissue Diseases

## Rheumatic Fever

## Week 13: Monday

Rheumatic fever is an acute or chronic disease marked by recurrent episodes due to Group A hemolytic streptococcal infection which involves the general connective tissues. The disease primarily affects the joints, heart, skin, vascular serous membrane and brain tissues. Clinically, it is characterized by fever and migrating, symmetrical and multiple inflammations of the large joints, erythema annulare, subcutaneous nodules, carditis (i.e., chronic rheumatic valvular disease of the heart, which is covered in Chapter 3 on cardiovascular system diseases) and chorea. Acute rheumatic fever commonly afflicts children and teenagers, with the first episode occurring the ages of 5 and 15. Both males and females are equally susceptible. The disease may return during the first 3~5 years after the initial episode, particularly in winter or early spring because cold and dampness are key factors that cause the disease. It has a negative correlation with age in terms of relapse rate, i.e., the younger the children, the higher the rate. In the acute stage, there may be complications of marked enlargement of the heart, heart failure or endomyopericarditis, all of which point to an unfavorable prognosis. In TCM, rheumatic fever is closely associated with "warm-heat disease", "bi-syndrome" or "heart bi-syndrome".

### Etiology and Pathology

TCM holds that rheumatic fever is caused by either endogenous or exogenous factors. The former refers to predominance of yang or weakness of

573

the body in children, while the latter refers to the invasion of pathogenic wind, cold and dampness into the interior from the exterior, which accumulate in the meridians and obstruct the circulation of qi and blood, eventually creating a predisposition to this disease.

The pathological changes are discussed as follows: Children with predominance of yang and accumulation of heat in the interior, when invaded by pathogenic wind, cold and dampness, can present with disorders of the joints, muscles, qi and blood due to migration of internal heat. If the children are already deficient in qi and weak in defense, the pathogenic wind, coupled with cold or dampness, will invade the body and affect the joints, tendons and vessels, congealing qi and blood and manifesting as wind-cold or wind-dampness bi-syndromes. When the disease persists, it may develop from the exterior to the interior, or from the meridians to the viscera. If it involves the skin and tendons, there will be subcutaneous nodules; the ying-blood and vessels, subcutaneous erythema; and cardiac vessels, heart bi-syndrome. Moreover, if the pathogenic factors turn into heat and consume qi and yin, there will be deficiency of qi and yin.

## Diagnostic Key Points

1. Migrating, symmetrical and multiple inflammations of the large joints accompanied by pain or soreness, redness, heat and limited movements. Besides, there are also manifestations of fever, erythema annulare, subcutaneous nodules, carditis and chorea.
2. Raised antistreptococcal antibody (ASO), accelerated blood sedimentation, elevated mucoprotein and enhanced white blood cell count.

## Syndrome Differentiation

### 1. Wind-heat bi-syndrome

Symptoms: High fever, sore throat, polydipsia, redness, swelling, heat and migrating pain of the joints and erythema marginatum; red tongue with yellow coating and slippery and rapid pulse. This pattern is common in acute rheumatic fever.

Analysis of symptoms: The patient is young with predominance of yang and exuberance of both pathogenic factors and healthy qi which combat fiercely, leading to impairment of fluid in the lungs and stomach, this is marked by high fever, sore throat and excessive drinking; stagnated wind, cold and dampness is transformed into heat, which affects the meridians and the joints, giving rise to redness, swelling, heat and migrating pain of the joints; the red tongue with yellow coating and slippery and rapid pulse are manifestations of the struggle between abundant pathogenic heat and healthy qi.

## 2. Wind-cold bi-syndrome

Symptoms: No fever or only low grade fever, no sensation of heat and redness of the joints but a feeling of cutting pain, aggravated by cold; pale complexion, subcutaneous nodules, slightly dark tongue with white and thin or white and greasy coating and taut and tense pulse. This pattern is common in chronic rheumatic arthritis.

Analysis of symptoms: Since wind-cold is predominant, there is no fever or only low grade fever; pathogenic cold invades the meridians and congeals qi and blood, so there is no sensation of heat and redness of the joints but instead, a cutting pain aggravated by cold; exuberance of cold with deficiency of yang is responsible for the pale complexion; cold congeals blood, so there are subcutaneous nodules; the slightly dark tongue with white and thin or white and greasy coating and the floating, taut and tense pulse are symptomatic of predominant wind-cold.

## 3. Wind-dampness bi-syndrome

Symptoms: Swollen, numb and painful joints possibly coupled with cold, white and greasy tongue coating and deep and soggy pulse; or dull fever and hot pain in the joints, thirst, profuse sweating, yellow and greasy tongue coating and rapid and soggy pulse. This pattern is common in chronic rheumatic arthritis.

Analysis of symptoms: Pathogenic wind, accompanied by wind, remains in the joints and blocks the circulation of qi and blood, this is marked by swollen, numb and painful joints; if it is accompanied by cold, there will be cold pain in the joints, white greasy tongue coating and deep soggy pulse; if dampness transforms into heat, there can be dull fever and hot pain in the joints, thirst, profuse sweating, yellow and greasy tongue coating and rapid and soggy pulse.

## 4. Obstruction of heart vessels by pathogenic factors

Symptoms: Painful and slightly swollen joints, possibly coupled with throat soreness, chest distress or ache, shortness of breath, spontaneous perspiration, or palpitations and insomnia; enlarged tongue in red or dark red thin and rapid or knotted and intermittent pulse. This pattern manifests itself commonly when rheumatism involves the heart valves.

Analysis of symptoms: Pathogenic wind, cold and dampness stagnate into heat and progress into the interior from the exterior, or into the viscera from the meridians. If it is in the interior, there will be a sore throat; in the meridians, swollen and painful joints; in the cardiac vessels, chest distress or ache. If the pathogens remain for a long time, there will be simultaneous impairment of qi and yin and disquietude of the heart spirit, marked by shortness of breath, spontaneous perspiration, palpitations and insomnia; the enlarged tongue in red or dark red and the thin and rapid or knotted and intermittent pulse are both attributable to the obstruction of heart vessels by pathogens, leading to deficiency of qi and yin.

## Differential Treatment

### 1. Wind-heat bi-syndrome

Treatment principle: Dispelling wind and dispelling heat, unblocking the collaterals and removing obstruction.

Prescription and herbs: Modified Baihu Decoction and Guizhi Decoction.

Shengshigao (Raw Gypsum) 30 g (decocted first), Zhimu (Common Anemarrhena Rhizome) 12 g, Guizhi (Cassia Twig) 9 g, Chishao (Red Peony Root) 15 g, Shengdi (Dried Rehmannia Root) 15 g, Sangzhi (Mulberry Twig) 20 g, Qinjiao (Largeleaf Gentian Root) 9 g and Rendongteng (Honeysuckle Stem) 20 g.

Modification: If there is a sore throat, Jinyinhua (Honeysuckle Flower) 15 g and Lianqiao (Weeping Forsythia Capsule) 15 g can be added to dispel heat and remove toxins; for marked subcutaneous erythema circinatum due to heat in the blood, Danpi (Cortex Moutan) 12 g can be added to dispel heat and cool blood; for transformation of toxic heat into fire with ardent fever and acute pain, Shuiniujiao (Buffalo Horn) 30 g (decocted first), Lingyangjiaofen (Antelope Horn Powder) 0.6 g (infused in water), Zhiruxiang (Prepared Boswellin) 6 g and Zhimuoyao (Prepared Myrrh) 6 g can be added to dispel heat and cool blood, as well as dredge the collaterals and relieve pain.

## 2. Wind-cold bi-syndrome

Treatment principle: Dispersing wind and dissipating cold, unblocking the collaterals and relieving pain.

Prescription and herbs: Supplementary Dawudou Decoction.

Zhichuanwu (Prepared Common Monkshood Mother Root) 9 g (decocted first), Mahuang (Ephedra) 9 g, Guizhi (Cassia Twig) 9 g, Gancao (Liquorice Root) 3 g, Baishao (White Peony Alba) 12 g, Weilingxian (Chinese Clematis Root) 12 g, Duhuo (Doubleteeth Pubesscent Angelica Root) 9 g and Fengmi (Honey) 12 g (infused in water).

Modification: If there is intolerance of cold and lack of warmth in the limbs, Danggui (Chinese Angelica) 9 g and Xixin (Manchurian Wildginger) 3 g are used to activate blood and dredge the meridians; for subcutaneous nodules, Taoren (Peach Seed) 9 g and Baijiezi (White Mustard Seed) 6 g can be added to warm, unblock and activate blood and dissipate nodules; if accompanied by swollen joints, Fangji (Fourstamen Stephania Root) 12 g and Yiyiren (Coix Seed) 30 g are employed to expel wind-dampness.

## 3. Wind-dampness bi-syndrome

Treatment principle: Dispelling wind and eliminating dampness, dredging the collaterals and removing obstruction.

Prescription and herbs: Modified Zhuobi Decoction.

Qianghuo (Incised Notoptetygium Rhizome or Root) 9 g, Duhuo (Doubleteeth Pubesscent Angelica Root) 9 g, Guizhi (Cassia Twig) 9 g, Qinjiao (Largeleaf Gentian Root) 9 g, Weilingxian (Chinese Clematis Root) 12 g, Sangzhi (Mulberry Twig) 20 g, Danggui (Chinese Angelica) 9 g, Zhiruxiang (Prepared Boswellin) 6 g and, Zhimuoyao (Prepared Myrrh) 6 g.

Modification: If there is cold pain in the joints with pathogenic cold, Mahuang (Ephedra) 9 g and Zhichuanwu (Prepared Common Monkshood Mother Root) 9 g (decocted first) can be added to warm and dredge the meridians; for hot pain in the joints with dull fever due to transformation of dampness into heat, Huangbai (Amur Cork-tree) 10 g, Cangzhu (Atractylodes Rhizome) 10 g, Yiyiren (Coix Seed) 30 g and Fangji (Fourstamen Stephania Root) 12 g can be added to dispel heat and resolve dampness.

## 4. Obstruction of heart vessels by pathogenic factors

Treatment principle: Replenishing qi and nourishing yin, expelling pathogenic factors and unblocking vessels.

Prescription and herbs: Supplementary Shengmai Potion.

Taizishen (Heterophylly Falsesatarwort Root) 15 g, Maidong (Dwarf Lilyturf Tuber) 15 g, Wuweizi (Chinese Magnolivine Fruit) 6 g, Danshen (Radix Salviae Miltiorrhiae) 15 g, Danggui (Chinese Angelica) 10 g, Chishao (Red Peony Root) 15 g, Fangji (Fourstamen Stephania Root) 10 g, Mugua (Papaya) 10 g, Qinjiao (Largeleaf Gentian Root) 10 g and Haitongpi (Erythrinae) 10 g.

Modification: If there is a sore throat, Jinyinhua (Honeysuckle Flower) 12 g and Lianqiao (Weeping Forsythia Capsule) 12 g can be added to dispel heat and remove toxins; for shortness of breath and spontaneous perspiration, Huangqi (Milkvetch Root) 30 g and Fuxiaomai (Blighted Wheat) 15 g can be added to nourish qi and reduce sweating; for palpitations and insomnia, Suanzaoren (Spine Date Seed) 12 g, Baiziren (Chinese Arborvitae Kernel) 12 g and Longgu (Os Draconis) 30 g (decocted first) can be added to nourish the heart and tranquilize the spirit.

## Chinese Patent Medicine

1. Xiaohuoluo Pill: 3 g for each dose, twice a day.
2. Xitong Pill: 5 g for each dose, 3 times a day.

## Simple and Handy Prescriptions

1. Laoguancao (Common Herons Bill Herb) 30 g and Xixiancao (Herba Siegesbeckiae) 30 g are boiled in water and administered once a day to treat rheumatism with obstruction of wind, cold and dampness.
2. Luxiangcao (Pyrolae) 30 g and Yiyiren (Coix Seed) 30 g are boiled in water and administered once a day to treat rheumatism in the chronic stage with weak constitution and painful joints.

## Other Therapies

External therapy: Dahuang (Rhubarb) 15 g and Shengnanxing (Raw Rhizoma Arisaematis) 15 g are ground up into fine powders, blended with vinegar and applied to the reddened, feverish and painful joints present during the acute stage.

Dietary therapy: Huangqi (Milkvetch Root) 15 g, Taizishen (Heterophylly Falsesatarwort Root) 10 g, Maidong (Dwarf Lilyturf Tuber) 15 g, Yiyiren (Coix Seed) 30 g and Hongzao (Red Date) 15 g are boiled together with a pig's heart and light seasonings for taste. Both the soup and the pig's heart can be consumed to treat repeated rheumatic fever involving the heart which is due to weakness of the body.

## Cautions and Advice

1. Rheumatic fever is marked by repeated episodes and tends to involve the heart and lead to rheumatic valvular disease. For this reason, prompt treatment is advisable.
2. Patients should take precautions against contracting wind-cold and avoid long-term residence in damp and cold places.

3. They should also engage in active physical exercise and modify their diets so as to strengthen their constitutions and improve their immune systems.

## Daily Exercises

1. List the pathological changes of rheumatic fever.
2. Recall the diagnostic key points of rheumatic fever.
3. Explain how rheumatic fever due to wind-heat bi-syndrome, wind-cold bi-syndrome and wind-dampness bi-syndrome can be differentiated and treated.

# Rheumatoid Arthritis
# Week 13: Tuesday

Rheumatoid arthritis (RA) is an autoimmune disease that causes chronic inflammation of the joints and the adjacent tissues, clinically marked by stiffness of the joints in the morning, symmetrical swelling and pain of multiple joints, impaired range of their movements or even deformity and loss of function. RA can be present in any age group and in male patients the disease progresses with age. The occurrence is three times more common in women than in men. Cold, dampness, fatigue, malnutrition, trauma and emotional disorder may all contribute to this disease. It is chronic and repetitive in nature, often bringing about disorders of the lungs, heart and nervous system as well as destruction and dysfunction of the joints. In TCM, RA is considered to be closely associated with "bi-syndrome", "joint-wind" and "crane's knee wind".

## Etiology and Pathology

TCM holds that this disease is caused by either endogenous or exogenous factors. The former refers to innate deficiency or lack of postnatal nourishment, while the latter refers to the invasion of pathogenic wind, cold, dampness and heat, which obstruct the meridians and impede the flow of qi and blood, consequently leading to this disease.

The pathological changes are discussed as follows: Pathogenic wind, cold and dampness invade the body while it is weak, affecting the meridians and joints primarily, inhibiting the flow of qi and blood and presenting as bi-syndrome of wind, cold and dampness. The combined invasion of wind, heat and dampness may also create a predisposition to this disease. If the patient usually has hyperactivity of yang or deficiency of yin with production of heat, the disease may demonstrate heat manifestations once there are exogenous pathogenic invasion. In addition, the prolonged retention of wind, cold and dampness in meridians and joints may produce heat and eventually result in heat-type arthritis. Prolonged affliction by this disease will cause retention of phlegm and blood stasis, gradual consumption of qi, blood and essence, deficiency of the liver and kidneys, malnutrition of the muscles, joints and meridians and lingering of wind, cold and dampness, characterized by swelling, pain, stiffness and even deformity and dysfunction of the joints.

## Diagnostic Key Points

1. Stiffness of the joints in the morning lasting more than an hour, with symmetrical swelling of multiple joints, especially the carpal and meta-carpophalangeal joints.
2. Rheumatoid factor (RF) test: positive; X-ray findings: Osteoporosis, or destruction of bones, subcutaneous nodule over the bony prominences or extensor surface of the joints and narrowed joint space.

## Syndrome Differentiation

### 1. Bi-syndrome due to wind, cold and dampness

Symptoms: Severe cold pain in the joints with swelling; pale tongue with white coating and taut and tense pulse.

Analysis of symptoms: A retention of wind, cold and dampness in the meridians leads to impeded flow of qi and blood, so there iscold pain in the joints; cold is congealing by nature, so exuberance of cold is mani-fested as stagnation of qi and blood in the meridians and severe pain; dampness is sticky by nature, so retention of wind, cold and dampness in the joints is responsible for persistent swelling; the pale tongue with white coating and taut and tense pulse are all manifestations of predominant wind, cold and dampness.

### 2. Bi-syndrome due to wind, dampness and heat

Symptoms: Red, swollen and painful joints with inability to extend and alleviation by cold; fever and aversion to wind may also be present; red tongue with yellow coating and taut, rapid and slippery pulse.

Analysis of symptoms: Retention of wind, dampness and heat in meridians and joints brings about stagnation of qi and blood, so the joints are red, swollen, painful and even impalpable; the pathogenic factors invade the muscles and skin, marked by fever and aversion to wind; the red tongue with yellow coating and taut, rapid and slippery pulse are all manifestations of predominant wind, heat and dampness.

### 3. Deficiency of the liver and kidneys with phlegm and stasis obstructing the collaterals

Symptoms: Prolonged swelling and pain in the joints with stiffness, deformity and restricted movements, as well as subcutaneous nodules, emaciation, listlessness, lusterless complexion, sore and painful waist and knees, dizziness and blurred vision; slightly dark tongue with thin coating and thin or thin-unsmooth pulse.

Analysis of symptoms: Prolonged affliction weakens healthy qi, retains blood stasis and phlegm in the collaterals or vessels and impedes circulation of qi and blood, marked by long-term swelling and pain in the joints with stiffness, deformity and inhibited movements; internal accumulation of phlegm and stasis is manifested as subcutaneous nodules; obstruction of vessels with deficiency of qi, blood and essence is responsible for emaciation, listlessness and lusterless complexion; deficiency of the liver and kidneys is marked by soreness in the lumbar vertebrae, dizziness and blurred vision; the slightly dark tongue with thin coating and thin or thin-unsmooth pulse are attributable to deficiency of the liver and kidneys with phlegm and stasis obstructing the collaterals.

### Differential Treatment

### 1. Bi-syndrome due to wind, cold and dampness

Treatment principle: Expelling wind and dissipating cold, removing dampness and dredging the collaterals.

Prescription and herbs: Modified Zhuobi Decoction.

Qianghuo (Incised Notoptetygium Rhizome or Root) 9 g, Duhuo (Doubleteeth Pubesscent Angelica Root) 9 g, Guizhi (Cassia Twig) 9 g, Qinjiao (Largeleaf Gentian Root) 9 g, Weilingxian (Chinese Clematis Root) 15 g, Danggui (Chinese Angelica) 9 g, Chuanxiong (Szechwan Lovage Rhizome) 9 g, Zhiruxiang (Prepared Boswellin) 9 g and Zhimuoyao (Prepared Myrrh) 9 g.

Modification: For predominance of wind with migrating pain of the joints, Fangfeng (Divaricate Saposhnikovia Root) 9 g and Baizhi (Dahurian Angelica Root) 9 g are added to control wind; for predominance of cold with severe pain in the joints, Fuzi (Prepared Common Monkshood Daughter) 9 g, Zhichuanwu (Prepared Common Monkshood Mother Root) 9 g and Xixin (Manchurian Wildginger) 3 g are added to unblock obstruction, dissipate cold and alleviate pain; for predominance of damp-ness with swelling and pain in the joints, Fangji (Fourstamen Stephania Root) 12 g, Bixie (Rhizoma Dioscoreae Hypoglaucae) 12 g and Yiyiren (Coix Seed) 30 g are used to expel pathogenic wind-dampness.

## 2. Bi-syndrome due to wind, dampness and heat

Treatment principle: Expelling wind and removing dampness, dispelling heat and dredging the collaterals.

Prescription and herbs: Modified Guizhi Shaoyao Zhimu Decoction.

Guizhi (Cassia Twig) 6 g, Baishao (White Peony Alba) 15 g, Zhimu (Common Anemarrhena Rhizome) 10 g, Fangfeng (Divaricate Saposhnikovia Root) 9 g, Fangji (Fourstamen Stephania Root) 12 g, Haitongpi (Erythrinae) 12 g, Sangzhi (Mulberry Twig) 20 g and Rendongteng (Honeysuckle Stem) 20 g.

Modification: If there are red, swollen and painful joints with aggravation at night, Shengdi (Dried Rehmannia Root) 15 g, Chishao (Red Peony Root) 15 g and Lingyangjiaofen (Antelope Horn Powder) 0.6 g (infused in water) can be added to dispel heat and cool blood, as well as calm the mind and alleviate pain; if there is abundant heat with fluid consumption marked by feverish dysphoria, thirst, red tongue with scanty fluid and rapid and taut pulse, Shengshigao (Gypsum) 30 g (decocted first) and Xuanshen (Figwort Root) 10 g can be added to dispel heat and promote fluid production.

## 3. Deficiency of the liver and kidneys with phlegm and stasis obstructing the collaterals

Treatment principle: Nourishing the liver and kidneys, expelling pathogenic factors and dredging the collaterals.

Prescription and herbs: Modified Duhuo Jisheng Decoction.

Dangshen (Radix Codonopsis) 15 g Fuling (Indian Bread) 12 g Danggui (Chinese Angelica) 10 g Chuanxiong (Szechwan Lovage Rhizome) 10 g Baishao (White Peony Alba) 12 g Shudi (Prepared Rhizome of Rehmannia) 12 g Sangjisheng (Chinese Taxillus Herb) 12 g Duzhong (Eucommia Bark) 10 g Niuxi (Twotoothed Achyranthes Root) 10 g Duhuo (Doubleteeth Pubesscent Angelica Root) 9 g Qinjiao (Largeleaf Gentian Root) 12 g Xixin (Manchurian Wildginger) 3 g Fangfeng (Divaricate Saposhnikovia Root) 9 g and Rougui (Cassia Bark) 3 g (decocted later).

Modification: For deficiency of yin with heat that is marked by dry mouth and constipation, Xixin (Manchurian Wildginger) and Rougui (Cassia Bark) can be replaced with Shengdi (Dried Rehmannia Root) 15 g, Xuanshen (Figwort Root) 9 g and Zhimu (Common Anemarrhena Rhizome) 12 g so as to dispel heat and nourish yin; for spasms of limbs with dragging pain, Dilong (Angle Worm) 12 g and Quanxie (Scorpion) 5 g are used to search out wind, relieve convulsions, dredge the collaterals and alleviate pain; for subcutaneous nodules, Chuanshanjia (Pangolin Scale) 9 g and Baijiezi (White Mustard Seed) 6 g can be added to resolve stasis and dissipate stagnation.

## Chinese Patent Medicine

1. Wangbi Infusion Powder: 1 bag for each dose, twice a day.
2. Kunmingshan Haitang Tablet: 1~2 tablets (0.25 g/tablet) for each dose 2~3 times per day.

## Simple and Handy Prescriptions

Guizhi (Cassia Twig) 10 g, Zhichuanwu (Prepared Common Monkshood Mother Root) 10 g (decocted first), Danggui (Chinese Angelica) 10 g,

Wushaoshe (Black-tail Snake) 10 g, Yinyanghuo (Epimedium Herb) 15 g, Shudi (Prepared Rhizome of Rehmannia) 15 g, Luxiangcao (Pyrolae) 30 g and Gancao (Liquorice Root) 5 g are boiled in water and administered once a day. It is used to treat chronic rheumatoid arthritis with retention of wind, cold and dampness.

## Other Therapies

Wasp-stinging therapy: To sting the affected area with a wasp every day for 7 days which constitutes a complete course of treatment.

Medicated wind therapy: Huangqi (Milkvetch Root) 10 g, Danggui (Chinese Angelica) 10 g, Honghua (Safflower) 10 g, Weilingxian (Chinese Clematis Root) 10 g, Shengdi (Dried Rehmannia Root) 10 g and Qishe (Long-noded Pit Viper) 10 g are immersed in 500 ml of distillated spirist for a month. It is administered (5 ml for each dose), twice a day.

## Cautions and Advice

1. Rheumatoid arthritis is a refractory disease, but if it is actively treated and controlled, the deformity or disability may be prevented.
2. Patients should avoid long-term residence in humid and cold environments.
3. They should also maintain a positive attitude towards life, pay attention to nutrition and strengthen their constitutions.

## Daily Exercises

1. Concisely describe the pathological changes of rheumatoid arthritis.
2. Recall the diagnostic key points of rheumatoid arthritis.
3. Explain how rheumatoid arthritis due to wind, cold and dampness can be diagnosed and treated.
4. Describe how Duhuo Jisheng Decoction can be applied to treat this disease.

# Systemic Lupus Erythematosus
# Week 13: Wednesday

Systemic lupus erythematosus (SLE) is an autoimmune connective tissue disease which affects many organs of the body; it is clinically marked by fever in varying degrees, edematous erythema on the exposed skin, joint pain and mouth or pharyngeal sores. If it involves the heart, there may be pericarditis, myocarditis, endocarditis, or even cardiac failure; the kidneys, nephritis, nephrotic syndrome and renal inadequacy; respiratory system, pleurisy, interstitial pneumonia; digestive system, hepatitis, gastric and intestinal ulcers or bleeding; nervous system, epilepsy, meningitis and cerebrovascular accident. SLE occurs primarily in young females. The acute type is characterized by a sudden onset, a poor prognosis and severe toxic symptoms, as well as damage to or dysfunction of many organs. The chronic type is marked by discoid lesions restricted to the skin (and rarely the internal organs), a slow progress and a relatively favorable prognosis. In TCM, it is closely associated with "yin-yang toxication", "butterfly rash", "horse-tassel erysipelas", "palpitations", "fever due to internal damage", "bi-syndrome", "edema" and "deficiency consumption".

## Etiology and Pathology

TCM believes that SLE is caused by either endogenous or exogenous factors. The former refers to innate deficiency of the body, while the latter to excessive lifestyles, exposure to strong sunlight, contraction of toxins, impairment by the seven emotions, overstrain and excessive sexual life, which lead to imbalance of yin, yang, qi and blood and endogenous production of toxins, heat and blood stasis.

The pathological changes are discussed as follows: Exuberant heat and toxins scorch the ying-blood and damage the vessels, this is marked by fever, mouth or pharyngeal ulcers, skin erythema and bloody vomitus, urine or stools; heat scorches the yin phase, leading to deficiency of yin, retention of blood and damage to the vessels, which incurs invasion of exogenous pathogenic factors, giving rise to joint pain due to obstruction of the collaterals; deficiency of yin with consumption of qi and obstruction of the heart by toxins is responsible for palpitations, shortness of breath, chest distress or pain and purplish lips; deficiency of yin also brings about blood stasis, resulting in low-grade fever and dark-red patches on the skin; deficiency of kidney yin is responsible for dizziness and hair loss; deficiency of yin can also affect the spleen yang and kidney yang, with such signs as edema in the lower limbs and soreness in the lumbar vertebrae. Furthermore, internal impairment by emotional disorders, stagnation of liver qi, unsmooth flow of blood and internal accumulation of toxins can create a predisposition to pain in the hypochondria and nodules below the costal region.

## Diagnostic Key Points

1. Butterfly or discoid red patches on the exposed skin which is sensitive to light, mouth ulcers and arthritis without deformity.
2. Proteinuria, cylindruria or bloody urine, low white blood cell or platelet count, or hemolytic anemia, accelerated blood sedimentation, positive antinuclear antibody; anti-DS DNA antibody (+), or LE (lupus) cell (+); skin (unaffected area) lupus band test (+) or renal biopsy (+).

## Syndrome Differentiation

## 1. Exuberance of heat and toxins

Symptoms: High fever, facial erythema or purpura, blood blister, or hematemesis, hemorrhinia, bloody urine, hemafecia, articular or muscular soreness, restlessness, thirst, or coma and delirium; red or purplish tongue with thin and yellow coating and slippery and rapid pulse. This syndrome is an acute type that is rare.

Analysis of symptoms: Abundance of heat and toxins is manifested as high fever; intense heat in the interior scorches the ying-blood, leading to facial erythema; blazing heat also causes blood stasis which is marked by suggillation; stagnated toxins areresponsible for blood blisters; heat damages the blood vessels, bringing about hematemesis, hemorrhinia, bloody urine and hemafecia; blood stasis debilitates the vessels, causing obstruction of the meridians by wind, dampness and heat which is marked by articular or muscular soreness; abundant heat consumes body fluid, giving rise to restlessness and thirst; heat enters the heart ying, resulting in coma and delirium; the red tongue with thin and yellow coating and slippery and rapid pulse are all manifestations of intense toxic heat in the blood and the purplish tongue is a sign of blood stasis due to heat.

## 2. Deficiency of yin with blood stasis

Symptoms: Low-grade hectic fever or feverish dysphoria, skin purpura, muscular soreness, vague pain in the joints, or migrating pain in the joints with redness, swelling and sensation of warmth; dark-red tongue with thin and yellow coating and thin and rapid pulse. These symptoms are characteristic of the subacute or chronic type of SLE.

Analysis of symptoms: Heat consumes yin and results in blood stasis, giving rise to low-grade hectic fever or skin suggillation; the collaterals are deficient, so there is vague pain in the joints; pathogenic wind, dampness and heat invade the collaterals from the exterior and then obstruct the circulation of qi and blood, causing muscular soreness and migrating pain in the joints with redness, swelling and sensation of warmth; the dark-red tongue with thin and yellow coating and thin and rapid pulse are all manifestations of blood stasis due to deficiency of yin and collateral obstruction caused by invasion of pathogens.

## 3. Deficiency of qi and yin

Symptoms: Palpitations, shortness of breath, chest distress or pain, dark skin with suggillation, cyanosed lips, spontaneous perspiration, insomnia, coma or mania; dark purple tongue with yellow coating, thin and rapid or knotted and intermittent pulse. These symptoms occur in cases with damage to the heart and lungs or to the central nervous system.

Analysis of symptoms: Prolonged retention of toxins leads to deficiency of qi and yin as well as malnourishment of the heart which is marked by spontaneous perspiration and insomnia; pathogenic toxins obstructing the heart manifest as palpitations, shortness of breath and chest distress or pain; blood stasis in the vessels is responsible for dark skin with suggillation and cyanosed lips; pathogenic toxins attacking the heart result in coma or mania; the dark purple tongue with yellow coating and the thin and rapid or knotted and intermittent pulse are attributable to deficiency of qi and yin with pathogenic toxins obstructing the heart.

## 4. Stagnation of liver qi with blood stasis

Symptoms: Hypochondriac pain, chest distress, gastric stuffiness, or masses below the costal region, dark skin, subcutaneous ecchymosis and menstrual disorder; purplish tongue with possible ecchymosis, thin and yellow tongue coating and thin and taut or unsmooth pulse. These symptoms occur when there is functional lesion of the liver or enlargement of the liver and spleen.

Analysis of symptoms: Stagnation of liver qi with blood stasis is manifested as hypochondriac pain, chest distress, gastric stuffiness, or masses below the costal region, dark skin and subcutaneous ecchymosis; internal accumulation of stagnated stasis results in masses forming below the costal region; liver blood is essential to women, so stagnation of liver qi with blood stasis can result in dysfunction of the thoroughfare vessel and conception vessel, marked by menstrual disorders; the purplish tongue with possible ecchymosis, thin and yellow coating and thin and taut or unsmooth pulse are due to stagnation of liver qi with blood stasis and accumulation of toxins in the interior.

## 5. Deficiency of yin and yang

Symptoms: Slightly dark erythema, waist soreness, dizziness, dark eyes, calvities, pale complexion, poor appetite, abdominal distension or loose stools, listlessness, edema, intolerance of cold and cold limbs; dark and enlarged tongue with thin coating and thin and feeble pulse. This syndrome is characteristic of lupus nephritis.

Analysis of symptoms: Retention of pathogenic factors leads to deficiency of healthy qi, insufficiency of yin blood of the liver and kidneys and malnutrition of the viscera and meridians, characterized by waist soreness, dizziness, dark eyes, calvities and pale complexion; deficiency of yin involving yang, as well as deficiency and unsmooth flow of blood, is responsible for the slightly dark erythema; deficiency of spleen yang and kidney yang is marked by poor appetite, abdominal distension or loose stools, listlessness, edema and intolerance of cold with cold limbs; the dark and enlarged tongue with thin coating and thin and feeble pulse are due to deficiency of yin and yang.

## Differential Treatment

### 1. Exuberance of heat and toxins

Treatment principle: Dispelling heat and removing toxins, cooling blood and resolving stasis.

Prescription and herbs: Modified Qingwen Baidu Powder.

Shengshigao (Raw Gypsum) 30 g (decocted earlier), Shuiniujiao (Buffalo Horn) 30 g (decocted earlier), Zhimu (Common Anemarrhena Rhizome) 12 g, Huanglian (Golden Thread) 5 g, Huangqin (Baical Skullcap Root) 15 g, Zhizi (Cape Jasmine Fruit) 12 g, Lianqiao (Weeping Forsythia Capsule) 12 g, Shengdi (Dried Rehmannia Root) 15 g, Danpi (Cortex Moutan) 15 g, Chishao (Red Peony Root) 15 g, Rendongteng (Honeysuckle Stem) 30 g and Qinjiao (Largeleaf Gentian Root) 12 g.

Modification: For persistent fever with coma and delirium, Lingyangjiaofen (Antelope Horn Powder) 0.6 g (infused in water) can be used to dispel heat and tranquilize the mind; for ecchymosis with severe bleeding, Oujie (Lotus Rhizome Node) 15 g, Baimaogen (Lalang Grass Rhizome) 30 g and Zicao (Arnebia Root) 15 g can be added to reinforce the action of cooling blood and stopping bleeding; for dry stools, Dahuang (Rhubarb) 9 g (decocted later) can be used to purge heat and dredge the intestine.

### 2. Deficiency of yin with blood stasis

Treatment principle: Nourishing yin and resolving stasis, expelling pathogenic factors and dredging the collaterals.

Prescription and herbs: Modified Dabuyin Pill, Siwu Decoction and Xuanbi Decoction.

Shengdi (Dried Rehmannia Root) 15 g, Guiban (Tortoise Shell) 15 g, Huangbai (Amur Cork-tree) 10 g, Zhimu (Common Anemarrhena Rhizome) 10 g, Danggui (Chinese Angelica) 10 g, Chishao (Red Peony Root) 15 g, Guizhi (Cassia Twig) 9 g, Fangji (Fourstamen Stephania Root) 12 g, Yiyiren (Coix Seed) 30 g, Lianqiao (Weeping Forsythia Capsule) 15 g, Chansha (Excrementum Bombycis) 12 g (wrapped) and Rendongteng (Honeysuckle Stem) 30 g.

·Modification: For incessant low-grade fever, Yinchaihu (Starwort Root) 15 g, Qinghao (Sweet Wormwood Herb) 15 g and Digupi (Chinese Wolfberry Root-Bark) 15 g can be added to dispel deficient heat; for severe joint pain, Sangzhi (Mulberry Twig) 20 g, Qinjiao (Largeleaf Gentian Root) 12 g, Jixueteng (Henry Magnoliavine Stem or Root) 15 g and Baihuashen (Agkistrodon)10 g or Quanxie (Scorpion) 6 g and Wugong (Centipede) 2 are added to reinforce the action of expelling pathogenic factors, dredging the collaterals and alleviating pain.

## 3. Deficiency of qi and yin

Treatment principle: Replenishing qi and nourishing yin, clearing the heart and removing toxins, activating blood and unblocking vessels.

Prescription and herbs: Modified Zhigancao Decoction and Qinggong Decoction.

Zhigancao (Liquorice Root) 9 g, Renshen (Ginseng) 9 g, Guizhi (Cassia Twig) 9 g, Shengdi (Dried Rehmannia Root) 15 g, Xuanshen (Figwort Root) 12 g, Maidong (Dwarf Lilyturf Tuber) 15 g, Lianzixin (Lotus Plumule) 6 g, Lianqiao (Weeping Forsythia Capsule) 13 g, Baihuashecao (Hedyotic Diffusa) 30 g, Danshen (Radix Salviae Miltiorrhiae) 15 g, Honghua (Safflower) 9 g and Yanhusuo (Corydalis) 12 g.

Modification: If there is deficiency of qi and spontaneous perspiration, Huangqi (Milkvetch Root) 30 g and Wuweizi (Chinese Magnolivine Fruit) 6 g can be added to nourish qi and reduce sweating; for vexation and insomnia, Suanzaoren (Spine Date Seed) 10 g and Baiziren (Chinese Arborvitae Kernel) 10 g are used to nourish the heart and calm the spirit; for coma or mania, Cishi (Magnetite) 30 g and Longgu (Os Draconis) 30 g (decocted first) can be added to tranquilize the mind and calm the spirit.

## 4. Stagnation of liver qi with blood stasis

Treatment principle: Soothing the liver qi, resolving stasis and removing toxins.

Prescription and herbs: Modified Xuefu Zhuyu Decoction Simiao Yongan Decoction.

Chaihu (Chinese Thorowax Root) 9 g, Danggui (Chinese Angelica) 9 g, Chishao (Red Peony Root) 15 g, Shengdi (Dried Rehmannia Root) 15 g, Zhiqiao (Orange Fruit) 15 g, Xuanshen (Figwort Root) 15 g, Jinyinhua (Honeysuckle Flower) 15 g, Baihuashecao (Hedyotic Diffusa) 30 g, Sanleng (Common Burreed Tuber) 12 g, Ezhu (Zedoray Rhizome) 12 g, Chuanlianzi (Szechwan Chinaberry Fruit) 12 g and Gancao (Liquorice Root) 3 g.

Modification: For apparent enlargement of the liver and spleen, Guiban (Tortoise Shell) 15 g and Biejia (Turtle Shell) 15 g can be used to soften and dissolve masses; for a weakened spleen due to hyperactive liver qi or fire, coupled with poor appetite, abdominal distension or loose stools, Dangshen (Radix Codonopsis) 15 g, Baizhu (Largehead Atractylodes Rhizome) 15 g, Shanyao (Common Yan Rhizome) 15 g and Chenpi (Dried Tangerine Peel) 9 g can be used to nourish the spleen and regulate qi.

## 5. Deficiency of yin and yang

Treatment principle: Nourishing yin and invigorating yang, rejuvenating the kidneys and removing toxins.

Prescription and herbs: Modified Zuogui Pill and Erxian Decoction.

Shudi (Prepared Rhizome of Rehmannia) 15 g, Shanyao (Common Yan Rhizome) 15 g, Shanzhuyu (Asiatic Cornelian Cherry Fruit) 9 g, Gouqizi (Barbary Wolfberry Fruit) 12 g, Tusizi (Dodder Seed) 15 g, Xianmao (Common Curculigo Rhizome) 12 g, Yinyanghuo (Epimedium Herb) 12 g, Danggui (Chinese Angelica) 9 g, Danpi (Cortex Moutan) 12 g, Luxiangcao (Pyrolae) 20 g, Liuyuexue (Junesnow) 30 g and Baihuashecao (Hedyotic Diffusa) 30 g.

Modification: For waist soreness, Duzhong (Eucommia Bark) 12 g and Bajitian (Mornda Root) 12 g can be used to nourish the kidneys and strengthen the waist; for swelling of the feet and proteinuria, Huangqi (Milkvetch Root) 30 g, Baizhu (Largehead Atractylodes Rhizome) 15 g, Buguzhi (Malaytea Scurfpea Fruit) 15 g and Fuling (Indian Bread) 30 g can be used to invigorate the spleen and nourish the kidneys, as well as promote urination to relieve edema; for calvities, Shouwu (Fleeceflower Root) 15 g and Baishao (White Peony Alba) 15 g can be added to nourish blood and regrow hair; for intolerance of cold with cold limbs, Fupian (Radix Aconitilateralis Preparata) 12 g and Rougui (Cassia Bark) 3 g (infused in water) can be used to warm yang and dissipate cold.

## Chinese Patent Medicine

1. Fufang Jingqiaomai Tablet: 6~8 tablets for each dose, 2~3 times per day.
2. Leigongteng Tablet: 1~2 tablets for each dose, 2~3 times per day.

## Simple and Handy Prescriptions

Santeng Syrup: Equal quantities of Leigongteng (Tripterygium Root), Hongteng (Sargentgloryvine Stem) and Jixueteng (Henry Magnoliavine Stem or Root) are made into syrup. It is administered (10~15 ml for each dose) 3 times a day for 2 months and can be used to treat different types of SLE.

## Other Therapies

External therapy: Qiancao (Indian Madder Root) 30 g and Dahuang (Rhubarb) 30 g are decocted into liquid and applied to the skin erythema several times a day.

Dietary therapy: 150 g of fresh Indian kalimeris herb are boiled in water and then cut into morsels, which are mixed with 150 g of fragrant beancurd. Seasonings may be added before consumption.

## Cautions and Advice

1. This disease can be controlled by long-term proper use of glucocorticoids and TCM.

2. Patients should avoid strong sunlight, overstrain and emotional stimulation; they should also keep a regular lifestyle and engage in physical exercise to improve their constitutions.
3. It is advisable for patients to avoid spicy food, cigarettes and alcohol.
4. Any infection should be treated promptly but without the use of drugs which may induce or aggravate the disease.

## Daily Exercises

1. List the etiological factors of systemic lupus erythematosus.
2. Recall the diagnostic key points of systemic lupus erythematosus.
3. Explain how the five syndromes of systemic lupus erythematosus can be differentiated and treated.

# Dermatomyositis

# Week 13: Thursday

Dermatomyositis refers to an autoimmune connective tissue disease primarily affecting the skin, muscles and vessels. Clinically, it is marked by slightly lilac-colored edematous erythema on the skin (the face, neck and the region around the eyes), myosalgia and myasthenia. It may also involve other organs of the body. Those with only muscular lesions rather than dermal damages are called polymyositis. Dermatomyositis mainly afflicts people between the ages of 40 and 60, with the ratio of males to females being 1:2. Most of the cases are chronic and progressive ones with favorable prognosis and can be treated within 2~3 years, while a few cases are acute ones and often accompanied by infection (which may lead to death) or tumor (which also points to an unfavorable prognosis). In TCM, this disease is closely associated with "muscular bi-syndrome", "flaccidity syndrome" and "deficiency consumption".

## Etiology and Pathology

TCM believes that this disease can be caused by either endogenous or exogenous factors. The former refers to innate deficiency of the body, while the latter to invasion of pathogenic factors or immersion of damp-heat, resulting in simultaneous impairment of the spleen and kidneys.

The pathological changes are discussed as follows: The deficient qi fails to resist the invasion of pathogenic factors, which accumulate in the skin and muscles. In addition, immersion of damp-heat in the skin and muscles leads to stagnation of qi and blood, marked by lilac-colored swollen patches on the skin and muscular pain; intense heat in the interior impairs the lung fluid. Damp-heat encumbers the spleen, bringing about deficiency of the spleen and stomach. Deficiency of liver yin and kidney yin is responsible for dysfunction of the tendons and muscles, characterized by flaccidity of the hands and feet.

## Diagnostic Key Points

1. Clinical manifestations are primarily typical skin lesions, such as edematous lilac erythema on the eyelid and its adjacent region, scaly

erythema on the extensor aspect of the fingers, or erythema on the limbs or trunk. Besides, there are also myasthenia, myosalgia and myogelosis, or slow movement and marked atrophy of the proximal end of the limbs.

2. Laboratory examination indicates elevation of serum creatine phosphokinase, aldolase, lactic acid dehydrogenase and lanine transaminase. Electromyogram and muscular biopsy show the presence of myositis.

## Syndrome Differentiation

### 1. Lung heat impairing fluids

Symptoms: Sudden onset, mostly with fever, erythema on the skin, dry throat with cough, vexation, thirst, lassitude, yellowish or reddish urine and dry stools; red tongue with thin and yellow coating, thin and rapid pulse.

Analysis of symptoms: Virulent warmth and heat invade the lungs and accumulate in the skin, this is marked by acute fever and erythema on the skin; heat in the lungs consumes body fluid and prevents it from moistening the whole body, giving rise to dry throat with cough, vexation, thirst, lassitude, yellowish or reddish urine and dry stools; abundant heat consumes body fluid and exhausts qi, resulting in lassitude; the red tongue with thin and yellow coating and thin and rapid pulse are manifestations of impaired fluid due to exuberance of heat.

### 2. Immersion of damp-heat

Symptoms: Edematous lilac erythema on the skin, muscular soreness, heavy sensation and flaccidity in the limbs; fever, chest and epigastric fullness and distress, poor appetite and loose stools may also be present; red tongue with yellow and greasy coating and slippery and rapid pulse.

Analysis of symptoms: Immersion of damp-heat in the skin and muscles with obstruction of qi and blood is responsible for red swollen patches on the skin, muscular soreness, or heavy sensation and flaccidity in the limbs; damp-heat inhibits qi movements, marked by fever, or chest and epigastric fullness and distress; damp-heat encumbers the spleen and impairs its function of transportation and transformation, leading to poor appetite and loose stools; the red tongue with yellow and greasy coating and slippery and rapid pulse are attributable to abundance of dampness and heat in the interior.

## 3. Weakness of the spleen and stomach

Symptoms: Flaccidity of the limbs aggravating gradually, poor appetite and loose stools, dull facial edema and lassitude; pale tongue with white and thin coating and thin and feeble pulse.

Analysis of symptoms: Long-term affliction of disease debilitates the spleen and stomach, which fail to produce enough cereal essence to nourish the four limbs and muscles, marked by flaccidity of the limbs aggravating gradually; dysfunction of the spleen and stomach is responsible for poor appetite and loose stools; deficiency of qi and blood with retention of dampness is characterized by dull facial edema and lassitude; the pale tongue with white and thin coating and thin and feeble pulse are due to weakness of the spleen and stomach with deficiency of qi and blood.

## 4. Yin deficiency of the liver and kidneys

Symptoms: Slow development in the late stage, vague muscular pain, flaccidity of the limbs, gradual muscular atrophy, flaccidity of limbs, soreness in the lumbar vertebrae, inability to stand for a long time; dizziness, calvities and tinnitus may also be present; red tongue with scanty coating and thin and rapid pulse.

Analysis of symptoms: The disease is marked by slow development when it enters into the late stage, so there is vague pain in the muscles; prolonged deficiency of qi and blood results in simultaneous insufficiency of the liver and kidneys, with inadequate essence and blood to nourish the tendons and bones, giving rise to flaccidity of the limbs, or even muscular atrophy; the waist is the "house of the kidneys", which controls the bones, so if the kidney essence is deficient, there will be soreness of lumbar vertebrae with inability to stand for long; the eye is the orifice of the liver, the ears are the orifices of the kidneys and the hair is "surplus of blood", so deficiency of the liver, kidneys and blood is characterized by dizziness, tinnitus and calvities; the red tongue with scanty coating and thin and rapid pulse are attributable to deficiency of liver yin and kidney yin.

## Differential Treatment

### 1. Lung heat impairing fluids

Treatment principle: Dispelling heat and moistening dryness, nourishing the lungs to produce fluid.

Prescription and herbs: Supplementary Qingzao Jiufei Decoction.

Shengshigao (Gypsum) 30 g (decocted first), Shashen (Root of Straight Ladybell) 12 g, Maidong (Dwarf Lilyturf Tuber) 12 g, Sangye (Mulberry Leaf) 9 g, Xingren (Almond) 9 g, Maren (Edestan) 9 g, Zhimu (Common Anemarrhena Rhizome) 9 g, Jinyinhua (Honeysuckle Flower) 12 g, Lianqiao (Weeping Forsythia Capsule) 12 g, Tianhuafen (Trichosanthin) 12 g, Rendongteng (Honeysuckle Stem) 20 g and Qinjiao (Largeleaf Gentian Root) 12 g.

Modification: If there are apparent lilac patches on the skin, Shengdi (Dried Rehmannia Root) 15 g and Danpi (Cortex Moutan) 12 g can be added to dispel heat, cool blood and resolve macula.

### 2. Immersion of damp-heat

Treatment principle: Dispelling heat, resolving dampness and soothing the collaterals.

Prescription and herbs: Modified Simiao Pill.

Huangbai (Amur Cork-tree) 10 g, Cangzhu (Atractylodes Rhizome) 10 g, Baizhu (Largehead Atractylodes Rhizome) 12 g, Fangji (Fourstamen Stephania Root) 12 g, Chuanmutong (Armand Clematis Stem) 6 g, Yiyiren (Coix Seed) 30 g, Chansha (Excrementum Bombycis) 12 g and Niuxi (Twotoothed Achyranthes Root) 12 g.

Modification: For chest and epigastric fullness, Huoxiang (Agastache Rugosa) 9 g, Peilan (Queen of the Meadow) 9 g and Houpu (Magnolia Bark)

9 g can be added to resolve dampness and turbidity; damp-heat impairs yin, leading to emaciation, low-grade fever, reddish tongue with scanty coating and thin and rapid pulse, in this case, Cangzhu (Atractylodes Rhizome) can be replaced with Shengdi (Dried Rehmannia Root) 15 g and Guiban (Tortoise Shell) 9 g so as to nourish yin and dispel heat; for numbness in the limbs with inhibited movement and purple or spotty tongue, Sumu (Sappan Wood) 9 g and Jixueteng (Henry Magnoliavine Stem or Root) 30 g can be added to activate blood and dredge the collaterals.

## 3. Weakness of the spleen and stomach

Treatment principle: Invigorating the spleen and supplementing qi, nourishing blood and strengthening tendons.

Prescription and herbs: Modified Shengling Baizhu Powder.

Dangshen (Radix Codonopsis) 15 g, Baizhu (Largehead Atractylodes Rhizome) 12 g, Biandou (Hyacinth Bean) 12 g, Fuling (Indian Bread) 12 g, Sharen (Villous Amomum Fruit) 3 g (decocted later), Chenpi (Dried Tangerine Peel) 6 g, Shanyao (Common Yan Rhizome) 15 g, Yiyiren (Coix Seed) 30 g, Lianzirou (Lotus Seed) 12 g, Sangjisheng (Chinese Taxillus Herb) 15 g, Bajitian (Mornda Root) 12 g and Niuxi (Twotoothed Achyranthes Root) 12 g.

Modification: For intolerance of cold with cold limbs, Fupian (Radix Aconitilateralis Preparata) 9 g and Ganjiang (Dried Ginger) 5 g can be added to warm and activate yang; for deficiency of qi and blood in the late stage, Huangqi (Milkvetch Root) 30 g, Shudi (Prepared Rhizome of Rehmannia) 15 g and Danggui (Chinese Angelica) 10 g can be added to invigorate qi and nourish blood.

## 4. Yin deficiency of the liver and kidneys

Treatment principle: Nourishing the liver and kidneys, supplemented by dispelling heat.

Prescription and herbs: Modified Huqian Pill.

Shengdi (Dried Rehmannia Root) 12 g, Shudi (Prepared Rhizome of Rehmannia) 12 g, Baishao (White Peony Alba) 15 g, Niuxi (Twotoothed Achyranthes Root) 12 g, Sangjisheng (Chinese Taxillus Herb) 15 g, Luxiangcao (Pyrolae) 30 g, Duzhong (Eucommia Bark) 12 g, Lujiaojiao (Deerhorn Glue) 9 g (melted in decoction), Guibanjiao (Tortoise Shell) 9 g (melted in decoction), Huangbai (Amur Cork-tree) 9 g and Zhimu (Common Anemarrhena Rhizome) 9 g.

Modification: For sallow and lusterless complexion and palpitations, Huangqi (Milkvetch Root) 30 g and Danggui (Chinese Angelica) 9 g can be added to invigorate qi and nourish blood; in the late stage, deficiency of yin will impair yang, marked by intolerance of cold, impotence, clear and profuse urine, pale tongue and thin and deep pulse, so Shengdi (Dried Rehmannia Root), Huangbai (Amur Cork-tree), Zhimu (Common Anemarrhena Rhizome) and Guibanjiao (Tortoise Shell Jelly) can be replaced with Yinyanghuo (Epimedium Herb) 12 g and Buguzhi (Malaytea Scurfpea Fruit) 12 g to invigorate the kidneys and warm yang.

## Chinese Patent Medicine

1. Dahuoluo Dan: 1 pill for each dose, twice a day.
2. Kunmingshan Tablet: 1 tablet (0.25 g/tablet), 3 times a day.

## Simple and Handy Prescriptions

Jinyinhua (Honeysuckle Flower) 15 g, Lianqiao (Weeping Forsythia Capsule) 15 g, Huercao (Saxifrage) 15 g, Qiancao (Indian Madder Root) 15 g, Chishao (Red Peony Root) 15 g, Zexie (Oriental Waterplantain Rhizome) 12 g, Cheqianzi (Plantain Herb) 12 g and Gancao (Liquorice Root) 10 g are boiled in water and administered once a day. It is used to treat marked lilac patches on the skin.

## Other Therapies

Dietary therapy: Zihechefen (Human Placenta Powder) and boiled pig (or cow) marrow are mixed in the ratio of 1 : 3 and then pounded. They are further mixed with rice flour and blended with refined sugar. Patients with a relatively good appetite can also take boiled fresh marrow with soyabean to treat dermatomyositis, flaccidity in the legs and muscular atrophy.

## Cautions and Advice

1. Dermatomyositis is mostly marked by chronic development and may spread to the internal organs, resulting in damage to the respiratory, digestive and cardiac systems, or complication of tumor. Clinically, the various complications should be actively treated.
2. Patients should avoid spicy food and alcohol; they should also balance work and rest in order to complement treatment.

## Daily Exercises

1. List the pathological changes of dermatomyositis.
2. Explain how dermatomyositis due to lung heat impairing fluids and dermatomyositis due to yin deficiency of the liver and kidneys can be differentiated and treated.

# Scleroderma

# Week 13: Friday

Scleroderma refers to an autoimmune disease characterized by colla-gen fibrosclerosis of the skin and various systems, with such clinical manifestations as lamellar, girdle-shaped or guttiform sclerosis on the skin of the face, neck, chest, abdomen or limbs. There are two main types: Localized scleroderma affects only the skin and muscles, while systemic scleroderma affects the internal organs, as well as the skin and muscles. Scleroderma mostly afflicts people 20~60 years of age. Localized scleroderma has a favorable prognosis, while systemic scle-roderma has a relatively poor prognosis, once it spreads to the lungs, heart and kidneys, due to the rapid deterioration. In TCM, scleroderma belongs to the category of "muscular bi-syndrome" and "skin bi-syndrome".

## Etiology and Pathology

TCM believes that scleroderma is caused by either endogenous or exog-enous factors. The former refers to innate deficiency of the body, the latter to pathogenic wind, cold and damp-heat, which obstruct the meridians and result in disorder of qi and blood.

The pathological changes are discussed as follows: Pathogenic wind, heat and toxins invade the lung-defense, causing dysfunction of the lungs in dispersion, imbalance between ying and wei, unsmooth circula-tion of qi and blood and obstruction of the collaterals, marked by mus-cular soreness of the joints and firmness of the skin. Qi is the "commander of blood", so stagnated qi hinders smooth blood flow; yang is in charge of warming and transporting, so deficiency of yang will lead to blood stasis and skin malnutrition, characterized by thick-ness and hardening of the skin. If the pathogenic factors linger for a long time, the healthy qi will be seriously damaged, with consumption of essence blood spreading from the exterior to the interior and eventu-ally to the five zang-organs.

## Diagnostic Key Points

1. In the initial stage: Agnogenic edema and symmetrical diffuse sclerosis on the dorsum of the hands and upper eyelids; in the late stage: Sclerosis of the skin, flexion contracture of the fingers. Raynaud phenomenon at the extremities of the four limbs, refractory ulcers and scar formation, multiple arthralgia and arthritis may also be present, coupled with dysphagia and dyspnea.
2. Skin biopsy of the extensor aspect of the forearm: Enlargement or fibrosis of the collagen fiber (which is also seen in the vessel wall).

## Syndrome Differentiation

### 1. Obstruction of the collaterals by toxic heat

Symptoms: Fever, cough, panting, pain and numbness in the muscles and joints, moist or dry necrosis of the toe tips; red tongue with yellow and dry or little coating, rapid pulse.

Analysis of symptoms: Pathogenic wind-heat invades the lung-defense and causes dysfunction of the lungs in dispersion, giving rise to fever, cough and panting; stagnation of pathogenic factors in the muscles and collaterals prevents smooth flow of qi and blood, leading to pain and numbness in the muscles and joints; pathogenic heat enters the ying-blood and putrefies the tissues, resulting in moist or dry necrosis of the toe tips; red tongue with yellow and dry or little coating and rapid pulse are manifestations of toxic heat entering the ying phase and damaging the body fluid.

### 2. Stagnation of qi with blood stasis

Symptoms: Dark complexion, muscular wasting, unnatural firmness of the skin and difficulty in swallowing; dark purple tongue with thin coating and thin and taut pulse.

Analysis of symptoms: Qi is in charge of blood circulation, so if qi is stagnated, there will be blood stasis in and malnutrition of, the muscles and collaterals, marked by a dark complexion, muscular emaciation and unnatural firmness of the skin; since qi is supposed to be in constant movement by nature, stagnated qi creates difficulty in swallowing; the dark purple tongue with thin coating and thin and taut pulse are due to stagnation of qi with blood stasis.

## 3. Retention of cold with blood stasis

Symptoms: Intolerance of cold, cold limbs, joint pain, tight, stiff and swollen; enlarged and slightly dark tongue with gray and slippery coating and thin and deep pulse.

Analysis of symptoms: Deficiency of yang qi incurs cold that congeals the meridians and vessels, hampering smooth blood circulation, this is marked by intolerance of cold, cold limbs, joint pain and tight, stiff and swollen muscles; the corpulent and slightly dark tongue with gray and slippery coating and thin and deep pulse are attributable to deficiency of yang, congealing of cold and stasis of blood.

## 4. Deficiency of healthy qi with lingering pathogens

Symptoms: Emaciation, lassitude, palpitations, shortness of breath, dizziness, pale complexion, muscular pain, lusterless and hardened skin akin to stiff paper and hair loss; pale tongue with thin coating and thin and feeble pulse.

Analysis of symptoms: A long-term retention of pathogenic factors leads to extreme deficiency of the healthy qi, deficiency of qi and blood and malnutrition of the five zang-organs. The heart controls blood, while the lungs govern qi, so malnutrition of the heart and lungs is manifested as pale complexion, palpitations and shortness of breath; the spleen dominates the muscles as well as the four limbs, while the kidneys store essence, produces marrow and supplements the brain, so malnutrition of the spleen and kidneys is manifested as emaciation, lassitude, palpitations, dizziness and loss of hair; long-term malnutrition of the skin and muscles by qi and blood leads to stasis, marked by muscular pain and lusterless, hardened skin; the pale tongue, thin coating and thin and feeble pulse are due to extreme deficiency of healthy qi coupled with deficiency of qi and blood.

## Differential Treatment

### 1. Obstruction of the collaterals by toxic heat ✦

Treatment principle: Dispelling heat and removing toxins, cooling ying and dredging the collaterals.

Prescription and herbs: Modified Yinqiao Powder and Qingying Decoction.

Jinyinhua (Honeysuckle Flower) 15 g, Lianqiao (Weeping Forsythia Capsule) 12 g, Jiegeng (Platycodon Root) 6 g, Niubangzi (Great Burdock Achene) 12 g, Shengdi (Dried Rehmannia Root) 15 g, Xuanshen (Figwort Root) 12 g, Chishao (Red Peony Root) 15 g, Danpi (Cortex Moutan) 12 g, Zicao (Arnebia Root) 15 g, Zihuadiding (Tokyo Violet Herb) 15 g, Rendongteng (Honeysuckle Stem) 30 g and Yiyiren (Coix Seed) 30 g.

Modification: If there is cough with yellow sputum, Beimu (Fritillariae Tuber) 9 g and Huangqin (Baical Skullcap Root) 15 g can be added to dispel heat and dissolve phlegm; for painful and stiff muscles, Guizhi (Cassia Twig) 6 g, Zhimu (Common Anemarrhena Rhizome) 9 g, Danggui (Chinese Angelica) 9 g and Luoshiteng (Chinese Starjasmine Stem) 15 g can be added to regulate ying (nutrient phase) and wei (defense phase), activate blood and dredge the collaterals.

### 2. Stagnation of qi with blood stasis

Treatment principle: Regulating qi and activating blood, resolving stasis and dredging the collaterals.

Prescription and herbs: Modified Shengtong Zhuyu Deoction.

Chuanxiong (Szechwan Lovage Rhizome) 9 g, Taoren (Peach Seed) 9 g, Honghua (Safflower) 9 g, Danggui (Chinese Angelica) 9 g, Wulingzhi (Faeces Trogopterorum) 9 g (wrapped), Xiangfu (Nutgrass Galingale Rhizome) 9 g, Niuxi (Twotoothed Achyranthes Root) 9 g, Qinjiao (Largeleaf Gentian Root) 9 g, Qianghuo (Incised Notoptetygium Rhizome or Root) 9 g and Dilong (Angle Worm) 12 g.

Modification: If there is muscular emaciation, Jixueteng (Henry Magnoliavine Stem or Root) 15 g and Huangqi (Milkvetch Root) 30 g can be added to invigorate qi and nourish blood; for blood stasis, Zhidahuang (Prepared Rhubarb) 9 g and Danpi (Cortex Moutan) 9 g can be added to resolve stasis and dispel heat.

### 3. Retention of cold with blood stasis

Treatment principle: Warming yang and dissipating cold, dredging the collaterals and resolving stasis.

Prescription and herbs: Modified Yanghe Decoction.

Danggui (Chinese Angelica) 9 g, Zhimahuang (Prepared Ephedra) 9 g, Shudi (Prepared Rhizome of Rehmannia) 15 g, Lujiaojiao (Deerhorn Glue) 9 g (melted in decoction), Baijiezi (White Mustard Seed) 9 g, Paojiang (Prepared Dried Ginger) 6 g, Rougui (Cassia Bark) 3 g (decocted later) and Honghua (Safflower) 9 g.

Modification: For relatively severe intolerance of cold and weakness and soreness of the waist and legs, Fupian (Radix Aconitilateralis Preparata) 15 g (decocted first) and Duzhong (Eucommia Bark) 12 g can be added to warm the kidneys and strengthen the waist; for loose stools and greasy tongue coating, Shudi (Prepared Rhizome of Rehmannia) 10 g can be replaced with Cangzhu (Atractylodes Rhizome) 10 g and Yiyiren (Coix Seed) 30 g to invigorate the spleen and resolve dampness; for localized stiffness of the skin, Cubiejia (Vinegar-prepared Turtle Shell) 9 g, Kunbu (Kelp or Tangle) 15 g and Haizao (Seaweed) 15 g can added to soften and resolve stasis.

### 4. Deficiency of healthy qi with lingering pathogens

Treatment principle: Invigorating qi and nourishing blood, activating blood and dredging the collaterals.

Prescription and herbs: Sijunzi Decoction and Taohong Siwu Decoction.

Huangqi (Milkvetch Root) 30 g, Dangshen (Radix Codonopsis) 15 g, Baizhu (Largehead Atractylodes Rhizome) 12 g, Fuling (Indian Bread)

15 g, Danggui (Chinese Angelica) 10 g, Chuanxiong (Szechwan Lovage Rhizome) 10 g, Taoren (Peach Seed) 9 g, Honghua (Safflower) 9 g, Jixueteng (Henry Magnoliavine Stem or Root) 15 g and Dilong (Angle Worm) 9 g.

Modification: If there is apparent soreness of the muscles and joints, Qinjiao (Largeleaf Gentian Root) 15 g, Weilingxian (Chinese Clematis Root) 15 g, Zhiruxiang (Prepared Boswellin) 6 g and Zhimuoyao (Prepared Myrrh) 6 g can be added to expel wind and dredge the collaterals, as well as resolve stasis and alleviate pain.

## Chinese Patent Medicine

1. Quanlu Pill: 6 g for each dose, 3 times a day.
2. Xiaohuoluo Dan: 6 g for each dose, 3 times a day.
3. Shiquan Dabu Pill: 1 pill for each dose, 3 times a day.

## Simple and Handy Prescriptions

Huangqi (Milkvetch Root) 30 g, Danggui (Chinese Angelica) 9 g, Guizhi (Cassia Twig) 9 g, Jixueteng (Henry Magnoliavine Stem or Root) 30 g and Lujiaopian (Sliced Cornus Cervi) 12 g are boiled in water and taken once a day. It is used to treat scleroderma with insufficiency of qi, blood and yang, as well as blood stasis.

## Other Therapies

External therapy: Equal quantities (20~45 g each) of Guizhi (Cassia Twig), Chuanxiong (Szechwan Lovage Rhizome), Sumu (Sappan Wood), Honghua (Safflower), Xixin (Manchurian Wildginger) and Aiye (Argy Wormwood Leaf) are boiled in water. The decoction is used to bathe or wash the affected limbs, including the feet and hands, for 20~40 minutes, 1~2 times a day, for a month. Take note that the decoction should be kept warm throughout.

Massage therapy: To palpate, palm-press, stroke, push, finger-press and pluck the related acupoints on the four limbs 30 times, once a day. The manipulations should be performed with a tolerable force.

## Cautions and Advice

1. Currently, there is no specific treatment for scleroderma, so long-term TCM therapy should be administered.
2. The disease may be aggravated during pregnancy, which should be avoided if possible.
3. It is advisable to keep the body (especially the extremities) warm and avoid cold stimulation.
4. The inflammation foci should be removed in addition to preventing overstrain and dramatic emotional fluctuation.

## Daily Exercises

1. List the main clinical characteristics of scleroderma.
2. Explain how scleroderma due to cold retention causing blood stasis and scleroderma due to deficient healthy qi with lingering pathogens can be differentiated and treated.

# Behcet Disease

# Week 13: Saturday

Behcet disease refers to an autoimmune disease marked by multisystem lesions due to the inflammation of minute blood vessels. Clinically, there is a trilogy of purulent iridocyclitis, oral sores and genitalia ulcers with alternated occurrence and remission. Behcet disease is mostly seen in females 16~40 years of age. It is generally not severe and has a favorable prognosis. If the larger vessels of the heart, alimentary tract and nervous system are affected, the prognosis will depend on the severity of the damage. In TCM, Behcet disease is closely associated with "fox-creeper disease".

## Etiology and Pathology

TCM holds that Behcet disease is mainly caused by either endogenous or exogenous factors. The former refers to deficiency of yin with internal heat, while the latter to toxic heat which putrefies the tissues and produces blood stasis.

The pathological changes are discussed as follows: Deficiency of yin produces internal heat which, coupled with exogenous toxic heat, accumulates in the interior and scorches the ying-blood; consequently the tissues began to putrify and the blood becomes stagnated, presenting as eye and mouth sores in the upper body and genital and anal sores in the lower body; eventually there will be deficiency of liver yin and kidney yin, or deficiency of spleen yang and kidney yang, with a weakening of healthy qi and lingering of pathogens, as well as simultaneous depletion of qi and blood; culminating in blood stasis, phlegmatic accumulation and refractory ulcers.

## Diagnostic Key Points

1. Recurrent ulcer(s) in the oral membrane, purulent iritis in the anterior chamber, genital ulcer(s), or joint pain and erythema nodosum.
2. Accelerated blood sedimentation, positive serum C reactive protein, positive human white blood cell antigen HLA-B5.

## Syndrome Differentiation

### 1. Exuberance of heat and toxins

Symptoms: Chills, fever, ulcers in the mouth, eyes, external genitalia and the anus, apparent erythema and acne on the skin, polydipsia, scanty reddish urine and dry stools; red tongue with thin and yellow coating and slippery and rapid pulse.

Analysis of symptoms: Pathogenic toxic heat combats with the healthy qi, bringing about intolerance of cold and fever; toxic heat scorches the vessels and putrefies the tissues, presenting as eye and mouth sores in the upper body and genital and anal sores in the lower body, as well as apparent erythema and acne on the skin; toxic heat consumes fluid, marked by polydipsia, scanty reddish urine and dry stools; the red tongue with thin coating and slippery and rapid pulse are due to abundance of heat and toxins.

### 2. Yin deficiency of the liver and kidneys

Symptoms: Dry, red and painful eyes, mouth and tongue sores, genital and anal ulcers, feverish sensations over the five centers, dizziness, tinnitus, forgetfulness, weakness and soreness in the waist and knees, or insomnia and night sweats; red tongue with scanty fluid, thin coating or no coating and thin and rapid pulse.

Analysis of symptoms: Deficiency of liver yin and kidney yin produces intense deficient fire in the heart and liver, which is marked by dry, red and painful eyes, mouth and tongue sores and feverish sensations over the five centers; deficient heat scorches the lower energizer, resulting in ulcers in the external genitalia and the anus; deficiency of liver yin and kidney yin leads to upward disturbance of deficient yang, giving rise to dizziness and tinnitus; the brain marrow is inadequate, so there is forgetfulness; deficiency of the kidneys is manifested as weakness and soreness in the waist and knees; deficient heat in the interior is responsible for insomnia and night sweats; the red tongue with scanty fluid, thin coating or no coating and thin and rapid pulse are attributable to deficiency of liver yin and kidney yin with an abundance of deficient heat in the interior.

## 3. Yang deficiency of the spleen and kidneys

Symptoms: Oral and genital sores without apparent redness and severe pain, scattered nodules with vague pain in the leg, intolerance of cold, cold limbs, poor appetite, loose stools, weakness and soreness in the waist and knees and edema in the lower limbs; pale and enlarged tongue with teeth marks, white greasy coating and thin and deep pulse.

Analysis of symptoms: The disease is a protracted one marked by transformation of yang into yin in the late stage. Deficiency of spleen yang and kidney yang results in unsmooth blood circulation and putrefied skin, characterized by oral and genital sores without apparent redness and severe pain due to decline of yang; deficiency of yang gives rise to phlegmatic accumulation and blood stasis, producing sparse nodules with vague pain in the leg; deficiency of spleen yang is responsible for poor digestion which is marked by a poor appetite and loose stools; deficiency of kidney yang is responsible for dysfunction in warming and transporting, causing an intolerance of cold, cold limbs, weakness and soreness of the waist and knees and edema in the lower limbs; the pale and enlarged tongue with teeth marks, white greasy coating and thin and deep pulse are due to deficiency of spleen yang and kidney yang.

## 4. Deficiency of qi and blood

Symptoms: Alternated refractory ulceration of the mouth, eyes, external genitalia and anus and skin, dizziness, blurred vision, pale complexion, palpitations, insomnia, lassitude, liability to sweat, shortness of breath and unwillingness to speak; pale tongue with white and thin coating, thin and soggy pulse.

Analysis of symptoms: Prolonged retention of pathogenic factors results in deficiency of qi and blood as well as a weakening of healthy qi, this is marked by refractory ulcers occurring everywhere; the lucid qi and blood fail to ascend, causing dizziness and pale complexion; the heart blood and spirit are malnourished, giving rise to palpitations and insomnia; deficiency of lung qi and spleen qi is marked by lassitude, liability to sweat and shortness of breath; the pale tongue with white and thin coating and thin and soggy pulse are attributeable to deficiency of qi and blood.

## Differential Treatment

### 1. Exuberance of heat and toxins

Treatment principle: Dispelling heat and removing toxins, purging fire and protecting yin.

Prescription and herbs: Modified Gancao Xiexin Decoction and Wuwei Xiaodu Potion.

Shenggancao (Raw Liquorice Root) 9 g, Huangqin (Baical Skullcap Root) 12 g, Huanglian (Golden Thread) 5 g, Zhizi (Cape Jasmine Fruit) 9 g, Jinyinhua (Honeysuckle Flower) 12 g, Lianqiao (Weeping Forsythia Capsule) 12 g, Pugongying (Dandelion) 15 g, Yejuhua (Wild Chrysanthemum Flower) 9 g, Zihuadiding (Tokyo Violet Herb) 15 g and Xuanshen (Figwort Root) 12 g.

Modification: If there is sweating and thirst due to intense heat, Shigao (Gypsum) 30 g (decocted earlier) and Zhimu (Common Anemarrhena Rhizome) 9 g can be added to dispel heat and promote fluid production; for joint pain and subcutaneous erythema, Shengdi (Dried Rehmannia Root) 15 g, Danpi (Cortex Moutan) 12 g, Rendongteng (Honeysuckle Stem) 15 g and Qinjiao (Largeleaf Gentian Root) 12 g are used to cool blood and dredge the collaterals; for dry stools, Dahuang (Rhubarb) 6 g (decocted earlier) can be added to purge heat and dredge the intestine.

### 2. Yin deficiency of the liver and kidneys

Treatment principle: Tonifying the liver and kidneys, activating blood and removing toxins.

Prescription and herbs: Modified Qiju Dihuang Pill.

Gouqizi (Barbary Wolfberry Fruit) 15 g, Juhua (Chrysanthemum Flower) 9 g, Shengdi (Dried Rehmannia Root) 12 g, Shudi (Prepared Rhizome of Rehmannia) 12 g, Shanyao (Common Yan Rhizome) 12 g, Shanzhuyu (Asiatic Cornelian Cherry Fruit) 9 g, Zexie (Oriental Waterplantain Rhizome) 12 g, Danpi (Cortex Moutan) 12 g, Xuanshen (Figwort Root) 12 g, Huangbai (Amur Cork-tree) 9 g, Danshen (Radix Salviae Miltiorrhiae) 12 g and Danggui (Chinese Angelica) 12 g.

Modification: If there are red, swollen eyes, Qingxiangzi (Feather Cockscomb Seed) 12 g and Xiakucao (Common Selfheal Fruit-Spike)

12 g can be added to purge liver fire; for genital sores with severe swelling and pain, Longdancao (Radix Gentianae) 9 g and Huzhang (Giant Knotweed Rhizome) 15 g can be added to dispel heat and resolve dampness in the liver meridians; for patients with irregular menstruation, Yimucao (Motherwort Herb) 15 g can be added to activate blood and regulate menstruation.

## 3. Yang deficiency of the spleen and kidneys

Treatment principle: Warming and nourishing the spleen and kidneys, dredging yang and activating blood.

Prescription and herbs: Modified Shenqi Pill and Lizhong Pill.

Fupian (Radix Aconitilateralis Preparata) 9 g, Rouguifen (Cassia Bark Powder) 3 g (infused in water), Shudi (Prepared Rhizome of Rehmannia) 12 g, Shanyao (Common Yan Rhizome) 15 g, Shanzhuyu (Asiatic Cornelian Cherry Fruit) 9 g, Fuling (Indian Bread) 12 g, Dangshen (Radix Codonopsis) 12 g, Baizhu (Largehead Atractylodes Rhizome) 10g, Paojiang (Prepared Dried Ginger) 5 g, Zhigancao (Liquorice Root) 5 g, Danggui (Chinese Angelica) 9 g and Chaopuhuang (Pollen Typhae) 15 g (wrapped during decoction).

Modification: For pale and unhealed ulcers, Huangqi (Milkvetch Root) 30 g and Lujiaopian (Sliced Cornus Cervi) 12 g (decocted first) can be added to nourish qi and invigorate yang, as well as to generate muscle and heal ulcers; for severe edema, Zhuling (Polyporus) 15 g and Yiyiren (Coix Seed) 30 g are added to reinforce the action of relieving edema; for persistent diarrhea, Buguzhi (Malaytea Scurfpea Fruit) 12 g and Roudoukou (Nutmeg) 6 g are added to warm the kidneys and consolidate the contents of the intestine.

## 4. Deficiency of qi and blood

Treatment principle: Invigorating qi and nourishing blood, removing toxins and healing ulcers.

Prescription and herbs: Modified Bazhen Decoction.

Huangqi (Milkvetch Root) 30 g, Dangshen (Radix Codonopsis) 15 g, Baizhu (Largehead Atractylodes Rhizome) 12 g, Fuling (Indian Bread) 12 g, Zhigancao (Stir-baked Liquorice Root) 6 g, Danggui (Chinese Angelica) 10 g, Chuanxiong (Szechwan Lovage Rhizome) 10 g, Baishao (White Peony Alba) 12 g, Shudi (Prepared Rhizome of Rehmannia) 12 g, Jinyinhua (Honeysuckle Flower) 12 g, Lianqiao (Weeping Forsythia Capsule) 15 g and Xuanshen (Figwort Root) 12 g.

Modification: For severe deficiency of blood, Ejiao (Donkey-hide Glue) 9 g (melted in decoction), Dazao (Chinese Date) 10 dates and Jixueteng (Henry Magnoliavine Stem or Root) 15 g can be added to nourish blood; for swollen and painful sores, Pugongying (Dandelion) 15 g and Zihuadiding (Tokyo Violet Herb) 15 g can be added to reinforce the action of dispelling heat and removing toxins.

## Chinese Patent Medicine

1. Leigongteng Tablet: 1~2 tablets for each dose, 3 times a day.
2. Xilei Powder: Applied in a small quantity to the affected area, several times a day.

## Simple and Handy Prescriptions

Jinyinhua (Honeysuckle Flower) 9 g and Yejuhua (Wild Chrysanthemum Flower) 9 g are soaked in hot water to serve as tea. It is administered several times a day for the treatment of Behcet disease with oral sores.

## Other Therapies

External therapy: For pudendal ulcers, Kushen (Lightyellow Sophora Root) 30 g, Dahuang (Rhubarb) 30 g and Huanglian (Golden Thread) 30 g are boiled in water and the decoction is later used to wash the affected areas once a day. Besides, Xilei Powder and Zhuhuang Powder can also be used for external application on the oral or pudendal sores.

## Cautions and Advice

1. During the occurrence of Behcet disease, patients should keep the affected area clean in addition to avoiding overstrain and emotional stimulation.
2. They should also eliminate the inducing factors from their lifestyle, i.e., to prevent infection, avoid drugs to which they have allergy and refrain from cigarettes and alcohol as well as spicy and stimulating food.

## Daily Exercises

1. Recall the main clinical characteristics of Behcet disease.
2. Describe the pathological changes of Behcet disease.
3. Explain how Behcet disease due to exuberance of toxic-heat and Behcet disease due to deficiency of qi and blood can be differentiated and treated.

# Sjogren's Syndrome
## Week 14: Monday

Sjogren's syndrome is an autoimmune disease leading to chronic inflammation in the exocrine glands that produce tears or saliva, clinically characterized by dry eyes and mouth. Sjogren's syndrome with gland inflammation (resulting in dry eyes and mouth) that is not associated with another connective tissue disease is referred to as primary Sjögren's syndrome. Sjögren's syndrome that is also associated with a connective tissue disease, such as rheumatoid arthritis, is referred to as secondary Sjögren's syndrome. This disease can afflict people of any age, but middle-aged females are most susceptible. It is marked by a slow progress and a favorable prognosis. However, if the lungs, kidneys and lymph nodes are affected, the prognosis may be unfavorable. In TCM, Sjogren's syndrome is associated with "dryness syndrome" and "dryness bi-syndrome".

### Etiology and Pathology

TCM believes that Sjogren's syndrome is caused by deficiency of yin coupled with invasion of pathogenic fire, heat, warmth and dryness; or by indulgence in spicy food; or by over consumption of yang-invigorating and dryness-producing herbs; or by excessive sexual activity. All the conditions can lead to consumption of body fluid, deficiency of yin and predominance of dryness (Sjogren's syndrome).

The pathological changes are discussed as follows: pathogenic heat, fire, warmth and dryness, or pathogenic dampness, toxins and heat, consume the body fluid and result in insufficiency of yin fluid and dryness in the viscera, this is marked by dry eyes with blurred vision if the liver yin is insufficient and dry throat with hoarseness or dry cough with constipation if the lung yin or stomach yin is insufficient. Deficiency of yin also produces internal heat, characterized by feverish sensation over the five centers (the palms, the soles and the heart). Dryness, combined with heat, can also damage the yin phase, leading to blood stasis or collateral obstruction with subcutaneous suggillation and joint pain. In the final stage, both yin and qi are exhausted, so there is deficiency of qi and yin.

## Diagnostic Key Points

1. Keratoconjunctivitis sicca, reduced secretion of tears or even absent lacrimation irresponsive to external stimuli; dry mouth with marked decrease in saliva production, or persistent swelling of the parotid; Alternatively, nonthrombocytopenic purpura in the ptosis position, joint pain, Raynaud phenomenon and leucoma may be present.
2. High levels of rheumatic factor and antinuclear antibody, natural flow rate of saliva $\leq 0.03$ ml/minute and abnormal findings on labial gland biopsy.

## Syndrome Differentiation

### 1. Deficiency of yin due to dryness and heat

Symptoms: Dry eyes, mouth and throat, feverish sensations over the five centers, scanty reddish urine, dry stools, or dry cough and absence of sputum; red tongue with little or no coating and thin pulse.

Analysis of symptoms: Dryness damages yin, marked by dry eyes if the liver yin is insufficient; dry throat, dry cough with no sputum and dry stools if the lung yin or stomach yin is insufficient. Deficiency of yin also produces internal heat, characterized by feverish sensation over the five centers and scanty reddish urine; the red tongue with little or no coating and the thin pulse are both manifestations of deficient yin due to dryness and heat.

### 2. Stasis of blood due to dryness and heat

Symptoms: Dry mouth and eyes, red eyes or sensation of a foreign body within the eye(s), swollen, warm and painful parotid, subcutaneous purpura, or joint pain; dark red tongue with possible ecchymosis, absence of coating or thin, yellow and dry tongue coating and thin, unsmooth pulse.

Analysis of symptoms: Dryness and heat consume fluid, leading to a dry mouth and eyes, or sensation of foreign body in the eye(s); dryness and heat scorches the blood, marked by reddened eyes; blood heat, stasis and toxins are responsible for the swollen, warm and painful parotid; blood dryness and stasis lead to subcutaneous suggillation; the collaterals are blocked, so there is joint pain; the dark red tongue with possible ecchymosis, absence of coating or thin, yellow and dry coating and thin, unsmooth pulse are symptomatic of blood stasis due to dryness and heat.

## 3. Transformation of damp-toxins into dryness

Symptoms: Bitter, dry and sticky sensation in the mouth, excessive secretion of turbid substances in the eyes with dry sensation, swollen and sore parotid, swollen and painful gums, thoracic and epigastric distress and stuffiness, poor appetite, foul breath, thirst, scanty reddish urine, loose or dry stools, red, swollen and painful joints; red tongue with yellow and greasy coating and slippery and rapid pulse are manifestations of abundant dampness, heat and toxins.

Analysis of symptoms: Pathogenic dampness and toxic heat scorch the body fluid and produce dryness. If the pathogens are in the liver meridian, there will be excessive secretion of turbid substances in the eyes with dry sensation; if the pathogens are in the stomach, there will be swelling and soreness of the parotid glands as well as swollen and painful gums; if the pathogens are in the middle energizer, there will be thoracic and epigastric distress and stuffiness, poor appetite, foul breath and thirst; if pathogens are in the lower energizer, there will be scanty reddish urine and loose or dry stools; if pathogenic dampness and heat are in the joints, there will be red, swollen and painful joints; the red tongue with yellow and greasy coating and slippery and rapid pulse are manifestations of abundant dampness and toxic heat in the interior.

## 4. Depletion of qi and yin

Symptoms: Lassitude with unwillingness to speak, dry mouth and throat, hoarseness, dry eyes with blurred vision, nasal discomfort and feverish sensations in the palms and soles; red and enlarged tongue, scanty and dry coating and thin and rapid or thin and weak pulse.

Analysis of symptoms: Prolonged retention of dryness and heat damages yin and consumes qi, marked by lassitude with unwillingness to speak in the case of deficient qi; marked by dry mouth and throat, hoarseness, dry eyes with blurred vision and nasal discomfort in the case of impaired fluid; deficiency of yin produces internal heat, causing feverish sensations in the palms and soles; the red and enlarged tongue with scanty and dry coating and thin and rapid or thin and weak pulse are due to simultaneous depletion of qi and yin.

## Differential Treatment

### 1. Deficiency of yin due to dryness and heat

Treatment principle: Dispelling heat to nourish yin, promoting fluid production to reduce dryness.

Prescription and herbs: Modified Yangyin Qingfei Decoction.

Shengdi (Dried Rehmannia Root) 15 g, Maidong (Dwarf Lilyturf Tuber) 12 g, Xuanshen (Figwort Root) 12 g, Baishao (White Peony Alba) 12 g, Danpi (Cortex Moutan) 9 g, Beimu (Fritillariae Tuber) 6 g, Shihu (Dendrobium) 15 g and Gancao (Liquorice Root) 3 g.

Modification: If there are feverish sensations over the five centers, sleeplessness and reddish urine, Huanglian (Golden Thread) 3 g and Zhimu (Common Anemarrhena Rhizome) 10 g can be added to clear the heart, purge fire and nourish yin.

### 2. Stasis of blood due to dryness and heat

Treatment principle: Nourishing yin to reduce dryness, dispelling heat and cooling blood.

Prescription and herbs: Modified Qingying Decoction.

Shuiniujiao (Buffalo Horn) 30 g, Xuanshen (Figwort Root) 12 g, Shengdi (Dried Rehmannia Root) 15 g, Maidong (Dwarf Lilyturf Tuber) 12 g, Danshen (Radix Salviae Miltiorrhiae) 15 g, Danpi (Cortex Moutan) 12 g, Chishao (Red Peony Root) 15 g, Jinyinhua (Honeysuckle Flower) 12 g, Lianqiao (Weeping Forsythia Capsule) 12 g and Zhuye (Henon Bamboo Leaf) 6 g.

Modification: For dry and painful eyes, Gouqizi (Barbary Wolfberry Fruit) 15 g, Shihu (Dendrobium) 15 g and Juhua (Chrysanthemum Flower) 6 g can be added to nourish the liver and dispel fire; for swollen and painful parotid glands, Pugongying (Dandelion) 30 g and Jiangcan (Stiff Silkworm) 10 g can be added to reinforce the action of dispelling heat and removing toxins, as well as subduing swelling and removing nodules; for joint pain, Qinjiao (Largeleaf Gentian Root) 12 g, Sangzhi (Mulberry Twig)15 g and Luoshiteng (Chinese Starjasmine Stem) 15 g are used to dredge the collaterals and alleviate pain.

## 3. Transformation of damp-toxins into dryness

Treatment principle: Dispelling toxins and resolving dampness, nourishing yin and reducing dryness.

Prescription and herbs: Modified Ganlu Xiaodu Dan.

Huoxiang (Agastache Rugosa) 10 g, Yinchen (Virgate Wormwood Herb) 15 g, Huangqin (Baical Skullcap Root) 15 g, Jinyinhua (Honeysuckle Flower) 15 g, Lianqiao (Weeping Forsythia Capsule) 15 g, Baikouren (Fructus Amomi Rotundus) 5 g Huashi (Talc) 15 g (wrapped during decoction), Chuanmutong (Armand Clematis Stem) 6 g, Nanshashen (Fourleaf Ladybell Root) 12 g, Shihu (Dendrobium) 12 g, Lugen (Reed Rhizome) 30 g and Tianhuafen (Trichosanthin) 15 g.

Modification: If there are dry and painful eyes, Juhua (Chrysanthemum Flower) 6 g and Gouqizi (Barbary Wolfberry Fruit) 12 g can be added to clear the liver and moisten the eyes; for a bitter taste in the mouth with foul breath, Huanglian (Golden Thread) 3 g and Zhuru (Bamboo Shavings) 9 g are used to clear the stomach and reduce adverseness. For constipation, Shengdi (Dried Rehmannia Root) 15 g and Xuanshen (Figwort Root) 12 g are used to nourish yin, moisten the intestine and promote defecation.

## 4. Depletion of qi and yin

Treatment principle: Replenishing qi and nourishing yin, reducing dryness and supplementing deficiency.

Prescription and herbs: Modified Zengye Decoction and Buzhong Yiqi Decoction.

Shengdi (Dried Rehmannia Root) 15 g, Xuanshen (Figwort Root) 12 g, Maidong (Dwarf Lilyturf Tuber) 12 g, Huangqi (Milkvetch Root) 20 g, Taizishen (Heterophylly Falsesatarwort Root) 15 g, Baizhu (Largehead Atractylodes Rhizome) 12 g, Danggui (Chinese Angelica) 9 g, Chenpi (Dried Tangerine Peel) 6 g, Gouqizi (Barbary Wolfberry Fruit) 15 g, Shihu (Dendrobium) 15 g, Shengma (Rhizoma Cimicifugae) 6 g and Zhigancao (Stir-baked Liquorice Root) 6 g.

Modification: If there is low fever, Biejia (Turtle Shell) 10 g and Qinghao (Sweet Wormwood Herb) 10 g can be added to dispel deficient heat.

## Chinese Patent Medicine

1. Qiju Dihuang Pill: 6 g for each dose, twice a day.
2. Shengmaiyin Oral Liquid: 10 ml for each dose, twice a day.

## Simple and Handy Prescriptions

Equal quantities (15 g each) of Shengdi (Dried Rehmannia Root), Shudi (Prepared Rhizome of Rehmannia), Tiandong (Cochinchinese Asparagus Root), Maidong (Dwarf Lilyturf Tuber), Shanyao (Common Yan Rhizome) and Roucongrong (Desertliving Cistanche) are boiled in water. The decoction is infused with 250 ml of milk and drunk for Sjogren's syndrome with dry mouth, tongue, skin and stools.

## Other Therapies

Dietary therapy: Pear juice, Chinese water chestnut juice, fresh reed rhizome juice, lotus root juice (or sugarcane juice) and dwarf lilyturf tuber juice are mixed evenly to serve as tea. It can be taken frequently for Sjogren's syndrome with dry mouth and tongue.

External therapy: To rinse the mouth with lemon juice.

## Cautions and Advice

1. Sjogren's syndrome, with a relatively high incidence rate, should be promptly treated. It is also important to adopt a regular lifestyle when receiving treatment for this disease.
2. Patients are advised to avoid using warm and dry herbs, consuming spicy food and alcohol, as well as cigarette smoke.
3. Patients should also avoid long-term negative emotional stimulation, overstrain and excessive sexual activities.

## Daily Exercises

1. Concisely describe the etiology and pathology of Sjogren's syndrome.
2. Explain how Sjogren's syndrome due to dry-heat consuming yin and Sjogren's syndrome due to dry-heat causing blood stasis can be differentiated and treated.

# CHAPTER 10

# Metabolic Diseases

## Diabetes
## Week 14: Tuesday

Diabetes is an endocrine metabolic disease due to absolute or relative insufficiency of insulin inside the body and it marked by metabolic disturbances of glucose, fat and protein. Clinically, there are manifestations such as polydipsia, polyuria, polyphagia and bulimia, emaciation or obesity, fatigue, as well as hyperglycemia. According to the difference in etiological factors, most cases of diabetes fall into four broad categories: Type 1, Type 2, special and gestational diabetes (1997ADA/WHO diabetes taxonomic revision standard). Type 1 diabetes is characterized by a lack of insulin production, an early onset in childhood and a tendency towards ketoacidosis. Type 2 diabetes (insulin resistance coupled with insulin insufficiency, or marked insulin deficiency with insulin resistance) occurs in over 90% of diabetes patients, primarily in senile patients (with an increasing incidence in younger ones who also obese). With the progress of diabetes, there may be chronic complications of the eyes, nerves, heart, brain and kidneys, which are the leading factors responsible for disability and death. In TCM, diabetes is also known as "wasting-thirst".

### Etiology and Pathology

TCM believes that diabetes is caused by either endogenous or exogenous factors. The former refers to innate deficiency of the body, whereas the latter refers to indulgence in fatty and sweet food, emotional disorder, overstrain, excessive sexual life, or contraction of toxic heat, all of which lead to consumption of yin fluid by fire and predominance of dry heat.

The pathological change is mainly a predominance of dry heat and deficiency of yin. The lungs are in charge of regulation and serve as the upper source of water; if dryness in the lungs depletes yin, body fluid will fail to moisten the stomach and kidneys; predominance of stomach heat is responsible for the consumption of lung fluid and kidney yin; insufficiency of kidney yin leads to exuberant fire, which scorches the lungs and stomach, causing polydipsia, polyuria and polyphagia. In the late stage, there will be simultaneous impairment of qi and yin, marked by fatigue and emaciation. If deficiency of yin affects yang, there can be deficiency of yin and yang, impairment of the spleen and kidneys and retention of water and dampness in the skin and muscles (edema). Predominance of dry heat with deficiency of yin is often characterized by the following complications: tuberculosis resulting from prolonged dryness in the lungs; cataract and deafness resulting from deficiency of yin blood or essence of the kidneys and liver, which fails to nourish the eyes and ears; furuncle resulting from external invasion of wind-heat, which scorches the ying-yin, obstructs the collaterals and transforms the toxins into pus; chest bi-syndrome resulting from obstruction of phlegm and blood stasis in the chest collaterals due to dryness and heat scorching fluid into phlegm and blood into stasis; and hemiplegia due to stroke resulting from obstruction of the meridians and heart orifices.

## Diagnostic Key Points

1. Clinically the disease is characterized by polydipsia, polyuria, polyphagia, reduced body weight, fatigue and weariness; in some cases, the symptoms may be atypical.
2. Laboratory examination: Fasting plasma glucose levels taken on two different days ay7.0 mmol/L, or random blood sugar (at any time after meals) ru ≥ 11.1 mmol/L. For those who are suspected to have this disease yet without elevated levels of blood sugar, a sugar tolerance test is recommended. Besides, insulin releasing test and glycosylated hemoglobin examination are also conducive to further diagnosis and clinical observation of the disease.

## Syndrome Differentiation

### 1. Dryness and heat in the lungs and stomach

Symptoms· Polydipsia, dry mouth and tongue, frequent micturition, polyphagia or bulimia, emaciation and dry stools; red tongue with yellow and
dry coating and slippery and rapid pulse. These symptoms present in the
early stage of diabetes.

Analysis of symptoms: Intense heat in the lungs consumes body fluid,
so there is polydipsia and dry mouth and tongue; dryness and heat
impair the regulative function of the lungs, bringing about disturbance
of water metabolism which is marked by profuse and frequent urination; blazing fire in the stomach is responsible for polyphagia or
bulimia; dryness and heat consumes body fluid and blood, leading to
emaciation; insufficient stomach fluid fails to moisten the large intestine, resulting in dry stools; the red tongue with yellow and dry coating
and slippery and rapid pulse are manifestations of abundant heat in the
lungs and stomach.

### 2. Deficiency of qi and yin

Symptoms: Dry mouth and lips, turbid and profuse urine, lassitude, dizziness, blurred vision, weakness and soreness in the waist and knees; red
tongue with thin or scanty coating and thin or thin-rapid pulse. These
symptoms occur in the middle stage of diabetes.

Analysis of symptoms: Prolonged retention of dryness and heat creates
a predisposition to deficiency of qi and yin, this is marked by a dry
mouth and lips, as well as lassitude; deficiency of the kidneys, the
fundamental cause of the disease, leads to the unchecked discharge of
fluid and essence, causing turbid, profuse urination; deficiency of
kidney yin also affects the liverpreventing sufficient essence and blood
from reaching the head and eyes, with such signs as dizziness and
blurred vision; the waist and knees are malnourished, giving rise to
weakness and soreness in the waist and knees; the red tongue with thin
or scanty coating and thin or thin-rapid pulse are due to deficiency of
qi and yin.

## 3. Deficiency of yin and yang

Symptoms: Frequent urination, or even immediate urination after drinking, with aggravation at night, dry mouth, withered complexion, weakness and soreness in the waist and knees, impotence, cold body and limbs, edema on the dorsum of the foot; pale and enlarged tongue with white and thin coating and thin, weak and deep pulse. These symptoms appear in the middle and late stages of diabetes.

Analysis of symptoms: The kidneys store essence and discharge turbid substances, so if the kidneys function improperly in this regard, there will be leakage of essence and impairment of yang due to deficiency of yin; the deficient yang fails to condense the urine, so there will be profuse and frequent urination; yang qi is declined at night, so the condition becomes aggravated at night; kidney essence is discharged out of the body with water and fluid, causing the dry mouth and withered face, as well as soreness in the waist and knees; deficient kidney yang fails to warm the body and transport water, bringing about impotence, cold body and limbs and retention of water and dampness in the back of the foot; the pale and enlarged tongue with white and thin coating and thin, weak and deep pulse are all attributable to deficiency of kidney yin and kidney yang.

## 4. Stagnant blood obstructing the collaterals

Symptoms: Dry tongue, inadequate drinking, pain or numbness in the extremities or limbs, hemiplegia, chest distress and pricking pain, or blindness; cyanosed tongue, thin and unsmooth pulse. This syndrome is common in Type 2 or special diabetes.[1]

Analysis of symptoms: Dryness and heat impair the body fluid, which fails to carry blood, bringing about retention of blood in the meridians of the four limbs, giving rise to numbness or pain in the limbs, or partial paralysis; obstruction of the chest collaterals is responsible for chest distress or pricking pain; obstruction of the liver collaterals leads to

---

[1] Also known as Type 3 diabetes and to refer to Alzheimer's Disease which results from insulin resistance in the brain.

malnourishment of the eyes and the resultant blindness; the cyanosed tongue and the thin and unsmooth pulse are both symptomatic of blood stasis in the collaterals.

## Differential Treatment

### 1. Dryness and heat in the lungs and stomach

Treatment principle: Clearing and moistening the lungs and stomach, promoting fluid production to quench thirst.

Prescription and herbs: Supplementary Xiaoke Fang and Zengye Decoction.

Huanglian (Golden Thread) 5 g, Tianhuafen (Trichosanthin) 12 g, Shengdi (Dried Rehmannia Root) 12 g, Xuanshen (Figwort Root) 12 g, Maidong (Dwarf Lilyturf Tuber) 12 g, Yuzhu (Fragrant Solomonseal Rhizome) 12 g, Zhimu (Common Anemarrhena Rhizome) 9 g and Lugen (Reed Rhizome) 12 g.

Modification: If there is polydipsia, shortness of breath, weariness, yellow and dry tongue coating and surging pulse, Renshen (Ginseng) 9 g and Shigao (Gypsum) 30 g (decocted first) are added to replenish qi and nourish yin, as well as dispel stomach fire; for polyphagia and bulimia, Huangqin (Baical Skullcap Root) 12 g and Zhizi (Cape Jasmine Fruit) 9 g can be added to dispel stomach fire; for skin ulcers, Pugongying (Dandelion) 15 g, Zihuadiding (Tokyo Violet Herb) 15 g and Zicao (Arnebia Root) 15 g can be used to dispel heat, remove toxins and resolve stasis.

### 2. Deficiency of qi and yin

Treatment principle: Replenishing qi and nourishing yin, invigorating the spleen and nourishing the kidneys.

Prescription and herbs: Supplementary Yuye Decoction and Zicui Potion.

Huangqi (Milkvetch Root) 30 g, Zhimu (Common Anemarrhena Rhizome) 9 g, Gegen (Kudzuvine Root) 9 g, Wuweizi (Chinese Magnolivine Fruit) 6 g, Shanyao (Common Yan Rhizome) 12 g, Shengdi (Dried Rehmannia Root) 12 g, Shudi (Prepared Rhizome of Rehmannia) 12 g, Shanzhuyu (Asiatic Cornelian Cherry Fruit) 12 g and Gouqizi (Barbary Wolfberry Fruit) 12 g.

Modification: For fatigue and emaciation, Renshen (Ginseng) 9 g can be added to supplement qi and invigorate the spleen; for weakness and soreness in the waist and knees, Sangjisheng (Chinese Taxillus Herb) 15 g and Roucongrong (Desertliving Cistanche) 15 g are added to nourish the kidneys and strengthen the waist; for turbid urine, Yizhiren (Bitter-seed Cardamn) 6 g and Sangpiaoxiao (Egg Capsule of Mantid) 9 g can be added to reduce the essence; for restlessness, insomnia, nocturnal emissions and red tongue with thin and rapid pulse, Huangbai (Amur Cork-tree) 9 g, Guiban (Tortoise Shell) 9 g (decocted first), Longgu (Os Draconis) 30 g and Muli (Oyster Shell) 30 g (decocted first) are used to purge fire and nourish yin, as well as secure the essence and subdue yang.

### 3. Deficiency of yin and yang

Treatment principle: Warming yang and nourishing the kidneys.

Prescription and herbs: Jingui Shenqi Pill.

Fupian (Radix Aconitilateralis Preparata) 9 g, Rouguifen (Cassia Bark Powder) 2 g (infused in water), Shengdi (Dried Rehmannia Root) 12 g, Shudi (Prepared Rhizome of Rehmannia) 12 g, Shanyao (Common Yan Rhizome) 12 g, Shanzhuyu (Asiatic Cornelian Cherry Fruit) 12 g, Fuling (Indian Bread) 15 g, Danpi (Cortex Moutan) 9 g and Zexie (Oriental Waterplantain Rhizome) 12 g.

Modification: For mental and physical strain, Huangqi (Milkvetch Root) 30 g and Renshen (Ginseng) 6~15 g can be added to drastically supplement the primordial qi; for edema with proteinuria, Baizhu (Largehead Atractylodes Rhizome) 15 g, Zhuling (Polyporus) 15 g, Buguzhi (Malaytea Scurfpea Fruit) 15 g and Luxiangcao (Pyrolae) 15 g are used to invigorate the spleen and relieve edema, as well as nourish the kidneys and remove protein from urine.

### 4. Stagnant blood obstructing the collaterals

Treatment principle: Replenishing qi and nourishing yin, activating blood and dredging the collaterals.

Prescription and herbs: Buyang Huangwu Decoction and Zengye Decoction.

Huangqi (Milkvetch Root) 15 g, Danggui (Chinese Angelica) 9 g, Chuanxiong (Szechwan Lovage Rhizome) 9 g, Chishao (Red Peony Root) 15 g, Dilong (Angle Worm) 9 g, Shengdi (Dried Rehmannia Root) 12 g, Maidong (Dwarf Lilyturf Tuber) 12 g and Xuanshen (Figwort Root) 12 g.

Modification: If there is pricking pain in the extremities, Chuanshanjia (Pangolin Scale) 9 g and Quanxie (Scorpion) 5 g can be added to dredge the collaterals and alleviate pain; for stroke with hemiplegia, Shuizhi (Leech) 9 g and Dibiechong (Eupolyphaga Seu Steleophaga) 9 g are used to reinforce the action of resolving stasis and dredging the collaterals; for chest distress and pricking pain, Taoren (Peach Seed) 9 g, Honghua (Safflower) 9 g, Danshen (Radix Salviae Miltiorrhiae) 15 g and Yanhusuo (Corydalis) 9 g can be used to regulate qi, activate blood, resolve stasis and alleviate pain; for blindness due to disorder of the eye ground, Huanliancao (Ecliptae Herba) 12 g, Shengdiyu (Garden Burnet Root) 12 g and Qingxiangzi (Feather Cockscomb Seed) 15 g can be added to clear the liver and cool blood.

## Chinese Patent Medicine

1. Jinqi Jiangtang Tablet: 7 tablets for each dose, 3 times a day.
2. Tangmaikang Infusion Powder: 1 small bag for each dose, twice a day.

## Simple and Handy Prescriptions

1. Equal quantities (30 g each) of Shengdi (Dried Rehmannia Root), Tianhuafen (Trichosanthin), Huangqi (Milkvetch Root) and Shanyao (Common Yan Rhizome) are boiled in water and administered once a day. It is suitable for diabetes with lassitude and dry mouth.
2. A pig's pancreas is dried at a low temperature and then ground into powder and subsequently made into honeyed pills. The pills are administered (6 g for each dose) twice a day. People at risk of diabetes should take these pills frequently.
3. Yumixu (Stigmata Maydis) 30 g and Jixuecao (Asiatic Pennywort Herb) 30 g are boiled in water and served as tea to treat diabetes with proteinuria.

## Other Therapies

Dietary therapy: A pig's pancreas, Shengyiyiren (Coix Seed) 30 g and Shanyao (Common Yan Rhizome) 30 g are boiled in a decoction of Huangqi (Milkvetch Root) 30 g (the gruffs should be removed). Seasonings of ginger, wine and salt can be added for taste. Both the soup and pancreas can be consumed to treat diabetes with polydipsia polyuria and lassitude.

## Cautions and Advice

1. Diabetes is a lifetime disease caused by multiple factors. Patients are advised to adhere to a comprehensive treatment approach incorporating both Chinese and Western medicines, so as to control levels of blood sugar, blood pressure and blood fat, as well as prevent or alleviate various complications.
2. They should adhere to a strict diet, engage in regular physical exercise, prevent obesity and avoid stress, overstrain and excessive sexual activities.

## Daily Exercises

1. List the criteria for classification and diagnosis of diabetes.
2. Concisely describe the etiology and pathology of diabetes.
3. Explain how diabetes due to deficiency of qi and yin and diabetes due to stagnant blood obstructing the collaterals can be differentiated and treated.

# Osteoporosis
# Week 14: Wednesday

Osteoporosis refers to a group of bone diseases due to various factors and marked by reduced bone mineral density, thinned cortical bone and weakened loading function of the bone, which cause a predisposition to pain in the waist, back and four limbs, deformity of the spine, or even bone fracture. This disease is mostly caused by aging and decrease in sexual gland function and, in less common cases, by endocrine disease and reduced rate of nutrient absorption. Women above 40, especially those who have passed menopause, have a higher rate of susceptibility. In TCM, this disease is closely associated with "bone bi-syndrome" and "bone atrophy".

## Etiology and Pathology

TCM holds that osteoporosis is caused by gradual decline of kidney qi after middle age, or by inadequate nutrient intake due to long-term deficiency of the spleen, or by frequent use of hormones. All these conditions can lead to this disease because of the insufficient essence and blood and the malnourished bone marrow.

The pathological changes are discussed as follows: Deficiency of kidney qi depletes essence and marrow; deficiency of the spleen depletes essence and blood; medicinal heat also consumes essence and blood. The above-mentioned conditions are all marked by insufficient essence and blood, which affect the sufficient production of marrow. The kidneys control the bones, store essence and produce marrow. The marrow is used to fill the bone cavity, but if the marrow and essence is in short supply, they will fail to supplement the bones as well as collaterals, leading to blood stasis. Hence, there will be manifestations of general bone pain or deformity, or even bone fracture and limb paralysis.

## Diagnostic Key Points

1. There is general bone ache and weariness and the pain is persistent, localized to the spine, pelvis and the fractured region; it is aggravated

when climbing or changing postures. In addition, such factors as gender, age, nutritional state and history of hormone administration should be taken into account.

2. Positive indication of blood serum bone alkaline phosphatase, bone gla protein and empty stomach urine calcium/creatinine ratio, as well as characteristic change in bone architecture (osteoporosis) on X-ray examination.

## Syndrome Differentiation

### 1. Insufficiency of marrow due to kidney deficiency

Symptoms: Vague pain and flaccidity in the waist and lower limbs, or even bone fracture, dizziness and tinnitus; for those with relative deficiency of kidney yin, the manifestations are emaciation, dry eyes, red and thin tongue with scanty coating and thin and taut pulse; for those with relative deficiency of kidney yang, the manifestations are general edema, profuse and frequent nocturnal urination, intolerance of cold on the back, slightly red tongue with thin or slippery coating and thin and deep pulse. This syndrome is mainly observed in middle-aged and old patients.

Analysis of symptoms: The kidneys control the bones and produce marrow and the waist is the "house of the kidneys", so if the kidney qi is insufficient, there will be inadequate essence and marrow, malnutrition of the waist and lower limbs, voidness of the collaterals and stasis of blood, giving rise to vague pain and flaccidity in the waist and lower limbs, or even bone fracture. The kidney qi is connected to the brain, so if the brain marrow is insufficient, there will be dizziness and tinnitus. For those with relative deficiency of kidney yin, the essence and blood are too deficient to nourish the body, resulting in emaciation with dry eyes. For those with relative deficiency of kidney yang, there is often dysfunction of qi transformation and retention of water and dampness, marked by general edema; yang qi is declined at night, giving rise to clear, profuse nocturnal urine. The governor vessel, pertaining to yang, spans the length of the spine, so if yang qi is too weak to warm the body, there will be intolerance of cold in the back. A red tongue with scanty coating and thin and taut pulse are manifestations of deficient kidney yin whilst a slightly red tongue with thin or slippery coating and thin and deep pulse are manifestations of deficient kidney yang.

## 2. Insufficiency of essence due to spleen deficiency

Symptoms: General bone ache, pale complexion, lassitude, poor appetite, loose stools, poor sleep, pale and enlarged tongue with white and thin coating, soggy and thin pulse. This syndrome is mostly seen in patients with malnutrition.

Analysis of symptoms: Weakness of the spleen and stomach leads to exhaustion of the source for qi and blood and consequently deficiency of essence and marrow, malnutrition of the bones and voidness of the collaterals with blood stasis, giving rise to general bone ache; the deficient qi and blood fail to nourish the face, so there is a pale complexion; the blood fails to transform into qi, bringing about lassitude; the deficient blood also fails to nourish the heart, resulting in poor sleep at night; a deficient spleen is unable to transform food properly, marked by a poor appetite with loose stools; the pale and enlarged tongue with white and thin coating and soggy and thin pulse are manifestations of insufficient essence due to deficiency of the spleen.

## 3. Consumption of essence and blood by heat

Symptoms: Occasional pain in the feet, hands, waist and legs, dry mouth with foul breath, constipation, corpulent body, feverish complexion, red tongue with thin and yellow coating and thin and slippery pulse. This syndrome is seen in those who receive long-term administration of hormones.

Analysis of symptoms: Long-term administration of hormones creates heat in the interior, which consumes essence and blood, resulting in deficiency of essence and marrow, malnutrition of the bones and voidness of the collaterals with blood stasis, marked by occasional pain in the feet, hands, waist and legs. Heat in the stomach consumes body fluid, leading to dry mouth, foul breath and constipation. Abundant heat condenses body fluid into phlegm, resulting in a corpulent body and feverish complexion due to accumulation of phlegmatic heat in the interior; the red tongue with thin and yellow coating and thin and slippery pulse are attributable to consumption of essence and blood by heat.

## Differential Treatment

### 1. Insufficiency of marrow due to kidney deficiency

Treatment principle: Tonifying the kidneys and strengthening the bones, supplementing essence and producing marrow.

Prescription and herbs: Modified Bushen Yangxue Decoction.

Shudi (Prepared Rhizome of Rehmannia) 15 g, Buguzhi (Malaytea Scurfpea Fruit) 12 g, Yinyanghuo (Epimedium Herb) 12 g, Tusizi (Dodder Seed) 12 g, Duzhong (Eucommia Bark) 12 g, Lujiaojiao (Deerhorn Glue) 9 g, Danggui (Chinese Angelica) 9 g, Baishao (White Peony Alba) 12 g, Gouqizi (Barbary Wolfberry Fruit) 12 g, Honghua (Safflower) 5 g, Hetaorou (Walnut) 12 g and Dangshen (Radix Codonopsis) 12 g.

Modification: If there is apparent lumbago, Gouji (Cibot Rhizome) 12 g and Zhichuanwu (Prepared Common Monkshood Mother Root) 6 g can be added to dredge the collaterals and stop pain; for bone fracture, Liujinu (Artemisiae Anomale) 15 g, Zhiruxiang (Prepared Boswellin) 6 g and Muoyao (Myrrh) 6 g can be added to activate blood and alleviate pain; for deficiency of kidney yin with dry eyes and emaciation, Nuzhenzi (Glossy Privet Fruit) 12 g and Huanliancao (Ecliptae Herba) 12 g are used to nourish yin and supplement blood; for deficiency of kidney yang with intolerance of cold in the back and clear, profuse urine, Zhifupian (Radix Aconitilateralis Preparata) 6 g and Rouguifen (Cassia Bark Powder) 2 g (swallowed) are used to warm yang and transform qi .

### 2. Insufficiency of essence due to spleen deficiency

Treatment principle: Invigorating the spleen and nourishing blood, supplementing essence and strengthening the bones.

Prescription and herbs: Modified Guipi Decoction.

Shenghuangqi (Raw Milkvetch Root) 30 g, Dangshen (Radix Codonopsis) 15 g, Baizhu (Largehead Atractylodes Rhizome) 12 g, Fuling (Indian Bread) 12 g, Danggui (Chinese Angelica) 9 g, Chuanxiong (Szechwan

Lovage Rhizome) 9 g, Baishao (White Peony Alba) 12 g, Shudi (Prepared Rhizome of Rehmannia) 15 g, Buguzhi (Malaytea Scurfpea Fruit) 15 g, Bajitian (Mornda Root) 12 g, Huainiuxi (Twotoothed Achyranthes Root) 15 g and Jixueteng (Henry Magnoliavine Stem or Root) 30 g.

Modification: If there is poor appetite and loose stools, Jiaoshanzha (Scorch-fried Hawthorn Fruit) 15 g and Shanyao (Common Yan Rhizome) 15 g can be added; for poor sleep, Chaozaoren (Semen Ziziphi Spinosae) 15 g and Longyanrou (Longan Aril) 10 g are used to nourish the heart and calm the spirit.

### 3. Consumption of essence and blood by heat

Treatment principle: Nourishing essence and blood, strengthening tendons and bones.

Prescription and herbs: Modified Huqian Pill.

Shudi (Prepared Rhizome of Rehmannia) 15 g, Guiban (Tortoise Plastron) 9 g, Chenpi (Dried Tangerine Peel) 9 g, Zhimu (Common Anemarrhena Rhizome) 6 g, Huangbai (Amur Cork-tree) 9 g, Baishao (White Peony Alba) 15 g, Suoyang (Songaria Cynomorium Herb) 12 g and Qiannianjian (Obscured Homalomena Rhizome) 15 g.

Modification: For dry mouth and stools, Zengye Decoction (Shengdihuang 15 g, Xuanshen 12 g, Maidong 12 g) can be used to nourish yin and promote defecation; for damage to the stomach collaterals by drugs, resulting in stomachache, Xiangfu (Nutgrass Galingale Rhizome) 9 g and Baiji (Common Bletilla Tuber) 9 g are added to regulate qi and protect the stomach.

## Chinese Patent Medicine

Xianling Gubao: 2 pills for each dose, twice a day.

## Simple and Handy Prescriptions

Shudihuang (Prepared Rhizome of Rehmannia) 12 g, Yinyanghuo (Epimedium Herb) 15 g, Longgu (Os Draconis) 30 g and Muli (Oyster Shell) 30 g are boiled in water. The decoction is administered twice a day for osteoporosis without predominance of yin or yang.

## Other Therapies

External therapy: Dog-skin plaster (in substitution for warm-moxibustion plaster), coupled with miraculous light physical therapy, is applied to the painful area.

Tuina therapy: Treat the painful joint and produce feverish sensation in the adjacent area by one-finger scrubbing, pressing and kneading. The force should be gentle so as not to trigger bone fracture.

Dietary therapy: Pig bone (mainly flat bone) 500 g, soyabean 250 g and seasonings of onion and ginger are boiled together till the bone is crisp and brittle.

## Cautions and Advice

1. Osteoporosis is a common disease in old people. Although it is slow in development, it has great impact on daily life and should be treated from different aspects. These include maintaining a diet with sufficient protein, calcium, salt and vitamins, increasing outdoor activities and reducing weight loading exercises. For patients who are bedridden, it is advisable to perform suitable passive as well as active exercises of the muscles in the limbs and back, so as to avoid muscular atrophy.
2. If there are definite etiological factors, such as hypercortisolism, they should be addressed immediately.

## Daily Exercises

1. List the diagnostic key points of osteoporosis.
2. Explain how osteoporosis due to deficiency of the kidneys and marrow can be diagnosed and treated.

# Simple Obesity
# Week 14: Thursday

Simple obesity is a condition of excessive accumulation of fat inside the body due to over-consumption of calories; it is marked by a fat and clumsy body (specifically, a body weight that is 20% more than the healthy weight recommended for one's height). Obesity is linked to hyperlipemia, hypertension, diabetes, coronary artery disease and fatty liver. In TCM, this disease is closely associated with "phlegm syndrome", "edema" and "deficiency consumption".

## Etiology and Pathology

This disease is caused by either endogenous or exogenous factors. The former refers to congenital deficiency of the spleen, while the latter refers to excessive intake of fatty and sweet food and inadequate physical exercise or a sedentary lifestyle, resulting in deficiency of spleen qi and production of phlegm and heat in the interior; or deficiency of the kidneys due to senility, which causes imbalance between yin and yang as well as accumulation of phlegm and stasis inside the body, thus leading to obesity.

The pathological changes are discussed as follows: Deficiency of spleen qi with excessive food intake and inadequate physical exercise lead to the transformation of water and food into phlegm and dampness instead of nutrients. In addition, excessive intake of fatty and sweet food, coupled with inadequate physical exercise or a sedentary lifestyle, results in deficiency of spleen qi, production of phlegm and heat and eventually obesity due to accumulation of phlegm and stasis inside the body. Moreover, after middle age, there is deficiency of the kidneys, imbalance between yin and yang and accumulation of water, dampness and turbid phlegm, or blood stasis in the next stage and finally obesity due to retention of turbid pathogens inside the body. Turbid phlegm produces heat, with such signs as intolerance of heat and excessive sweating. The spleen dominates the muscles and the four limbs, so if the spleen qi is deficient, turbid phlegm obstructs the channels through which the nutrients from water and food are transported to muscles and the four limbs, resulting in lassitude (especially in the limbs), shortness of breath upon physical exertion and sweating.

## Diagnostic Key Points

Body weight is 20% more than the healthy weight recommended for one's height, body mass index is more than 26, and the patient is not suffering from endocrine diseases such as hypercortisolism, hypothyroidism and multicystic ovary.

## Syndrome Differentiation

### 1. Accumulation of phlegm due to qi deficiency

Symptoms: Corpulent body, shortness of breath upon physical exertion, sweating, lusterless skin, listlessness, lethargy, poor appetite, gastric distension, or loose stools, puffy limbs and heavy head or body; enlarged tongue with white coating and thin and slippery pulse.

Analysis of symptoms: Deficiency of the spleen qi leads to accumulation of phlegm and dampness inside the body, marked by corpulence; disorder of the mother organ involves the child organ, bringing about deficiency of the lungs and spleen, with such manifestations as shortness of breath upon exertion and sweating; transformation of water and food into phlegm and dampness instead of nutrients results in malnourishment of the body, resulting in lusterless skin; failure of lucid yang to ascend gives rise to listlessness and lethargy; deficiency of the spleen leads to stagnation of qi and dysfunction in transportation and transformation, with such signs as poor appetite, gastric and abdominal distension, as well as loose stools; deficiency of the spleen also results in the retention of dampness, so there are puffy limbs and a heavy head or body; the enlarged tongue with white coating and thin and slippery pulse are all manifestations of phlegmatic accumulation due to deficiency of qi.

## 2. Accumulation of phlegm and heat

Symptoms: Corpulent body, oily complexion, good appetite, intolerance of heat, restlessness, a bitter taste in the mouth and dry throat, or presence of yellowish urine with constipation; red tongue with thin and yellow coating and taut and slippery pulse.

Analysis of symptoms: Fatty, greasy and sweet food enters the stomach and is subsequently scorched by the stomach fire, producing an accumulation of phlegm and heat inside the body which manifests as corpulence and an oily complexion; intense stomach fire is responsible for polyorexia, intolerance of heat and restlessness; stomach fire also consumes body fluid, bringing about the bitter taste in the mouth and dry throat, or yellowish urine and constipation; red tongue with thin and yellow coating and taut and slippery pulse are due to accumulation of phlegm and heat.

## 3. Accumulation of phlegm and stasis in the interior

Symptoms: Corpulent body, weariness and shortness of breath upon exertion, liability to sweat, dizziness, chest distress, gastric and hypochondriac distension or pain and masses below the costal region; dark and enlarged tongue with white and thin coating and greasy, soggy and thin pulse.

Analysis of symptoms: Weakness of the body with deficiency of spleen qi and kidney qi due to senility leads to internal accumulation of phlegm and stasis, which is marked by corpulence, weariness and shortness of breath on exertion, as well as a liability to sweat; phlegm and stasis obstruct the collaterals, resulting in malnourishment of the upper orifices and dizziness; retention of turbid phlegm in the thoracic region is responsible for chest distress; stagnation of liver qi and stomach qi is manifested as gastric and hypochondriac distension or pain; accumulation of stasis in the liver collaterals brings about the formation of masses below the costal region (fatty liver); the dark and enlarged tongue with white and thin coating and greasy, soggy and thin pulse are symptomatic of phlegm and stasis accumulating in the interior due to deficiency of spleen qi and kidney qi.

## 4. Imbalance between yin and yang

Symptoms: Corpulent body, restlessness, intolerance of heat, or occasional intolerance of cold, cold limbs, emotional depression or excitement, lethargy, soreness in the lumbar vertebrae, edema in the lower limbs, with aggravation in the afternoon and irregular menstruation in women; slightly red tongue with thin coating and thin and feeble or thin and taut pulse.

Analysis of symptoms: After middle age, the kidney qi is deficient in its function of steaming and transforming water and fluid, thus leading to an accumulation of water, dampness and turbid phlegm in the interior, marked by a corpulent body; deficiency of kidney yin produces internal heat, with such signs as restlessness and intolerance of heat; malnutrition of the liver is responsible for emotional depression and excitement; the liver fire disturbs the heart, bringing about insomnia; deficiency of the liver and kidneys with malnutrition of the thoroughfare vessel and governor vessel is manifested as irregular menstruation in women; deficiency of kidney yang may affect the spleen yang, bringing about retention of phlegm and dampness, lethargy, soreness in the lumbar vertebrae and edema in the lower limbs; the slightly red tongue with thin coating and the thin and feeble or thin and taut pulse are due to imbalance between kidney yin and kidney yang.

## Differential Treatment

### 1. Accumulation of phlegm due to qi deficiency

Treatment principle: Replenishing qi, invigorating the spleen and dissolving phlegm.

Prescription and herbs: Fangji Longgu Decoction and Liujunzi Decoction.

Fangji (Fourstamen Stephania Root) 12 g, Huangqi (Milkvetch Root) 15 g, Dangshen (Radix Codonopsis) 12 g, Fuling (Indian Bread) 15 g, Zhuling (Polyporus) 9 g, Baizhu (Largehead Atractylodes Rhizome) 12 g, Chenpi (Dried Tangerine Peel) 6 g, Banxia (Pinellia Tuber) 9 g, Jiaoshanzha (scorch-fried Hawthorn Fruit) 12 g and Heye (Lotus Leaf) 9 g.

Modification: If there is scanty urine, Zexie (Oriental Waterplantain Rhizome) 15 g and Cheqianzi (Plantain Seed) 15 g (wrapped during decoction) can be used to promote urination; for gastric and abdominal distension, Zhiqiao (Orange Fruit) 9 g and Xiangfu (Nutgrass Galingale Rhizome) 9 g are used to regulate qi and remove stagnation.

## 2. Accumulation of phlegm and heat

Treatment principle: Clearing the stomach, dissolving phlegm and eliminating turbidity.

Prescription and herbs: Modified Sanhuang Shigao Decoction and Xiaochengqi Decoction.

Huanglian (Golden Thread) 3 g, Huangqin (Baical Skullcap Root) 9 g, Zhizi (Cape Jasmine Fruit) 9 g, Shigao (Gypsum) 15 g (decocted first), Dahuang (Rhubarb) 5 g (decocted later), Houpu (Magnolia Bark) 9 g, Banxia (Pinellia Tuber) 9 g and Gancao (Liquorice Root) 5 g.

Modification: If there is frequent occurrence of furuncles or acne on the skin, Pugongying (Dandelion) 15 g and Zicao (Arnebia Root) 12 g can be added to dispel heat, remove toxins and cool blood; for thirst with polydipsia and reddish tongue with scanty coating, Shengdi (Dried Rehmannia Root) 15 g, Xuanshen (Figwort Root) 12 g and Maidong (Dwarf Lilyturf Tuber) 15 g are used to nourish yin and produce fluid.

## 3. Accumulation of phlegm and stasis in the interior

Treatment principle: Activating blood and resolving stasis, eliminating phlegm and reducing body weight.

Prescription and herbs: Modified Taoren Honghua Decoction.

Danshen (Radix Salviae Miltiorrhiae) 15 g, Chishao (Red Peony Root) 15 g, Taoren (Peach Seed) 9 g, Honghua (Safflower) 9 g, Chuanxiong (Szechwan Lovage Rhizome) 9 g, Yanhusuo (Corydalis) 9 g, Qingpi (Green Tangerine Peel) 6 g, Zelan (HerbaLycopi) 12 g, Zexie (Oriental Waterplantain Rhizome) 12 g, Fuling (Indian Bread) 12 g, Laifuzi (Radish Seed) 9 g and Heye (Lotus Leaf) 9 g.

Modification: If there is obesity with high fat level in the blood, Puhuang (Pollen Typhae) 20 g (wrapped during decoction) and Huzhang (Giant Knotweed Rhizome) 30 g can be used to activate blood and reduce fat; for fatty liver, Sanleng (Common Burreed Tuber) 15 g, Ezhu (Zedoray Rhizome) 15 g and Haizao (Seaweed) 30 g are used to resolve stasis, expel phlegm and soften the hard tissue.

## 4. Imbalance between yin and yang

Treatment principle: Regulating yin and yang, discharging water and dissolving phlegm.

Prescription and herbs: Modified Erxian Decoction.

Xianmao (Common Curculigo Rhizome) 9 g, Yinyanghuo (Epimedium Herb) 12 g, Bajitian (Mornda Root) 9 g, Tusizi (Dodder Seed) 15 g, Danggui (Chinese Angelica) 9 g, Zhimu (Common Anemarrhena Rhizome) 9 g, Huangbai (Amur Cork-tree) 9 g, Fuling (Indian Bread) 15 g, Zhuling (Polyporus) 15 g and Zexie (Oriental Waterplantain Rhizome) 15 g.

Modification: In cases of mental uneasiness and insomnia, Baihe (Lily Bulb) 15 g and Yejiaoteng (Caulis Polygoni Multiflori) 30 g can be added to clear the liver and tranquilize the mind; for severe waist soreness, Duzhong (Eucommia Bark) 9 g and Gouji (Cibot Rhizome) 9 g can be added to nourish the kidneys and strengthen the waist; for chest distress, Puhuang (Pollen Typhae) 20 g (wrapped during decoction) and Yujin (Turmeric Root Tuber) 9 g can be used to activate blood and regulate qi.

## Chinese Patent Medicine

Fangfeng Tongshen Pill: 6 g for each dose, twice a day.

## Simple and Handy Prescriptions

1. Equal quantities of Huangqi (Milkvetch Root), Fangji (Fourstamen Stephania Root), Zexie (Oriental Waterplantain Rhizome), Shanzha (Hawthorn Fruit) and Danshen (Radix Salviae Miltiorrhiae) are ground up into fine powders and then made into tablets, with each tablet containing 1g of the crude drug. The tablets should be taken 3 times a day, with 5 tablets constituting 1 dose. It is used to treat obesity with deficiency of qi and accumulation of phlegm.

2. Caojueming (Semen Cassia) is fried and then ground up into powder for infusion. It is administered (3~5 g for each dose) 2~3 times a day for the treatment of obesity with hyperlipemia.
3. Weight-reducing tea: Heye (Lotus Leaf) 6 g, Suye (Beef-steak Plant Leaf) 6 g, Shanzha (Hawthorn Fruit) 10 g and green tea 3 g are infused in hot water to be drunk once a day.

## Other Therapies

Dietary therapy:

(1) Baifuling (White Indian Bread) 30 g, Yiyiren (Coix Seed) 30 g, Shanzha (Hawthorn Fruit) 15 g and Jiangmi (Rice Fruit) 50 g are made into porridge for obesity due to deficiency of the spleen with exuberant phlegm.
(2) Celery 250 g and mushroom 50 g are fried with seasonings for obesity with hypertension and hyperlipemia.

Exercise therapy: Patients should engage in various exercises, such as weight training, running, swimming or ball sports, based on their interest.

## Cautions and Advice

1. Obesity is a common disease in modern society and its harmfulness must be fully understood before preventive measures can be successfully adopted.
2. Patients should exercise strict control over what they consume and at the same time refrain from alcohol and tobacco.
3. They should also cultivate a regular lifestyle and participate more actively in physical exercise.

## Daily Exercises

1. List the etiological factors of simple obesity.
2. Explain how obesity due to qi deficiency with phlegm accumulation and obesity due to accumulation of phlegm-heat can be differentiated and treated.

# Gout

# Week 14: Friday

Gout is a disease due to disorders of purine metabolism, marked by hyperuricemia and the recurrence of the resultant acute gouty arthritis, deposition
of arthritic calculus, chronic tophaceous arthritis or joint deformity and,
when the kidneys are involved, chronic interstitial nephritis or uric acid
renal ithiasis. The disease can be divided into two major categories according to etiological factors: primary gout and secondary gout. The causes of
the former are still unknown, although in a few cases it is caused by enzyme
deficiency; primary gout is often accompanied by hyperlipemia, obesity,
diabetes, hypertension, arteriosclerosis and coronary artery disease. The
latter is mainly due to renal disorders, blood diseases and improper use of
drugs. This disease mainly afflicts males who are over 40 years old but
females who have passed menopause may also be susceptible. Excessive
intake of alcohol and food, overstrain and contraction of cold or infection
can often lead to recurrence of this disease. In the late stage, this disease is
often accompanied by renal inadequacy. In TCM, gout is closely associated
with "bi-syndrome", "joint-wind disorder" and "waist pain".

## Etiology and Pathology

TCM believes that gout is caused by excessive intake of fatty and sweet
food, alcohol abuse, overstrain, tension, or contraction of wind, cold,
dampness and heat, which result in obstruction of the meridian qi due to
stagnation of qi and blood, as well as retention of phlegm and blood in
the joints.

The pathological changes are discussed as follows: Pathogenic wind-
heat, coupled with dampness creates a predisposition for the disease; in
addition, predominance of yang, hyperactivity of the liver and excessive
intake of alcohol and food can all lead to retention of pathogenic wind,
dampness and heat, or pathogenic wind, phlegm and heat in the meridians
and joints, obstructing the flow of qi and blood and bringing about bi-
syndrome due to wind, dampness and heat; pathogenic wind-cold, combined with dampness, invades the meridians and obstructs the flow of qi

and blood, bringing about bi-syndrome due to wind, dampness and cold. If the bi-syndrome persists, the flow of qi and blood will become even more sluggish, giving rise to an obstinate adhesion of turbid phlegm and blood stasis to the joints and meridians, marked by pricking pain, nodules and even deformity of the joints. The prolonged lingering of pathogens will inevitably impair the healthy qi, so there is often deficiency of spleen yang and kidney yang and fatigue or weakness due to unchecked discharge of essence in the late stage.

## Diagnostic Key Points

1. Sudden simple joint pain with redness in the big toe, foot plate, ankle and knee after middle age, accompanied by restricted movements, or articular calculus in metatarsophalangeal, interphalangeal and metacarpophalangeal joints.
2. Urate crystal detected by polarimicroscopic examination on bursa mucosa obtained through joint puncture; increase in blood uric acid and sometimes renal uric acid calculus or proteinuria, as well as renal hypofunction.

## Syndrome Differentiation

### 1. Bi-syndrome due to wind, dampness and heat

Symptoms: Redness, warmth and pain in the joints of the toes, or migratory pain, sweating, fever with restlessness and sore throat; red tongue with thin and greasy coating and taut and slippery pulse.

Analysis of symptoms: Pathogenic wind, dampness and heat invade the body and damage the defensive qi in the exterior, giving rise to fever, sweating and sore throat; if they enter the meridians and impede the flow of qi and blood, there will be redness, warmth and pain in the joints of the toes; pathogenic wind drags damp-heat through the meridians, causing the migratory pain; the red tongue with thin and greasy coating and the taut and slippery pulse are manifestations of bi-syndrome due to wind, dampness and heat.

## 2. Bi-syndrome due to wind, dampness and cold

Symptoms: Cold pain and swelling in the joints of the toes that is aggravated by cold and alleviated by warmth, slightly red or normal skin in the affected area; slightly red tongue with thin coating and taut and tense pulse.

Analysis of symptoms: Pathogenic wind, dampness and cold invade the meridians and congeal qi and blood, causing a cold pain and swelling in the joints of the toes which is aggravated by cold and alleviated by warmth; dampness impairs yang qi and impairs the smooth circulation of blood, so there may be a slight redness of the skin in the affected area; the slightly red tongue with thin coating and taut and tense pulse are manifestations of bi-syndrome due to wind, dampness and cold.

## 3. Obstinate retention of phlegm and stasis

Symptoms: Frequent pricking pain in the joints that is aggravated at night, along with nodules, swelling, deformity and inhibited movements; darkish red tongue with possible ecchymosis and thin-taut or unsmooth pulse.

Analysis of symptoms: Phlegm and stasis combine and remain in the meridians, obstructing qi and blood in the joints, giving rise to pricking pain and multiple nodules; phlegm and stasis are yin pathogens so the obstruction and pain is aggravated at night when yang qi begin to decline; if left unaddressed, the nodules increase and are accompanied by swelling, deformity and inhibited movements; darkish red tongue with possible ecchymosis and thin-taut or unsmooth pulse are due to obstinate retention of phlegm and stasis.

## 4. Yang deficiency of the spleen and kidneys

Symptoms: Pale complexion, lack of warmth in the feet and hands, weakness and soreness in the waist and legs that is aggravated upon physical exertion, profuse nocturnal urination, lassitude and occasional joint pain; pale tongue with white and thin coating and thin and deep pulse.

Analysis of symptoms: Prolonged lingering of pathogenic factors will inevitably impair the healthy qi, leading to deficiency of spleen yang and kidney yang, which fail to warm and transport qi and blood, resulting in a pale complexion and lack of warmth in the feet and hands; deficiency of the kidneys is responsible for weakness and soreness in the waist and legs; deficiency of the spleen is manifested as intolerance of strain and aggravation upon exertion; deficiency of kidney qi and kidney yang leads to uncondensed and unchecked urine, marked by profuse nocturnal urination; loss of essence results in physical weariness and weakness; obstinate retention of phlegm and stasis in the meridians brings about joint pain; the pale tongue with white and thin coating, or thin and deep pulse are all attributable to yang deficiency of the spleen and kidneys.

## Differential Treatment

### 1. Bi-syndrome due to wind, dampness and heat

Treatment principle: Dispelling wind and heat, resolving dampness and dredging obstruction in the collaterals.

Prescription and herbs: Supplementary Simiao Powder.

Cangzhu (Atractylodes Rhizome) 9 g, Huangbai (Amur Cork-tree) 12 g, Niuxi (Twotoothed Achyranthes Root) 12 g, Yiyiren (Coix Seed) 30 g, Haitongpi (Erythrinae) 12 g, Sangzhi (Mulberry Twig) 30 g, Weilingxian (Chinese Clematis Root) 12 g, Rendongteng (Honeysuckle Stem) 15 g, Lucao (Cairo Morningglory Root or Leaf) 20 g and Qinjiao (Largeleaf Gentian Root) 10 g.

Modification: If there is gout with red, warm and painful joints, Shengdi (Dried Rehmannia Root) 15 g, Chishao (Red Peony Root) 15 g and Dilong (Angle Worm) 12 g can be added to dispel heat, cool blood and dredge the collaterals.

### 2. Bi-syndrome due to wind, dampness and cold

Treatment principle: Warming the meridians to dissipate cold, dispelling wind to resolve dampness.

Prescription and herbs: Supplemented Wutou Decoction.

Zhichuanwu (Prepared Common Monkshood Mother Root) 9 g, Mahuang (Ephedra) 9 g, Baishao (White Peony Alba) 12 g, Huangqi (Milkvetch Root) 15 g, Fupian (Radix Aconitilateralis Preparata) 9 g, Guizhi (Cassia Twig) 9 g, Baizhu (Largehead Atractylodes Rhizome) 12 g, Fangfeng (Divaricate Saposhnikovia Root) 9 g, Fangji (Fourstamen Stephania Root) 12 g and Gancao (Liquorice Root) 6 g.

Modification: For gout with nodules, Taoren (Peach Seed) 9 g and Baijiezi (White Mustard Seed) 9 g can be added to activate blood, dredge the collaterals and dissipate stagnation.

## 3. Obstinate retention of phlegm and stasis

Treatment principle: Dissolving phlegm and expelling stasis, dredging the meridians and dissipating stagnation.

Prescription and herbs: Modified Taohong Siwu Decociton.

Taoren (Peach Seed) 9 g, Honghua (Safflower) 9, Danggui (Chinese Angelica) 9 g, Chuanxiong (Szechwan Lovage Rhizome) 9 g, Weilingxian (Chinese Clematis Root) 12 g, Chuanshanjia (Pangolin Scale) 12 g, Baijiezi (White Mustard Seed) 9 g, Dannanxing (Bile Arisaema) 9 g, Quanxie (Scorpion) 3 g and Wugong (Centipede) 1.

Modification: If there is severe joint pain, Zhichuanwu (Prepared Common Monkshood Mother Root) 6 g, Zhicaowu (Prepared Kusnezoff Monkshood Root) 6 g and Xixin (Manchurian Wildginger) 3 g can be added to warm the meridians and stop pain; for increased blood uric acid, Huangbai (Amur Cork-tree) 9 g, Cangzhu (Atractylodes Rhizome) 9 g, Yiyiren (Coix Seed) 30 g and Fangji (Fourstamen Stephania Root) 15 g can be used to dispel pathogenic factors.

## 4. Yang deficiency of the spleen and kidneys

Treatment principle: Warming and invigorating the spleen and kidneys.

Prescription and herbs: Modified Yougui Pill.

Shudi (Prepared Rhizome of Rehmannia) 15 g, Shanyao (Common Yan Rhizome) 15 g, Shanzhuyu (Asiatic Cornelian Cherry Fruit) 10 g, Tusizi (Dodder Seed) 15 g, Gouqizi (Barbary Wolfberry Fruit) 12 g, Duzhong (Eucommia Bark) 12 g, Fupian (Radix Aconitilateralis Preparata) 10 g, Rouguifen (Cassia Bark Powder) 2 g (infused in water), Huangqi (Milkvetch Root) 20 g, Dangshen (Radix Codonopsis) 12 g, Baizhu (Largehead Atractylodes Rhizome) 12 g and Zhigancao (Liquorice Root) 3 g.

Modification: For calculus in the urinary tract, Jinqiancao (Christina Loosestrife) 20 g, Haijinshao (Lygodium) 10 g (wrapped during decoction) and Jineijin (Corium Stomachium Galli) 9 g are used to dispel the stones; for loose stools and joint pain, Ruxiang (Boswellin) 6 g, Muoyao (Myrrh) 6 g, Baijiezi (White Mustard Seed) 6 g and Yiyiren (Coix Seed) 30 g can be added to activate blood and dredge the collaterals.

## Chinese Patent Medicine

Haitong Tablet: 6 g for each dose, 3 times a day.

## Simple and Handy Prescriptions

Cangzhu (Atractylodes Rhizome) 10 g, Huangbai (Amur Cork-tree) 10 g, Yiyiren (Coix Seed) 30 g and Niuxi (Twotoothed Achyranthes Root) 10 g are boiled in water and administered once a day for the treatment of gout with red, warm and painful joints.

## Other Therapies

External therapy: Jinhuang Plaster is applied on the swollen and painful areas of the joints and changed once every 2~3 days. A course of treatment lasts 10 days. This therapy is suitable for gout with obstruction by wind, dampness and heat.

Dietary therapy: Fresh grapes 30 g and rice 50 g are boiled together. The porridge is eaten each day to promote excretion of uric acid.

## Cautions and Advice

1. Gout is often accompanied by obesity, hyperlipemia, hypertension, coronary artery disease and diabetes. In some cases, hyperuricemia affects the kidneys, leading to renal inadequacy. For this reason, hyperuricemia should be treated promptly.
2. It is advisable for patients to control their intake of certain foods, avoid consumption of alcohol as well as animal viscera or broth which is rich in purine. Food or products made from bean or fish which are rich in protein and fat should also be avoided.

## Daily Exercises

1. Concisely describe the etiology and pathology of gout.
2. Recall the diagnostic key points of gout.
3. Explain how gout due to wind, dampness and heat and gout due to obstinate retention of phlegm and stasis can be differentiated and treated.

# Hyperlipemia
# Week 14: Saturday

Hyperlipemia is a disease marked by abnormally elevated levels of lipids in blood plasma due to metabolic disturbance of lipids. Because lipids are mostly combined with proteins in blood plasma, this disease is also known as hyperlipoproteinemia. Clinically, it may be associated with obesity and xanthoma, but may also have no specific symptoms. It can be divided into two categories according to etiological factors: primary and secondary. The former is a congenital defect of lipid or lipoprotein metabolism, while the latter is secondary to certain diseases, such as diabetes, hepatic diseases, renal diseases and thyroid diseases, as well as excessive diets or lifestyles such as overconsumption of alcohol or food. Long-term hyperlipemia is liable to speed up arteriosclerosis and, in particular, trigger and aggravate coronary artery disease and cerebrovascular diseases. In TCM, this disease is closely associated with "phlegm syndrome", "consumptive disease", "chest bi-syndrome" and "dizziness".

## Etiology and Pathology

TCM holds that this disease is caused by deficiency of the spleen with profuse phlegm; or by abundant stomach fire and excessive intake of fatty and sweet food which gives rise to turbid phlegm in the interior; or by weakness of the body in old age when the visceral qi declines, bringing about deficiency of yin and transformation of the retained phlegm and blood stasis into turbid lipids which stays inside the body and forms a predisposition to this disease.

The pathological changes are discussed as follows: Deficiency of the spleen results in profuse phlegm and dampness as well as the retention of turbid lipids due to poor transformation; in addition, patients usually have predominant yang and abundant stomach fire and if they consume too much fatty and sweet food, there will be accumulation of phlegm and heat which will then transform into turbid lipids; if the phlegm accumulates in the interior over a long period of time, it may eventually enter the collaterals and cause blood stasis; furthermore, when the patients get old, their bodies will become weak and the visceral qi will become deficient, marked by deficiency of liver yin and kidney yin which transform into turbid phlegm instead of blood; in addition, the retained blood and phlegm can also turn into turbid lipids which stay inside the body and create a predisposition to this disease.

## Diagnostic Key Points

1. Laboratory examination findings: Abnormally elevated levels of total cholesterol, low density lipoprotein and cholesterol, or triglyceride (triacylglycerol).
2. Patients with xanthoma usually have a family history of this disease.

## Syndrome Differentiation

### 1. Accumulation of phlegm due to spleen deficiency

Symptoms: Fat body with loose muscles, lassitude, stuffiness and fullness in the chest, dizziness, heavy or swollen limbs, poor appetite or loose stools; enlarged tongue with white and thick coating and soggy pulse.

Analysis of symptoms: Deficiency of the spleen leads to abundant dampness and accumulated phlegm, marked by a fat body with loose muscles as well as lassitude; obstruction of phlegm and dampness in the interior results in a feeling of stuffiness and fullness in the chest; upward disturbance of turbid phlegm is manifested as dizziness; retention of water and dampness in the four limbs is characterized by heavy or swollen limbs; deficiency of the spleen and stomach with abundant dampness and phlegm is marked by poor appetite and loose stools; the enlarged tongue with white and thick coating and soggy pulse are manifestations of accumulated phlegm due to spleen deficiency.

### 2. Obstruction of the intestine with heat in the stomach

Symptoms: Corpulent body, fever with restlessness, voracious appetite, thirst and constipation; yellow-greasy or yellow-thin tongue coating and slippery or slippery-rapid pulse.

Analysis of symptoms: Hyperactivity of yang with abundant heat in the stomach is marked by fever with restlessness and voracious appetite; indulgence in fatty and sweet food results in the accumulation of phlegm and heat, characterized by a corpulent body; intense stomach fire consumes fluid, so there is thirst and constipation; the yellow-greasy or yellow-thin tongue coating and the slippery or slippery-rapid pulse are due to obstruction of the intestine with heat in the stomach, as well as accumulation of phlegm and heat.

## 3. Retention of phlegm and stasis

Symptoms: Occasional xanthoma at the eyelids, intermittent chest distress, dizziness, distending pain in the head, numb limbs or partial paralysis; dark tongue with possible ecchymosis, white greasy or turbid greasy tongue coating and deep and slippery pulse.

Analysis of symptoms: Persistently retained phlegm enters the collaterals and causes obstruction with blood stasis, marked by xanthoma at the eyelids; obstruction of the chest collaterals by phlegm and stasis is responsible for intermittent chest distress; obstruction of the brain collaterals by phlegm and stasis gives rise to dizziness and distending pain in the head; retention of phlegm and stasis in the meridians is characterized by numb limbs or partial paralysis; the dark tongue with possible ecchymosis, white greasy or turbid greasy tongue coating and deep and slippery pulse are attributable to retention of phlegm and stasis.

## 4. Yin deficiency of the liver and kidneys

Symptoms: Thin body with elevated levels of blood fat, dizziness, blurred vision, forgetfulness, weakness and soreness in the waist and knees, insomnia, or feverish sensations over the five centers (the palms, the soles and the heart); red tongue with thin or scanty coating and thin pulse or thin, rapid pulse.

Analysis of symptoms: When the patient gets old, the body will become weak and the liver and kidneys will be deficient in yin, which in turn transforms into turbid phlegm instead of essence, marked by body thinness with elevated levels of blood fat; deficiency of yin in the upper energizer and failure of lucid yang to reach the head causes malnutrition of the brain, with such signs as dizziness, blurred vision and forgetfulness; deficiency of yin in the lower energizer leads to malnutrition of the kidneys which is characterized by weakness and soreness in the waist and knees; insufficient kidney yin fails to rise and coordinate the heart, resulting in disturbance of the heart spirit by hyperactive heart fire, manifesting as insomnia; deficiency of yin brings about exuberant fire, marked by feverish sensations over the five centers; the red tongue with thin or scanty coating and thin pulse or thin, rapid pulse are due to deficiency of liver yin and kidney yin, or deficiency of yin with exuberant fire.

## Differential Treatment

### 1. Accumulation of phlegm due to spleen deficiency

Treatment principle: Replenishing qi and invigorating the spleen, removing dampness and dissolving phlegm.

Prescription and herbs: Modified Shenling Baizhu Powder and Erchen Decoction.

Dangshen (Radix Codonopsis) 15 g, Huangqi (Milkvetch Root) 15 g, Fuling (Indian Bread) 12 g, Baizhu (Largehead Atractylodes Rhizome) 12 g, Biandou (Hyacinth Bean) 12 g, Shanyao (Common Yan Rhizome) 12 g, Banxia (Pinellia Tuber) 10 g, Chenpi (Dried Tangerine Peel) 6 g, Yiyiren (Coix Seed) 15 g, Shengshanzha (Raw Hawthorn Fruit) 15 g, Heye (Lotus Leaf) 9 g and Zexie (Oriental Waterplantain Rhizome) 15 g.

Modification: If there are greasy sensations or a bitter taste in the mouth with greasy yellow tongue coating, Yinchen (Virgate Wormwood Herb) 15 g and Pugongying (Dandelion) 15 g can be added to dispel heat and resolve dampness; for edema in the limbs, Zhuling (Polyporus) 15 g and Guizhi (Cassia Twig) 9 g can be added to warm and transport water and dampness, as well as relieve edema.

## 2. Obstruction of the intestine with heat in the stomach

Treatment principle: Clearing the stomach and purging heat, dredging the intestines and removing stagnation.

Prescription and herbs: Supplementary Xiexin Decoction.

Huanglian (Golden Thread) 3 g, Huangqin (Baical Skullcap Root) 9 g, Dahuang (Rhubarb) 6 g (decocted later), Binglang (Areca Seed) 9 g, Caojueming (Semen Cassia) 15 g and Laifuzi (Radish Seed) 15 g.

Modification: If there is impairment of fluid due to abundant heat, fever with restlessness and thirst, Shengdi (Dried Rehmannia Root) 15 g and Maidong (Dwarf Lilyturf Tuber) 12 g can be added to nourish yin and produce fluid.

## 3. Retention of phlegm and stasis

Treatment principle: Activating blood and removing stasis, dissolving phlegm and decreasing blood fat.

Prescription and herbs: Modified Tongyu Decoction.

Danggui (Chinese Angelica) 9 g, Honghua (Safflower) 9 g, Taoren (Peach Seed) 9 g, Shanzha (Hawthorn Fruit) 15 g, Danshen (Radix Salviae Miltiorrhiae) 15 g, Zexie (Oriental Waterplantain Rhizome) 15 g, Zelan (Herba Lycopi) 15 g, Puhuang (Pollen Typhae) 20 g (wrapped during decoction), Sanleng (Common Burreed Tuber) 12 g, Ezhu (Zedoray Rhizome) 12 g, Haizao (Seaweed) 15 g and Kunbu (Kelp or Tangle) 15 g.

Modification: For coronary artery disease with intermittent chest distress, Yanhusuo (Corydalis) 9 g and Yujin (Turmeric Root Tuber) 9 g can be added to reinforce the action of regulating qi, activating blood and resolving stasis; for dizziness, distending pain in the head and high blood pressure, Tianma (Tall Gastrodis Tuber) 9 g, Gouteng (Gambir Plant) 15 g (decocted later) and Shijueming (Sea-ear Shell) 30 g (decocted first) can be added to subdue the liver and extinguish wind; for stroke with lingering effects, Huangqi (Milkvetch Root) 30 g, Chuanxiong (Szechwan Lovage Rhizome) 12 g, Chishao (Red Peony Root) 12 g and Dilong

(Angle Worm) 9 g are used to supplement qi, activate blood and dredge the collaterals; for fatty liver, Pianjianghuang (Wenyujin Concise Rhizome) 9 g, Yinchen (Virgate Wormwood Herb) 15 g and Huzhang (Giant Knotweed Rhizome) 15 g can be added to clear the liver, activate blood and regulate qi.

## 4. Yin deficiency of the liver and kidneys

Treatment principle: Tonifying the liver and kidneys, nourishing yin and decreasing blood fat.

Prescription and herbs: Modified Erzhi Pill and Liuwei Dihuang Pill.

Nuzhenzi (Glossy Privet Fruit) 15 g, Huanliancao (Ecliptae Herba) 15 g, Shengdi (Dried Rehmannia Root) 15 g, Shanzhuyu (Asiatic Cornelian Cherry Fruit) 10 g, Fuling (Indian Bread) 12 g, Zexie (Oriental Waterplantain Rhizome) 15 g, Zelan (Herba Lycopi) 15 g, Shanzha (Hawthorn Fruit) 15 g, Sangjisheng (Chinese Taxillus Herb) 15 g, Huangjing (Solomonseal Rhizome) 15 g, Gouqizi (Barbary Wolfberry Fruit) 15 g and Shouwu (Fleeceflower Root) 15 g.

Modification: If there is severe soreness in the lumbar vertebrae, Duzhong (Eucommia Bark) 9 g and Chuanduan (Shichuan Radix Dipsaci) 9 g can be used to nourish the kidneys and strengthen the waist; for nocturnal insomnia, Suanzaoren (Spine Date Seed) 12 g and Wuweizi (Chinese Magnolivine Fruit) 6 g are added to nourish the liver and calm the heart.

## Chinese Patent Medicine

Xuezhikang: 2 pills for each dose, twice a day.

## Simple and Handy Prescriptions

1. Caojueming (Semen Cassia) 15 g and Dahuang (Rhubarb) 3 g are boiled in water and served as tea to be drunk once a day. It is suitable for hyperlipemia with a strong body, good appetite and constipation.
2. Equal quantities (15 g each) of Nuzhenzi (Glossy Privet Fruit), Huanliancao (Ecliptae Herba), Shouwu (Fleeceflower Root), Huangjing

(Solomonseal Rhizome), Yuzhu (Fragrant Solomonseal Rhizome) and Shanzha (Hawthorn Fruit) are boiled in water and administered once a day. It is used to treat hyperlipemia with a thin body and deficient yin.

## Other Therapies

Dietary therapy: The following three combinations can be seasoned, fried and frequently eaten for the treatment of hyperlipemia: Fresh mushroom 250 g and heart of cabbage 500 g; winter bamboo shoot 300 g and shepherd's purse 150 g; celery 250 g and mushroom 50 g.

External therapy: Cheqianzi (Plantain Seed) 9 g, Puhuang (Pollen Typhae) 9 g and Zaojiaomo (Gleditsiae Powder) 1.5 g are blended with vinegar and consumed once a day.

## Cautions and Advice

1. Apart from congenital factors, hyperlipemia is also closely associated with diet. Hence, the high-fat and high-glucose diets should be avoided.
2. Physical exercise is an effective way to reduce obesity and hyperlipemia, so it is highly recommended.
3. The patient should quit smoking and alcohol, cultivate a healthy lifestyle, control hyperlipemia and reduce complications.

## Daily Exercises

1. Recall the pathological changes of hyperlipemia.
2. Concisely describe the different patterns of hyperlipemia.
3. Explain how hyperlipemia due to retained phlegm and stasis and hyperlipemia due to yin deficiency of the liver and kidneys can be differentiated and treated.

# Index

acupuncture and moxibustion 针灸 531

alternate chills and fever 寒热往来 291

apoplexy 中风 525

calming the heart and tranquilizing the mind 宁心安神 160, 552

channels and collaterals 经络 527, 529, 535

Chinese herbs 中草药 505

coma and delirium 神昏谵语 101, 298, 308, 315, 402, 404, 588, 589, 591

concretions and conglomerations 症瘕 270

consumptive worms 痨虫 113, 114, 264

deficiency of the primary aspect 本虚 178, 270, 280

depressive psychosis 癫病 550

diarrhea before dawn 五更泻 55, 56, 116, 119, 242, 257, 265

dispel heat and purge fine 36–38, 53, 286, 292, 293, 328, 521, 613

dissolve phlegm and relieve cough 化痰止咳 69, 79, 80, 109, 117, 159

drum belly 鼓胀 270, 280

drying dampness and eliminating phlegm 燥湿祛痰 28

endogenous pathogenic factors 内邪 16, 52, 72, 91

excess of the secondary aspect 标实 178, 270, 280

flaccidity syndrome 痿证 501, 507, 510, 596

healthy qi 正气 49, 56, 66, 91, 92, 98, 101, 105–107, 110, 113, 122, 130, 132, 148, 155–157, 165, 179, 180, 207, 240, 264, 266, 267, 283, 291, 296, 311, 329, 333, 348, 360, 377, 380, 406, 408, 410, 411, 413, 452, 519–521, 526, 529, 535, 536, 575, 583, 590, 603, 605–607, 609–612, 647, 649

hypochondriac pain 胁痛 16, 19, 188, 190, 274, 280, 282, 289, 291, 303, 305, 311–313, 316, 365, 560, 590

improper diet 饮食不节 31, 45, 54, 69, 83, 85, 86, 105, 155, 157, 170,

186, 221, 240, 254, 257, 270, 280, 420, 426, 486, 525, 533, 542, 565

inactivation of yang qi 阳气不振 272

internal injury due to overstrain 劳倦内伤　61, 399

invigorating qi and nourishing blood 益气养血　144, 166, 402, 403, 442, 443, 496, 607, 614

jaundice due to blood accumulation 淤血黄疸　270, 272, 273, 298, 305

life cultivation 养生　163, 269
liver accumulation 肝积　280, 311
liver syncope 肝厥　296

middle energizer 中焦　19, 23, 32, 34, 46, 47, 57, 58, 60, 70, 151, 157, 214, 217, 224, 225, 229–231, 249, 254, 271, 275, 282, 284, 285, 296, 313, 317, 325, 329, 362, 397, 416, 417, 472, 476, 488, 501, 503, 569, 619

night sweats 盗汗　38–40, 43, 44, 71, 73, 94, 108, 113–116, 118, 119, 124, 126, 158, 161, 173, 176, 179, 181, 183, 191, 209, 243, 250, 252, 257, 264, 266, 297, 336, 354, 369–371, 380, 407–409, 414, 416, 421–423, 427, 428, 454, 457, 470, 476, 503, 611

nourishing the heart to calm the mind 养心安神　35

pathogenic factor 病邪　14, 16, 20, 52, 59, 60, 69, 65, 66, 72, 73, 83, 85, 90–92, 98, 105–107, 110, 113, 122, 130, 148, 154–157, 163, 165, 170, 179, 185, 235, 248, 266, 267, 270, 283, 291, 296, 311, 333, 350, 360, 377, 399, 402, 406, 426, 446, 447, 452, 472, 479, 525, 526, 574–578, 583, 585, 587, 590–592, 596, 603–605, 612, 649, 650

poor appetite 纳差　15, 19, 28, 32, 33, 47, 53–55, 58, 62, 63, 75–77, 81, 85, 86, 119, 124, 125, 127, 134, 141–143, 151, 160, 175, 188, 198, 203, 215, 216, 227, 229–232, 235, 236, 242, 248, 249, 254–257, 265, 266, 268, 270, 273–275, 305, 312–314, 316, 325, 326, 335, 336, 342, 343, 345, 354, 361–363, 366, 379, 385–388, 394, 400, 422, 428, 440–442, 463, 468, 473, 474, 488, 494, 495, 520, 521, 551, 552, 567, 569, 590, 591, 593, 597, 598, 612, 619, 635, 637, 640, 654

primary aspect 本　23, 123, 171, 178, 207, 270, 280

qi stagnation and blood stasis 气滞血瘀　125, 143, 256, 264, 280, 283, 369, 372, 374, 377, 408, 487, 489, 491, 571

relieve convulsions and extinguish wind 止痉熄风　103

replenishing qi to invigorate the spleen 益气健脾　74, 211, 284, 317, 429

secondary aspect 标　23, 171, 178, 207, 270, 280

soothing the liver and regulating qi 疏肝理气   203, 217, 225, 250, 317, 454, 559

stagnation of liver qi 肝气郁结   38, 63, 186, 194, 195, 202, 234, 254, 281, 284, 304, 314, 315, 379, 433, 435, 447, 451, 457, 487, 493, 544, 551, 556, 557, 570, 588, 590, 593, 641

summer-heat   暑热   42, 44, 45, 47, 66, 69, 70, 254

sweating syndrome 汗证   26

syndrome differentiation 辨证   xi, xii, 14, 24, 32, 39, 44, 46, 53, 62, 66, 70, 73, 84, 92, 99, 106, 114, 124, 132, 141, 149, 156, 164, 171, 181, 188, 195, 202, 208, 215, 222, 230, 233, 235, 239, 241, 249, 255, 265, 271, 281, 288, 290, 297, 304, 310, 312, 324, 334, 342, 351, 361, 370, 378, 386, 394, 400, 407, 414, 421, 427, 434, 441, 447, 452, 455, 457, 462, 466, 468, 473, 480, 485, 487, 493, 502, 508, 513, 515, 520, 526, 534, 544, 551, 556, 564, 566, 574, 582, 588, 597, 604, 611, 618, 627, 634, 640, 647, 654

tuina 推拿疗法   638

water attacking the heart 水气凌心   165

yang deficiency of the spleen and kidney 脾肾阳虚   76, 80, 134, 136, 173, 176, 242, 244, 257, 261, 265, 266, 273, 276, 353, 357, 386, 387, 389, 395, 396, 401, 403, 415, 417, 441–443, 445, 457, 459–461, 463, 464, 466–471, 488, 490, 612, 614, 648–650